CW01368017

Handbook of
Work Group Psychology

To Gillian Hardy, who has taught me most about working with others

Handbook of Work Group Psychology

Edited by
Michael A. West
*Institute of Work Psychology,
University of Sheffield, UK*

JOHN WILEY & SONS
Chichester · New York · Brisbane · Toronto · Singapore

Copyright © 1996 by John Wiley & Sons Ltd,
Baffins Lane, Chichester,
West Sussex PO19 1UD, England

National 01243 779777
International (+44) 1243 779777

All rights reserved.

No part of this book may be reproduced by any means, or transmitted, or translated into a machine language without the written permission of the publisher.

Other Wiley Editorial Offices

John Wiley & Sons, Inc., 605 Third Avenue,
New York, NY 10158-0012, USA

Jacaranda Wiley Ltd, 33 Park Road, Milton,
Queensland 4064, Australia

John Wiley & Sons (Canada) Ltd, 22 Worcester Road,
Rexdale, Ontario M9W 1L1, Canada

John Wiley & Sons (Asia) Pte Ltd, 2 Clementi Loop #02-01,
Jin Xing Distripark, Singapore 0512

British Library Cataloguing in Publication Data

A catalogue record for this book is available from the British Library

ISBN 0-471-95790-9

Typeset in 10/12pt Times by Best-set Typesetter Ltd., Hong Kong
Printed and bound in Great Britain by Bookcraft (Bath) Ltd
This book is printed on acid-free paper responsibly manufactured from sustainable forestation, for which at least two trees are planted for each one used for paper production.

Contents

About the Editor		ix
List of Contributors		xi
About the Authors		xv
Acknowledgements		xxiii
Preface	Introducing Work Group Psychology *Michael A. West*	xxv

SECTION I	**INTRODUCTION**	
Chapter 1	Fundamental Consideration about Work Groups *Richard A. Guzzo*	3

SECTION II	**THE CONTEXTS OF GROUPS**	
Chapter 2	Temporal Issues in Work Groups *Joseph E. McGrath and Kathleen M. O'Connor*	25
Chapter 3	The Consequences of Diversity in Multidisciplinary Work Teams *Susan E. Jackson*	53
Chapter 4	Group Affective Tone *Jennifer M. George*	77
Chapter 5	Group Task Structure, Processes and Outcome *Franziska Tschan and Mario von Cranach*	95

SECTION III	**GROUP PROCESSES**	
Chapter 6	Making Work Groups More Effective: the Value of Minority Dissent *Charlan Nemeth and Pamela Owens*	125

Chapter 7	Unconscious Phenomena in Work Groups *Mark Stein*	143
Chapter 8	Interaction and Decision-making in Project Teams *Marjolein van Offenbeek and Paul Koopman*	159
Chapter 9	Group Leadership: a Levels of Analysis Perspective *Francis J. Yammarino*	189
Chapter 10	Autonomous Work Groups and Quality Circles *John L. Cordery*	225
Chapter 11	Dimensions, Criteria and Evaluation of Work Group Autonomy *Eberhard Ulich and Wolfgang G. Weber*	247
SECTION IV	**GROUP OUTCOMES**	
Chapter 12	Criteria for the Study of Work Group Functioning *Felix C. Brodbeck*	285
Chapter 13	Innovation and Creativity in Work Groups *Anders Agrell and Roland Gustafson*	317
Chapter 14	Work Group Factors and Individual Well-being *Sabine Sonnentag*	345
SECTION V	**GROUPS IN ORGANIZATIONS**	
Chapter 15	Affective Reactions to the Group and the Organization *Natalie J. Allen*	371
Chapter 16	Intergroup Relations in Organizations *Jean F. Hartley*	397
Chapter 17	Work Group Socialization *Neil Anderson and Helena D.C. Thomas*	423
Chapter 18	Approaches to Communication Structure: Applications to the Problem of Information-seeking *J. David Johnson*	451
SECTION VI	**CROSS-CULTURAL ASPECTS OF WORK GROUP FUNCTIONING**	
Chapter 19	Cultural Differences in Group Processes *Peter B. Smith and Julia Noakes*	477
Chapter 20	Promoting Team Effectiveness *Scott I. Tannenbaum, Eduardo Salas and Janis A. Cannon-Bowers*	503

Chapter 21	Facilitating Group Development: Interventions for a Relational and Contextual Construction *René Bouwen and Ron Fry*	531
SECTION VII	**CONCEPTUAL INTEGRATION**	
Chapter 22	Reflexivity and Work Group Effectiveness: a Conceptual Integration *Michael A. West*	555
Indexes		580

About the Editor

Michael West is Professor of Work and Organizational Psychology at the Institute of Work Psychology, University of Sheffield, and co-Director of the Corporate Performance Programme at the Centre for Economic Performance, London School of Economics. He received his PhD from the University of Wales (UWIST) in 1977 for work on the psychology of meditation. He is the author or co-author of seven books, including *Effective Teamwork* (1994), *Innovation and Creativity and Work* (with Farr, 1990) and *Managerial Job Change* (with Nicholson, 1988). He has also published more than 100 scientific journal articles, chapters and articles in practitioner publications, many of them in the areas of work group psychology and innovation. He is former editor of the *Journal of Occupational and Organizational Psychology*.

Contributors

Professor Anders Agrell, *Department of Psychology, University of Orebro, PO Box 923, Orebro, Sweden.*

Professor Natalie J. Allen, *Centre for Administrative and Information Studies, The University of Western Ontario, London, Ontario, Canada.*

Dr Neil Anderson, *Psychology Department, Goldsmiths College, University of London, New Cross, London, UK.*

Professor René Bouwen, *Katholieke Universiteit of Leuven, Department Psychologies, Arbeids-en Organisatiepsychologie, Tiensestraat 102, Leuven, Belgium.*

Dr Felix C. Brodbeck, *Experimental and Applied Social Psychology Unit, Department of Psychology, University of Munich, Leopoldstr 13, D-80802, Munich, Germany.*

Dr Janis A. Cannon-Bowers, *Naval Air Warfare Center, Training Division, USA.*

Dr John L. Cordery, *Department of Organisational and Labour Studies, The University of Western Australia, Nedlands, Australia.*

Professor Ron Fry, *Weatherhead School of Management of Case Western Reserve University, Ohio, USA.*

Professor Jennifer M. George, *Department of Mangement, Texas A & M University, College Station, Texas, USA.*

Professor Roland Gustafson, *Department of Psychology, University of Orebro, PO Box 923, Orebro, Sweden.*

Professor Richard A. Guzzo, *Department of Psychology, University of Maryland, College Park, Maryland, USA.*

Dr Jean F. Hartley, *Department of Organizational Psychology, Birkbeck College, University of London, Malet Street, London, UK.*

Professor Susan E. Jackson, *New York University, 40 West 4th Street, Suite 7–23, New York, USA.*

Professor J. David Johnson, *Department of Communication, Michigan State University, East Lansing, Michigan, USA.*

Professor Paul Koopman, *Department of Work and Organisational Psychology, Vrije Universiteit, De Boelelaan, 1081 HV Amsterdam, The Netherlands.*

Professor Joseph E. McGrath, *Psychology Department, University of Illinois, USA.*

Professor Charlan Nemeth, *Department of Psychology, University of California, Berkeley, California, USA.*

Julia Noakes, *Sheppard, Moscow Ltd, London, UK.*

Kathleen M. O'Connor, *Psychology Department, Rice University, USA.*

Pamela Owens, *Department of Psychology, University of California, Berkeley, California, USA.*

Dr Eduardo Salas, *Naval Air Warfare Center, Training Division, USA.*

Dr Peter B. Smith, *Centre for Research into Cross-Cultural Organisation and Management, University of Sussex, and Roffey Park Management Institute, Brighton, UK.*

Dr Sabine Sonnentag, *Justus-Liebig-Universitat Giessen, Fachbereich 06 Psychologie, Otto-Behagel-Strabe 10/F, Giessen, Germany.*

Dr Mark Stein, *South Bank University, London, UK.*

CONTRIBUTORS

Professor Scott I. Tannenbaum, *School of Business, University at Albany, State University of New York, Albany, New York, USA.*

Helena D.C. Thomas, *Psychology Department, Goldsmiths College, University of London, New Cross, London, UK.*

Dr Franziska Tschan, *Institute of Psychology, University of Bern, Switzerland.*

Professor Eberhard Ulich, *Swiss Federal Institute of Technology, Lehrstuhl Fur Arbeits und Organizations Psycologie der ETH, Nelkenstrasse 11, CH-8092, Zurich, Switzerland.*

Professor Marjolein von Offenbeek, *Faculty of Management and Organization, Rijksuniversiteit Groningen, Groningen, The Netherlands.*

Dr Mario von Cranach, *Institute of Psychology, University of Bern, Switzerland.*

Professor Wolfgang G. Weber, *Swiss Federal Institute of Technology, Lehrstuhl Fur Arbeits und Organizations Psychologie der ETH, Nelkenstrasse 11, CH-8092, Zurich, Switzerland.*

Professor Michael A. West, *Institute of Work Psychology, The University of Sheffield, Sheffield S10 2TN, UK.*

Professor Francis J. Yammarino, *Center for Leadership Studies and School of Management, State University of New York at Binghamton, PO Box 6015, Binghamton, New York, USA.*

About the Authors

Anders Agrell earned his Doctor's degree in psychology at the University of Uppsala, Sweden. He is a trained clinical and work and organizational psychologist and he has worked as an applied psychologist for many years. Since 1981 he has been on the faculty of the University of Örebro, Sweden, currently as Senior Lecturer and director for the Human Resource Management Program. He has published research in the fields of traffic safety, behavioural toxicology and work and organizational psychology.

Natalie J. Allen received her PhD in psychology from the University of Western Ontario (London, Canada). She is an Associate Professor and Director of the Centre for Administrative and Information Studies, a multidisciplinary teaching and research unit at UWO. Much of her research focuses on the development and consequences of employee commitment to the organization and other work-related domains. Other areas of research interest include cross-cultural issues within organizational behaviour and the composition of, and processes within, work teams. Her work appears in the *Journal of Applied Psychology*, *Journal of Occupational and Organizational Psychology* and the *Academy of Management Journal*.

Neil Anderson is Senior Lecturer in Occupational Psychology at Goldsmiths' College, University of London, UK. His current research interests include organizational socialization, recruitment and selection, and innovation at work. He is Co-editor (with Peter Herriot) of the handbook *Assessment and Selection in Organizations* (Wiley) and is Editor of the *International Journal of Selection and Assessment*.

René Bouwen is Professor in Group Dynamics and Organizational Psychology at the Catholic University of Leuven in Belgium. His research concentrates around three major topics: effectiveness and development of groups; conflict analysis and conflict management; and innovation and change processes in organizations. The development of a social constructionist reading and approach of these dynamic organizational contexts is the common thread in his work. He is also involved in social change projects in organizations, especially through the professional training of process consultants. He is Co-author with Paul Salipante of a book, *The Social Construction of Conflict in the Workplace*, and has published several articles about organizational innovation and change.

Felix Claus Brodbeck has a Master's degree (Diplom) in Clinical Psychology from the University of Munich (Germany), and a Doctorate in Work and Organizational Psychology from the University of Giessen (Germany). He is Assistant Professor and Senior Research Psychologist in the Psychology Department of the University of Munich. His research interests include team development and performance, minority influence in decision making groups, process gains and process losses in task performing groups, cross-cultural issues of leadership and performance, human–computer interaction and computer–supported cooperative work. He is currently Country Co-Investigator in the Global Organizational Behavior and Effectiveness Research Programm (GLOBE) conducting research on cross-cultural differences in implicit theories of leadership.

Janis A. Cannon-Bowers is Senior Research Psychologist in the Science and Technology Division of the Naval Air Warfare Center, Training Systems Division, USA. She holds an MSc and PhD in Industrial/Organizational Psychology from the University of South Florida, Tampa, FL. Her research interests include team training and performance, crew coordination training, training effectiveness and tactical decision-making. She is currently Principal Investigator for the Tactical Decision-Making Under Stress (TADMUS) project, conducting research concerned with improving individual and team decision-making in the Navy tactical environment.

John Cordery has a Master's degree in Industrial/Organizational Psychology from the University of Canterbury, and a Doctorate in Occupational Psychology from the University of Sheffield. He is currently Associate Professor in the Department of Organisational and Labour Studies at the University of Western Australia, where he has been since 1991. His research interests relate to work redesign and its impact on employee performance and well-being, and he has carried out a number of longitudinal studies of autonomous work groups. Recently he has been researching work redesign in the context of the introduction of advanced manufacturing technology within meat-processing firms.

Ron Fry is Associate Professor of Organizational Behavior and Director of the Executive MBA Program at the Weatherhead School of Management of Case Western Reserve University, Ohio, USA. His research domains include the functioning of executives, the development of effective groups, fundamental change in organizations, and appreciative ways of knowing. He is actively involved in management and organizational development efforts with corporate, non-profit, and global change organizations. He is Co-editor with Suresh

Srivastva of a recent book, *Executive and Organization Continuity: Balancing the Paradoxes of Stability and Change*, and has published numerous articles on team development and organization change.

Jennifer M. George is an Associate Professor in the Department of Management at Texas A&M University, USA. She received a PhD in 1987 from the Department of Management and Organizational Behavior at New York University. Her research on topics such as the nature, antecedents and consequences of affect at work for both individuals and groups has been widely published in leading journals such as the *Journal of Applied Psychology, Psychological Bulletin, Journal of Personality and Social Psychology*, and the *Academy of Management Journal*. In 1989 she was a recipient of the Outstanding Competitive Paper Award from the Organizational Behavior Division of the Academy of Management. She is currently on the editorial review boards of the *Journal of Applied Psychology* and the *Journal of Management* and has previously served on the editorial review board of the *Academy of Management Journal*.

Roland Gustafson earned his Doctor's degree in psychology at the University of Uppsala, Sweden. He is a trained clinical and work and organizational psychologist and has worked as an applied psychologist for many years. Since 1980 he has been on the faculty of the University of Örebro as a Professor and Senior Researcher in Psychology. He has published extensively in international scientific journals, book chapters and conference reports. His research has mainly been focused on the acute effects of alcohol on psychological and social variables, such as aggression and violence, attention and cognition, on psychotherapeutic methods, and on work and organizational problems.

Richard A. Guzzo is professor of Psychology at the University of Maryland, USA. He earned his PhD in 1979 from Yale University in Administrative Sciences. Prior to joining the University of Maryland, he was on the faculties of New York University and McGill University. His primary research interests include team effectiveness in organizations and human productivity, and he has published numerous articles and three books on these topics. Other research interests include employer practices toward expatriate employees and employee loyalty and commitment.

Jean Hartley is Senior Lecturer in Organizational Psychology at the Department of Organizational Psychology, Birkbeck College, University of London. Her current research interests are in the areas of employment relations and organizational change. She has published a variety of articles on psychological aspects of personal and organizational change, including unemployment and job insecurity, as well as on conflict in labour–management relations. She is also researching and writing about organizational change in large public sector organizations. She is the author of *Steel Strike* (with J. Kelly & N. Nicholson, 1983), and *Job Insecurity: Coping with Jobs at Risk* (with D. Jacobson, B. Klandermans & T. van Vuuren, 1991). She co-edited (with G. Stephenson) the major text on psychological aspects of employment relations, entitled *Employment Relations: The Psychology of Influence and Control at Work.*

Susan E. Jackson is Professor of Management and Psychology at New York University, USA. She received her MA and PhD degrees from the University of California at Berkeley and her undergraduate degree from the University of Minnesota. Her work on the topic of workforce diversity emphasizes the consequences of diversity for teamwork in organizations and the importance of linking diversity issues to strategic business issues. In addition to her research, other activities include serving as Editor of the *Academy of Management Review*, a scholarly journal published for a global audience of readers interested in organizational science, and serving on the Board of Governors for the Center for Creative Leadership, a non-profit organization dedicated to improving leadership capabilities through research, education and training.

J. David Johnson gained his PhD at the Michigan State University in 1978 and is currently Professor and Chairperson of the Department of Communication at Michigan State University. He has authored numerous publications in such journals as *Human Communication Research, Communication Research, Communication Monographs, Academy of Management Review, Science Communication, Journal of Business Research, Journal of Business Communication*, and the *Journal of Social Psychology*. Recently, his book *Organizational Communication Structure*, was published by ABLEX, and he has a forthcoming book, *Information Seeking*, to be published by Quorum Books. His major research interests focus on organizational communication structure, information seeking, and health communication.

Paul Koopman is Professor of the Psychology of Management and Organization in the Department of Work and Organizational Psychology at the Vrije Universiteit, Amsterdam, The Netherlands. In 1980 he finished his PhD study at the same university on the subject "Decision-making in Organizations". He is Co-author (with F.A. Heller, P.J.D. Drenth and V. Rus) of *Decisions in Organisations: A Three-country Comparative Study* (Sage, 1988). Other domains of his research interest are: automation, leadership, motivation, and organizational culture.

Joseph E. McGrath is Professor of Psychology at the University of Illinois, Urbana-Champaign, USA. He received his PhD in social psychology from the University of Michigan in 1955. His research interests include small group processes and performance, temporal and gender issues in social psychology, and research methodology.

Charlan Jeanne Nemeth is Professor of Psychology at the University of California, Berkeley, USA. Having trained in the USA, England and France, she completed her PhD in Psychology with a minor in Statistics at Cornell University. She professor of work and organizational psychology and director of the Institute of Work Psychology at the Swiss Federal Institute of Technology (ETH) in Zurich, Switzerland. His main interests are in work and organizational design, appropriate use of advanced technology and human–computer interaction. He published twelve books as author or co-author, and about 400 contributions to books and journals and edited another 50 books. He is head of the ETH-Center for Integrated Production Systems. He received an honorary doctorate from the Technical University of Dresden.

Marjolein van Offenbeek is Associate Professor of Organization Studies at the Faculty of Management and Organization at the University of Groningen, The Netherlands. She studied organizational psychology at the Free University of Amsterdam and received her PhD from the same university in 1993. The title of her thesis was "From Method to Scenarios: Matching Context and Strategy in Information System Development". Her current research interests include the management of information technology-supported change, such as business process re-engineering; the role, position and quality of working life of middle management in changing organizations; and applying social constructivism to organizational diagnosis and change.

Mario von Cranach was born in 1931, and studied Law and Psychology, being awarded the Dr Phil in 1956. He has held various research and teaching positions at the Universities of Mannheim and Munich, the Max-Planck-Institut for Psychiatry in Munich and the Max-Planck-Institut for Educational Research in Berlin (all Germany). Since 1971 Von Cranach has been Full Professor for Psychology at the University of Berne (Switzerland), with guest professorships at the Ecole des Hautes Etudes en Science Social in Paris (France), the University of Erlangen-Nuremberg (Germany), Visiting Fellow of the British Psychological Society, Visiting Professor at the University of Bologna (Italy), Wilhelm-Wundt-Professor at the University of Leipzig (Germany), and Visiting Professor at the UNAM, Mexico City. Van Cranach has conducted research and has authored and edited books and articles in the fields of Social Attitudes, Human Ethology, Nonverbal Communication, Goal Directed Action, Social Representations. Group Action. Forthcoming edited volume on the Psychological Aspects of Freedom of the Will.

Wolfgang G. Weber, born in 1957, graduated in psychology (1985) and received the PhD (1991) from the Technological University of Berlin. He worked as a research assistant at the Institute for Human Science in Work and Education of the Technological University of Berlin from 1985 till 1991. Since 1992 he has been working as research assistant, project leader (Cooperation in Computer-Supported Work), and part-time lecturer at the Swiss Federal Institute of Technology (ETH) in Zurich (Work and Organizational Psychology Unit / Center for Integrated Production Systems). His activities include research projects and publications on psychological work analysis, applications of action regulation and activity theory, designing jobs with CNC machine tools and jobs in flexible manufacturing systems, and on analysis and evaluation of semi-autonomous group work.

Francis J. Yammarino gained his PhD at the State University of New York (at Buffalo) is a Professor of Management and Fellow of the Center for Leadership Studies at the State University of New York at Binghamton, USA. He is Senior Editor of *Leadership Quarterly* and a Fellow of the American Psychological Society. Professor Yammarino is co-author of two books and has published articles in journals such as *Journal of Applied Psychology*, *Personnel Psychology*, *Leadership Quarterly, Journal of Occupational Psychology, Human Relations, Public Opinion Quarterly*, and *Research in Personnel & Human Resources Management*. His research interests include superior–subordinate relationships, leadership, and multiple levels of analyses issues.

Sabine Sonnentag is Assistant Professor in the Work & Organizational Psychology Unit at the University of Amsterdam. Her research interests include expertise in individual and cooperative work settings, individual and team-related working strategies, and work situation in research and development.

Mark Stein, PhD, has degrees from the universities of Warwick, Cambridge, Brunel, and the London School of Economics. He has also studied psychodynamic phenomena at the Tavistock Clinic for over a decade. Following six years of public sector work experience, Mark Stein was a Research Fellow in Organisation Development at Brunel University, where he worked predominantly in the service sector. This was followed by his appointment as a Researcher and Consultant at the Tavistock Institute, working mainly in the manufacturing sector, where much of the research for his chapter was undertaken. Mark Stein is now Senior Lecturer in Human Resource Management at South Bank University, London, and a member of OPUS consultancy services.

Scott I. Tannenbaum is President of the Executive Consulting Group Inc, a management consulting firm, and an Associate Professor in the School of Business, State University of New York at Albany. He holds a PhD from Old Dominion University in industrial/organizational psychology. His applied work has been with clients such as American Express, Swiss Bank, Tiffany & Co., PepsiCo, and SEFCU. He has served as Principal Investigator on several US Navy and Air Force research projects. He has over 50 articles, chapters, and presentations and has published in such journals as *Journal of Applied Psychology*, *Human Factors*, *Academy of Management Journal*, *Personnel Psychology*, and the *Human Resource Planning Journal*.

Helena Thomas is currently a PhD candidate working with Neil Anderson at Goldsmiths College, London, UK. Her research interests include organizational socialization, the implementation of equal opportunities, and wellness at work.

Franziska Tschan gained her Dr. phil. hist. at the Department of Psychology, Sub-department of Social Psychology at the University of Bern, Switzerland, in 1986 and pursued studies in psychology, paedagogics and psychopathology at the University of Bern. She undertook postdoc total studies at Texas A&M University and LRDC, University of Pittsburgh. Her main research interests are action theories, small group processes, work teams, group and organizational productivity, and training.

Eberhard Ulich graduated in psychology from the University of Munich in 1954, and received the PhD in 1955 from the same university. He has been with the Max-Planck-Institute for Work Physiology in Dortmund from 1955 to 1957. From 1958 until 1967 he was lecturer and senior researcher at the University of Munich. He was professor of psychology at the Technical University of Berlin from 1967 to 1969, in Cologne from 1969 to 1972. Since 1972 he has been taught at the University of Chicago, the University of Virginia, the University of British Columbia and held visiting professorships in Bristol, Mannheim and Paris before coming to the University of California, Berkeley. Her research interests have been primarily in the field of influence and, more particularly, how minority ideas come to prevail and how influence processes serve originality. She has conducted numerous studies on jury decision-making, served as a consultant to lawyers and courts and, more recently, has turned to organizational issues as she continues her interests in the "trade-offs" of social control and social change. Her most recent project involves interviews with Nobel laureates in an attempt to further understanding of processes in creativity.

Julia Noakes is a Consultant in Organization Development with Sheppard, Moscow Ltd and a part-time doctoral candidate at the University of Sussex.

Kathleen M. O'Connor is Assistant Professor of Psychology at Rice University Houston, Texas, USA. She received her PhD in industrial / organizational psychology from the University of Illinois, Urbana-Champaign, in 1994. Her current research interests include: an examination of the social and cognitive processes that lead to effective team negotiation outcomes; the antecedents and consequences of conflict in organizational work groups; and the impact of affect on conflict resolution between and within groups.

Pamela Owens is a graduate student in the Social Psychology Program at the University of California, Berkeley, USA. Having completed her BA in Economics, she worked for several years in various organizations, primarily in the advertising field. Her interests include influence processes, quality of decision-making, organizational commitment and, more generally, organizational behavior. Her most recent projects involve applying the groupthink model to corporate decision-making and an investigation of the scope of minority influence.

Eduardo Salas is Manager of the Training Systems Development Branch of the Science and Technology Division, Naval Air Warfare Center Training Systems Division, USA. He earned his PhD from Old Dominion University in industrial/organizational psychology in 1984. He is on the editorial board of *Human Factors* and *Personnel Psychology*. He has co-authored over 50 journal articles and book chapters and has co-edited four books. Dr. Salas' research interests include team training and performance, training effectiveness, tactical decision-making under stress, team decision-making, human performance measurement and modelling, and learning strategies for teams.

Peter B. Smith is Professor of Social Psychology at the University of Sussex, and Director of the Centre for Research Into Cross-Cultural Organisation and Management (CRICCOM), which is jointly located at the University of Sussex and Roffey Park Management Institute, Horsham, UK.

Preface: Introducing Work Group Psychology

Living and working together in groups is a fundamental element of our experience. Family groups potentially provide the social support, safety and security necessary for human development, adjustment and mental health. Within work groups people pursue shared objectives by integrating diverse skills, ideally to achieve an optimal use of their resources. It is not surprising, therefore, that psychologists have been fascinated by the study of groups for more than half a century. Social psychologists have focused particularly upon intragroup behaviour such as racial prejudice, while organizational psychologists have devoted most attention to work group processes such as decision-making and to outcomes such as group productivity.

Despite considerable progress made in both these fields of psychology and in the understanding of intragroup processes and group performance, there are few clear and authoritative overviews available which describe what is known and what is not known about human behaviour in groups in work settings. At the same time there have been important advances in understanding about factors influencing work group effectiveness, group development, group structure, group climate, group innovation, intergroup processes and relationships between groups and their wider organizations.

The main purpose of this book is to provide a clear overview of psychological knowledge about groups at work, drawing principally from the literatures of social and industrial/organizational psychology to provide a cogent, comprehensive and stimulating account of the state of knowledge in this area. The second purpose is to present the ideas of researchers in this field about important alternative perspectives on work group development which will shape research in this area in the future.

WHAT IS A WORK GROUP?

It is useful to distinguish between formal and informal work groups, the latter being groups which have no formal organizational identity or function but which are nevertheless present in organizations. They may be social groups, such as people who play sport together, who come together to share their common religious orientation, or who come together to discuss shared grievances about the organization. In this book, the contributors focus primarily on formal groups, those which have an identity and set of functions derived from and contributing to the achievement of organizational objectives. Such groups come in many forms. They include project groups, such as a research and development group exploring new ways of putting plastic cabling onto wheels; multidisciplinary groups, such as a nurse, physiotherapist and counsellor collaborating to plan treatment for victims of road traffic accidents; cross-functional groups, for example, representatives from marketing, production, sales and research and development; semi-autonomous work groups who are largely responsible for their own work planning and processes; quality improvement groups, such as a group trying to reduce the level of customer complaints; and functional groups, such as surgical groups and airline flight crews.

What characterizes formal groups or teams (the terms "group" and "team" will be used interchangeably in this chapter)? First, members of the group have shared objectives in relation to their work. They depend on and must interact with each other in order to achieve those objectives. Group members have more or less well defined roles, some of which are differentiated from one another (for example, in the primary health care team: doctors, nurses, receptionists) and they have an organizational identity as a work group with a defined organizational function (for example, a public relations group for a pharmaceutical company)— i.e. they see themselves, and others in the organization see them, as a defined and bounded group. Finally, they are not so large that they would be defined more appropriately as an organization with an internal structure of vertical and horizontal relationships, characterized by sub-groups. In practice this is likely to mean that the work group will be smaller than about 20 members, though clearly there would be exceptions to this.

WHY DO WE ORGANIZE WORK IN GROUPS?

Work groups are formed because of a belief that, in some circumstances, having people work on shared goals interdependently will lead to synergy—the aggregate of individuals' performance will be exceeded by work group performance. Also, it is believed that by bringing together diverse skills and integrating them, the achievement of organizational goals may be more successful. For example, the skills of nurses, administrators and doctors in a primary health care group will better meet the health needs of the local population if they are integrated and combined, rather than distributed and perhaps competing. Moreover, groups enable organizations to maintain memories. If one person leaves the group, important information is not necessarily lost, but continues to be maintained in the group memory. A similar argument can be applied to the experience of the group. Knowledge and skills of functioning are retained even if one member is absent or leaves the group.

As organizations have grown in size and become structurally more complex, the need for groups of people to work together in coordinated ways to achieve objectives which contribute to the overall aims of the organization has become increasingly clear. Indeed, groups are a response to the complexity of modern organizations which often now have an international dimension. Organizations may engage in production, marketing and sales internationally, not simply within the borders of the country of origin. Similarly, technology has changed within the last 50 years, with the development of advanced manufacturing technologies and the burgeoning of information technology. Such complexity requires more complex structures or groupings of people in response.

Conceptually, too, organizations have become more complex. Conversations and language used by organizations reveal ever-increasing conceptual sophistication. Culturally, organizations have become richer and more varied as legislation, psychological contracts and management techniques have altered. Clearly, the environments within which organizations operate have also evidenced rapid and often catastrophic change, with ever greater competition and the internationalization of markets and production. At the same time nation states are being transformed and new economic blocks have developed, such as the EEC. Groups are, in one sense, an organizational response to that increasing complexity.

Psychologists have much to offer to further understanding of work group behaviour, and the long histories of research in social and work and organizational psychology reveal the considerable knowledge construction which has been achieved as a result of research and theoretical development over the last 100 years. The aims of this book are therefore:

1. To provide an authoritative overview of empirical evidence in relation to the various areas covered by the Handbook.
2. To present clear models of groups at work.
3. To integrate the ideas of researchers from the fields of social and work and organizational psychology.
4. To provide a substantial theoretical base for research in the future.
5. To offer the views of leading researchers in the area about future directions and understanding of groups at work.
6. To articulate applications of existing knowledge of processes and functioning of groups at work for those involved in practical interventions in organizational settings.

The success of the book is to be judged by how well these aims are met.

This edition of the Handbook incorporates eight sub-sections, including 22 chapters by leading researchers in the field. The contributors largely come from social and organizational psychology backgrounds and represent the orientations of researchers in Europe, Australia and North America. Of particular importance is that the separate traditions of research into group functioning of European and North American psychologists are combined in this Handbook.

Section I is an **Introduction** to what follows and, apart from this introductory chapter, includes a broad, authoritative historical overview by *Richard Guzzo* (Chapter 1). He links work group psychology research to the organizational change and effectiveness literatures, and provides a helpful analysis of trends in approaches to understanding. Of particular significance is his analysis of the future of work group psychology and the identification of two factors which may impede development—that the boundaries of work groups are changing very rapidly within organizations, and that the diversity of multidisciplinary research could produce a fractionated, disintegrated and incoherent body of research and theory.

Section II concerns **The Contexts of Groups**. In Chapter 2 *Joe McGrath* and *Kathleen O'Connor* lucidly examine issues to do with group development, temporal phasing of group tasks and temporal patterning in group functioning and processes. The importance of considering temporal issues has often been ignored, with work groups treated as static entities. This chapter will enlighten those who have not considered how fundamental time is, in work group functioning.

Susan Jackson considers group structure in Chapter 3, giving particular attention to the concept of group composition, and how it impacts upon interpersonal relationships, team turnover and performance. Her analysis suggests that multidisciplinary teams offer particular promise in terms of their creativity and effectiveness, but that problems of potential conflict and high turnover have to be overcome. She also examines power and status issues within such teams and considers how cohesiveness can be developed in the face of diversity. This is a major challenge for those examining work groups and her cogent analysis reveals the real difficulty of achieving effective, coordinated and rich teamworking in multidisciplinary teams.

In Chapter 4, *Jennifer George* examines the concept of group affective tone as the context for work groups. She considers the extent to which positive vs. negative affect in groups impacts upon group functioning and well-being. She distinguishes between interested, excited, strong, enthusiastic, pro-social, alert, inspired, determined, attentive and active groups and those which are distressed, upset, guilty, scared, hostile, irritable, ashamed, nervous, jittery and afraid. Her analysis provides an alternative view to understanding the experience of those who work in groups and illustrates how work group effectiveness may be promoted by considering the dimension of affective tone.

The last chapter in this section (Chapter 5), by *Franziska Tschan* and *Mario von Cranach*, views group tasks as the crucial element of the context of groups, determining processes and outcomes. They present sequential and hierarchical descriptions of tasks, based on action theory. This enables a detailed and logical account of the processes groups engage in to achieve goals, by deconstructing sequences of actions, hierarchies of actions and the cyclical regulation of actions in work groups. Many researchers have identified the group task as being a fundamental force in shaping work group processes, and the analysis provided by Franziska Tschan and Mario von Cranach offers a structured and accessible way for exploring this thesis further.

Section III focuses on **Group Processes** and forms the largest single subsection of the book. It begins with an examination of minority dissent presented by *Charlan Nemeth* and *Pamela Owens* (Chapter 6). This theoretical perspective within social psychology has been much neglected within industrial/organizational psychology. The central thesis is that minorities stimulate conflict and divergent thinking within groups and organizations, despite group and organizational pressures on members to conform. Charlan Nemeth and Pamela Owens offer those working in organizational domains the opportunity to understand how this theoretical orientation can contribute to a deeper understanding of conflict, power and innovation processes within groups and in relation to groups within organizations.

Mark Stein (Chapter 7) also presents an important and neglected perspective in work and organizational psychology, that of unconscious phenomena in work groups. Drawing on the seminal work of Bion, which has had great influence in family therapy orientations towards group functioning, he explores splitting, projection, unchallenged basic assumptions, and envy as phenomena which have powerful impacts upon group and individual processes and outcomes in the work place.

Marjolein van Offenbeek and *Paul Koopman*, in Chapter 8, present a cogent analysis of decision-making and interaction processes, which goes well beyond simple stage models. They describe how to manage decision-making and interaction in innovative project teams. In particular, they confront the political process involved for groups working within organizations and indicate that decision-making and interaction involve continuous consideration of strategic, tactical and operational choices in work groups. The chapter offers particularly useful insights for practitioners seeking to promote effectiveness in project groups.

In Chapter 9, *Francis Yammarino* squarely confronts the challenge of examining group leadership, about which a great deal has been written but from which little clear understanding has developed. This chapter presents a penetrating analysis of approaches to group leadership. It offers a comprehensive framework which considers group leadership at multiple levels of analysis considering groups as a whole, parts of groups, and dyads within groups. It also examines the three principle orientations to leadership—inspirational, instrumental and informal leadership—and presents a clear research agenda for researchers.

In Chapter 10, *John Cordery* describes research on autonomous work groups and quality circles. His examination reveals that quality circles seem to produce a honeymoon effect, but that organizational realities limit their long-term success. He explores the possibility that quality circles may be a "false empowerment" of work groups since management control is largely retained. On the other hand, autonomous work groups tend to have more power. Consideration of the effects of autonomous group working on well-being and productivity exposes some common misunderstandings. There are clear implications in this chapter about how autonomous group working can be developed more effectively within organizations.

Eberhard Ulich and *Wolfgang Weber* (Chapter 11) also focus on work group autonomy considering dimensions, criteria and evaluations of work group autonomy. They give clear and precise definitions of groups before exploring the concept of autonomy and considering how, in practical terms, researchers can determine the real extent of autonomy within work groups. The conflict between management control and the devolution of responsibility has been evidenced sharply in the difficulty with which popular notions of empowerment and teamworking are operationalized in practice. The contribution of this chapter, therefore, in defining precisely how autonomy can be measured, is helpful. The authors conclude that implementing group work requires a comprehensive, socio-technically oriented concept of production.

Section IV considers **Group Outcomes** and begins with analyses of the concepts of performance and effectiveness in work group functioning by *Felix Brodbeck* (Chapter 12). Work group performance is considered to include processes such as motivation, knowledge and skills; internal and external relationships; and collective strategies. Outcomes are defined as productive outputs, personal criteria (e.g. well-being), social criteria (e.g. group social climate) and innovations. Felix Brodbeck implies a multifaceted concept of effectiveness and his analysis of conceptual and measurement issues provides a coherent overview, enabling researchers to make reasoned choices about the measurement of group performance and effectiveness.

In Chapter 13, *Anders Agrell* and *Roland Gustafson* examine the individual, group and organizational factors influencing processes and outcomes in innovation. They examine group diversity, climate, psychodynamics and the organizational context of groups. Their thorough analysis of the literature combined with case studies enables them to develop a model of the relationship between individual, group climate and organizational context factors and group innovation.

In Chapter 14, *Sabine Sonnentag* examines a much neglected area—the impact of work group factors upon individual well-being. There has been no sustained research thrust in this area, but a moderate amount of relevant data has been collected. There has long been a need for a coherent review of this area and Sabine Sonnentag provides just this, challenging and offering valuable guidance to those concerned with well-being at work. Her review suggests which factors influence group member well-being and implies how work groups can be vehicles for promoting employee well-being.

Section V focuses on **Groups in Organizations**. This section explores the organizational context of groups from a number of perspectives. In Chapter 15, *Natalie Allen* explores new terrain by examining the concept of dual identities, i.e. people's commitment to both their work group and their organization, and the extent to which employees distinguish affectively between these two entities. Natalie Allen reminds readers of the need to focus on the interplay between group and organizational variables, and encourages them to create work places in which employees feel positively towards both their work group and their organization. There has been no previous conceptual/theoretical work in this area and this chapter provides an important map for others to follow.

Chapter 16 examines intergroup relations in organizations. *Jean Hartley* takes a different perspective on work groups from other contributors, including within it "identity" groups such as gender groups, managers, trade unionists and the unemployed. Drawing on social psychology, management theory and views of conflict and power in organizations, Jean Hartley develops a conflict view of intergroup relations, in contrast to the more congruent orientation taken in the previous chapter. She describes relevant social psychological work, including Tajfel's social identity theory, Sherif's realistic conflict theory and Alderfer's embedded intergroup relations theory. Her critique of social identity theory for ignoring multiple and changing group memberships or identities suggests that the real world is more complex than the theory suggests. She explores group identification as a more useful notion, especially in the context of shifting membership boundaries (echoing the comments of Richard Guzzo in Chapter 1).

In Chapter 17, *Neil Anderson* and *Helena Thomas* reflect on the neglect of work group socialization processes. They explore the effects of the group on the individual, but also point out (as do McGrath and O'Connor in Chapter 2) the effects of newcomers on the work group. Neil Anderson and Helena Thomas present a stage model of anticipation, encounter and adjustment which can be used to describe the processes of work group socialization. Again, the first mapping of this new territory offers researchers important guidelines for how to explore these important changes and transitional issues in work groups.

Chapter 18 represents a contribution from the only non-psychologist among the contributors. *David Johnson* deals with a core aspect of work group behaviour—communication. He examines how information is applied to, and shared between, groups in organizations. Organizations, he indicates, are designed to encourage ignorance and groups must seek information and communicate with other groups. He offers three orientations to understanding such communication: hierarchies, networks and markets. The analysis suggests how an understanding of communication can enhance our knowledge about group climate, shared representations, intergroup relations, managing dual identities, socialization, minority influence processes, power relationships and multiple group memberships (which he refers to as "multiplexity"). David Johnson also explores strong and weak ties and the role of liaison links between groups.

Section VI considers **Cultural Aspects of Work Group Functioning**. In Chapter 19, *Peter Smith* and *Julia Noakes* sharply remind readers that studies of teams from different cultures reveal different behaviour patterns. Much work group research has taken place within the USA and individual vs. collectivist cultural orientations may help us to understand why some of this research may not be representative of work group behaviour internationally. Peter Smith and Julia Noakes consider how multi-national teams operate, and examine issues to do with cultural heterogeneity and the consequent diversity of viewpoints. They stress the importance of appropriate conflict management, but urge researchers and practitioners to encourage work group members to appreciate cultural relativity and to develop sensitivity to individuals and groups by "valuing difference". The significance of both language problems and different perspectives on preferred leadership styles are also emphasized.

In Chapter 20, *Scott Tannenbaum*, *Ed Salas* and *Janis Cannon-Bowers* review interventions for effectiveness in work groups. Expenditure on team interventions internationally is on a massive scale, but few empirical analyses of the effectiveness of these interventions have been offered. Given the gap that exists between the real and ideal of team functioning there is an enormous need for deeper understanding of how team effectiveness can be promoted. The authors consider three types of interventions: selection for teams, team-building, and team-training. The authors review the increasing research on selection for teams and offer new understanding about the impact of such selection processes. The limited impact of team-building upon productivity outcomes is also discussed. The authors finally consider team-training, which focuses on individuals, task issues and roles as ways of increasing effectiveness.

In Chapter 21, *Rene Bouwen* and *Ron Fry* adopt a view in contrast to the previous chapter. They focus on facilitating group development and review traditional conceptual orientations towards team development: task/instrumental, relational/developmental and contextual/organizational. Their chapter demands that group theory offer "an intelligible formulation amongst a welter of impressions", whereas they see previous theories as simply tools to engineer groups towards effectiveness. They claim that interventions are "co-authoring a history ... or narrative ... that involves the participants in co-enquiry and co-visioning with the intervenor(s)". Rene Bouwen and Ron Fry offer an important alternative perspective—the constructionist perspective—on work groups, which sees meaning as being made through conversation.

The final section of the book (Section VII) concerns **Conceptual Integration** and in Chapter 22 I offer a conceptual integration of some of the common threads which weave through the preceding chapters, focusing on processes and outcomes in complex decision-making groups. The chapter seeks to integrate some major themes and consistent streams of research findings in an understanding of how work groups should ideally be functioning in order to achieve greatest effectiveness. It also considers work groups and their relationships with organizations and the wider society. As in many of the chapters in the Handbook, one aim is to provide an alternative to the *status quo*, in order that debate can be enriched in the search for understanding about how people can collaborate effectively together in pursuit of their shared objectives.

Overall, my hope is that readers will find that the book has largely achieved its aims of providing a clear exposition of existing theoretical and empirical bases; integrating ideas from social and industrial organizational psychology; presenting both new and alternative models; offering views about future research directions and drawing out some of the applications of knowledge to date. In particular, I hope it will provide researchers, students and practitioners with an overview which will also stimulate their thinking to new understandings of the richness of human collaborative and conflict processes in work groups.

Michael A. West
Institute of Work Psychology
The University of Sheffield, UK

Section I

Introduction

Chapter 1

Fundamental Considerations about Work Groups

Richard A. Guzzo
Department of Psychology, University of Maryland, USA

Abstract

This chapter adopts an historical perspective in examining salient topics and themes in theory and research on groups at work. These themes include changes in how groups have been viewed in relation to organizations, changes in such things as the relative emphasis placed on intragroup processes and their influence on individual members, and changes in the course of theory and research. Changes in theory include a movement toward viewing groups as small social systems embedded in larger social systems. Changes in research include a movement toward interdisciplinary field-based studies, emphasizing effectiveness as a key variable. Recent research that focuses on the contributions of groups to overall organizational effectiveness is given special attention. The chapter also visits the question of whether groups and teams are different entities, since the latter term has become increasingly popular. The chapter concludes by looking to the future, raising the possibility that the nature of groups at work will soon be transformed due to a coming erosion of group boundaries, and speculates on the problems posed by interdisciplinary research and theorizing.

As this book attests, groups are important landmarks of contemporary organizational terrain. One cannot make a thorough, enlightened analysis of organizations without in some way accounting for the presence and impact of groups. Such was not always the case, and it seems unlikely that we will ever return to those times.

This chapter examines selected considerations fundamental to understanding work groups in organizations. It begins with a brief historical look at the changing

Handbook of Work Group Psychology. Edited by M.A. West.
© 1996 John Wiley & Sons Ltd.

nature of groups, how they have appeared in research and practice, especially how they have been regarded in the organizational sciences. Some of the more salient theoretical approaches to understanding teams are highlighted and an assessment is offered of the current states of practice, research, and theorizing regarding teams in organizations. The chapter concludes with a look toward the future of groups at work and of the organizational sciences studying them.

THE SLOW AND RECENTLY GRAND EMERGENCE OF GROUPS AT WORK

Groups became recognized as social entities critical to the productive efficiency of work organizations quite some time ago. Many people (e.g. Leavitt, 1975) point to the Hawthorne studies begun in the 1920s as the first large-scale, systematic social science effort to bring to light the importance of groups in organizations (e.g. see Roethlisberger & Dickson, 1939). The Hawthorne studies, so named for the place where they were done, surfaced several considerations of enduring importance, such as the relevance of relationships between groups in organizations, the strength of effects that groups have on their members, and the extent to which informal groups permeate organizations. Informal groups arise out of propinquity, friendships and other non-work bases. They are contrasted to formal groups, those intentionally created by organizations for the purpose of fulfilling organizational missions. In organizations, informal groups more often than not were seen as problems to be managed (Shea & Guzzo, 1987). Not being a formal part of the typical bureaucratic design, informal groups were thought to disrupt the efficiencies of the classical individually-centered bureaucracy. Apart from work gangs and crews that predominated in certain industries, groups were little relied on for task accomplishment. Although not embraced by organizations early on, groups were nonetheless intensively studied during the 1940s, 1950s and 1960s. However, the rate of research publications during the 1960s began to decline and that decline continued through the 1970s (Zander, 1979).

Group Process and Influence

Two characteristics of much of the early research on groups, especially true of research in the USA, were relative emphases on processes of interaction among members and the impact of those dynamics on individual members (Guzzo & Shea, 1992; Shea & Guzzo, 1987). The effectiveness of groups at tasks was a secondary concern, and the tasks studied were usually relatively simple tasks that could be performed in laboratory settings. Early textbooks in organizational psychology such as that by Viteles (1939) emphasized the need to understand group influences on individuals at work. Many significant research efforts focused on this general issue, as illustrated by Whyte's (1995) work on individual responses to incentive pay, as those responses are shaped by such things as peer pressure and group norms. The great depth and breadth of research on work-relevant group influences on individuals is synthesized and summarized more recently by Hackman (1992).

The focus on processes of group interaction took many forms. One indicator of the salience of this focus was the appearance of several analytic schemes for representing the nature of intragroup interaction, the most widely adopted being that of Bales (1950). This particular scheme relied on observers to classify interactions in terms of whether they were expressive or task-oriented, positive or negative, active or passive. Bales's categories, though reliably observable, bore little systematic relation to task performance (McGrath, 1984, 1991). Reviews and reconceptualizations offered by Hackman and Morris (1975) and Steiner (1972) were some of the later influential works attempting to further our understanding of the connections between groups process and performance. Each offered new ways of thinking about task interaction and each cited the nature of group tasks as important to that link.

For many years virtually all research and theorizing about groups reflected an underlying input–process–output model (Guzzo & Shea, 1992). Inputs were typically regarded as qualities members brought to the group, such as personality differences, expertise, strength. These inputs were then transformed into outputs through member interaction (exchange of information, coordination of efforts, attempts to exert leadership, and so on). According to Steiner (1972), these inputs largely determined the *potential* productivity of a group. *Actual* productivity, according to Steiner (1972), was determined by a group's potential productivity less decrements due to process losses. The bias is clear here: groups get in the way of potential productivity because they suffer process losses due to poor coordination or slackening effort among group members. While occasional departures from this paradigm emphasized the unique gains that could be attained through groups (the notion of synergy; Collins & Guetzkow, 1964), the dominant orientation in the research literature was one of understanding and fixing group process problems. And considerable research energy was invested in a related issue: whether group performance could exceed individual performance in relatively simple tasks (e.g. Hill, 1982).

Hackman and Morris (1975) examined a large body of literature conforming to the input-process-output paradigm. They found strong evidence that inputs were related to observable group processes. However, the connection between group processes and output effectiveness was weaker, and very few tests existed of the whole causal chain, according to Hackman and Morris (1975). Their review opened the possibility that the nature of group processes may indeed be a useful predictor of certain outcomes, such as individual affective reactions to a group, but not necessarily a powerful predictor of how well groups accomplish their work.

Groups as Performing Units

In addition to the study of group processes and their impact on individuals, groups have been studied as task-performing entities. The nature of group processes was indeed important to this line of work, but its relative emphasis was on the effective accomplishment of work, especially among groups in organizations. This line of thinking was advanced first in European literature as expressed, for example, in Bion's (e.g. 1961) writing and in scholarship within the sociotechnical systems framework (e.g. Trist, 1981). Bion saw the group as a small social system in existence to perform some primary task but in which the rational, planned task-performance activity was imbued with, and often displaced by, activity attributable to unconscious forces concerning such matters as dependence and conflict. Bion's group-as-whole perspective provided an early foundation for understanding how the formal work of groups relates to affective and social dynamics found in them. These contributions very much emphasized small groups as bounded, system-like social entities responsive to their environments (Homans, 1950, provides another early contribution along these lines, drawn in part on the Hawthorne studies).

Sociotechnical theory also emphasized groups as social systems. It is one of the few conceptually rich paradigms that has had a significant impact on organizational practices. The familiar distinction between task and social lines of activity in work groups is also a foundation of the sociotechnical framework. Another core premise of this framework is that both task and social goals can be jointly optimized, if the circumstances are properly structured. What the sociotechnical perspective offered were unique ideas about how to attain this joint optimization through groups. Specifically, it prescribed autonomy and self-regulation for work groups. That is, groups were to control their own task procedures and their transactions with others outside the group (i.e. boundary control). Autonomy also was thought to be enhanced by differentiating groups' tasks from the tasks of others in an organization. The theoretical principles of the sociotechnical perspective have been tested in several typically complex studies that have appeared from time to time over a prolonged period. The results have largely been supportive though sometimes unevenly so (see reviews by Beekun, 1989; Goodman, Devadas & Hughson, 1988; Pearce & Ravlin, 1987; and studies such as those by Cohen & Ledford, 1994; Cordery, Mueller & Smith, 1991; Wall et al., 1986).

Groups and Organizational Practices

Whether primarily regarded as sources of influence on individuals or as social entities capable of high levels of productivity, extensive research and theorizing about work groups had accumulated since the time of the Hawthorne studies. However, during this time there was only a slow growth of interest in, and application of, groups in work organizations. Then, in the 1970s but particularly in the 1980s, things changed: the glory period of the history of groups in organizations began. This widespread interest in groups was a response to several factors. Emphasizing groups in organizations was in part a response to worker alienation (e.g. Davis & Taylor, 1972). Groups not only provided camaraderie and means of social support at work but also carried with them the capacity to redefine the scope of jobs, making them more challenging and less stifling. Also, a few celebrated cases of experimentation with work teams, such as Volvo's implementation of teams in lieu of traditional assembly line automobile production (Gyllenhammar, 1977), set off a wave of interest and emulation. Further, forceful competition was encountered from Japanese-produced goods of high quality. The success of Japanese firms was attributed, in part, to management practices that emphasized the creation of groups—especially quality circles—responsible for purging errors and creating innovations in work processes. As Shea & Guzzo (1987) noted, the wave of interest in groups as productive entities in organizations was ignited more by practical concerns than by insights and appreciations derived from formal theory and research; practice and research at this time were quite disconnected. In fact, the practical interest in groups arose just about the time research interest in groups was fading (Zander, 1979), But by whatever route, groups were becoming popular solutions to organizational problems.

The current importance of groups to organizations has been most thoroughly documented in Western and in Japanese cultures (e.g. Cole, 1989). In the USA, for example, a steep growth curve in the use of teams was documented over a short time, 1987–1990, by Lawler, Mohrman & Ledford (1992). Gordon (1992) estimated that 80% of US organizations with 100 or more employees use teams in some way. Another indicator of the rapid emergence of teams in the workplace is the number of popular press articles and books appearing on the topic in the past few years.

In summary, the *idea* that groups are important to organizations was established about 70 years ago. However, only in the past 15 years or so has that idea been seized and widely acted on by large numbers of organizations. This grand emergence of groups on the organizational landscape has brought about many changes and complications. One of those in need of resolution is a matter of terminology.

GROUPS OR TEAMS?

The rapid emergence of groups in the workplace has brought with it a change in terminology: the word "team" has largely supplanted the word "group" in the language of the organizational sciences, especially among practitioners (Guzzo & Dickson, 1996). The connotation is clear: teams are superior to and more desirable than mere groups. These days it seems that teams, not groups, are taken seriously (cf. Leavitt, 1975).

What is a work group? Following the definitional work of Alderfer (1977) and

Hackman (1987), work groups are defined by the joint presence of the following attributes:

- They are social entities embedded in larger social systems (i.e. organizations).
- They perform one or more tasks relevant to their organization's mission.
- Their task performance has consequences that affect others inside or outside the organization.
- They are made up individuals whose work roles require them to be, to some appreciable degree, interdependent.
- They have membership that is identifiable not only to those in the group but also to those outside it.

This is a very encompassing definition. It applies to groups that provide services to customers internal or external to the organization, that manufacture things, that sell, that make decisions, that provide health care, and so on. It also applies to groups that are temporary or permanent, successful or unsuccessful, large or small. Embeddedness in a larger social system is a key property of groups. How an organization treats groups embedded in it can greatly influence the other properties. For example, organizations that recognize group accomplishments with visible celebrations and monetary rewards heighten the distinction between employees in and those not in the rewarded groups. The nature of any one work group very much is a function of its embeddedness in its surrounding organization.

Are teams of a different nature than groups? For Katzenbach & Smith (1993), for example, the distinction between teams and groups "turns on performance results" (p. 112). They go on to say that a group's performance is a function of what members do as individuals, whereas a team's performance includes individual and collective or joint work products. To make the distinction between teams and groups in this way harks of long-known types of group tasks. Namely, *additive* tasks are those for which the group product is the sum of individual members' contributions (Steiner, 1972). There is no task-based interdependence in groups performing additive tasks as members *co-act* rather than *interact* to produce outcomes. Katzenbach & Smith (1991) attempt to restrict, in order to make room for the term "teams," the use of the term "group" to that set of circumstances in which additive tasks exist. But in doing so they relegate groups to a very narrow set of circumstances for, according to Steiner, "outside the laboratory, complete additivity is probably rather rare" (1972, p. 33). Certainly distinguishing between groups and teams by confining the term "group" to infrequently encountered conditions is quite unsatisfactory.

Distinctions like that offered by Katzenbach & Smith (1993) also imply that substantial bodies of empirical research and theory on groups would somehow become irrelevant to teams. Would we ignore previous theory and data on, say, intergroup relations because groups are not teams? Would prior knowledge of the group influences on individuals be rendered insignificant with regard to teams? And what about autonomous work groups? Teams and groups share too many dynamics to make any grand distinction between them. I suggest the following convention: what can be said is that all teams are groups but that not all groups are teams. Not all groups are teams because the term group has indeed been used very expansively in general social science, for example to describe social aggegrates in which there is no interdependence of members. But this has not been the case in the organizational sciences. The definition of a *work group* easily accommodates the term "team." Consequently, in this chapter I make no real distinction between "groups" and "teams" in organizations, regarding the two terms as synonyms.

CHANGES IN GROUP RESEARCH

The emergence of teams in organizational settings is connected to changes in more than just terminology. Changes in theoretical orientations, in dependent variables and research methods also have occurred. It is not the case that, for example, certain long-standing interests have abruptly disappeared from the literature. Rather, these shifts of interest are a matter of the relative degree of interest and activity.

Interdisciplinary Interests

One notable change concerns who are the most active researchers of groups. Levine & Moreland (1990) asserted that research activity among social psychologists, who for decades were the leaders of group research, has been eclipsed by the research activity of organizational psychologists. While other fields also traditionally active in group research (communication, education, and sociology) have remained so, organizational psychologists indeed have placed themselves among the pre-eminent researchers of groups. But interest in organizations, and thus interest in groups, comes from many fields in addition to psychology. The organizational sciences busy with group research now reflect many disciplines, including economists (e.g. research on group incentives; Nalbantian, 1987), anthropologists (e.g. analyses of the construction of meaning from group meetings; Schwartzman, 1986), political scientists (e.g. understanding group decision making at the highest levels of government; Hermann, 1994), information science researchers (e.g. the effects of computer-assisted group meetings; Poole et al., 1993), engineers (e.g. the role of groups in quality assurance systems; Deming, 1986), and management generalists. Group research is today a highly interdisciplinary enterprise.

Effectiveness as a Key Variable

As the discipline base of group research shifted substantive and methodological changes became discernible. One visible change concerned the primary phenomena of interest. In the decades of that stream of group research dominated by social psychologists, the greatest interest was in the impact of the group on individual members and in intragroup dynamics and processes. That is, what happens within a group, and the consequences of intragroup action for individuals (e.g. individuals' attitude change, individuals' identification with the group) remained the center of research attention. Early research on conformity and, more recently, research on influence processes between members in the minority and those in the majority within groups illustrate this. What has changed is not so much the disappearance of an interest in intragroup processes but the dominance of a new focus, that of group performance effectiveness defined in terms of the products and consequences of group action. This new focus is not surprising, since most of the organizations in which groups are studied are businesses where the pressures of competition can be great and the relative performance of an enterprise can have substantial consequences. Typical dependent variables in group research now include such things as sales, speed of service, defects in products, the volume of goods produced and other aspects of output.

Methodological Changes

Group research also has changed by virtue of how it is done. In years past the social psychological experiment, usually conducted in a laboratory, reigned as the favored tactic of research. McGrath & Altman (1966) estimated that only 5% of the studies in existence at the time of their review were studies of groups in natural settings. In the organizational research literature laboratory experiments also appear, though probably at a lower rate. One area where experiments do predominate as a research tactic is that of computer mediation of group work. Hollingshead & McGrath (1995) reviewed 50 research reports investigating computer-assisted group decision-making and communication. Of these, 80% were laboratory experiments. The remainder were a mixture of field experiments and case studies (see Exhibit 1, Hollingshead & McGrath, 1995). Placing research on computer-mediated groups aside for the moment, there are now larger numbers of field research projects than ever before. In contrast to laboratory investigations that examine the influence of one or a few variables, recent field research on groups tends to investigate multiple variables simultaneously. Sometimes this multivariate work is highly quantitative. Gladstein (1984) provides an early example; Campion, Medsker & Higgs (1993) provide a more recent one. Other field research analyzes its multiple variables rather qualitatively. Ancona & Caldwell's (1992) research on how teams cross their boundaries and act on their environments is an example, as are the reports contained in Hackman (1990). Simply put, there are many methods in use in group research in the organizational sciences, and that methodological diversity represents a significant departure from past practice.

Emphasis on the Context

As the organizational sciences increased their level of research activity intragroup processes remained of interest but often became secondary to an emphasis placed on the importance of groups' organizational *context* (Guzzo & Shea, 1992). This emphasis on context coincided with a clarifying focus on performance effectiveness as the critical dependent variable of interest in group research in the organizational sciences. Hackman (1987, 1990), for example, offered a theoretical model of group performance that stressed as causal factors such things as reward systems, information flows and training opportunities in organizations. Such contextual factors were seen to influence intragroup processes relevant to team effectiveness. Similarly, Sundstrom, De Meuse & Futrell (1990) cited the organizational context as a principal influence on group effectiveness. Campion, Medsker & Higgs (1993) offered evidence that a variety of what they refer to as "group design" variables related to group effectiveness. Many of the group design variables they investigate (e.g. managerial support) directly reflect the impact of the organizational context in which groups work and only secondarily reflect aspects of intragroup processes. These examples represent the broader theoretical movement toward an emphasis on groups vis-à-vis their organizational context and the sharpened focus on performance effectiveness as a key dependent variable. This emphasis on context has renewed the attention given to organizations as social systems, as the following section discusses.

Teams in Organizational Systems

Some of the most recent literature on team effectiveness at work has not only addressed the impact of contextual influences on teams but has also addressed the part teams play in the overall effectiveness of organizations. Teams embedded in organizational systems are both subject to the influences of those systems and are sources of influence on them. So, for example, it is possible to question what role teams play in overall organizational effectiveness. This is a meaningful though not easily answered question.

The sources of difficulty of answering the question of teams' impact on organizational effectiveness are parallel to those explored in the book by Harris (1994). That book explores the apparent paradox that large investments in information technology have not resulted in often-promised gains in organizational productivity. Whether one accepts the paradox as factual or not, the book explores the many pitfalls and problems of establishing connections between elements of a system (e.g. computer equipment, teams) and the overall organizational system (e.g. its productivity and effectiveness). Problems and pitfalls relate to the many uncertainties of measurement, the ambiguity about the strength of linkages among the various components of an organization (McGrath, 1991, for example, speaks of groups as being loosely coupled to their embedding organizations), the often-questionable wisdom of expecting to observe effects at one level of analysis (e.g. the total organization) resulting from changes made at some other level (e.g. in the design department where new computer technology was installed), and the likely presence of multiple moderators and mediators of the transmission of effects from one part of an organization to another. Cognizant of the complications, it is nonetheless instructive to examine recent research on the potential link between teams and broader organizational effectiveness. Most of this relevant research is made up of studies—typically case histories, but some controlled and some quantitative investigations—of targeted interventions and of large-scale organizational change efforts.

Macy & Izumi (1993) located nearly 1800 North American organizational change studies reported over three decades. They subjected 131 of them (those providing sufficient statistical information) to a meta-analysis seeking to estimate the extent to which variance in dependent variables of interest (e.g. financial indicators of effectiveness, employee attitudes, behaviors such as turnover and absenteeism) related to the types of interventions made. In general, Macy & Izumi found that organizational change efforts had greater effects on financially-related measures of effectiveness and fewer effects on other indicators, such as attitudes. In fact, employee attitudes showed little systematic change in response to the interventions studied.

Macy & Izumi (1993) also report that the greater the number of changes made in an intervention, the greater the impact on effectiveness. That is, the organizational change efforts most likely to be successful are those that make multiple changes rather than, say, implementing a single new practice. Many types of interventions were analyzed, including job redesign, employee involvement, changes in organizational structure, changes in workflow, and team-oriented interventions such as the creation of autonomous work groups and team development activities. Those interventions with the greatest effects on financially-related measures were team-related interventions. These also appeared to influence turnover and absenteeism more strongly than did other interventions. These results demonstrate that the effects of team-oriented practices can have positive broader effects in organizations.

Applebaum & Batt (1994) offer convergent evidence. They reviewed the results of a dozen extensive surveys of organizational practices in the USA as well as 185 case studies of innovations in management practices. They find the evidence compelling that teams contribute to improved organizational effectiveness, especially in terms of increased efficiency and quality. Their evidence largely concerns increases in effectiveness following the introduction or diffusion of team-based work arrangements where no or few such arrangements previously existed.

Applebaum & Batt (1994) also noted that the implementation of team-based work practices was accompanied in some organizations by changes in hiring, compensation, decision-making, technology and other practices. They suggest that these organizations, rather than those making more limited changes, will experience enduring gains. Like Macy & Izumi (1993) and others (e.g. Guzzo, Jette & Katzell, 1985; Schnelder & Klein, 1994), Applebaum & Batt (1994) point to the power of multiple interventions. Mohrman, Cohen & Mohrman (1995) agree. They prescribe many simultaneous changes required of organizations seeking to become successful team-based systems.

Other researchers provide evidence of the favorable impact of team-based work practices on organizational performance. Kalleberg & Moody (1994) studied over 700 work establishments in the USA and found that those in which teams were relied on were rated as more effective on certain performance dimensions (e.g. product quality, employee relations) than were organizations in which teams were not an important part of the design of the organization. Levine & D'Andrea Tyson (1990) reviewed research from several disciplines and found that employee participation has a modest effect on organizational productivity and that teams are a chief mechanism of employee participation (also see Cotton, 1993), thus giving teams a share of the credit for productivity gains.

Conclusion

Group research has taken on some new characteristics in the hands of organizationally-interested scholars. The number of disciplinary perspectives applied to teams has expanded; the frequency with which various methods of research are used has changed; performance effectiveness as a key dependent variable has become dominant; and there has arisen a vigorous interest in understanding teams *vis-à-vis* their organizational context. This interest in context has followed two courses. One course addresses how factors outside the team influence the team and its effectiveness. The other course addresses teams as components of larger social systems and seeks to understand the impact teams have on the well-being and effectiveness of those systems. So far, the evidence about teams' impact on organizational effectiveness is positive. With these considerations as background, the next section examines anticipated developments in group research and management practices.

THE PROBLEMATIC FUTURE OF TEAMS AND TEAM RESEARCH

There are reasons to believe that the grand emergence of groups at work may run a short course. Broadly, these reasons have to do with the continually changing nature of organizations and of organizational research. Because of technological, social and other developments, teams in organizations of the near future may be quite different from teams as they are now. These changes will mount new challenges to group researchers and theorists. Two problematic developments examined below are (1) the erosion and weakening of team boundaries in organizations and (2) the potential for discord in the group research enterprise of the organizational sciences.

The Coming Erosion of Team Boundaries

As Sundstrom, De Meuse & Futrell (1990), summarizing a long line of group theorizing, have clearly maintained, the existence of group boundaries is crucial. Boundaries "are difficult to describe concisely" (Sundstrom, De Meuse & Futrell, 1990, p. 121). They serve the functions of demarcating a group from its environment (e.g. from other groups, from other parts of the organization) while also serving as the gateways of exchange with others (customers, other members of the organization). Boundaries have many aspects. Some are physical, such as might occur when each team in an organization is given its own unique space in which to work, and some are temporal, maintained, for example, by prescribed cycles of activity. Boundaries also have psychological aspects, such as when stereotyping creates subjective but sometimes insurmountable distinctions between in-group and out-group. Qualifications and credentials required to enter a group are also an aspect of boundaries, as are differences between groups in rights, responsibilities and obligations. Boundaries have many facets, but all groups have them; they make it possible for groups to have integrity as social entities.

If team boundaries change then the nature of teams will change. As Sundstrom, De Meuse & Futrell (1990) point out, if boundaries become too open or indistinct a team risks losing its essence. If boundaries become too exclusive teams can become isolated. It is easy to imagine how boundaries matter. For example, the identification of members with their groups surely must be affected by the strength and permeability of those groups' boundaries. Intragroup processes such as majority and minority influence and task coordination also appear to depend on the nature of a team's boundaries. Changes in team boundaries are not necessarily bad, but they do portend many things for research and theorizing on teams at work. In this section I explore forces in organizations that could change the nature of team boundaries—mostly making them less distinct—and the implications of such changes for future research and theory on teams at work.

Computers

What forces might erode team boundaries? Perhaps the paramount force is computer technology. Computers can indeed serve a decision *support* function for groups, as originally conceived. But the technology has evolved to the point today where it profoundly changes the nature of groups. Computer-mediated teleconferencing, for example, links individuals from disparate places for a real-time, non-face-to-face meeting. The electronic medium can carry audio and video as well as text information, and the combination of the hardware and software govern how a meeting transpires (e.g. how communication unfolds, how information is managed, etc.). Further, technology exists ("groupware") for individuals to work as teams via the exchange of electronic communications and documents without ever meeting in real time.

Evidence indicates that the procedures of communicating, decision-making and so on in groups are materially changed by computer technology. Compared to face-to-face groups, computer-assisted groups tend to have more equal rates of communication while having less overall communication (i.e. fewer communicative acts), less argumentation, "more uninhibited communication ('flaming'), especially in computer conferences, and more positive socioemotional communication" (Hollingshead & McGrath, 1995, p. 74). More than just surface characteristics of group interaction are different: the very nature of the team-as-entity seems to be changed. For such teams there are no physical boundaries, neither are there strong temporal boundaries (except those that exist during a real-time computer conference). Surely the psychological boundaries of such teams are diluted because members are remote from one another and communicate in restricted ways.

Multiple Team Memberships

Alderfer (1977) pointed out that most people in organizations carry memberships in multiple groups. Mostly those multiple groups are what Alderfer referred to as identity groups, those based on shared characteristics thought to be central to one's own understanding of one's self, such as age, ethnicity and gender. Alderfer also referred to membership in a task group, such as one's department. Since Alderfer's writing a change has occurred, one that has accompanied the emergence of groups in the workplace. It is that employees increasingly are members of more and more teams. For example, Gordon's (1992) survey results indicated that it is not uncommon for employees to be members of more than one work team. Multiple work team memberships would seem especially prevalent in organizations characterized by high levels of employee participation in decision-making and by the use of project teams. Thus the number of task groups in which individuals are members appears to be rising, and so the total number of group memberships (identity plus task) rises.

One of the consequences of multiple group memberships, according to Weick (1969), is the resulting *partial inclusion* of members. As a result of belonging to many groups, individuals allocate their resources (time, attention, energy, identity) to those groups, with the consequence that in several groups an individual can be less than a fully-fledged member. Put another way, the boundaries of groups are diluted as individuals spread themselves across several groups rather than investing fully in one. Although there may be positive consequences of multiple group memberships for individuals and for their employing organizations—an intriguing possibility worthy of investigation—it does appear that the strength of any one group's boundaries for an individual is influenced by the number and importance of other groups in which that individual holds membership.

Flexible Work Practices

Many organizations currently seek flexibility in their work arrangements. Rather than insisting on a standard, "one-size-fits-all" approach to work rules, organizations are accommodating to the demands of commuting, of family, and of employees' personal preferences by implementing such practices as telecommuting, contract workers, job sharing, increased reliance on part-time employees, and variable work schedules. Some of the attractive features of flexible work practices, from the organization's perspective, are that a workforce with ample part-time and contract employees can be grown and shrunk more rapidly and with less difficulty than a work-force of all full-time career employees. Further, desirable employees who might otherwise have left the employer can be retained through flexible practices. From the employee's side, flexibility may serve personal needs (e.g. childcare) and personal preferences very well, though there seem to be risks associated with each specific practice (e.g. unemployment, out-of-sight out-of-mind risks for telecommuters). As regards the nature of teams in the workplace, flexible practices appear to be another force that could reduce the strength and clarity of team boundaries. Are the membership boundaries of teams staffed only by full-time career employees different from those of teams staffed in part by contract workers? Are the boundaries of on-site teams of a different character than those of teams with members who telecommute? Although few data exist with which to answer such questions, it is plausible that the increased use of flexible work practices can have the unintended consequence of changing the nature of teams in organizations by weakening team boundaries.

Implications

Information technology, multiple group memberships, and flexible work practices present forces that can erode the strength of team boundaries. Assuming that team boundaries in organizations in fact become less distinct, what are the possible consequences for groups and what are the possible responses by group researchers?

Because teams have attained a permanent place in organization architecture they will not disappear. Rather, the *nature* of teams may change significantly. With less distinct boundaries teams can be expected to be less cohesive. That is, confronted with multiple team memberships and weak links to fellow members, levels of cohesiveness are likely to decline. Similarly, the strength of individuals' identification with any one team is likely to diminish. Together, these factors make it probable that the amount of influence groups in organizations have over their individual members will shrink. Under these circumstances groups will be less able to extract compliance with norms, for example, and individuals will less often rely on a primary group for information or support.

As described earlier, understanding group influences on individuals has been a core research concern for many years. But this research endeavor will need to adapt in order to be faithful to the changing nature of groups in organizations. It is clear that the field is adapting in part to these changes, as the growth of research on the dynamics of computer-assisted groups shows. However, additional research is needed on the consequences of multiple group memberships and on the impact of flexible work practices on teams. Also, groups with weaker boundaries may rely on different forms of influence tactics than groups with stronger boundaries, and research that directly investigates the links between the boundary strengths and mechanisms of influence is needed.

It is also the case that the changing nature of teams in organizations has implications for research and theory on team effectiveness. Sundstrom, De Meuse & Futrell, (1990) assert that boundaries, though infrequently studied in past small-group research, may be critical to team effectiveness in organizations. More specifically, they suggest that group boundaries must be managed so that the internal coherence of teams can be sufficiently preserved, while at the same time a team's integration into the larger organization can be accomplished with the degree of synchronization and coordination required for the team to contribute to organizational effectiveness. Could the gains in organizational effectiveness attributable to teams in the Applebaum & Batt (1994) review have been realized if team boundaries were weak? As important as boundaries may be to team effectiveness, Sundstrom, De Meuse & Futrell, admit that "practitioners can hope for little guidance from current research evidence" (1990, p. 130) regarding how to manage them. They cite a great need for such research. More generally, theories that explicitly recognize boundary management activities as among the important determinants of team effectiveness are required. Perhaps the prospects here are good. A theoretical emphasis on boundary management would appear to be an easy outgrowth of the attention given in recent theories to the group in its context. Further, because boundary management has consequences both for internal dynamics in teams and their performance effectiveness, future theorizing on this issue may provide a means of integrating two sometimes separate streams of groups research, those on group influences on individuals and those on group effectiveness.

In closing, it is worth noting that certain organizational practices may in fact be countervailing forces against those that weaken team boundaries. For example, the implementation of new pay practices that reward team accomplishments could strengthen team boundaries, because they would heighten the tangible consequences of being a member of a team and participating in its work. As Applebaum & Batt (1994) note, some organizations seem to adopt such team-supporting practices more than others. Such between-organization differences in their team-related practices are to be expected. Consequently, the erosion of team boundaries will be more visible in some organizations than in others.

The Potential for Discord

One other development in group research is its high potential for discord and disarray. Two realities, already discussed, that could drive future group research in this direction are its highly interdisciplinary and multi-method character. These differences play themselves out in many ways. Consider, for example, the topic of group decision-making. Decision-making in groups is studied from many diverse disciplines and methods, as evident in the works compiled by Guzzo & Salas (1995). In that book decision-making is addressed as it occurs in all sorts of groups, from tactical weapons teams on naval ships to top management teams. It is studied in teams of diverse membership, in teams under stress, in teams operating under varying degrees of competition and cooperation, in computer-assisted teams, and in teams in a variety of other settings. The disciplines involved in its study include various fields of psychology (organizational, military, social), management, engineering, communication, political science, and others. The methods by which group decision-making are studied are disparate. Data examined in the Guzzo & Salas (1995) work come from laboratory experiments, naturalistic observations, simulations, interviews and surveys, analyses of archives and transcripts, and other sources. New methods for modeling team decision-making and performance are emerging, too. Coovert, Craiger & Cannon-Bowers (1995) explore the applicability of Petri nets, fuzzy sets, neural networks and other tools for research on teams. And the topic of decision-making is studied from several levels of analysis, including that of the individual (e.g. how individuals in groups use information), the dyad (e.g. how prior experience of a leader with an individual member affects the leader's use of information from that member), team decision processes, and the organizational support system for group decision-making. Are these circumstances catalysts of discord in group research?

It is unrealistic to expect that at any time soon will there appear a consolidated theory of group decision-making that encompasses the abundance of variables, data and conceptual orientations now in the literature. And decision-making is but one topic in research on groups. This scenario of multi-discipline, multivariate literatures exists for many topics in group research. The question seems not to be whether convergence will soon occur in group research. Rather, the question is whether the enterprise of group research will be pulled apart by its own heterogeneity, collapsing into a jumble of unrelated research reports and unused knowledge.

The danger of a disparate, unintegrated research literature should not be taken lightly; it appears to me as a real possibility. Yet there are many positive qualities inherent to the current state of group research, such as its energy. That energy is generated by the current importance of groups to organizations, the appearance of fresh methods and ideas, and the rubbing together of different disciplines. In the end, I am a guarded optimist about the future of group research. Even if organizations change and teams become less fashionable, teams will always be a part of organizations. And too much already has been learned about work groups, with too many researchers participating in generating that knowledge, for group research to dwindle. The grand emergence of groups in organizational practice and research has created waves of research activity that will be felt for a long time to come. Hopefully, that activity will be well orchestrated.

REFERENCES

Ancona, D.G. & Caldwell, D.F. (1992). Bridging the boundary: external activity and performance in organizational teams. *Administrative Science Quarterly*, **37**, 634–665.

Alderfer, C.P. (1977). Group and intergroup relations. In J.R. Hackman & J.L. Suttle (eds), *Improving the Quality of Work Life*. Pallisades, CA: Goodyear, pp. 227–296.

Applebaum, E. & Batt, R. (1994). *The New American Workplace*. Ithaca, NY: ILR Press.

Bales, R.F. (1950). A set of categories for the analysis of small group interaction. *American Sociological Review*, **15**, 257–263.

Beekun, R.I. (1989). Assessing the effectiveness of socio-technical interventions: antidote or fad? *Human Relations*, **47**, 877–897.

Bion, W.R. (1961). *Experience in Groups*. New York: Basic Books.

Campion, M.A., Medsker, G.J. & Higgs, A.C. (1993). Relations between work group characteristics and effectiveness: implications for designing effective work groups. *Personnel Psychology*, **46**, 823–850.

Cohen, S.G. & Ledford, G.E. Jr (1994). The effectiveness of self-managing teams: a field experiment. *Human Relations*, **47**, 13–43.

Cole, R.E. (1989). *Strategies for Learning: Small-group Activities in American, Japanese, and Swedish Industry*. Berkeley, CA: University of California Press.

Collins, E.B. & Guetzkow, H. (1964). *A Social Psychology of Group Processes for Decision Making*. New York: Wiley.

Coovert, M.D., Craiger, J.P. & Cannon-Bowers, J.A. (1995). Innovations in modeling and simulating team performance: implications for decision making. In R.A. Guzzo & E. Salas (eds), *Team Effectiveness and Decision Making in Organizations*. San Francisco: Jossey-Bass, pp. 149–203.

Cordery, J.L., Mueller, W.S. & Smith, L.M. (1991). Attitudinal and behavioral effects of autonomous group working: a longitudinal field study. *Academy of Management Journal*, **34**, 464–476.

Cotton, J.L. (1993). *Employee Involvement*. Newbury Park, CA: Sage.

Davis, L.E. & Taylor, J.C. (eds) (1972). *Design of Jobs*. Harmondsworth: Penguin.

Deming, W.E. (1986). *Out of the Crisis*. Cambridge, MA: Center for Advanced Engineering Study, Massachusetts Institute of Technology.

Gladstein, D. (1984). Groups in context: a model of task group effectiveness. *Administrative Science Quarterly*, **29**, 499–517.

Goodman, P.S., Devadas, R. & Hughson, T.L.G. (1988). Groups and productivity: analyzing the effectiveness of self-managing teams. In J.P. Campbell & R.J. Campbell (eds), *Productivity in Organizations*. San Francisco: Jossey-Bass, pp. 295–327.

Gordon, J. (1992). Work teams—How far have they come? *Training*, **29**, 59–65.

Guzzo, R.A. & Dickson, M.D. (1996). Teams in organizations: recent research on performance and effectiveness. *Annual Review of Psychology*, **46**, 307–338.

Guzzo, R.A. & Shea, G.P. (1992). Group performance and intergroup relations in organizations. In M.D. Dunnette & L.M. Hough (eds), *Handbook of Industrial and Organizational Psychology*, 2nd Edn, Vol. 3. Palo Alto, CA: Consulting Psychologists Press, pp. 269–313.

Guzzo, R.A. & Salas, E. (eds) (1995). *Team Effectiveness and Decision Making in Organizations*. San Francisco: Jossey-Bass.

Guzzo, R.A., Jette, R.D. & Katzell, R.A. (1985). The effects of psychologically based intervention programs on worker productivity: a meta-analysis. *Personnel Psychology*, **38**, 275–291.

Gyllenhammar, P.G. (1977). How Volvo adapts work to people. *Harvard Business Review*, July–August, 102–113.

Hackman, J.R. (1992). Group influences on individuals in organizations. In M.D. Dunnette & L.M. Hough (eds), *Handbook of Industrial and Organizational Psychology*, 2nd Edn, Vol. 3. Palo Alto, CA: Consulting Psychologists Press, pp. 269–313.

Hackman, J.R. (ed.) (1990). *Groups That Work and Those That Don't*. San Francisco: Jossey-Bass.

Hackman, J.R. (1987). The design of work teams. In J.W. Lorsch (ed.), *Handbook of Organizational Behavior*. Englewood Cliffs, NJ: Prentice-Hall, pp. 315–342.

Hackman, J.R. & Morris, C.G. (1975). Group tasks, group interaction process, and group performance effectiveness: a review and proposed integration. In L. Berkowitz (ed.), *Advances in Experimental Social Psychology*, Vol. 8. New York: Academic Press, pp. 1–55.

Harris, D.H. (ed.) (1994). *Organizational Linkage: Understanding the Productivity Paradox*. Washington, D.C.: National Academy Press.

Hermann, C.F. (1994). Avoiding pathologies in foreign policy decision groups. In D. Caldwell & T. McKeown (eds), *Force, Diplomacy, and Leadership*. Boulder, CO: Westview Press.

Hill, G.W. (1982). Group versus individual performance: Are $n + 1$ heads better than one? *Psychological Bulletin*, **91**, 517–539.

Hollingshead, A.B. & McGrath, J.E. (1995). Computer-assisted groups: a critical review of the empirical research. In R.A. Guzzo & E. Salas (eds), *Team Effectiveness and Decision Making in Organizations*. San Francisco: Jossey-Bass, pp. 46–78.

Homans, G.C. (1950). *The Human Group*. New York: Harcourt Brace.

Kalleberg, A.L. & Moody, J.W. (1994). Human resource management and organizational performance. *American Behavioral Scientist*, **37**, 948–962.

Katzenbach, J.R. & Smith, D.K. (1993). The discipline of teams. *Harvard Business Review*, March–April, 111–120.

Lawler, E.E., Mohrman, S.A. & Ledford, G. (1992). *Employee Involvement and TQM: Practice and Results in Fortune 5000 Companies*. San Francisco: Jossey-Bass.

Leavitt, H. (1975). Suppose we took groups seriously... In E.L. Cass & F.G. Zimmer (eds), *Man and Work in Society*. New York: Van Nostrand Reinhold, pp. 67–77.

Levine, J.M. & Moreland, R.L. (1990). Progress in small group research. *Annual Review of Psychology*, **41**, 585–634.

Levine, D.I. & D'Andrea Tyson, L. (1990). Participation, productivity, and the firm's environment. In A.S. Blinder (ed.), *Paying For Productivity*. Washington, D.C.: The Brookings Institution, pp. 183–237.

Macy, B.A. & Izumi, H. (1993). Organizational change, design, and work innovation: a meta-analysis of 131 North American field studies—1961–1991. *Research in Organizational Change and Development*, Vol. 7. Greenwich, CT: JAI Press, pp. 235–313.

McGrath, J.E. (1984). *Groups: Interaction and Performance*. Englewood Cliffs, NJ: Prentice-Hall.

McGrath, J.E. (1991). Time, interaction, and performance: a theory of groups. *Small Group Research*, **22**, 147–174.

McGrath, J.E. & Altman, I. (1966). *Small Group Research: A Synthesis and Critique of the Field*. New York: Holt, Rinehart and Winston.

Mohrman, S.A., Cohen, S.G. & Mohrman, A.M. (1995). *Designing Team-based Organizations*. San Francisco: Jossey-Bass.

Nalbantian, H. (ed.) (1987). *Incentives, Cooperation, and Risk Sharing*. Totowa, NJ: Rowman & Littlefield.

Pearce, J.A. & Ravlin, E.C. (1987). The design and activation of self-regulating work groups. *Human Relations*, **40**, 751–782.

Poole, M.S., Holmes, M., Watson, R. & DeSanctis, G. (1993). Group decision support systems and group communication: a comparison of decision-making in computer-supported and non-supported groups. *Communication Research*, **20**, 176–213.

Roethlisberger, F.J. & Dickson, W.J. (1939). *Management and the Worker*. Cambridge, MA: Harvard University Press.

Schneider, B. & Klein, K.K. (1994). What is enough? A systems perspective on individual–organizational performance linkages. In. D.N. Harris (ed.), *Organizational Linkages:*

Understanding the Productivity Paradox. Washington, D.C.: National Academy Press, pp. 81–104.

Schwartzman, H.B. (1986). Research on work group effectiveness: an anthropological critique. In P.S. Goodman (ed.), *Designing Effective Work Groups*. San Francisco: Jossey-Bass, pp. 233–276.

Shea, G.P. & Guzzo, R.A. (1987). Groups as human resources. In K.M. Rowland & G.R. Ferris (eds), *Research in Personnel and Human Resources Management*, Vol. 5. Greenwich, CT: JAI Press, pp. 323–356.

Steiner, I.D. (1972). *Group Process and Productivity*. New York: Academic Press.

Sundstrom, E., De Meuse, K.P. & Futrell, D. (1990). Work teams: applications and effectiveness. *American Psychologist*, **45**, 120–133.

Trist, E. (1981). *The Evolution of Sociotechnical Systems: A Conceptual Framework and Action Research Program*. Toronto: Ontario Quality of Working Life Centre.

Viteles, M.S. (1939). *Industrial Psychology*. New York: Norton.

Wall, T.D., Kemp, N.J., Jackson, P.R. & Clegg, C.W. (1986). Outcomes of autonomous work groups: a field experiment. *Academy of Management Journal*, **29**, 280–304.

Weick, K.E. (1969). *The Social Psychology of Organizing*. Reading, MA: Addison Wesley.

Whyte, W.F. (1955). *Money and Motivation*. New York: Harper.

Zander, A. (1979). The study of group behavior during four decades. *Journal of Applied Behavioral Science*, **15**, 272–282.

Section II

The Contexts of Groups

Chapter 2

Temporal Issues in Work Groups

Joseph E. McGrath
and
Kathleen M. O'Connor*
*Psychology Department, University of Illinois, and
Psychology Department, Rice University, USA

Abstract

Many temporal issues can have an impact on the effective functioning of work groups. This chapter identifies and discusses a number of the key temporal issues that can arise within each of four facets of a group's life cycle, namely: the origins and subsequent development of the group as a socio-technical systems; the processes by which the group performs its tasks; changes that come about in the group as a function of its own developmental and task performance experience; and dynamic changes that occur in groups as a function of changes in their constituent parts and in their environments. Those four facets constitute the four main sections of the chapter. Each section discusses the nature of the temporal issues, presents a selective review of existing theory and evidence about them, and identifies some key questions for which further research and theory are needed.

Groups are continuing and dynamic systems that develop and change over time. Temporal issues arise within several facets of a group's life cycle. First, there are temporal issues involved in the *origins and subsequent development* of the group as a socio-technical system. Second, there are temporal issues involved in *how groups go about performing whatever tasks they perform*. Third, there are temporal issues pertaining to *how groups change, as a function of their own developmental and task performance experience*. Finally, there are temporal issues regarding

Handbook of Work Group Psychology. Edited by M.A. West.
© 1996 John Wiley & Sons Ltd.

the dynamic changes that occur in groups as a function of changes in their constituent parts and in their environments. Those four sets of temporal issues correspond, roughly, to the four generic CORE processes (Construction processes, Operations processes, Reconstruction processes and External Relations processes) that Argote & McGrath (1993) have proposed as descriptive of the interconnected recurrent cycle of activities that constitutes a work group's life cycle. We will use these sets of temporal issues as the frame for organization of this chapter.

Accordingly, the first section of the chapter deals with temporal issues that have to do with the *origination and development of work groups*. It addresses various questions concerning types of work groups and stages of group development. The second section deals with temporal issues that have to do with *group task performance*: planning, synchronization and scheduling, as well as phases of group problem-solving. The third section deals with *effect of experience over time*, under conditions of continuity. It treats issues of group and organizational learning and of the development of norms, procedures and routines. The fourth section addresses a number of issues regarding *change, especially membership change*. That section concludes with a discussion of some models of change in the structure of participation, influence and leadership in groups, which connects some of the temporal issues raised in all four sections.

THE ORIGINS AND DEVELOPMENT OF WORK GROUPS

Work groups come about in an organization when a set of people, tools and purposes are selected, recruited or created, and then organized and adapted so as to become the members, the technology and the projects of a multiperson task-performance system. "Members" refers to the humans who "belong to" the group, in their own and other's perceptions. "Projects" refers to focused activities in pursuit of purposes or goals; they consist of tasks, steps and actions. "Technology" refers not only to physical implements but also to rules, procedures and other resources that guide and enable the conduct of instrumental activities.

Multiple Paths by which Work Groups Originate

There are at least three kinds of work groups, distinguished from one another in terms of the developmental "paths" by which they come about.

1. Some work groups come about when an organization has a specific project that it wishes to have done, and it therefore selects some individuals to be members of a *task force*—which then selects and makes use of tools, rules, resources and procedures by which it will carry out that project.

2. Other work groups come about when an organization selects individuals who have a particular array of knowledge, skills and abilities, and then trains, equips and organizes those individuals into a *team* that will have responsibility, on a continuing basis, for carrying out projects of a particular class.
3. Still other work groups come about when an organization establishes a focused technology designed to carry out a class of projects, and then recruits personnel to provide a *crew* for that project–technology system.

Those three types of work groups—task forces, teams and crews—differ in terms of which constituent element is primary (the project, the members or the technology, respectively), and which elements, thereby, become less central and hence more subject to adaptation. They offer different potential strengths and are differentially vulnerable to particular kinds of problems, including temporal ones, over time (e.g. Arrow & McGrath, 1994).

Stages in Group Development over Time

The study of group development has enjoyed a long history in social psychology. Typically, researchers have characterized group development in terms of a relatively fixed series of stages. (There is a parallel idea, equally long-lived, about a fixed series of stages of individual growth and development, within child-developmental psychology.) But the idea of fixed stages of group development has always been controversial.

Stages of Group Development vs. Phases of Group Problem-solving

We are drawing a sharp distinction here between ideas about a sequence of stages of development of a group as a socio-technical system (which will be a central topic of this section) and ideas about a sequence of phases by which such a group carries out a particular task (which will be a topic of the second section). The two have not always been clearly distinguished and separated in past group research and theory. In fact, Hare (1973) deliberately interweaves the two in his recounting of the history of study of group processes. We think it is important to distinguish the two, at least in the context of this chapter, for at least two reasons. First, stages of group development and phases of group problem-solving have different referents. The former refers to a group as a continuing social system; the latter refers to a group as a performance unit engaged in a particular task. Second, stages of development and phases of problem-solving also have drastically different temporal features, as will be described in the discussions to follow. Stages of group development are discussed here; phases of group problem-solving will be discussed in the next section.

Formulations of Stages of Group Development

Tuckman (1965) did the classic work on stages of group development, and his theoretical formulation continues to have a major impact. Based on an extensive review of studies of a number of training groups, therapy groups, laboratory groups and natural groups, he postulated four stages that became paraphrased as: "forming, storming, norming and performing". Each stage involved both interpersonal activity and task activity (hence subsuming both what we here call "stages of group development" and "phases of problem-solving"). Later, after a review of studies exploring stages of development dating from the presentation of the earlier model, Tuckman & Jensen (1977) added a fifth stage—adjourning. In that later review, they found only one study that had directly tested the original Tuckman model, but found a number of studies that seemed to give *post hoc* support for it—with the exception of the addition of a termination phase.

More recently, Worchel and colleagues (Worchel, 1994; Worchel, Coutant-Sassic & Grossman, 1992) have presented a six-stage model that is very similar to Tuckman & Jensen's five-stage model. Other examinations of stages of development (e.g. Handfinger, 1984) have shown results that can be interpreted as partially supporting, or at least not disconfirming, the modified Tuckman five-stage model or similar systems. Practitioners have also been influenced by that work, incorporating the Tuckman stages into organizational interventions (e.g. Bunning, 1991; Heinen & Jacobson, 1976; Smith, 1993).

Hare (1973) has reviewed a number of research efforts involving developmental stage theories and systems for coding and analyzing group interaction data. Hare does not sharply distinguish between stages of group development and phases of group problem-solving as we are doing here. In fact, he integrates the two topics with one another by means of a four-function schema (Latent Pattern Maintenance, Adaptation, Integration, and Goal Attainment) based on earlier theoretical formulations by Parsons (1961). Hare uses that schema to show relations among stages and phases as proposed by Bales & Strodtbeck (1951), Tuckman (1965), Mann (1967), Bion (1961), and other researchers.

Some Questions about Group Development over Time

Group development over time is an exceedingly complex topic. Any exploration of it must untangle, and deal with, a whole series of related and partially nested questions that too often have been ignored and/or confounded with one another. These questions include:

1. Do groups change over time, or do they function pretty much the same early, later, and still later in their life spans? Or, to put the question in a more complex form: which facets of groups change over time and which do not?
2. If groups change, do all groups change in the same way or is the pattern of changes over time unique to individual groups or types of groups? If the

latter, then what types of groups (e.g. task forces, teams, crews) are there, in terms of differences in patterns of development? Are group types to be identified in terms of: (a) their overall group purposes (e.g. therapy groups vs. work groups vs. social groups), (b) their specific group purposes (e.g. steel puddling groups vs. basketball teams vs. product development teams), (c) their formative paths (e.g. task forces, teams, crews), or (d) in even more specific terms (such as size, diversity of group composition, available technology and the like)?
3. If all groups (or all types of groups) change in the same way, can that pattern be characterized as a series of stages of development, with the changes patterned so that the same kinds of structures and processes occur in the same fixed sequence for all groups (of the relevant kinds)?
4. If there is a fixed sequence of stages of development, are the stages of equal or differential durations in time, and do all groups go through the stages at the same rate? Is that pattern of stages immutable, or is it subject to alteration by unique circumstances and/or external events in the group's embedding context?
5. Can the pattern of stages be expressed in different specific behaviors by group members?

Most research in this domain has assumed that there is a fixed sequence of stages that is the same for all groups, that the stages are of equal duration, and that groups go through them at uniform rates. These assumptions are usually not made on the basis of theory, but rather made tacitly, by means of methodological choices that facilitate data processing (e.g. by dividing group interaction up into arbitrary time periods of equal duration), rather than explicitly by theoretical postulate.

Cissna (1984) has carried out an excellent review that deals directly with the first of the questions listed above, namely: do groups change? He concludes that most groups do change in many ways. He further concludes that the evidence regarding the universality of phases across groups is not definitive, neither is the exact number and content of the phases, although he seems to accept Tuckman's modified five-stage model as an acceptably good first approximation. He urges (and we agree) that future research should stop asking whether groups change over time and instead examine the more complicated questions involved in this topic (such as the ones outlined above).

Group Development vs. Group Socialization of Members

There also has been some work exploring stages of socialization of members into groups, and on the relationship of those socialization stages to stages of group development (Moreland & Levine, 1982, 1988, 1989; Wanous, Reichers & Malik, 1984). Moreland & Levine consider five stages of relationship of member and group, each marked by evaluation of the potential "reward value" of the relationship by both member and group. The stage are: recruitment, socialization, maintenance, resocialization, remembrance. Role transitions from one stage to the next take place when those evaluations pass the member's and groups's criterion threshold. Thus, individuals begin as potential members and as they move through the socialization process may become, in turn, new members, "regular" members, marginal members and ex-members.

Wanous, Reichers & Malik (1984) also lay out a schema regarding socialization, couching their discussion in terms of organizational socialization rather than socialization to a group. They (a) suggest a four-stage socialization model, (b) accept the Tuckman four-stage model of group development, (c) regard both of those models as fixed sequences of stages necessary for full socialization or development, and (d) suggest several schemata and research approaches that can help link the two.

Summary

There are a number of temporal features involved in the origination and development of work groups; some have received some research attention while others have not. These issues merit further consideration, but should not be treated in the oversimplified ways they have been in the past. Rather, they should be examined in ways that reflect the considerable complexity involved in the dynamics of groups over time.

SOME TEMPORAL FACETS OF GROUP TASK PERFORMANCE

Whenever people set out to work together to achieve common goals, they must deal with at least three key temporal problems:

1. They must find ways to match available resources (including temporal resources) with demands of the task and situation—that is, they need some way to *allocate temporal* (and other) *resources.*
2. They must find ways to coordinate both the content and the timing of the actions of multiple individuals with one another—that is, they need to *synchronize actions within and between members.*
3. They must find ways to be able to anticipate what events and actions will take place and when they will occur—that is, they need some way to *schedule task activities.*

It is worth noting that although allocation, synchronization and scheduling are all temporally related concepts, they each make use of different *time-reckoning systems*. Allocation is typically done in terms of "staff hours" or the equivalent. Synchronization has to do with *when* specific activities are to take place *with respect to each other*—reckoned in terms of an "internal" or system-defined time.

Scheduling is done in reference to *clock and calendar* time, a time-reckoning system "external" to the group.

Allocation, synchronization and scheduling are responses to key temporal problems of collective action. They will provide the frame for our examination of temporal issues in relation to group task performance in the first parts of this section. Then, we offer a brief discussion of some of the temporal issues raised by the use of electronic media for communication within groups, and an examination of the idea of a fixed set of phases by which groups carry out their task performances—an idea already introduced in the previous section on stages of group development.

Planning as the Allocation of Temporal Resources

When a work group or organization attempts to deal in advance with the allocation of time, effort and materials to member–task–technology complexes, that effort is typically referred to as *planning*. There is much rhetorical literature, and some research literature, about the importance of planning in work organizations. Virtually all of that work treats planning, and allocation of time more generally, at individual, organizational or societal levels; there is relatively little research on planning at a group level.

At the individual level, there has been limited but very interesting work on how individuals allocate their time among activities. Much of that work has relied on the use of time diary methods (e.g. de Chalendar, 1976; Robinson, 1977, 1988; Robinson & Converse, 1972); that is, self-reports of allocations of time to various classes of activities. These are usually coded into categories reflecting classes of concrete activities (e.g. going to and from work, doing household chores, preparing and eating meals). Elchardus and Glorieux (1988) have challenged this approach, arguing that time allocation data should be interpreted at more general, and theoretically more meaningful, levels rather than at epiphenomenal levels of concrete behavior. In their own empirical work (Elchardus & Glorieux, 1994), they show that time use is patterned differently, in both work and non-work domains, as a function of gender, socioeconomic class and occupation.

There also is a literature on organizational planning, although more of it is rhetorical than empirical. One key idea in that literature is that a future orientation (and, especially, a long "planning horizon") is a prerequisite for effective long-range planning (Das, 1991, 1993), at least among high-level managers. Hay & Usunier (1993) examined the relation of such time perspectives to strategic planning, taking a cross-cultural comparative view of strategic time perspectives within the international banking industry. They argue that strategic time perspective is influenced by "corporate cognitive styles", which in turn are influenced by national cultures, as well as by the time horizons of various constituencies. They question the common belief that success of Japanese banks (compared to US, UK and German banks) has arisen in part because Japanese have a future orientation. They see the difference, rather, as due to the Japanese corporations (and their controlling constituencies) having a long-term rather than a short-term time horizon. Furthermore, they see the Japanese as following what they term "Makimono time"—a conception of time in which both the past and the future are represented, cognitively, in the present—in contrast to the linear-directional conception of time so ubiquitous in western European and US culture.

Whipp (1994) takes that latter argument further. He recognizes that there has been a recent surge of interest in temporal matters by both organizational researchers and organizational practitioners, but notes that that work is based almost exclusively on Western culture's constraining conception of time—as abstract, clock-reckoned, linear and homogeneous. That resurgence of interest in time in organizations, Whipp argues, has totally ignored the conceptual developments that have considered more complex conceptions of time, in organizations and in society generally. That latter work regards time as constructed rather than objectively "given". Furthermore, it regards organizations as developing "... structural and temporal repertoires"—that is, sets of rules and activities—by which those organizations construct time-ordering arrangements to deal with event-based, recursive, irregular cycles of organizational activity.

There are many key questions in this area for which we do not yet have either theoretical or empirical answers. For example: how do different members of the same culture come to have different temporal orientations? How do those orientations affect the strategies used for temporal planning? How do they vary among individuals, across situations, among cultures and subcultures and over time? How do they affect subsequent patterns of group interaction and task performance?

Synchronization as the Coordination of Multiple Activities in Time

Synchronization is a rather complicated concept. It involves ideas of simultaneity, succession and coordination, themselves quite complicated concepts. Synchronization can be defined as the coordination of two or more actions in time. The synchronized actions may be similar or complementary; they may be carried out simultaneously or in a fixed sequence with a pre-ordained timing; and they may be carried out by the same individual (or group) or by different ones. Synchronization means ensuring that the appropriate person (or group) carries out the intended action at the appropriate time.

Synchronization can be considered at each of several levels. Intra-individual synchronization involves time-sharing across tasks by a single individual. Interindividual or intragroup synchronization involves coordination of the actions of two or more members. External synchronization involves the temporal coordination of group actions with actions or events external to the group (e.g. an externally imposed deadline). Finally, scheduling, which involves matching sets of activities to specific social units and to specific periods of time, can be regarded both as a macro-level of synchronization and as a micro-level of planning.

Those levels of synchronization and scheduling are discussed, in turn, below, followed by a brief discussion of how work groups' technology—and in particular the communication technology—may both aid and hinder synchronization efforts. This section ends with a discussion of phases of group task performance.

Intra-individual Synchronization: Doing More Than One Thing at a Time

Although there is a cultural prescription that "you can't do more than one thing at a time (and do it well)", people violate that prescription all the time. They deliberately fill relatively "empty" intervals—waiting for a bus, riding a bus, waiting for an appointment time—by doing a second task (e.g. reading a book, making lists). (People *can* walk and chew gum at the same time!)

Beyond these somewhat trivial examples, group members often are faced with the need to carry out two or more tasks at the same time. What are the conditions under which individuals or groups can do more than one thing at a time and still do them both well (or well enough)?

There has been much human engineering work on time-sharing for motor tasks, and some cognitive science work on parallel processing. Most of this has been at the individual level. For instance, M.R. Jones (1985, 1986) has done especially interesting work on what she terms the "interleaving" of multiple simultaneous tasks.

In general, doing more than one activity in the same block of time—e.g. business–golf, business–lunch, reading on a trip—works well when and if the activities: (a) don't use the same input and output modalities (e.g. one requires talking and the other is a motor task such as driving a car); (b) have interspersable temporal patterns (e.g. reading while waiting for a bus, because the latter requires only intermittent attention); and (c) are helped (or at least not harmed) by the ambient conditions (e.g. talking business during lunch in a restaurant that is not too noisy). However, as in other temporal topics, there has been much more work on these issues at the level of individual psychological processes than at the group level (McGrath & Rotchford, 1983).

Intra-group Synchronization: Mutual Entrainment and Coordinated Action

One way to state the key question addressed here is: how is the flow of interaction in groups patterned over time? Temporal patterning has to do with the frequency, duration, periodicity, sequences and temporal locations of various interactive events. For example, many behavioral processes are cyclical. Often, such cycles are very stable for a given individual over time but show substantial and stable individual differences (in cycle length, phase and magnitude). Circadian rhythms (that is, cyclic patterns of behavior with near-daily periodicity) are relatively well known examples of such cycles, but there are many rhythmic processes with a cycle lengths of hours and minutes, on the one hand, and days, week, months and longer, on the other. Considerable work has been done on these issues, some of it involving social-psychological processes relevant to organizations. (e.g. Bodenhausen, 1990; Cappella, 1981; Chapple, 1970; Gottman, 1979; Hayes & Cobb, 1979; Jaffe & Feldstein, 1970; J.M. Jones, 1988; Kelly, 1988; Kelly, Futoran & McGrath, 1990; Kelly & McGrath, 1985; R. Levine, 1988; McGrath & Kelly, 1986; Smoll, 1975; Warner, 1979, 1988, 1991; Werner et al., 1988).

Furthermore, under some conditions, these individual behavior cycles become mutually entrained for interacting partners. Mutual entrainment refers to the synchronization, in phase and periodicity (and sometimes in magnitude), of some particular behavior or pattern of action by two or more interacting partners. Evidence of entrainment comes from a variety of contexts in which entrainment has involved quite different behaviors. For example: in the context of interpersonal behavior, Warner (1988) found that interacting dyads entrained (i.e. synchronized the timing of) both their conversation and their respiration. With regard to longer-term interpersonal relationships. Chapple (1970) holds that smoothly entrained cycles provide more pleasant interpersonal relationships for the participants. In contrast, Gottman's (1979) work on marital couples suggests that high predictability (which should follow from close entrainment) may be associated with negative interpersonal affect for long-term relationships. Perhaps long-term relationships are best when there is a loose coupling between interacting partners, which would be indicated by a curvilinear relation between "tightness" of the synchronization (entrainment) among interacting partners, on the one hand, and pleasantness of the relationship, on the other.

Here, too, there are many crucial questions for which we do not yet have either theoretical or empirical answers. For example: under what circumstances, and by what processes, do behaviors of interacting partners become mutually entrained? What are the consequences of such mutual entrainment for subsequent interaction, for task performance, for the quality of interpersonal relationships and for individual satisfaction and well-being?

External Synchronization: Entrainment to Deadlines and Other Temporal Markers

People use deadlines to regulate their own and others' work. Such deadlines function as "time-markers" to help structure behavioral fields. The temporal structuring of behavior so as to fit with an external deadline or temporal signal is a form of entrainment. Just as the behaviors of interacting individuals become mutually entrained to one another, they also become entrained to external time-markers and deadlines. Much of the research referred to in our discussion of mutual entrainment, above, also involves entrainment to external signals, hence it is germane to the present topic as well.

Research on external entrainment raises a number of questions. How do specific deadlines/endpoints affect the flow of work in groups? Under what conditions (and in what pattern) can they entrain the timing of interaction and task performance? These is some research pertinent to these. For example: Gersick (1988, 1989) has shown that project deadlines pace group work in a pattern she calls "punctuated equilibrium". One way to interpret her results, in part, is that it is "the time remaining", not "the amount of work already done", that defines "phases" of work on a project. More research is needed to explore the scope and boundaries of her findings. On a related topic, Valex and Sarocchi (1989) have studied "temporal stops"—time-markers defining endpoints of recurrent behavior (cycles)—as a basis for the planning of multiple simultaneous work activities. Kelly, Futoran & McGrath (1990) have shown that deadlines on early trials entrain both the rate of productivity and the pattern of interaction on that trial and on later trials. They found two patterns of entrainment: (a) response to problems of capacity (how much can the system do in a given time?); and (b) response to problems of capability (how much task difficulty can the system handle?). When early trials pose problems of capacity, individuals and groups speed up their rates on subsequent trials of the same task even if time demands have been relaxed; when early trials pose problems of capability, individuals and groups slow down their rate of performance on later trials, presumably to accomplish "deeper" cognitive processing.

It is not clear how persistent and robust these entrainment phenomena are. There is evidence that they may be very robust in some respects, but very fragile in others. For example, some of M.R. Jones' work suggests that external entrainment patterns persist for several days for performance of the same task, when there have been no interpolated activities related to the same stimuli. But some of the work of McGrath and colleagues suggests that interpolated activity in the form of a task of a different type may dis-entrain performance even on later trials of the same experimental session. Future research should explore these issues, as well as addressing additional questions that may link this area with other areas in organizational psychology. For instance, we need to examine how closely deadlines are related to goals. If they are close kin, then we can expand the goal-setting concepts beyond the issues of *quantity* of production (to which most past goal-setting research has been addressed) to include quality and timing issues as well.

Scheduling as a Time/Activity Match

Scheduling is the matching of specific periods of time to specific sets of activities and to specific social units (i.e. individuals and groups) that are to perform those activities. It is, in a sense, a combination of the allocation and synchronization processes. Scheduling is by no means a simple or straightforward task. Periods of time of the same "objective" size are not totally interchangeable; neither are bundles of activities or sets of task-performing units. Therefore, one very critical set of questions regarding temporal issues in work groups has to do with how this time/activity match is accomplished.

It is clear that time as experienced is epochal rather than homogeneous. That as, all time periods of equal clock and calendar lengths are not equivalent and interchangeable in terms of human experience (cf: McGrath, Kelly & Machatka, 1984). Some sets of activities are inflexible with respect to time; if they are not done at certain time periods they cannot be done at all, or can be done only at a high cost in efficiency. Similarly, some periods of time are not very versatile with regard to what activities can be done (efficiently) in them.

Moreover, there are differences among sets of activities in their modularity— that is, in how efficiently or effectively the activities can be combined into larger bundles to be done in a single large block of time, and/or divided up into smaller bundles to be done in each of a number of small time intervals that are spread over longer periods of clock and calendar time. Important sets of activities (e.g. child care, leisure activities) are not very modular. For example: a parent cannot "save up" a fall week's worth of child care, to be done by devoting all day Sunday to it. Neither is it practical in most cases to write a report that ordinarily takes 2 hours by doing it in convenient 2-minute time segments spread over a couple of days. Thus, time/activity matches are particularistic with regard to both times and activities.

Furthermore, the "size" of both time periods and sets of activities does not remain constant over all conditions. There is a certain amount of *elasticity* regarding the amount of time it takes a given individual or group to do a certain set of activities. For example, stringent time limits often lead to faster rates of task performance (perhaps with a sacrifice in quality). Some of these elasticity issues have already been discussed in this section, in relation to the cluster of issues dealing with deadlines and with entrainment.

Temporal Patterning of Communication in Work Groups: some Effects of Technology

Our presentation in this chapter is based on the assumption that there is a complex interplay among features of the project tasks being performed, features of the technology by which those tasks are carried out, features of the group and its members, and features of the temporal context in which that action is taking place. With the widespread use of computers, the technology component has begun to get more attention.

There has been some research on the broad question of how complex technology, in general, alters temporal features of task performance systems (e.g. Barley, 1988, deals with the temporal consequences of introduction of hi-tech medical systems). There has been much more research on the more focused topic of the use of computer technology in groups. That topic has spawned a vast literature, but only a small part of that research has given much attention to temporal issues. Several researchers (e.g. Hesse, Werner & Altman, 1990; McGrath, 1989; McGrath & Hollingshead, 1993, 1994; Jessup & Valacich, 1993)) have laid out many of those temporal issues and have summarized the current body of knowledge on them.

Electronic media, used in either an individual or a group context, can have pervasive temporal effects, some desirable and some not. Compared to face-to-face groups, communication in computer-mediated work groups involves:

1. Different transmission and feedback time lags.
2. Different rates at which various communication activities can be carried out (e.g. typing is slower than talking, but reading is faster than listening).
3. Different timing of components of the communication process (e.g. composition, editing, transmission and reception times are distinguishably separate for computer conferences but are intertwined for face-to-face groups).
4. Different degrees of turbulence in the flow of information in interaction.
5. Different constraints on the channels or modalities by which information can be transmitted (e.g. non-verbal and paraverbal cues are absent in computer-mediated communication).

Overall, computer-mediated communication reduces the richness of the information that can flow, which makes achieving consensus, in work groups whose members have different perspectives at the outset, both more problematic and slower.

The matter becomes more complex still. Many of these media effects are interactive functions of task type, group composition, the individual member's past experience both with that group and with that medium, and a number of task and temporal operating conditions such as time deadlines, task difficulty and the degree to which the task requires consensus. Furthermore, many of these effects changes over time with continued experience (Hollingshead, McGrath & O'Connor, 1993).

Phases of Group Task Performance

Earlier, we made the distinction between temporal regularities that are stages in the development of a group-as-a-system (discussed in the section on origins and development of groups) and temporal regularities that reflect a sequence of phases in a group's execution of a particular task or project. The belief that all groups go through a set sequence of phases as they carry out problem-solving or other task performances is another idea of long standing in group research. This, too, has long been controversial, and the controversy is gaining intensity. Several related temporal issues are involved.

First, we can ask about what regularities there generally are in the paths by which groups perform tasks (solve problems, make decisions, etc.) and to what degree those regularities are contingent on the kind of group involved (e.g. task forces, teams, crews) and on the group's composition, its task, its technology and its operating context.

The classic work on problem-solving phases was done by Bales & Strodtbeck (1951). They postulated regularities in the form of a fixed sequence of problem-solving phases (orientation, evaluation, control). Other early work on phases of group problem-solving was carried out by Bion (1961), Mann (1967), Mills (1964) and their colleagues (see Hare, 1973, for a good review of all of that work). Much of that early research proposed a fixed sequence of phases as *normative*—that is, as the *most efficient* path for group task performance. Steiner's (1972) concept of "process losses" implies a similar notion—that there is a normatively most efficient path for group task performance on any given type of task, and that all departures from that path constitute "error".

However, others have questioned various assumptions of such phase models, including: the universality of *any* set of phases over groups and conditions; the stability of the sequence in which such phases occur; and the validity of such a sequence as a normative prescription. Recent work by Poole and colleagues, based on adaptive structuration theory (Poole, 1983; Poole & Roth, 1998a, 1998b), poses the phase question in a much more sophisticated form and, not surprisingly, arrives at a much more complex set of answers. They postulate a contingency theory view, which holds that there are multiple paths along each of three concurrent streams of behavior—task activity, group relations and content—by which groups can do tasks; and that groups generate different alternative paths, as a function of features of the group's composition and structure, its task, its context and its own past history. These authors also find much unorganized (chaotic) behavior that fits no phase sequence at all. But that work still retains the normative notion that some of the paths are more efficient and effective than others.

Alternatively, McGrath (1991) has challenged both the idea of a temporally fixed sequence of phases and the idea that such a sequence, if it did exist, would carry some privileged normative status. He postulates that there are four "modes of activity" by which groups carry out whatever work they are doing. These four modes, which apply in somewhat varying forms to task performance activities and to activities directed at maintaining group well-being and providing member support, are: Mode I, *inception* (acquisition, acceptance) of a project (goal choice); Mode II, *solving technical problems* (means choice); Mode III, *resolving conflicting views and interests* (policy choice); and Mode IV, *execution* (goal attainment).

McGrath's modes are not a fixed sequence of phases. Rather, he argues, groups construct different patterns of activity by which they carry out their projects—time/activity paths, so to speak—and those paths/patterns are contingent on group, member, task and context conditions. The first and fourth modes of activity (inception and execution), with respect to the production function, must occur in all completed projects virtually by definition. Otherwise, these modes of activity are not a fixed sequence, neither are they all necessary to the conduct of any given project. Furthermore, at any given time actual work groups are often engaged in more than one project, and may or may not be actively engaged in production, group well-being and member support activities.

For example: if an established group is carrying out a single, well formulated task on which they have much past experience, they are likely to engage only in Mode I (inception) and Mode IV (execution) activities, in regard to their production function—and none at all in regard to the group well-being and member support functions. They do not need to delve into the solution of technical or political issues, since the task is routine; neither do they need to delve into group or interpersonal issues, because for an established group with a routine task those matters are not problematic. Hence, Mode I–Mode IV on the production function constitutes a "default path" for these unproblematic circumstances—not normatively best, but simply sufficient.

On the other hand, if and when any features of the group as a system become problematic (e.g. if there is change in membership, or in task type or difficulty, or in available resources), the work group will attempt to engage in other modes of the production function or modes of the other functions. Such departures from the default path are not to be regarded as "process losses", "biases", "heuristics", or any other pejorative term. Rather, they are to be regarded as the group's response to ambient circumstances.

Here, too, we can pose some complex questions about which we yet know relatively little: To what degree are regularities in task performance contingent on the group's composition, on the type of task, on the technology it is using, and on other features of its context? How does the group's own past experience with the task, and its expectations about future task performance, affect the group's current problem-solving process? How is that process affected by changes in the group? Some of these questions are addressed in the remaining sections of this chapter.

LEARNING FROM EXPERIENCE: CHANGES OVER TIME UNDER CONDITIONS OF CONTINUITY

Natural work groups exist over relatively long periods of time. At any given point in time, each such work group has a history and a potential future. Conditions affecting group behavior are cumulative over time. That is to say, groups change as a function of their own experience. Here, we are considering such experienced-based changes for relatively stable groups and situations—that is, the dynamic effects of experience under conditions of continuity (i.e. no major changes in the constituents of the group-as-a-system). In the next section of this chapter, we will consider the dynamic effects on groups that result from various kinds of changes in conditions.

Group and Organizational "Learning"

If experience is to have any effect, groups (and any other social unit) must have some way to "embed" the results of the experience they gain while performing tasks—that is, to exhibit something akin to what we regard as "learning" in individuals. If groups are composed of members, projects and technology, then logically such learning can be embedded in the members, the projects, the technology, or combinations of them. It is likely that those embedded knowledge structures will often appear in combinations: as member–technology combinations (e.g. habitual routines); as member–project combinations (e.g. a division of labor or role network); as project–technology combinations (e.g. project templates, norms, SOPs).

There has been considerable research done recently on what is termed organizational learning—explorations of whether, and how, organizations increase their production efficiency with continued production experience on the same product (Argote & McGrath, 1993 summarize much of that work). Some of it has been based on the problematic assumption that evidence of more efficient per unit production is, *ipso facto*, evidence of learning, without controlling for other factors (e.g. the scale of production, the mix of products) that may also affect productivity. Research in this domain needs to explore: (a) where in the system the results of that "learning" reside; hence (b) the conditions under which it might be lost or unretrievable (e.g. with member turnover); and (c) what kinds of interventions might be feasible to prevent such loss (e.g. cross-training).

Recently, too, there has been an upsurge in research on socio-cognitive processes in groups, including such topics as: group learning, group memory, transactive memory and other aspects of groups viewed as information-processing systems (e.g. Davis et al., 1989; Gruenfeld & Hollingshead, 1993; Harmon & Rohrbaugh, 1990; Hinsz, 1990; Liang, Moreland & Argote, 1995; Lazenga, 1990; Stasser, Taylor & Hanna, 1989; Stasser & Titus, 1985, 1987; Tindale, 1989; Wegner, 1986; Wegner, Erber & Raymond, 1991. See Argote & McGrath, 1993, and Levine & Moreland, 1991, for summaries of that work from different perspectives).

In general, research on socio-cognitive factors in groups—perhaps trying to avoid awakening the ghost of "group mind"—seems to finesse the question of *where* results of such "learning" or "memory" might reside in the "group-as-a-system". Furthermore, work done at a group level seldom addresses the quite obvious point that, in work organizations, much of the results of experience (though by no means all of it) resides in archival records—minutes of meetings, inter-office memos, correspondence, production and sales records, and the like. Research on group memory, transactive memory and similar topics needs to deal with how such "hard-copy" records of the past fit into work groups' sociocognitive activities.

Group Development of Norms, Procedures and Routines

Gersick & Hackman (1990) have begun the analysis of when and how groups develop habitual routines and the conditions under which those routines persist or change. Poole and colleagues (Poole & Desanctis, 1990; Poole & Roth, 1988a, 1988b), using adaptive structuration theory, explore the patterns that groups develop to carry out their work (see discussion under phases of group activity). Bettenhausen & Murnighan (1991), as well as Hulbert (1994), explore the development of normative structures in task groups. Besides these valuable contributions, there does not appear to be much other research on how work groups develop and change their ways of doing business, their norms, procedures, and even their "division of labor"—although it is clear that such development and change does take place. Nor is there much research available that considers the circumstances under which groups "embed" their learning in new standard operating procedures, new norms or new project-plans, rather than in changes in the members' knowledge and skills. These issues could be important in the successful functioning of work groups under conditions of change, especially change in membership. Effects of such changes are addressed in the next section.

ADAPTING TO CHANGE: THE IMPACT OF CHANGES IN GROUP MEMBERSHIP, TASKS, TECHNOLOGY, AND CONTEXT

As dynamic systems, groups are affected by both continuity and change over time. Learning from experience, discussed in the previous section, represents continuity—that is, changes *internal* to the system that result from the group's own experience in carrying out its projects, under conditions of relative stability of group membership, technology, tasks and context. This fourth section deals with the consequences for the group when there are changes in the group's constituent parts (i.e. its membership, its tasks and its technology) and/or in its environmental context.

Some Issues Regarding Change in Groups Over Time

Natural work groups frequently have changes in their basic constituent parts—in their membership, in the projects they undertake, in the technology by which they carry out those projects—as well as changes in their embedding systems. Such changes can produce dynamic effects dramatically different from those of continuity. In general, we would expect *continuity*, or increased experience of a group, over time, with the same basic constituents, to result in increased *routinization* of patterns of group behavior. In contrast, we would expect *change*—in members, in projects, in technology or in context—to result in *perturbation* of such patterns of group behavior. But such a sweeping general statement leaves many crucial questions unaddressed.

Regarding change, the state of affairs in research is in sharp contrast to the state of affairs in natural groups. Consider membership, for example. Frequently, natural groups show considerable variation in formal membership over time, as well as in actual attendance at any given "session". Yet group research, especially laboratory research, has dealt almost exclusively with groups of stable composition and structure. That is easily achieved in single-session studies, which represent the bulk of past group research. But even in the relatively few studies of groups over extended periods of time, researchers often have gone to great lengths (e.g. excluding the data of groups with imperfect attendance) to avoid membership variations in groups over the course of the study. Much of that emphasis on stable membership, of course, has been in the service of methodological rigor, as well as methodological convenience. Nonetheless, it leaves us with little systematic evidence or theory about the impact of membership change. There are some notable exceptions to this lack of empirical research on membership change, including early work by Trow (1960) and Weick & Gilfallen (1971) and more recent work by Insko and colleagues (Insko et al., 1982; Insko et al., 1980).

Some Issues Regarding Membership Change

Effects of changes in membership is a third-order question. To study it effectively, we must already know (or presume to know!) a great deal about which factors make a difference in the cross-sectional or static comparison case, and also about how these relationships change over time given continuity of membership. In the following paragraphs, we will address some key questions regarding the effects of change, with particular emphasis on membership change.

Group Boundary Issues

In a longitudinal study of work groups (Arrow & McGrath, 1993; McGrath et al., 1993), membership change appeared to have a much greater impact on group interaction process than changes in tasks, technology or operating conditions. There are several alternative hypotheses about why this was the case in that study: (a) because the groups were organized on the basis of membership, rather than on a task/purpose or technology basis—that is, they were teams, not task forces or crews; (b) because the membership changes were done much later in the group's life span than the experimentally imposed technology changes; (c) because the participants' perceptions of the reasons for that change (namely, the experimenter's manipulation) may have threatened the group's boundary control or autonomy.

Membership changes vary in whether they are perceived to be permanent or temporary; whether they are initiated by the member, by the group, or by outside forces (e.g. experimenter, supervisor); and whether the changes are perceived to be related to the needs of, or contributions by, the members who are changed. It seems likely that the strong impact of certain member changes in the study described above derived from such "boundary control" issues.

Relation of Membership Change to Prior Membership Stability

It is clear that the consequences of membership change interact with the length of past group history and the degree of membership continuity during that past time. But the particular pattern of this interaction is not clear, and may be quite complex. There are reasonable conceptual (and some empirical) bases for two opposite sets of predictions. On the one hand, past membership change may have an "inoculation" or "buffering" effect, and past membership stability may make a group more "brittle", so to speak, so that a later membership change has the least negative effects on groups that have already had considerable prior membership variation. On the other hand, past membership fluctuations may cumulate as "load" or unresolved "stress", and subsequent membership change may thereby function as a stress overload, so that membership change has the most negative effects on groups that have had prior membership variation. We need to explore these issues much more extensively than has been done to date.

The Particularity of Change

The impact of any given change in membership is always particular for that group and that occasion or context. Effects of member change depend on: the length and stability of the group's past history (including its history of membership stability); the "size" of the change relative to the size of the group; whether the changes involve adding, subtracting or substituting members; and how those changes relate to the particulars of the group's division of labor, the nature of its task and the roles played by the members involved in the changes (see Arrow & McGrath, 1994). We need to develop indices of membership change that take these different kinds of changes into account, and use them to explore effects of membership changes in detail.

Membership Change and System Restructuring

The theoretical and empirical analyses discussed above imply that change in membership of a group on a given occasion—a disruption of continuity—*predicts departures from typical patterns of performance of that group*. As already discussed, under particularity of change, some membership changes (e.g. loss of members whose individual contributions have been crucial to the group's task performance) can be expected to have more powerful effects on group process and task performance than other changes. The nature and degree of membership change (e.g. how central the missing member was in group process; how structured the group was prior to the change; whether a missing member is replaced or not) affects the degree of consequent change in group process and performance, via a complex set of relations involving member roles, division of labor and the like (Rao & Argote, 1992; Devadas & Argote, 1990).

However, there may be a complicated interplay between "size" of membership change and the fundamental form of the group's response to it. Minor changes in group membership (e.g. loss of a single, relatively inactive member) may only perturb the group's established patterns to a minor degree, and the group may re-establish its "equilibrium" (i.e. its typical patterns of process and performance) rather quickly and easily. Under some circumstances, however, a major change in group membership may function as if that system were what has been termed a "dissipative structure"—a system operating "far from equilibrium" (Smith & Gemmill, 1991). Changes for systems far from equilibrium may be dramatic and system-restructuring, and their exact pattern would be exceedingly hard to predict. We need to explore further the conditions under which membership or other kinds of changes function as "equilibrium-restoring" or as "system-restructuring" processes. This requires detailed pattern analysis of a complex of dependent variables (process, task performance and member reactions) for groups that have undergone a range of membership change. Arrow and her colleagues (e.g. Arrow, 1994; McGrath, Berdahl & Arrow, 1994) have begun such analyses.

The Impact of Changes on Group Task Performance Effectiveness

A change in group membership (or, for that matter, in its technology or other major aspects of the group's operation) necessarily disrupts some prior patterns of group process and task performance, making them more difficult or even impossible to enact. To the extent that those disrupted patterns had contributed to effective group task performance, such disruption will necessarily have a negative effect on speed and quality of task performance and on other outcome measures as well, at least in the short run.

At the same time, a change in one of the group's constituent parts (e.g. group membership) may not only force a change in some of the group's performance routines, but also may provide an opportunity for a group to view things from new perspectives, and to abandon routines that have been limiting performance potential. Doing so may help the group achieve more rapid and effective task performance.

But changes may not have the same effect on all groups—in particular, a given change may have different effects on previously successful vs. previously unsuccessful groups. There are different and somewhat conflicting perspectives on this question. One set of theoretical considerations would lead us to expect that such changes would reduce the variation among groups on measures of effectiveness. In that view, a major membership change can provide an opportunity for an ineffective group to give up its prior (ineffective) procedures and make major changes in how it functions, hence to make major improvements in efficiency of its process and effectiveness of its task performance. At the same time, such a major membership change may force effective groups to give up prior (effective?) procedures, and that may result in taking time and energy away from task performance, leading to deterioration of previously effective patterns of process and outcomes.

An alternative set of theoretical considerations would predict an opposite effect, namely that changes would increase the variation among groups rather than reduce it. Task goals are often attainable by multiple performance paths. Hence, even major changes in ways of functioning may not necessarily result in reduced levels of effectiveness of outcomes for previously effective groups. Furthermore, there is no reason to believe that a previously ineffective group, now altered in its membership, will automatically change from ineffective to effective ways of functioning and thereby improve its performance. Groups may be able to transcend even substantial changes in membership. Indeed, effective groups may be especially able to "make the most" of an altered set of membership capabilities, and ineffective groups may be especially likely to vitiate opportunities to alter process in ways that would have yielded improved performance. Indeed, effective groups may be successful in part because they have developed strategies for coping with changes in their constituent parts and in their task environments; ineffective groups may be ineffective in part because they lack strategies that would allow them to adapt to such changes. In this view, we would expect major membership changes to lead to major alterations in process that quickly stabilize into patterns of task performance that tend to amplify the range of variation in effectiveness among groups—good groups get even better, poor groups get worse or remain the same.

Which of these four models of change will hold in a given case may depend on a number of conditions. Does change operate in similar or different ways for different kinds of work groups (i.e. task forces, teams, crews)? Furthermore, it may be the case that different models of change hold for changes in different "panels" of factors—membership, task, technology, context. For example, data from our recent studies (Arrow & McGrath, 1993; Hollingshead, McGrath & O'Connor, 1993; McGrath et al., 1993) suggest that changes in technology appear to be disruptive, especially for high performance groups, at least in the short run. In contrast, task changes may simply amplify prior differences among groups, with effective groups being effective on new tasks and with ineffective groups being even further disrupted by task changes. Membership changes seem to pose even more complicated patterns. The "change model" that applies in a given case may depend on the centrality of the roles involved in the membership changes, the group's past experience with membership change and continuity, and the group's prior history of process and task performance success.

Models of Change in Group Process and Structure under Conditions of Continuity and of Change

We conclude this section with discussion of a topic that ties together some of the material considered in all of the sections of this chapter, namely: models of how groups develop and change their patterns of participation, influence and leadership over time, under conditions both of continuity and of change.

Arrow and her colleagues (Arrow, 1994; McGrath, Berdahl & Arrow, 1994) have drawn on prior theoretical presentations to identify five models of change in group structure, with emphasis on change in the structure of participation, influence and leadership (PIL) over time. Two of those models involve changes in structure that are expected to occur over time when the group's constituent parts and its relation to the external environment are relatively stable (continuity models). The other three models have reference to changes in structure that are expected to follow as a consequence of particular kinds of externally originated changes in major facets of the group (e.g. in its membership, its tasks, its technology or its context).

The Continuity Models

The first of the "continuity" models is a model based on the premise that group development follows a course of "robust equilibrium". In that view, although a given group may explore various PIL patterns for a short time at the outset of the group's existence, it will soon settle into a "natural" pattern and thereafter remain in that pattern throughout its life cycle. The second of the "continuity" models is a model based on the premise that a group's development follows a pattern that reflects the "inherent developmental form" of such groups. This type of model is the type implied in most schemata for "stages of group development" (e.g. Tuckman & Jensen, 1977). These two types of "continuity" model differ; the robust equilibrium model reflects an interplay between the group and its operating situation, whereas the inherent-developmental-form model reflects mainly an "internal" developmental force or pattern.

The Change Models

Arrow and colleagues have also identified three models that deal with changes in PIL structure that result from changes in the group and its embedding context. Both of the continuity models beg the question of how the PIL pattern would be altered over time if there were external change, and they also beg the question of whether all groups, of all varieties and under all circumstances, will develop the same PIL pattern over time. The three change models all speak to both of those issues.

The first of the change models is the "punctuated equilibrium" model (Gersick, 1988, 1989). This is a change-sensitive variant of the robust equilibrium model. It suggests that a given group more or less immediately adopts a pattern of participation, influence and leadership, and continues with that pattern until some critical external event occurs to "punctuate" the passage of time; that the group then restructures itself, often into dramatically different forms; and that the new pattern continues until some further critical event again punctuates the temporal structure.

A second change model, called the "crisis contingency model," also builds on the idea that external events produce major changes in the group. For this model, a group acquires a PIL pattern that persists as long as "normal" operating conditions prevail. When faced with a major change in crucial external conditions (i.e. a "crisis"), the group develops and rapidly shifts to a different PIL pattern. When the crisis is over, the group reverts back to the original pattern.

The final change model, called the "adaptive matching model", proposes that groups adopt PIL patterns that fit their situations, and those patterns will vary in ways that match variations in features of their operating situation—e.g. different tasks, different communication technologies. For such a model, variations in structure arise because of—and more or less adaptively match—variations in the environmental conditions under which the group is operating, rather than because of any internal conditions of the group.

McGrath, Berdahl & Arrow (1994) use those models to examine the potential dynamic effects of membership diversity in work groups (with special attention to diversity of gender composition) on development and change of group PIL structure. As noted above, this line of exploration brings together some of the temporal issues discussed under stages of group development, some topics considered in our treatment of continuity, and some of the issues raised regarding effects of change.

CONCLUDING COMMENTS

Groups are dynamic systems that get constructed, carry out their purposes, learn from their experience, and all the while adapt to changes in the environment. All of those involve temporal issues in several senses. The group's embedding context is eminently temporal. Group behavior is temporally patterned. The group's developmental history is at once both a record of group experience and an expression of its reactions to change.

We have drawn a rather complex picture of the ways in which a wide variety of temporal issues may have an impact on various aspects of the development and operation of work groups. Yet we are aware that both our theoretical formulations and our review of research have been far from complete. For example, for reasons of space we chose not to address the difficult questions surrounding the creation of a criterion system for measuring and interrelating the multiple important parameters of time (e.g. rate, duration, periodicity, etc.), even though several researchers have tackled those issues (see, for example: Arundale, 1978, 1980; Gamst, 1993; Kelly & McGrath, 1988; Zakay, 1990). So it is likely that the true picture, regarding time and groups, is even more complicated than we have drawn it.

But as we have indicated, to date research on work groups has not given very much attention to these temporal issues, and for good (pragmatic) reasons: those issues are enormously difficult and costly to study. Yet, if these temporal factors are as important in the operation of work groups as we have here argued, and if work groups are as central to effective performance of organizations as many have suggested, then we must begin to address these temporal issues more adequately in future theory and research. Even if we accept high difficulty and cost as sufficient reasons for not having studied temporal issues in the past, we cannot let them excuse continued neglect of these factors in the future—else we will continue to limit our understanding of work groups to the static case.

ACKNOWLEDGEMENTS

The research on which this chapter is based was supported in part by NSF grants BNS 91-06501 and IRI 91-07040 (Joseph E. McGrath, Principal Investigator).

REFERENCES

Argote, L. & McGrath, J.E. (1993). Group process in organizations: continuity and change. In C. Cooper & I.T. Robertson (eds), *International Review of Industrial & Organizational Psychology*. Chuchecker: Wiley.

Arrow, H. (1994). Mapping the structural dynamics of groups: patterns of leadership and influence over time in work groups with changing membership. Unpublished Masters Thesis, Department of Psychology, University of Illinois, Urbana, IL.

Arrow, H. & McGrath, J.E. (1993). Membership matters: how member change and continuity affect small group structure, process, and performance. *Small Group Research*, **24**, 334–361.

Arrow, H. & McGrath, J.E. (1994). Membership dynamics in groups at work: a theoretical framework. In B. Staw & L.L. Cummings (eds), *Research on Organizational Behavior*, Vol 17. New York: JAI Press, pp. 373–411.

Arundale, R.B. (1978). Sampling across time for communication research: a simulation. In R.M. Hersch, P.V. Miller & F.G. Cline (eds), *Strategies for Communication Research*. Beverly Hills, CA: Sage, pp. 257–285.

Arundale, R.B. (1980). Studying change over time: criteria for sampling from continuous variables. *Communication Research*, **7**(2), 227–263.

Bales, R.F. & Strodtbeck, F.L. (1951). Phases in group problem solving. *Journal of Abnormal and Social Psychology*, **46**, 485–495.

Barley, S.R. (1988). On technology, time, and social order: technologically induced change in the temporal organization of radiological work. In F.A. Dubinskas (ed.), *Marking Time: Ethnographies of High-Technology Organizations*. Philadelphia, PA: Temple University Press.

Bettenhausen, K.L. & Murnighan, J.K. (1991). The development of an intergroup norm and the effects of interpersonal and structural changes. *Administrative Science Quarterly*, **36**, 20–35.

Bion, W.R. (1961). *Experiences in Groups and Other Papers*. New York: Basic Books.

Bodenhausen, G.V. (1990). Stereotypes as judgmental heuristics: evidence of circadian variations in discrimination. *Psychological Science*, (4 pp; no page numbers).

Bunning, R.L. (1991). Smooth steps to transition meetings. *HR Magazine*, **August,** 59–64.

Cappella, J.N. (1981). Mutual influence in expressive behavior: adult–adult and infant–adult dyadic interaction. *Psychological Bulletin*, **89**, 101–132.

Chalendar, J. de (1976). *Lifelong Allocation of Time*. Report prepared for the Organization for Economic Cooperation and Development, Paris, France.

Chapple, E.D. (1970). *Culture and Biological Man: Explorations in Behavioral Anthropology*. New York: Holt, Rinehart & Winston.

Cissna, K.N. (1984). Phases in group development: the negative evidence. *Small Group Behavior*, **15**, 3–32.

Das, T.K. (1991). Time: the hidden dimension in strategic planning. *Long Range Planning*, **24**, 49–57.

Das, T.K. (1993). Time in management and organizational studies. *Time and Society*, **2**, 267–274.

Davis, J.H., Kameda, T., Parks, C., Stasson, M. & Zimmerman, S. (1989). Some social mechanics of group decision making: the distribution of opinion, polling sequence, and implications for consensus. *Journal of Personality and Social Psychology*, **57**, 1000–1012.

Devadas, R. & Argote, L. (1990). Learning and depreciation in work groups: the effects of turnover and group structure. Paper presented at the meetings of the *American Psychological Society*, Dallas, TX, June, 1990.

Elchardus, M. & Glorieux, I. (1988). The generalized meanings of the use of time: time budget applications. Paper prepared for International Meeting on Studies of Time Use Budapest, Hungary, Jun, 14–18, 1988.

Elchardus, M. & Glorieux, I. (1994). The search for the invisible 8 hours: the gendered use of time in a society with a high labour force participation of women. *Time and Society*, **3**, 5–28.

Gamst, F.C. (1993). "On time" and the railroader: temporal dimensions of work. In S. Helmers (ed.), *Ethnologie der Arbeitswelt: Beispiele aus europaischen und aussereuropaischen Feldern*. Bonn: Holos Verlag, pp. 105–131.

Gersick, C.J.G. (1988). Time and transition in work teams: toward a new model of group development. *Academy of Management Journal*, **31**, 9–41.

Gersick, C.J.G. (1989). Marking time: predictable transitions in task groups. *Academy of Management Journal*, **32**, 274–309.

Gersick, C.J.G. & Hackman, J.R. (1990). Habitual routines in task-performing groups. *Organizational Behavior and Human Decision Processes*, **47**, 65–97.

Gottman, J.M. (1979). *Marital Interaction: Experimental Investigations*. New York: Academic Press.

Gruenfeld, D.H. & Hollingshead, A.B. (1993). Sociocognition in work groups: the evolution of group integrative complexity and its relation to task performance. *Small Group Research*, **24**, 353–382.

Handfinger, R. (1984). The contextual organization model for processing and evaluating (COMPE). A theoretical tool for practitioners in the behavioral sciences. *Small Group Behavior*, **15**, 375–386.

Hare, A.P. (1973). Theories of group development and categories for interaction analysis. *Small Group Behavior*, **4**, 259–304.

Harmon, J. & Rohrbaugh, J. (1990). Social judgment analysis and small group decision making: cognitive feedback effects on individual and collective performance. *Organizational Behavior and Human Decision Processes*, **46**, 34–54.

Hay, M. & Usunier, J. (1993). Time and strategic action: a cross-cultural view. *Time and Society*, **2**, 313–334.

Hayes, D.P. & Cobb, L. (1979) Ultradian biorhythms in social interaction. In A.W. Siegman & S. Feldstein (eds), *Of Speech and Time: Temporal Speech Rhythms in Interpersonal Contexts*. Hillsdale, NJ: Erlbaum.

Heinen, J.S. & Jacobson, E. (1976). A model of task group development in complex organizations and a strategy of implementation. *Academy of Management Review*, **1**, 98–111.

Hesse, B.W., Werner, C.M. & Altman, I. (1990). Temporal aspects of computer mediated communication. *Computers in Human Behavior*, **4**, 147–165.

Hinsz, V. (1990). Cognitive and consensus processes in group recognition memory performance. *Journal of Personality and Social Psychology*, **59**(4), 705–718.

Hollingshead, A.B., McGrath, J.E. & O'Connor, K.M. (1993). Group task performance and computer technology: a longitudinal study of computer-mediated versus face-to-face work groups. *Small Group Research*, **24**, 307–333.

Hulbert, L. (1994). The Development and Persistence of Normative Standards in Small Groups. Unpublished doctoral dissertation. University of Illinois, Urbana-Champaign, IL.

Insko, C.A., Gilmore, R., Moehle, D., Lipsitz, A., Drenan, S. & Thibaut, J.W. (1982). Seniority in the generational transition of laboratory groups: the effects of social familiarity and task experience. *Journal of Experimental Social Psychology*, **18**, 557–580.

Insko, C.A., Thibaut, J.W., Moehle, D., Wilson, H., Diamond, W.D., Gilmore, R., Solomon, M.R. & Lipsitz, A. (1980). Social evolution and the emergence of leadership. *Journal of Personality and Social Psychology*, **39**, 431–448.

Jaffe, J. & Feldstein, S. (1970). *Rhythms of Dialogue*. New York: Academic Press.

Jessup, L.M. & Valacich, J.S. (1993). *Group Support Systems: New Perspectives*. New York: Macmillan.

Jones, J.M. (1988). Cultural differences in temporal perspectives: instrumental and expressive behaviors in time. In J.E. McGrath (ed.), *The Social Psychology of Time: New Perspectives*. Newbury Park, CA: Sage, pp. 21–38.

Jones, M.R. (1985). Structural organization of events in time: a review. In J.A. Michon & J.L. Jackson (eds), *Time, Mind, and Behavior*. Heidelberg, Germany: Springer-Verlag, pp. 192–214.

Jones, M.R. (1986). Attentional rhythmicity in human perception. In J.R. Evans & M. Clynes (eds), *Rhythm in Psychological, Linguistic, and Music Processes*. Springfield, IL: Charles C. Thomas, pp. 13–40.

Kelly, J.R. (1988). Entrainment in individual and group behavior. In J.E. McGrath (ed.), *The Social Psychology of Time: New Perspectives*. Newbury Park, CA: Sage, pp. 89–110.

Kelly, J.R., Futoran, G.C. & McGrath, J.E. (1990). Capacity and capability: seven studies of entrainment of task performance rates. *Small Group Research*, **21**(3), 283–314.

Kelly, J.R. & McGrath, J.E. (1985). Effects of time limits and task types on task performance and interaction of four-person groups. *Journal of Personality and Social Psychology*, **49**, 395–407.

Kelly, J.R. & McGrath, J.E. (1988). *On Time and Method*. Newbury Park, CA: Sage.

Liang, D.W., Moreland, R. & Argote, L. (1995). Group versus individual training and group performance: the mediating role of transactive memory. *Personality and Social Psychology Bulletin*, **21**(4), 384–393.

Lazenga, E. (1990). Internal politics and the interactive elaboration of information in workgroups: an expioratory study. *Human Relations*, **43**, 87–101.

Levine, J.M. & Moreland, R.L. (1991). Culture and socialization in work groups. In L. Resnick, J. Levine & S.D. Teasley (eds), *Perspectives on Socially Shared Cognition*. Washington, D.C.: American Psychological Association, pp. 257–279.

Levine, R.V. (1988). The pace of life across cultures. In J.E. McGrath (ed.), *The Social Psychology of Time: New Perspectives*. Newbury Park, CA: Sage pp. 39–60.

Mann, R.D. (1967). *Interpersonal Styles and Group Development*. New York: Wiley.

McGrath, J.E. (1989). Time matters in groups. In J. Galegher, R.E. Kraut & C. Egido (eds), *Intellectual Teamwork: Social and Technical Bases of Cooperative Work*. Hillsdale, NJ: Erlbaum, pp. 23–61.

McGrath, J.E. (1991). Time, interaction and performance (TIP): a theory of groups. *Small Group Research*, **22**(2), 147–174.

McGrath, J.E., Arrow, H., Gruenfeld, D.H., Hollingshead, A.B. & O'Connor, K.M. (1993). Groups, tasks, and technology: the effects of experience and change. *Small Group Research*, **24**, 406–420.

McGrath, J.E., Berdahl, J.L. & Arrow, H. (1996). Traits, expectations, culture and clout: the dynamics of diversity in work groups. In S.E. Jackson & M.M. Ruderman (eds), *Productivity and Interpersonal Relations in Work Teams Characterized by Diversity*. Washington D.C.: American Psychological Association.

McGrath, J.E. & Hollingshead, A.B. (1993). Putting the "group" back in group support systems: some theoretical issues about dynamic processes in groups with technological enhancements. In L.M. Jessup & J.E. Valacich (eds), *Group Support Systems: New Perspectives*. New York: Macmillan, pp. 78–96.

McGrath, J.E. & Hollingshead, A.B. (1994). *Groups Interacting with Technology.* Newbury Park, CA: Sage.

McGrath, J.E. & Kelly, J.R. (1986). *Time and Human Interaction.* New York: Guilford.

McGrath, J.E. & Kelly, J.R. (1992). Temporal context and temporal patterning: toward a time-centered perspective for social psychology. *Time and Society,* 1(3), 399–420.

McGrath, J.E., Kelly, J.R. & Machatka, D.E. (1984) The social psychology of time: entrainment of behavior in social and organizational settings. In S. Oskamp (ed.), *Applied Social Psychology Annual,* Vol. 5. Beverly Hills, CA: Sage.

McGrath, J.E. & Rotchford, N.L. (1983) Time and behavior in organizations. In L. Cummings & B. Staw (eds), *Research in Organizational Behavior,* vol. 5. Greenwich, CT: JAI Press, pp. 57–101.

Mills, T.M. (1964). *Group Transformation: An Analysis of a Learning Group.* Englewood Cliffs, NJ: Prentice-Hall.

Moreland, R.L. & Levine, J.M. (1982). Socialization in small groups: temporal changes in individual-group relations. In L. Berkowitz (ed.), *Advances in Experimental Social Psychology,* 15, 137–192.

Moreland, R.L. & Levine, J.M. (1988). Group dynamics over time: development and socialization in small groups. In J.E. McGrath (ed.), *The Social Psychology of Time: New Perspectives.* Newbury Park, CA: Sage.

Moreland, R.L. & Levine, J.A. (1989). Newcomers and oldtimers in small groups. In P.B. Paulus (ed.), *Psychology of Group Influence,* 2nd Edn, Hillsdale, NJ: Erlbaum.

Parsons, T.C. (1961). An artline of the social system. In T.C. Parsons, E. Shils, K.D. Naegele & J.R. Pitts (eds), *Theories of Society.* New York: Free Press, pp. 30–79.

Poole, M.S. (1983). Decision development in small groups II: a study of multiple sequences in decison making. *Communication Monographs,* 50, 206–232.

Poole, M.S. & DeSanctis, G. (1990). Understanding the use of decision support systems: the theory of adaptive structuration. In J. Fulk & C. Steinfield (eds), *Organizations and Communication Technology.* Newbury Park, CA: Sage, pp. 175–195.

Poole, M.S. & Roth, J. (1988a). Decision development in small groups IV: a typology of group decision paths. *Human Communication Research,* 15, 323–356.

Poole, M.S. & Roth, J. (1988b). Decision development in small groups V: test of a contingency model. *Human Communication Research,* 15, 549–589.

Rao, R. & Argote, L. (1992). Collective learning and forgetting: the effects of turnover and group structure. Paper presented at annual meeting of Academy of Management, Las Vegas, NV, 1992.

Robinson, J.P. (1977). *How Americans Use Time: A Social-Psychological Analysis of Everyday Behavior.* New York: Praeger.

Robinson, J.P. (1988). Time-diary evidence about the social psychology of everyday life. In J.E. McGrath (ed.), *The Social Psychology of Time: New Perspectives.* Newbury Park, CA: Sage, pp. 134–148.

Robinson, J.P. & Converse, P.E. (1972). Social changes reflected in the use of time. In A. Campbell & P.E. Converse (eds), *The Human Meaning of Social Change.* New York: Russell Sage Foundation.

Smith, R. (1993). No man is an island. *Management Accounting,* 71, 63–64.

Smith, C. & Gemill, G. (1991). Change in the small group: a dissipative structure perspective. *Human Relations,* 44, 697–716.

Smoll, F.L. (1975). Between-days consistency in personal tempo. *Perceptual and Motor Skills,* 41, 731–734.

Stasser, G., Taylor, L. & Hanna, C. (1989). Information sampling in structured and unstructured discussions of three- and six-person groups. *Journal of Personality and Social Psychology,* 57, 67–78.

Stasser, G. & Titus, W. (1985). Pooling of unshared information in group decision making: biased information sampling during discussion. *Journal of Personality and Social Psychology,* 48, 1467–1478.

Stasser, G. & Titus, W. (1987). Effects of information load and percentages of shared information on the dissemination of unshared information during group discussion. *Journal of Personality and Social Psychology*, **53**, 81–93.

Steiner, I.D. (1972). *Group Process and Productivity*. New York: Academic Press.

Tindale, R.S. (1989). Group vs. individual information processing: the effects of outcome feedback on decision making. *Organizational Behavior and Human Decision Making*, **44**, 454–471.

Trow, D.R. (1960). Membership succession and team performance. *Human Relations*, **13**, 259–269.

Tuckman, B.W. (1965). Developmental sequences in small groups. *Psychological Bulletin*, **63**, 384–399.

Tuckman, B.W. & Jensen, M.A.C. (1977). Stages of small group development revisited. *Group and Organizational Studies*, **2**, 419–427.

Valax, M-F. & Sarocchi, F. (1989). Structure of action plans and the notion of temporal stop. *European Bulletin of Cognitive Psychology*, **9**(2), 223–238.

Wanous, J.P., Reichers, A.E. & Malik, S.D. (1984). Organizational socialization and group development: toward an integrative perspective. *Academy of Management Review*, **9**, 670–683.

Warner, R.M. (1979) Periodic rhythms in conversational speech. *Language and Speech*, **22**, 381–396.

Warner, R. (1988). Rhythm in social interaction: In J.E. McGrath (ed.), *The Social Psychology of Time: New Perspectives*. Newbury Park, CA: Sage, pp. 63–88.

Warner, R. (1991). Incorporating Time. In B. Montgomery & S. Duck (eds), *Studying Interpersonal Interaction*. New York: Guilford, pp. 82–102.

Wegner, D.M. (1986). Transactive memory: a contemporary analysis of the group mind. In B. Mullen & George R. Goethals (eds), *Theories of Group Behavior*. New York: Springer-Verlag.

Wegner, D.M., Erber, R. & Raymond, P. (1991). Transactive memory in close relationships. *Journal of Personality and Social Psychology*, **61**, 923–929.

Weick, K.E. & Gilfallen, D.P. (1971). Fate of arbitrary traditions in a laboratory microculture. *Journal of Personality and Social Psychology*, **17**, 179–191.

Werner, C.M., Haggard, L.M., Altman, I. & Oxley, D. (1988). Temporal qualities of rituals and celebrations: a comparison of Christmas street and Zuni shalako. In J.E. McGrath (ed.), *The Social Psychology of Time: New Perspectives*. Newbury Park, CA: Sage, pp. 303–352.

Whipp, R. (1994). A time to be concerned: a position paper on time and management. *Time and Society*, **3**, 99–116.

Worchel, S. (1994). You can go home again: returning group research to the group context with an eye on developmental issues. *Small Group Research*, **25**, 205–223.

Worchel, S., Coutant-Sassic, D. & Grossman, M. (1992). A developmental approach to group dynamics: A model and illustrative research. In S. Worchel, W. Wood & J. Simpson (eds), *Group Process and Productivity*. Newbury Park, CA: Sage.

Zakay, D. (1990). The evasive art of subjective time measurement: some methodological dilemmas. In R.A. Block (ed.), *Cognitive Models of Psychological Time*. Hillsdale, NJ: Erlbaum, pp. 59–84.

Chapter 3

The Consequences of Diversity in Multidisciplinary Work Teams

Susan E. Jackson
New York University, USA

Abstract

As organizations pursue new business strategies to compete in the global marketplace, they often conclude that multidisciplinary teams are needed to develop innovative products and services and respond to customers interested in a broad range of products and services. Multidisciplinary teams provide a structure for bringing together employees with the diverse technical backgrounds needed for these tasks. The increasing popularity of team-based organizational structures reflects the widely shared belief that teamwork offers the potential to achieve outcomes that could not be achieved by individuals working in isolation.

As they restructure around multidisciplinary teams, however, many organizations are discovering that teams do not always produce the desired results. Even when teams fulfill their potential, team members and their organizations may experience unanticipated negative side-effects, such as unproductive conflict and high turnover. This chapter explores the interpersonal dynamics that arise within multidisciplinary teams, and the longer-term consequences of such dynamics. A description of the types of diversity likely to be present in multidisciplinary teams is presented first. This is followed by an overview of research that has investigated how diversity affects the way team members feel about each other and the ways they behave toward each other. The research reveals that members of multidisciplinary teams are likely to experience a variety of challenges. Communicating effectively with team-mates who do not share a common technical language or perspective is one such challenge, but it is perhaps not the most difficult one. Also on the team's agenda are issues of power and status, the struggle to develop a feeling of cohesiveness, and managing relationships beyond the team's boundary. How these challenges are addressed has implications for how individuals on the team feel about themselves and others, as well as for the performance and long-term survival of the team.

To succeed in increasingly competitive domestic and global markets, many organizations are pursuing new business strategies that emphasize the development of innovative products and services and responsiveness to customers who may be interested in a broad range of products and services offered by a firm. Achieving these new objectives requires coordination among employees who have dissimilar technical backgrounds and perspectives, so many organizations now are incorporating multidisciplinary teams as a basic form of organizing. For example, in the telecommunications and electronics industries, multidisciplinary R&D teams bring together experts with a variety of knowledge backgrounds, with the expectation that such teams will be more likely to generate innovative ideas for new products and services. In order to ensure that the new products or services appeal to customers, the teams may include representatives from marketing or even the eventual end-users. When manufactured products are to be produced, multidisciplinary design teams may also include suppliers, whose presence can ensure that materials and components needed for production meet quality standards and are available when needed. For service delivery, multidisciplinary teams often are designed to ensure that all of a customer's potential needs can be met by a single team. Regardless of whether the customer is a medical patient being served by a multidisciplinary medical team, or an insurance policy holder who holds many different types of insurance policies, multidisciplinary service teams simplify the customer–organization interface and may improve the service received.

The increasing popularity of team-based organizational structures reflects the widely shared belief that teamwork offers the potential to achieve outcomes that could not be achieved by individuals working in isolation. As many organizations are discovering, however, the pay-off from teamwork is not automatic. Although teams offer great potential for increased innovation, quality and speed, the potential is not always realized. Even when teams fulfill their potential, team members and their organizations may experience unanticipated negative side-effects, such as unproductive conflict and high turnover.

To be maximally effective, multidisciplinary teams must successfully manage the assets and liabilities associated with their diversity. To manage diversity, in turn, presumes an understanding of the types of diversity likely to be present in multidimensional teams and the consequences of various types of diversity for the behavior of team members. After describing in some detail the types of diversity likely to be present in multidisciplinary teams, this chapter provides an overview of research that shows how diversity affects the way team members feel about each other and the ways they behave toward each other. The composition of multidisciplinary teams is shown to have implications for problem-solving and decision-making processes, the development of status hierarchies, patterns of participation and communication, the development of cohesiveness, team performance, and, in the longer term, both the stability of the team and its ability to learn and develop over time. Because of the complexity of team composition and the important influences of organizational and societal context, the precise ways in which these dynamics will unfold in a specific team are impossible to fully control, or even accurately predict. Consequently, this chapter concludes by suggesting that, when relying on multidisciplinary teams to carry out significant tasks, an organization should be prepared to experiment and learn along the way. To be effective, experimentation and learning should be based upon an understanding of what is known to date, as reflected in the literature reviewed here and in the experiential knowledge of an organization's most skilled team leaders.

THE NATURE OF DIVERSITY IN MULTIDISCIPLINARY TEAMS

In this chapter, the term "diversity" is used to refer to the social *composition* of teams; "diversity" does not refer to the characteristic of an individual person. In order to fully describe the diversity of a team, both the content and structure of the team's composition must be considered.

The Content of Diversity

As we have seen, multidisciplinary teams are designed to be diverse in terms of the occupational backgrounds and functional areas of expertise of the team members. These teams are likely to be diverse in other ways as well. For example, in the everyday language of the popular press, the term diversity is widely used within the USA, and increasingly within Europe, to refer to the demographic (e.g. gender, ethnicity, age) composition of an organization's workforce. Throughout much of the world, organizations that previously employed a workforce that was mostly male and mostly from a single cultural or ethnic group now employ increasing numbers of women and people from many different ethnic and cultural backgrounds. Assuming these employment patterns continue, demographically diverse organizations will soon replace the relatively homogeneous organizations of the past.

In organizations that rely on work teams, other dimensions of diversity that are likely to become salient include status diversity, age diversity and educational diversity. Status diversity is introduced whenever teams are formed to include members from different levels of the organizational hierarchy. For example, in the USA, it is common to staff a task force by taking people from a "diagonal slice." which goes across functional groups and includes people from the top to the bottom of the organization. Because status in organizations tends to co-vary with age and education, teams created using this approach typically have high levels of age and educational diversity as well.

Another type of diversity present in many organizations reflects the restructuring that took place during the past decade of corporate mergers and acquisitions. These have created organizations populated by the combined workforces of previously distinct companies. Whereas the unmerged firms may each have had a monolithic corporate culture, embodied within the new firm are multiple corporate cultures; after a merger, diversity replaces homogeneity. Like national cultures, corporate cultures shape expectations for behavior and guide interactions among interdependent employees. Until corporate cultures began colliding, they often went unnoticed, but now the difficulties that arise in merging dissimilar corporate cultures are widely recognized by top level executives (Kanter, 1989).

Finally, rapid advances in electronic communications make it possible for organizations to create "virtual" teams, with members dispersed across neighboring cities, states or countries. In addition to the many other types of diversity that may be present in such teams, the geographic diversity of these teams creates some unique challenges, which must be carefully managed in order for the team to function effectively (e.g. see Armstrong and Cole, 1996).

As should now be apparent, the composition of any particular team is complex; the people who make up a team can differ from each other in many different ways. Diversity may be low for one content dimension (e.g. when everyone shares the same national culture) and high for another content dimension (e.g. when the team has three men and four women). Thus, it is not sufficient to say that a team is diverse or homogeneous; the content of diversity must be specified, also.

Because the term diversity can refer to so many different aspects of team composition, it is useful to organize the types of diversity found in multidisciplinary teams into the simple two-dimensional taxonomy shown in Figure 3.1. In this taxonomy, the individual attributes that create diversity within a team are categorized as either *readily detected or underlying*, and as either *task-related or relations-oriented*. Together, readily detected and underlying attributes contribute to the *total* diversity present in a team. To fully understand how diversity affects the functioning of multidisciplinary teams, team dynamics associated with task-related diversity *and* relations-oriented diversity must be considered.

Readily detected attributes can be determined quickly and consensually with only brief exposure to a target person. Generally, they are immutable. Readily detected task-related attributes include organizational and team tenure, department or unit membership, formal credentials and education level. Readily detected relations-oriented attributes include gender, race, ethnicity, national origin and age.

In comparison to readily-detected attributes, *underlying attributes* are less

	Task related attributes	Relations-oriented attributes
Readily detected attributes	Department/unit membership Organizational tenure Formal credential and titles Education level Memberships in professional association	Sex Age Nationality Ethnicity Religion Political memberships Physical appearance
Underlying attributes	Knowledge and expertise Skills Physical abilities Task experience	Socio-economic status Attitudes Values Personality

Figure 3.1 A taxonomy for describing the content of team diversity. The examples shown in each cell of the taxonomy are intended to be illustrative, not exhaustive. Adapted from Jackson, May & Whitney (1995), with permission

obvious, more difficult to verify, and subject to more interpretation and construal. Task-related underlying attributes include physical skills and abilities as well as cognitive knowledge, skills, abilities and job experience; relations-oriented underlying attributes include social status, attitudes, values and personality.

Managers and researchers alike often assume that readily detected attributes are associated with task-related underlying attributes (Hambrick & Mason, 1984; Lawrence, 1991). For example, an automotive design team that is occupationally diverse (e.g. a purchasing manager, a market researcher, an R&D engineer and a foreman from the manufacturing plant) would be expected to make better design decisions than a more homogeneous team *because* of the diversity of task-relevant knowledge, skills, and abilities they presumably would bring to the task.

What managers (and some researchers) often ignore are the possible effects of the relations-oriented diversity that might be present in such a team. Relations-oriented diversity can shape behavior even when there is no association between it and the team's task-related attributes, because it triggers stereotypes that influence the way team members think and feel—about themselves as well as others on the team. For example, data from several million US students indicates that cognitive ability differences between males and females are negligible (Hyde, Fennema & Lamon, 1990; Hyde & Linn, 1988), yet males are generally perceived as more intelligent than females (Wallston & O'Leary, 1981). Similarly, the evidence indicates that the deteriorating effects of age have little impact on intellectual capacity until the seventh decade of one's life (Labouvie-Vief,

1989), yet managers appear to denigrate employees who are older than the norm for a particular job or position (Lawrence, 1988; see also Tsui, Xin & Egan, 1996). Interpersonal relations and interaction patterns follow from stereotype-based thoughts and feelings, and ultimately these determine what information is available to the team, what information is attended to by the team, and who has the most influence in decision-making processes (e.g. see Berger & Zelditch, 1985; Devine, 1989; Stephan, 1985; Turner, 1987).

The Structure of Diversity

To this point, our discussion has treated diversity as a construct that varies from high to low. Much of the theoretical and empirical literature adopts this vocabulary also. But this is an oversimplification. Many different configurations of attributes can be present in a team. A few configurations of diversity have drawn special attention, however, because of their powerful consequences. One such configuration is the nearly homogeneous team that includes a "token" or "solo" member, such as a lone female in a team of males (see Kanter, 1977). Two other psychologically distinct configurations are (a) a homogeneous team that includes a small minority faction (i.e. two members who are similar to each other but distinctly different from the other members of a team), and (b) a bipolar team composition, which is characterized by the presence of two equal-size coalitions (e.g. a team composed of 50% employees from headquarters and 50% employees from a subsidiary). Such configurations can be particularly powerful determinants of how team members perceive themselves, their feelings toward each other as well as communication and influence processes within teams—processes which are central to team decision making.

THE CONSEQUENCES OF DIVERSITY

Diversity is of interest because it has important consequences, including how individuals feel about themselves and other members of the team, communication patterns within the team, communications across team boundaries, the distribution of resources among team members, team performance, and so on. Figure 3.2 lists the many types of outcomes that can be affected by diversity. The columns in Figure 3.2 distinguish between consequences that reflect effects observed as a team is performing its tasks (labeled short-term effects) and consequences that become apparent over longer periods of time or may even persist after the team has disbanded (labeled long-term outcomes).* The distinction between short-term and long-term is not as sharp as it appears in the Figure, however, for the time dimension that is used to separate these categories

---

*The consequences labelled "short-term" here are similar to what McGrath, Berdahl & Arrow (1996) refer to as "modes of activity", with the exception that McGrath et al. treat goal attainment as an activity mode, whereas here performance outcomes are treated as "longer-term outcomes".

	Short-term effects	Long-term outcomes
Individual members	Seeking, offering and receiving task information Initiating/responding to influence attempts Seeking, offering and receiving social support and information Seeking, offering, receiving tangible resources and aid	Performance (speed, creativity) Satisfaction with performance of self and team Acquisition of knowledge and skills (learning) Establishment of position in communication networks
Team	Task–related communication networks Resource distributions Influence networks Status hierarchy Friendship communications Cohesiveness	Establishment of external relations Balance of interpersonal accounts (political debts and credits) Friendship coalitions Performance (speed, solidity, creativity) Membership stability

Figure 3.2 The possible consequences of team diversity. The examples shown in each cell of the taxonomy are intended to be illustrative, not exhaustive. Adapted from Jackson, May & Whitney (1995), with permission

of outcomes is continuous. The rows in Figure 3.2 distinguish between consequences for individual team members and consequences for the team as a whole. Again, the distinctions among these types of outcomes are not as sharp as they appear in Figure 3.2. Many consequences experienced by individuals have implications for the team as a whole, and almost all consequences experienced by the team as a whole have implications for individuals in the team.

As the reader will soon discover, the implications of diversity are far-reaching. No single theory explains the full set of established empirical relationships between aspects of diversity and its consequences. Instead, a variety of theoretical interests and perspectives have guided the studies described, including expectation states theory (Berger & Zelditch, 1985), the "upper echelons" perspective and research on top management team composition (Hambrick & Mason, 1984; Hambrick, 1994), organizational demography (Pfeffer, 1983), relational demography (Tsui & O'Reilly, 1989), and social identity theory (Turner et al., 1987). These literatures reflect the varied interests of psychologists, sociologists and management scholars; each is limited, but together they offer many insights about how diversity affects multidisciplinary teams.

A full discussion of all research relevant to understanding how different types of diversity are related to these many consequences is more than can be accomplished in this chapter, so this review is necessarily selective. The focus is on well-established findings and draws most heavily on research that appears to have clear applicability in field settings. Short-term team effects are described first, including diversity's effects on internal team dynamics and diversity's effects on the team's external relationships. Then longer-term outcomes are considered, including longer-term consequences for individuals and the team as a whole.

Diversity Shapes Internal Dynamics within the Team

In the short term, diversity has many consequences for the way members of a team process information, make decisions and carry them out. Diversity also shapes the social dynamics within the team. This section describes some of these consequences in detail.

Decision-making and Problem-solving

Decision-making processes are central to the functioning of multidisciplinary teams. Indeed, it is often because diverse perspectives are presumed to improve decision processes that organizations employ multidisciplinary team structures.

If one adopts a rational view of the decision-making process, diverse perspectives seem to be beneficial on several counts. For example, during the environmental scanning that occurs in the earliest phase of decision-making, members with diverse perspectives should provide a more comprehensive view of the possible issues that might be placed on the team's agenda, including both threats and opportunities. Once potential threats and opportunities have been identified, discussion among members with diverse perspectives should improve the team's ability to consider a variety of alternative interpretations of the information gathered by the team and to generate creative solutions that integrate the diverse perspectives. As the team discusses alternative courses of action and solutions, diverse perspectives presumably will increase the team's ability to foresee all possible costs, benefits and side-effects (e.g. see Cowan, 1986; Haythorn, 1968; Hoffman, 1959; Hoffman & Maier, 1961; Pearce & Ravlin, 1987; Porac & Howard, 1990; Simon, 1987; Triandis, Hall & Ewen, 1965).

This view of the benefits of diversity during decision-making accurately reflects some of the potential benefits to be gained by creating diverse decision-making teams, but it is not the whole picture. Decision-making is not simply rational information processing. In particular, the availability of expertise does not guarantee the use of that expertise because information held by only one member of a team is often ignored.

Research on conformity and social influence indicates the value of having on a team at least two people who agree on a correct answer. The most well-known social influence studies are the classic experiments of Solomon Asch, who asked subjects to judge line lengths after hearing the erroneous judgments of several other people. This research revealed that when a person's private judgment was unlike the judgments expressed by others, the person soon abandoned his or her own judgment, even when their answer was verifiably correct. However, in the presence of just one other person who agreed, subjects persevered in the face of opposition (Asch, 1951, 1956; see also Allen, 1965; Sherif, 1935).

Just as a lone individual is likely to lack confidence, the team may lack confidence that a deviant opinion is correct. For typical problems, characterized by ambiguity, a team is much more likely to endorse the correct solution to a problem when at least two members of the team have the information or ability needed to determine the correct answer. This pattern of findings can be summarized as "truth *supported* wins" (Laughlin, 1980; Hill, 1982). This conclusion warns that if the correct answer is discovered by a sole person who has no ally in the team, the team is unlikely to adopt the correct answer as their solution to the problem. This is especially true if the person with the correct answer is of relatively low status (Torrance, 1959). Such evidence suggests that better decision-making and problem-solving should occur when team members have overlapping domains of expertise, instead of a sole expert for each relevant knowledge domain.

Status and Power

The texture of interactions observed within decision-making teams is not a function of task-based information alone. Observed behaviors also reflect status and power differentials. Surprisingly, there is little psychological or organizational research that empirically examines the consequences for decision-making teams of differences in *expertise-based* status or power, although everyday experiences indicate that these are relevant to communications, influence attempts, negotiations and resource allocation. The lack of empirical research may indicate that most scholars assume that the consequences of expertise-based status and power over resources are straightforward and obvious (i.e. rational).

In contrast, numerous studies have investigated the effects of socially defined status (e.g. status based on age and gender). Much of this research has been conducted to test hypotheses from expectation states theory, which emphasizes the formation and consequences of status hierarchies (Berger, Cohen & Zelditch, 1966, 1972). Although there is debate within this literature regarding the processes that lead to status hierarchies, there is agreement about the fact that status is usually correlated with demographic characteristics that are not relevant to performance (Ridgeway, 1987).

In the USA, decades of national opinion polls and psychological research on prejudice and discrimination show that the status attributed to individuals corresponds to their sex, age and ethnicity (Jaffe, 1987; Johnston & Packer, 1987; Katz & Taylor, 1988; Kraly & Hirschman, 1990; Chronicle of Higher Education, 1992). Unfortunately, the workplace is not immune from these status attributions. For example, in a study of 224 R&D teams in 29 large organizations, Cohen & Zhou (1991) found that even after controlling for performance, higher status was attributed to males than females. Demographic cues such as age, sex and ethnicity trigger status assignments quickly, and unfairly low (non-task) status assignments prove difficult to undo (Ridgeway, 1982).

The behavioral effects of initial status attributions are pervasive. Compared to those with lower status, higher status persons display more assertive non-verbal behaviors during communication; speak more often, criticize more, state more commands, and interrupt others more often; have more opportunity to exert influence, attempt to exert influence more, and actually are more influential (Levine & Moreland, 1990). Consequently, participation in task-related decision-making is likely to be unequal among members of teams characterized by demographic diversity, with lower status members participating less. At the team level, the presence of status differences among members (status diversity) is detrimental. Status differentiation inhibits creativity and appears to contribute to process losses (Steiner, 1972) because the expertise of lower-status members is not fully used (Silver, Cohen & Crutchfield, 1994).

Implementing Decisions

In the decision-making literature, a distinction often is drawn between *deciding* upon a course of action and *implementing* the decision. Whereas decision-making itself has been studied extensively, implementation has received less attention. Most of the evidence concerning the effects of diversity on decision processes comes from laboratory studies. In that setting, teams usually have responsibility only for generating new ideas and possible courses of action—they seldom actually implement their ideas. Work teams, on the other hand, usually take responsibility for both generating ideas and implementing them. Indeed, new management practices such as the use of multidisciplinary teams for concurrent engineering were specifically developed to ensure that idea generation and implementation were integrated. Thus, in field settings, team performance often requires being effective in two types of activities: creative decision-making *and* task execution or implementation.

Psychological research on the execution of well structured tasks with clearly specified goals provides some basis for predicting the consequences of diversity during implementation. On the one hand, studies show that teams with diverse abilities outperform teams with homogeneous abilities, assuming members are free to take responsibility for the tasks that match their abilities. On the other hand, teams composed of members who are homogeneous with respect to attributes that are not relevant to the task (e.g. demographic characteristics), perform better than diverse ones (Clement & Schiereck, 1973; Fenelon & Megaree, 1971). This effect has been found for tasks that require a great deal of interdependence as well as for tasks requiring relatively little interdependence.

One reason why diversity that is not relevant to the task may interfere with implementation is because all members of the team may be less strongly committed to whatever solution is eventually agreed upon. If diversity of perspectives makes reaching consensus difficult, teams may choose to resolve conflicts through compromise and majority rule instead of persisting to a creative resolution that is acceptable to everyone. Reliance on compromises or majority rule may decrease team members' acceptance of and enthusiasm for the team's resolution. Less acceptance of decisions is often assumed to be negative, but it is possible that an unexamined benefit of skepticism is the development and use of more elaborate mechanisms for obtaining feedback, greater attention paid to signals suggesting failure, and greater willingness to change the team's decision in the face of negative feedback.

Overall, then, diversity may slow down the processes of decision-making and implementation while increasing the team's vigilance in attending to feedback about the quality of their decisions. The trade-off between speed and vigilance suggests that diversity may be a very positive feature for teams engaged in high-risk decisions, especially when actions have irreversible effects (e.g. in medical or military settings).

Cohesiveness

For complex decision-making problems, the expression and discussion of conflicting opinions and perspectives ensures thorough discussion of a wide range of interpretations, possible solutions and alternative consequences that might follow the acceptance of a solution (see Cosier, 1981; Janis, 1972; Schweiger, Sandberg & Rechner 1989; Schwenk, 1983). Exposure to alternative views may improve the quality of thinking about the issue at hand. It may also stimulate learning, which should benefit the team as it works on new tasks in the future (Nemeth, 1986). Unfortunately, however, dissent and disagreement often arouse negative emotional reactions (Nemeth & Staw, 1989; Schmidt, 1974), which may be directed toward other individuals in the team.

Cohesiveness refers to the degree of interpersonal attraction and liking among team members. To assess cohesiveness, researchers almost always ask team members to indicate their personal feelings about other members and/or their liking of the team as a whole. Under most circumstances, members of homogeneous teams experience more positive affect than members of diverse teams (Levine & Moreland, 1990; Lott & Lott, 1965; O'Reilly, Caldwell & Barnett, 1989; Zander, 1979), and similarity among friendship pairs has been found for a variety of readily detected and underlying attributes, including age, gender, race, education, prestige, social class, attitudes and beliefs (e.g. Berscheid, 1985; Brass, 1984; Byrne, 1971; Cohen, 1977; Ibarra, 1992; McPherson & Smith-Lovin, 1987; Verbrugge, 1977; Zander & Havelin, 1960).

The way team members feel about each other is important for many reasons. In the long term, for example, these feelings determine whether members retain their membership in the team. More immediately, positive affect promotes helping behavior and generosity, cooperation and a problem-solving orientation during negotiations (for a review, see Isen & Baron, 1991). Helping is likely to be beneficial in many types of work situations, as when it takes the form of mentoring (Kram, 1985) or generally offering assistance to colleagues. When positive affect occurs in the form of attraction to team members, it may translate into greater motivation to contribute fully and perform well as a means of gaining approval and recognition (Festinger, Schachter & Back, 1950). Conversely, anxiety may inhibit a person's participation in team activities (Allen, 1965; Asch, 1956).

For decision-making teams, studies of how affect influences negotiations are of particular interest. In these problem-solving situations, where flexible and creative thinking can lead to more effective resolutions than compromise, positive affect is likely to be particularly beneficial for improving performance. For example, in a study of dispute resolution, negotiators induced to feel positive affect reached agreement more often, broke-off from discussions less often, cooperated more, obtained better outcomes, and evaluated the other negotiator more favorably, compared to negotiators in a control condition (Carnevale & Isen, 1986).

Communication

In the broadest sense, communications are the means through which a team manages information. Communication involves producing, transmitting (sending) and interpreting (receiving) symbols (Roloff, 1987)—through verbal as well as non-verbal channels, directly and indirectly, passively and proactively (e.g. see Miller & Jablin, 1991). Work-related communications involve descriptive and evaluative task information, exchanged primarily for instrumental purposes. In contrast, friendship communications involve social information (i.e. support) and carry their own intrinsic value (Brass, 1984; Ibarra, 1992).

Studies of communication networks in work organizations reveal that team composition predicts who talks to whom about what, as well as how much people talk to each other overall. In general, communication networks are characterized by demographic homogeneity (Brass, 1984; Hoffman, 1985; Lincoln & Miller, 1979). For example, work-related communications between men and women are less frequent in units that are more diverse with respect to sex (South et al., 1982). Formal and informal meetings among peers and with immediate subordinates are lower in racially diverse groups (Hoffman, 1985). And age and tenure similarities between co-workers predict levels of communication among project teams of engineers (Zenger & Lawrence, 1989).

Diversity Shapes External Relationships

Psychologists have traditionally adopted an internal perspective for studying groups. Consequently, little is known about how diversity impacts performance on tasks that require teams to adopt an external perspective (Ancona, 1987). An external perspective is adopted whenever a team interfaces with constituencies outside the team, including constituencies within the organization and those in the organization's external environment. Recent studies of new product teams indicate that these teams engage in several types of external contacts, including vertical communications aimed at managing the perceptions of higher level managers and obtaining feedback and horizontal communications aimed at obtaining information about markets and technologies (Ancona & Caldwell, 1992).

Consideration of the externally-oriented tasks of multidisciplinary teams suggests several avenues for future research. For example, it suggests the need to study how a team's composition influences its persuasive effectiveness in external negotiations. Externally oriented persuasion activities include winning the support and commitment of those inside the organization, image management and resource acquisition. These activities may be especially relevant to the successful implementation of decisions—a large, and largely ignored, aspect of team work in organizations.

Also, the external perspective shifts the focus of attention from intergroup analyses to intergroup analyses. This shift in focus raises the issue of how the composition of constituency groups shape the relationship between the team and their external constituencies. For example, teams may use different tactics when they interact with a constituency group that is homogeneous, compared to a diverse one. Or, composition effects may be more complex. For example, multidisciplinary teams may interact differently with constituencies whose compositions mirror their own team composition than they do with constituencies made up of people who are dissimilar to the team. Until additional research is conducted, such possibilities must remain within the realm of speculation.

Team Diversity and Longer-term Outcomes

For one team working on a specific task in a particular organizational setting, the short-term behavioral consequences of diversity are difficult to predict. Teams are dynamic and interaction patterns change during the course of task performance (McGrath, Berdahl & Arrow, 1996; Watson, Kumar & Michaelson, 1993). In the longer term, however, the eventual consequences of diversity are more predictable.

Individual Consequences

For individuals, the potential consequences of participating as a member of a diverse team are many. Here two are highlighted: team membership and performance enhancement or learning.

Ultimately, the probability of maintaining one's membership in the team may be partly determined by the team's diversity. This was illustrated in a study of 199 top management teams in US banks. Seven dimensions of team diversity were investigated: age, tenure, education level, curriculum, the college one attended, military experience and job experience. These indicators of diversity predicted the probability of turnover among team members over a 4-year period of time. Managers who were members of more diverse teams were more likely to leave the team during the 4 years, compared to managers who were members of homogeneous teams. This was true regardless of the characteristics of the individual managers, and regardless of how similar a manager was to other members of the team. Simply being a members of a diverse team increased the likelihood that a manager would leave the team (Jackson et al., 1991). Presumably, this effect occurred because the more diverse teams experienced greater conflict and were less cohesive (cf., Wagner, Pfeffer & O'Reilly, 1984), creating feelings of dissatisfaction and perhaps increasing the perceived desirability of other job offers.

Although diversity appears to make some people feel uncomfortable, some people find diversity stimulating. One of the positive individual consequences of working amidst diversity may be individual growth and learning. For example, an interesting phenomenon observed within problem-solving groups composed of a mix of experts and relative novices is the "assembly bonus effect", which occurs when people perform better within the team context than they would alone. Such effects would be expected for low ability members, but it is notable that assembly bonus effects also have been observed for expert members interacting with others who are less knowledgeable (see Laughlin & Bitz, 1975; Shaw & Ashton, 1976).

One explanation for assembly bonus effects in that experts learn during their interactions with non-experts, perhaps because they take on the role of "teacher". Serving in the role of teacher may lead high ability members to sharpen their own thinking. Another possibility is that the questions and inputs of more naive members encourage the expert members to unbundle the assumptions and rules they automatically use when dealing with issues and problems in their areas of expertise (Simon, 1979). This unbundling may increase the probability of discovering assumptions that warrant scrutiny and decision rules for which exceptions may be needed. For multidisciplinary teams, findings such as these suggest the counter-intuitive idea that performance is enhanced more when both experts in the problem domain and novices are represented in the team, compared to teams composed of experts only.

Team Performance

It is interesting to consider how diversity shapes the internal dynamics of teams and the consequences of diversity for individual team members, but ultimately team performance probably is the long-term consequence of most concern to organizations. Presumably, team performance partially determines the performance of the organization as a whole. A team's performance may also have implications for how the organization responds to the team and its members. For example, members of a high performance team may be individually rewarded through team incentive schemes. High performance teams may also accrue power in the organization, which they can then use in negotiations concerning the team's autonomy and to garner resources—including human resources, time, money and access to information. Clearly, the question of whether diversity relates to team performance is an important one.

Jackson (1992) provided a detailed review of research that examined the relationship between team diversity and performance outcomes. As that review makes clear, the effects of diversity on team performance are complex. Different effects are found depending on which attributes are studied (task-related or relations-oriented) and on the nature of the task being performed. For most types of tasks, there is simply too little evidence to draw any conclusions about the effects of diversity on team performance. Tasks involving creativity and judgmental decision-making are the exception, however.

Creative decision-making refers to the activities groups perform when they are faced with tasks that require formulating new solutions to a problem and/or resolving an issue for which there is no "correct" answer. Many tasks assigned to multidisciplinary teams can be characterized as creative decision-making tasks in that novel products, services or processes are being designed and there may be two, three, or many solutions that would be equally effective. For these types of tasks, the available evidence supports the conclusion that team diversity is associated with better quality team decision-making (Filley, House & Kerr, 1976; Hoffman, 1979; McGrath, 1984; Shaw, 1981). This effect has been found for diversity of many types, including personality (Hoffman & Maier, 1961), training background (Pelz, 1956), leadership abilities (Ghiselli & Lodahl, 1958), attitudes (Hoffman, Harburg & Maier, 1962; Triandis, Hall & Ewen, 1965; Willems & Clark, 1971) and gender (Wood, 1987), and for top management teams diversity with respect to occupational background (Bantel & Jackson, 1989) and education (Smith et al., 1994).

Membership Stability

As already described, members of diverse teams often express feelings of greater dissatisfaction and the team as a whole is often less cohesive. In the longer term, reactions such as these might be expected to result in members leaving the team, either voluntarily or because they feel pressured to leave by other team members.

During the past decade, several studies have examined the relationship between team diversity and team turnover rates. Many of these studies were stimulated by Pfeffer's (1983) discussion of organization demography. Most support the assertion that diversity is associated with higher turnover rates: In particular, several studies have shown that age and/or tenure diversity correlate with turnover rates (Jackson et al., 1991; McCain, O'Reilly & Pfeffer, 1983; O'Reilly, Caldwell & Barnett, 1989; Wagner, Pfeffer & O'Reilly, 1984). In addition, diversity in terms of college attended, curriculum studied and industrial experiences has been shown to predict turnover rates for top management teams (Jackson et al., 1991).

The higher turnover rates associated with team diversity have often been treated as a negative consequence of diversity. Under many circumstances, turnover can be disruptive to team functioning. Nevertheless, turnover can be beneficial, also. This is because, over time, the repeated exposure of team members to each other gradually results in the homogenization of their attitudes, perspectives and cognitive schemas; in the process, the team's creative capacity diminishes also. Thus, the turnover experienced by diverse teams may be a cloud with a silver lining that offers an opportunity for the continual addition of fresh ideas.

CONCLUSION

Diversity is a fundamental fact in today's business organizations, and it is the heart of multidisciplinary teams. Even in the most traditional company, employees differ from each other in terms of tenure, technical knowledge, educational background and organization status. Furthermore, throughout the world, many organizations are experiencing increasing workforce diversity along dimensions such as ethnicity, gender, and age. These and other aspects of diversity can have profound effects on the way one feels about oneself, as well as how one feels and behaves toward other members of the organization.

In organizations that rely on multidisciplinary teams, the effects of diversity extend beyond individuals to the team as a whole. As this chapter has described, the empirical evidence clearly indicates that in the longer term, diversity partly determines team performance and membership stability. Therefore, as companies restructure to take better advantage of multidisciplinary teams—whether at the level of top management or on the shop floor—understanding the dynamics of diversity becomes increasingly important.

The complexity of diversity and its myriad consequences means that a complete understanding of the phenomenon awaits many more years of research. This research must begin to consider how multiple attributes *in combination* create the texture of a team's life. Furthermore, we must consider more carefully the interplay between the specific nature of a team's diversity and the larger context that surrounds the team's activities. Context includes the nature of the tasks to be completed, the technologies used to complete the task, as well as the organizational and societal histories and cultures that serve as the backdrop for team activities. Although not discussed in detail in this chapter, all of these contextual factors can shape the unfolding dynamics of diversity for a specific work team (e.g. see McGrath, Berdahl & Arrow, 1996; Cox, 1996; Nkomo, 1996; Triandis, 1996).

The complexity of diversity's effects surely means that organizations will never be able to manage multidisciplinary teams effectively simply by following a few specified rules. For example, it is unlikely that researchers will ever produce meaningful answers to questions such as "What is the ideal composition for a seven-person team in country X working on task Y in an organization whose culture and climate can be describe as Z?" And even if researchers could provide answers to such questions (eventually), it would not be for a very long time. Given that diversity is already a fact of organizational life, and that teams are fast replacing individuals as the fundamental building blocks in organization structures, the practical task of effectively managing diverse teams will challenge many organizations. How should they proceed?

Faced with the complex and uncertain consequences of team diversity, the best advice for organizations may be to proceed in the mode of a learning organization. A learning organization recognizes that current actions should be informed by all available information (e.g. the results of past research), but it also accepts responsibility for creating new knowledge through its own actions. In order to learn more about the special challenges and benefits of diverse teams, organizations that rely on diverse teams to carry out significant tasks should be prepared to monitor the internal dynamics and longer-term outcomes of its teams, and learn from their experiences. Furthermore, organizations should be prepared to experiment with alternative ways of structuring the task and with alternative team compositions, relying on the input of team members for feedback about successes and failures.

For example, Brewer and her associates (see Brewer, 1996) have investigated a technique called "cross-cutting" for structuring teams that requires the input of people with diverse areas of expertise. The objective of cross-cutting is to ensure that task-related attributes (such as expertise) are not correlated with relations-oriented attributes (such as gender) within the task force. Because this concept of cross-cutting is a relatively new one, however, precise recommendations for how to design cross-cutting teams cannot be made. Experimentation is needed. Suppose a task required the expertise of market researchers and product design engineers. In the organization as a whole, it may be that the market research unit is populated mostly by women, while the product design engineers are likely to be men. Brewer's research suggests that, in composing a task force, it would be helpful to avoid assigning two female market researchers and two male engineers to the task. A cross-cutting design would suggest having one male and one female for each area of expertise. This type of team design is predicted to result in low levels of intergroup differentiation and bias, and relatively high levels of cooperation.

Although it sounds promising, the effectiveness of cross-cutting team designs has not been demonstrated in the field. Therefore, if organizations choose to follow Brewer's recommendation, it would be prudent to monitor teams designed according to cross-cutting principles in anticipation of making design adjustments, as needed. For a specific organization operating in a specific cultural context, a learning-based approach to managing diversity within work teams is perhaps the only way to maximize the potential benefits of diversity while simultaneously minimizing the potential costs (see also Jackson, 1993).

Organizations that choose to adopt a learning approach may be most likely to succeed if they have in place managers with strong leadership skills. Team members often tailor their behavior based on cues from the leader in order to avoid jeopardizing their own personal status. Therefore, leaders have a disproportionate influence on team dynamics; through their own attitudes and behavior, leaders may amplify, nullify or moderate some of the natural consequences of diversity. They can shape informal norms and structure the processes used for decision-making.

Inept leaders may squander the potential benefits of diversity by not allowing adequate time for a full discussion to occur; they may support norms that stifle the expression of disagreement in general, or the expression of dissent by a minority faction in particular (e.g. see Bourgeois, 1980). If they do allow a team to engage in open disagreements, inept leaders may be insensitive to the importance of moving from disagreement to consensus through the construction of new and genuinely shared understandings (Ginsberg, 1990), and instead encourage compromises to which no one feels committed.

In contrast, skillful leaders know how to use conflict-inducing decisions aids, such as devil's advocates and dialectical inquiry, to temporarily diversify a homogeneous team (Cosier & Schwenk, 1990; Quinn, 1980). When necessary, they know how to reduce dysfunctional conflict through the exploration of unstated assumptions and values, and thereby speed up the learning process that is often needed before a team is able to craft satisfying resolutions (see Cook & Hammond, 1982). When conflict has been intense, regardless of whether it arose naturally or was induced, skillful leaders attend to the aftermath, ensuring that cohesiveness is restored.

In order to reap the benefits of multidisciplinary teams, managers will need to rely on all of the resources they have at hand, including: (a) the large body of social science research and theory, which can be used to develop a deeper understanding of the many possible functional and dysfunctional dynamics that can arise within diverse teams; (b) the methods used by learning organizations to generate new knowledge that has immediate local applicability, which include systematic experimentation and monitoring; and (c) the conflict management skills of their most effective leaders. Alone, each of these would be inadequate, but used in combination, they should provide adequate guidance to ensure the effective use of multidisciplinary teams. Taking a longer-term perspective, social scientists can draw upon these same resources to improve the base of knowledge that will be available in the future.

REFERENCES

Allen, V.L. (1965). Situational factors in conformity. In L. Berkowitz (ed.), *Advances in Experimental Social Psychology*, Vol, 2. Orlando, FL: Academic Press, pp. 133–175.

Ancona, D.G. (1987). Groups in organizations: extending laboratory models. In C. Hendrick (ed.), *Annual Review of Personality and Social Psychology: Group and Intergroup Processes*. Beverly Hills, CA: Sage, pp. 207–231.

Ancona, D.G. & Caldwell, D.F. (1992). Bridging the boundary: external activity and performance for organizational teams. *Administrative Science Quarterly*, **37**, 634–665.

Armstrong, D.J. & Cole, P. (1996). Managing distances and differences in geographically distributed groups. In S.E. Jackson and M. Ruderman (eds), *Diversity in workteams: Paradigms for a changing workplace*. Washington, D.C.: American Psychological Association.

Asch, S.E. (1951). Effects of group pressure upon the modification and distortion of judgments. In H. Guetzkow (ed.), *Groups, Leadership, and Men*. Pittsburgh, PA: Carnegie Press, pp. 177–190.

Asch, S.E. (1956). Status of independence and conformity: a minority of one against a unanimous majority. *Psychological Monographs*, **70**(9), Whole No. 416.

Bantel, K.A. & Jackson, S.E. (1989). Top management and innovations in banking: does the composition of the top team make a difference? *Strategic Management Journal*, **10** (Special Issue), 107–124.

Berger, J., Cohen, B.P. & Zelditch, M. Jr (1966). Status characteristics and expectation states. In J. Berger, M. Zelditch Jr & B. Anderson (eds), *Sociological Theories in Progress*. Boston, MA: Houghton-Mifflin, pp. 47–73.

Berger, J., Cohen, B.P. & Zelditch, M. Jr (1972). Status characteristics and social interaction. *American Sociological Review*, **37**, 241–255.

Berger, J. & Zelditch, M. Jr (eds) (1985). *Status, Rewards, and Influence*. San Francisco: Jossey-Bass.

Berscheid, E. (1985). Interpersonal attraction. In G. Lindsey & E. Aronson (eds), *The Handbook of Social Psychology*, Vol. 2. New York: Random House, pp. 413–484.

Bourgeois, L.J. (1980). Performance and consensus. *Strategic Management Journal*, **1**, 227–248.

Brass, D.J. (1984). Being in the right place: a structural analysis of individual influence in an organization. *Administrative Science Quarterly*, **29**, 518–539.

Brewer, M.B. (1996). Managing diversity: can we reap the benefits without paying the costs. In S.E. Jackson & M. Ruderman (eds), *Diversity in workteams: Paradigms for a changing workplace*. Washington, D.C.: American Psychological Association.

Byrne, D. (1971). *The Attraction Paradigm*. New York: Academic Press.

Carnevale, P.J. & Isen, A.M. (1986). The influence of positive affect and visual access on the discovery of integrative solutions in bilateral negotiation. *Organizational Behavior and Human Decision Processes*, **37**, 1–13.

Chronicle of Higher Education (1992). The Chronicle of Higher Education Almanac. *Chronicle of Higher Education*, **39**, 15.

Clement, D.E. & Schiereck, J.J. Jr (1973). Sex composition and group performance in a visual signal detection task. *Memory and Cognition*, **1**, 251–255.

Cohen, J.M. (1977). Sources of peer group homogeneity. *Sociology of Education*, **50**, 227–341.

Cohen, B.P. & Zhou, X. (1991). Status processes in enduring work groups. *American Sociological Review*, **56**, 179–188.

Cook, R.L. & Hammond, K.R. (1982). Interpersonal learning and interpersonal conflict reduction in decision-making groups. In R.A. Guzzo (ed.), *Improving Group Decision Making in Organizations: Approaches from Theory and Research*. New York: Academic Press, pp. 63–81.

Cosier, R.A. (1981). Dialectical inquiry in strategic planning: a case of premature acceptance? *Academy of Management Review*, **6**, 643–648.

Cosier, R. & Schwenk, C. (1990). Consensus and thinking alike: ingredients for poor decisions. *Academy of Management Executive*, **4**, 69–74.

Cowan, D.A. (1986). Developing a process model of problem recognition. *Academy of Management Review*, **11**, 763–776.

Cox, T. Jr. (1996) The complexity of diversity challenges and directions for future research. In S.E. Jackson & R.N. Ruderman (eds.), *Diversity in workteams: Paradigms for a changing workplace*, pp 235–247. Washington, D.C.: American Psychological Association.

Devine, P.G. (1989). Stereotypes and prejudice: their automatic and controlled components. *Journal of Personality and Social Psychology*, **56**, 5–18.

Fenelon, J.R. & Megaree, E.I. (1971). Influence of race on the manifestation of leadership. *Journal of Applied Psychology*, **55**, 353–358.

Festinger, L., Schachter, S. & Back, K. (1950). *Social Pressures in Informal Groups: A Study of Human Factors in Housing*. New York: Harper.

Filley, A.C., House, R.J. & Kerr, S. (1976). *Managerial Process and Organizational Behavior*. Glenview, IL: Scott Foresman.

Ghiselli, E.E. & Lodahl, T.M. (1958). Patterns of managerial traits and group effectiveness. *Journal of Abnormal and Social Psychology*, **57**, 61–66.

Ginsberg, A. (1990). Connecting diversification to performance: a sociocognitive approach. *Academy of Management Review*, **15**, 514–535.

Hambrick. D.C. (1994). Top management groups: a conceptual integration and reconsideration of the "team" label. *Research in Organizational Behavior*, **16**, 171–213.

Hambrick, D.C. & Mason, P.A. (1984). Upper echelons: the organization as a reflection of its top managers. *Academy of Management Review*, **9**, 193–206.

Haythorn, W.W. (1968). The composition of groups: a review of the literature. *Acta Psychologica*, **28**, 97–128.

Hill, G.W. (1982). Group versus individual performance: are $N + 1$ heads better than one? *Psychological Bulletin*, **91**, 517–539.

Hoffman, E. (1985). The effect of race-ratio composition on the frequency of organizational communication. *Social Psychology Quarterly*, **48**, 17–26.

Hoffman, L.R. (1959). Homogeneity and member personality and its effect on group problem solving. *Journal of Abnormal Social Psychology*, **58**, 27–32.

Hoffman, L.R. (1979). Applying experimental research on group problem solving to organizations. *Journal of Applied Behavioral Science*, **15**, 375–391.

Hoffman, L.R. & Maier, N.R.F. (1961). Quality and acceptance of problem solutions by members of homogeneous and heterogeneous groups. *Journal of Abnormal and Social Psychology*, **62**, 401–407.

Hoffman, L.R., Harburg, E. & Maier, N.R.F. (1962). Differences and disagreement as factors in creative group problem solving. *Journal of Abnormal and Social Psychology*, **64**, 206–214.

Hyde, J.S., Fennema, E. & Lamon, S.J. (1990). Gender differences in mathematics performance: a meta-analysis. *Psychological Bulletin*, **107**, 139–155.

Hyde, J.S. & Linn, M.C. (1988). Gender differences in verbal ability: a meta-analysis. *Psychological Bulletin*, **104**, 53–69.

Ibarra, H. (1992). Homophily and differential returns: sex differences in network structure and access in an advertising firm. *Administrative Science Quarterly*, **37**, 422–447.

Isen, A.M. & Baron, R.A. (1991). Positive affect as a factor in organizational behavior. In L.L. Cummings & B.M. Staw (eds), *Research in Organizational Behavior*, Vol. 13. Greenwich, CT: JAI Press, pp. 1–53.

Jackson, S.E. (1992). Consequences of group composition for the interpersonal dynamics of strategic issue processing. *Advances in Strategic Management*, **8**, 345–382.

Jackson, S.E. (1993). Stepping into the future: guidelines for action. In S.E. Jackson & Associates, *Diversity in the Workplace: Human Resources Initiatives*. New York: Guilford Press.

Jackson, S.E., Brett, J.F., Sessa, V.I., Cooper, D.M., Julin, J.A. & Peyronnin, K. (1991). Some differences make a difference: individual dissimilarity and group heterogeneity as correlates of recruitment, promotions and turnover. *Journal of Applied Psychology*, **76**, 675–689.

Jackson, S.E., May, K.E. & Whitney, K. (1995). Dynamics of diversity in decision making teams. In Guzzo, R.A. & E. Salas (eds), *Team Decision Making Effectiveness in Organizations*. San Francisco: Jossey-Bass.

Jaffe, M.P. (1987, December). Workforce 2000: forecast of occupational change. Technical appendix to William B. Johnston et al., *Workforce 2000: Work and Workers for the 21st Century*. Washington, D.C.: Corporate Press.

Janis, I.L. (1972). *Groupthink: Psychological Studies of Policy Fiascoes*, 2nd Edn. Boston: Houghton-Mifflin.

Johnston, W.B. & Packer, A.E. (1987). *Workforce 2000: Work and Workers for the 21st Century*. Washington, D.C.: US Department of Labor.

Kanter, R.M. (1977). *Men and Women of the Corporation*. New York: Basic Books.

Kanter, R.M. (1989). *When Giants Learn to Dance*. New York: Simon & Schuster.

Katz, P.A. & Taylor, D.A. (1988). *Eliminating Racism: Profiles in Controversy*. New York: Plenum.

Kraly, E.P. & Hirschman, C. (1990). Racial and ethnic inequality among children in the United States—1940 and 1950. *Social Forces*, **69**, 33–51.

Kram, K.E. (1985). *Mentoring at Work: Developmental Relationships in Organizational Life*. Glenview, IL: Scott Foresman.

Labouvie-Vief, G. (1989) Intelligence and cognition. In J.E. Birren & K.W. Schaie (eds.), *Handbook of the psychology of aging* (pp. 500–530) (2nd edn.). New York: Van Nostrand Reinhold.

Laughlin, P.R. (1980). Social combination processes of cooperative problem-solving groups on verbal intellective tasks. In M. Fishbein (ed.), *Progress in Social Psychology*, Vol. 1. Hillsdale, NJ: Erlbaum, pp. 210–231.

Laughlin, P.R. & Bitz, D.S. (1975). Individual versus dyadic performance on a disjunctive task as a function of initial ability level. *Journal of Personality and Social Psychology*, **31**, 487–496.

Lawrence, B.S. (1988). New wrinkles in a theory of age: demography, norms, and performance ratings. *Academy of Management Journal*, **31**, 309–337.

Lawrence, B.S. (1991). The Black Box of Organizational Demography. University of California, Los Angeles. Unpublished manuscript.

Levine, J.M. & Moreland, R.L. (1990). Progress in small group research. *Annual Review of Psychology*, **41**, 585–634.

Lincoln, J.R. & Miller, J. (1979). Work and friendship ties in organizations: a comparative analysis of relational networks. *Administrative Science Quarterly*, **24**, 181–199.

Lott, A.J. & Lott, B.E. (1965). Group cohesiveness and interpersonal attraction: a review of relationships with antecedent and consequent variables. *Psychological Bulletin*, **64**, 259–302.

McCain, B.E., O'Reilly, C. & Pfeffer, J. (1983). The effects of departmental demography on turnover: the case of a university. *Academy of Management Journal*, **26**, 626–641.

McGrath, J.E. (1984). *Groups: Interaction and Performance*. Englewood Cliffs, NJ: Prentice-Hall.

McGrath, J.E., Berdahl, J.L. & Arrow, H. (1996). Traits, expectations, culture, and clout: the dynamics of diversity in work groups. In S.E. Jackson & M. Ruderman (eds), *Diversity in workteams: Paradigms for a changing workplace*. Washington, D.C.: American Psychological Association.

McPherson, J.M. & Smith-Lovin, L. (1987). Homophily in voluntary organizations: status distance and the composition of face-to-face groups. *American Sociological Review*, **52**, 370–379.

Miller, V.D. & Jablin, F.M. (1991). Information seeking during organizational entry: influences, tactics, and a model of the process. *Academy of Management Review*, **16**(1), 92–120.

Nemeth, C.J. (1986). Differential contributions of majority and minority influence. *Psychological Review*, **91**, 23–32.

Nemeth, C.J. & Staw, B.M. (1989). The tradeoffs of social control and innovation in groups and organizations. *Advances in Experimental Social Psychology*, **22**, 175–210.

Nkomo, S.M. (1996) Identities and the complexity of diversity. In S.E. Jackson & R.N.

Ruderman (eds.), *Diversity in workteams: Paradigms for a changing workplace*, pp. 247–254. Washington, D.C.: American Psychological Association.

O'Reilly, C.A., Caldwell, D.F. & Barnett, W.P. (1989) Work group demography, social integration, and turnover. *Administrative Science Quarterly*, **34**, 21–37.

Pearce, J.A. & Ravlin, E.C. (1987). The design and activation of self-regulating work groups. *Human Relations*, **40**(11), 751–782.

Pelz, D.C. (1956). Some social factors related to performance in a research organization. *Administrative Science Quarterly*, **1**, 310–325.

Pfeffer, J. (1983). Organizational demography. *Research in Organizational Behavior*, **5**, 299–357.

Porac, J.F. & Howard, H. (1990). Taxonomic mental models in competitor definition. *The Academy of Management Review*, **2**, 224–240.

Quinn, J.B. (1980). *Strategies for change: logical incrementalism*. Homewood, IL: Irwin.

Ridgeway, C.L. (1982). Status in groups: the importance of motivation. *American Sociological Review*, **47**, 76–88.

Ridgeway, C.L. (1987). Nonverbal behavior, dominance, and the basis of status in task groups. *American Sociological Review*, **52**(2), 683–694.

Roloff, M.E. (1987). *Interpersonal Communication: The Social Exchange Approach*. Beverly Hills, CA: Sage.

Schmidt, W.H. (1974). Conflict: a powerful process for (good or bad) change. *Management Review*, **63**, 4–10.

Schweiger, D.M., Sandberg, W.R. & Rechner, P.L. (1989). Experiential effects of dialectical inquiry, devil's advocacy, and consensus approaches to strategic decision making. *Academy of Management Journal*, **32**, 745–772.

Schwenk, C.R. (1983). Laboratory research on ill-structured decision aids: the case of dialectical inquiry. *Decision Sciences*, **14**, 140–144.

Shaw, M.E. (1981). *Group Dynamics: The Psychology of Small Group Behavior*. New York: McGraw-Hill.

Shaw, M.E. & Ashton, N. (1976). Do assembly effects occur on disjunctive tasks? *Bulletin of the Psychonomics Society*, **8**, 469–471.

Sherif, M. (1935). *The Psychology of Social Norms*. New York: Harper.

Silver, S.D., Cohen, B.P. & Crutchfield, J.H. (1994). Status differentiation in information exchange in face-to-face and computer mediated idea generation. *Social Psychology Quarterly*, **57**, 108–123.

Simon, H.A. (1979). *The Sciences of the Artificial*, 2nd Edn. Cambridge, MA: MIT Press.

Simon, H.A. (1987). Making management decisions: The role of intuition and emotion. *Academy of Management Executive*, **February**, 57–64.

Smith, K.G., Smith, K.A., Olian, J.D., Sims, H.P. Jr, O'Brannon, D.P. & Scully, J.A. (1994). Top management team demography and process. The role of social integration and communication. *Administrative Science Quarterly*, **39**, 412–438.

South, S.J., Bonjean, C.M., Markham, W.T. & Corder, J. (1982). Social structure and intergroup interaction: men and women of the federal bureaucracy. *American Sociological Review*, **47**, 587–599.

Steiner, I.D. (1972). *Group Process and Productivity*. New York: Academic Press.

Stephan, W.G. (1985). Intergroup relations. In G. Lindzey & E. Aronson (eds), *Handbook of Social Psychology*, Vol. II. New York: Random House, pp. 599–658.

Torrance, E.P. (1959). The influence of experienced members of small groups on behavior of the inexperienced. *Journal of Social Psychology*, **49**, 249–257.

Triandis, H.C. (1996) The importance of context in studies of diversity. In S.E. Jackson & R.N. Ruderman (eds.), *Diversity in workteams: Paradigms for a changing workplace*, pp. 225–234. Washington, D.C.: American Psychological Association.

Triandis, H.C., Hall, E.R. & Ewen, R.B. (1965). Member heterogeneity and dyadic creativity. *Human Relations*, **18**, 33–55.

Tsui, A.S. & O'Reilly, C.A. III (1989). Beyond simple demographic effects: the importance of relational demography in superior-subordinate dyads. *Academy of Management Journal,* **32,** 402–423.

Tsui, A.S., Xin, K.R. & Egan, T.D. (1996). Relational demography: The missing link in vertical dyad linkage. In S.E. Jackson & M. Ruderman (eds), *Diversity in workteams: Paradigms for a changing workplace,* pp. 97–130. Washington, D.C.: American Psychological Association.

Turner, J.C. (1987). *Rediscovering the Social Group: A Self-categorization Theory.* Oxford: Basil Blackwell.

Turner, J.C., Hogg, M., Oakes, P., Reicher, S. & Wetherell, M. (1987). *Rediscovering the Social Group: A Self-categorization Theory.* Oxford: Blackwell.

Verbrugge, L.M. (1977). The structure of adult friendship choices. *Social Forces,* **56,** 576–597.

Wagner, W.G., Pfeffer, J. & O'Reilly, C.A. (1984). Organizational demography and turnover on top-management groups. *Administrative Science Quarterly,* **29,** 74–92.

Wallston, B.S. & O'Leary, V.E. (1981). Sex and gender make a difference: differential perception of women and men. *Review of Personality and Social Psychology,* **2,** 9–18.

Watson, W.E., Kumar, K. & Michaelson, L.K. (1993). Cultural diversity's impact on interaction process and performance: comparing homogeneous and diverse task groups. *Academy of Management Journal,* **36,** 590–602.

Willems, E.P. & Clark, R.D. III (1971). Shift toward risk and heterogeneity of groups. *Journal of Experimental and Social Psychology,* **7,** 302–312.

Wood, W. (1987). Meta-analytic review of sex differences in group performance. *Psychological Bulletin,* **102,** 53–71.

Zander, A. (1979). The psychology of group processes. *American Review of Psychology,* **30,** 417–451.

Zander, A. & Havelin, A. (1960). Social comparison and interpersonal attraction. *Human Relations,* **13,** 21–32.

Zenger, T.R. & Lawrence, B.S. (1989). Organizational demography: the differential effects of age and tenure distributions on technical communications. *Academy of Management Journal,* **2,** 353–376.

Chapter 4

Group Affective Tone

Jennifer M. George
Department of Management, Texas A&M University, USA

Abstract

This chapter focuses on the affective tone of work groups. Affective tone is defined as consistent or homogeneous affective reactions within a group and can be described in terms of two dimensions, positive affective tone and negative affective tone. Affective tone is a theoretically-based construct supported by three complementary theoretical perspectives: interactionism, socialization and social influence, and group tasks and outcomes. Group affective tone does not necessarily exist for all groups. Potential antecedents of group affective tone include the dispositional composition of the group in terms of the personality traits of positive affectivity and negative affectivity, leader affect, key group members, and rewards and punishments. Group affective tone has the potential to impact team mental models, group decision-making, prosocial behavior performed by group members, withdrawal behaviors, and group member well-being.

Descriptions about what groups are like and characterizations of both high performing and low performing groups often allude to the importance of affect in groups. A high performing group or team might be characterized as enthusiastic, active and high-energy. A team in trouble may be thought of as fraught with crippling anxiety, mistrust and hostility. Descriptions of both the highs and lows of groups and teamwork also allude to the critical role of affect in groups.

Given that groups are fertile breeding grounds for affect, it is surprising that affect in groups (or as will be defined a little later, group affective tone) has not been the focus of scholarly theorizing and research until recently. This chapter focuses on the affective nature of groups, how it comes about and what are its consequences. I start by describing the construct of group affective tone, the theoretical rationale supporting the construct, and how it can be measured. I then move on to consider potential antecedents and consequences of group affective tone.

THE NATURE OF GROUP AFFECTIVE TONE

George (1990) coined the term group affective tone to refer to consistent or homogeneous affective reactions within a group. If members of a group experience similar kinds of affective states at work, then affect is meaningful not only in terms of their individual experiences but also at the group level. The group has its characteristic kinds of affect or affective tone. If, for example, members of a group tend to be excited, energetic and enthusiastic, then the group itself can be described as being excited, energetic and enthusiastic. As another example, if members of a group tend to be distressed, mistrustful and nervous, then the group also can be described in these terms.

What if members of a group do not experience similar kinds of affective states at work? For example, some members of a group might be enthusiastic while others are not, or some members might be distressed while others are relaxed. Under these circumstances, a group does not have an affective tone because of dissimilarity in the affective experiences of group members. When such dissimilarity exists, affect can be used to describe individual group members' experiences but not the group as a whole. The fact that group affective tone might not exist for some groups is not, in and of itself, problematic. Rather, it suggests that researchers cannot *a priori* assume that group affective tone is a relevant construct for all groups. As discussed below, however, theory and research indicate that group affective tone does exist for many groups.

In order to impart a better understanding of the nature of group affective tone, below I describe the dimensions that can be used to characterize group affective tone, the theoretical and empirical research which supports the existence and relevance of this construct, and how group affective can be ascertained and measured.

Dimensions of Group Affective Tone

A seemingly endless array of adjectives can be used to describe the varied affective states that individuals experience. While traditionally these traits tended to be viewed along a positive–negative continuum, a substantial body of literature indicates that affective states are best characterized by two major and independent dimensions, not a single dimension (e.g. Costa & McCrae, 1980; Meyer & Shack, 1989; Watson & Pennebaker, 1989; Watson & Tellegen, 1985).

These two dimensions of affective experience, positive affect and negative affect, are caused by different factors, have differential relationships with behaviors and life events, and have different consequences for individuals and organizations (e.g. Costa & McCrae, 1980; George, 1989, 1992; Watson & Clark, 1984; Zautra, 1983). Positive affective states are described by terms such as interested, excited, strong, enthusiastic, proud, alert, inspired, determined, attentive and active (Watson, Clark & Tellegen, 1988). Negative affective states are described by terms such as distressed, upset, guilty, scared, hostile, irritable, ashamed, nervous, jittery and afraid (Watson, Clark & Tellegen, 1988).

Given that group affective tone, as a construct, is derived from homogeneous individual affective experience within groups, it stands to reason that the two dimensions that can be used to describe individual affect, positive affect and negative affect, can also be used to describe group affective tone (George, 1990). A self-managed work team with a strong sense of involvement in and ownership over its activities, for example, may feel interested, excited, proud, determined and active. A top performing R&D team might feel, for example, proud, alert and inspired. Alternatively, a top management team carrying out a massive downsizing effort may feel distressed, upset, guilty and ashamed. As a final example, a team of law enforcement officers attempting to control an angry mob might feel hostile and afraid.

Why and When Does Group Affective Tone Exist?

Given that group affective tone is defined as relatively homogeneous affective reactions within a group, it is not a given that it will exist for a majority of groups or at least enough groups to cause it to be a meaningful construct. That is, if members of a group experience different kinds of affective states at work, then the group does not have an affective tone and affect is only meaningful at the individual level. As mentioned earlier, however, preliminary research suggests that a majority of groups may, in fact, have affective tones (George, 1990, 1995).

Importantly, group affective tone is a *theoretically-based* construct and the theoretical rationale underlying and justifying its existence is perhaps more important than, or at least equally important to, initial empirical confirmation of its presence in ongoing groups. There are at least three complementary theoretical rationales supporting the existence of group affective tone: interactionism, socialization and social influence, and group tasks and outcomes.

Interactionism

Interactionism, as a meta-theoretical perspective, grew, in part, out of Mischel's (1968) criticism of trait theories and research and advocacy of a situational perspective which views behavior as largely influenced by situational or contextual factors. (For ease of exposition, an all-encompassing view of behavior is adopted here, including such things as feelings or affect, thoughts and attitudes in addition to concrete actions.) For years, theorists and researchers have been polarized around this fundamental question of whether behavior is based in persons or situations under the rubrics of what has been come to be called the person–situation debate. Even though some of the most influential writings in the interactionist tradition appeared in print over 20 years ago (e.g. Argyle & Little, 1972; Bowers, 1973; Endler, 1975), the person–situation debate (called a pseudo-issue in 1966 by Endler & Hunt) continues occasionally to rear its ugly head (George & James, 1994). As Carson (1989, pp. 228–229) has indicated:

> I have been baffled for two decades by the debate about whether internal dispositions and external circumstances exclude and oppose each other in determining behavior... Mischel himself abandoned years ago any radical situationist propensities (e.g. Mischel, 1973) in favor of what appears to be a frankly interactionist perspective.

By now it should be evident that interactionism is a meta-theoretical perspective which proposes that behavior is the result of the interaction of person and situation factors. Just as personality traits alone cannot give an adequate account of behavior, neither can situational or organizational influences. While some researchers might be used to thinking about interactions in a statistical sense, interactionism adopts an all-encompassing view of the range of person–situation interactions ultimately responsible for behavior (Pervin & Lewis, 1978). In addition to the familiar statistical interactions, viewing person and situation factors as each having main effects on behavior, as well as complex reciprocal relations between person and situation factors ultimately culminating in behavior, are each consistent with interactionism (Pervin & Lewis, 1978).

A key premise of interactionism has been cogently stated by Bowers (1973, p. 152):

> Situations are as much a function of the person as the person's behavior is a function of the situation.

The fact that people can create situations which can consequently influence their behavior is one way in which behavior is a function of complex reciprocal relations between the person and the situation.

Important for the concept of group affective tone is the fact that members of a group are instrumental in creating the very nature of the group which in turn affects them. While originally articulated at the organizational level of analysis, Schneider's (1987) attraction–selection–attrition framework (ASA) posits that people with similar kinds of personalities will be attracted to and selected by work settings, and those with dissimilar personalities will tend to leave work settings, resulting in relative homogeneity in personality within a work setting. Consistent with the ASA model, research suggests that attraction to work settings is partially a result of personality (e.g. Holland, 1985; Tom, 1971) and that attrition can result from a lack of fit between a person and a work setting (e.g. Mobley, 1982).

At the work group level, it has been argued that ASA processes are likely to lead to similarity in personality within groups (George, 1990; George & Brief, 1992). There are several means through which these processes may operate, examples of which follow. First, prospective group members may be attracted to or repelled by groups dependent upon the extent to which their personality is similar to that of other group members, as similarity in personality is one of the bases for attraction (e.g. Bryne, Griffitt & Stefaniak, 1967; Griffitt, 1966). Second, groups (as in the case of some self-managed work teams) or group leaders or supervisors may select group members based upon their assessments of the extent to which a prospective group member will "fit in". Third, placement decisions in organizations may be impacted by decision-makers' judgments of who will get along well together. As a final example, group members who find themselves at odds with the modal personality type of their group might seek a transfer to another, more compatible group. These are just some examples of the ways in which ASA processes may operate to produce similarity in personality within work groups (George, 1990).

Particularly relevant to the concept of group affective tone is the fact that positive and negative affect at the individual level are partially determined by the personality traits of positive affectivity and negative affectivity, respectively. Positive affectivity and negative affectivity are general and broad-based dimensions of personality which predispose people to experience positive and negative affective states (Tellegen, 1985). Positive affectivity corresponds to what is commonly called extraversion, and negative affectivity corresponds to what is commonly called neuroticism, in the robust Big Five Model of personality (Church & Burke, 1994; Digman, 1990; McCrae, 1989; Norman, 1963). Research in organizations has demonstrated that individuals who are high on positive affectivity are more likely to experience positive affective states at work and individuals who are high on negative affectivity are more likely to experience negative affective states at work (e.g. George, 1989, 1991a, 1991b; George et al., 1993).

Interactionism and ASA processes suggest that there will be similarity in global dimensions of personality like positive affectivity and negative affectivity within groups. If group members are similarly predisposed to experience certain levels of positive and negative affect (due to their similar standing on the traits of positive and negative affectivity), then it is likely that the group as a whole has a characteristic positive and negative affective tone. Consistent with this reasoning, George (1990) found that characteristic levels of positive affectivity in groups of salespersons were significantly and positively related to the positive affective tones of the groups, and characteristic levels of negative affectivity were significantly and positively related to the negative affective tones of the groups.

Socialization and Social Influence

A second theoretical perspective supportive of the group affective tone construct comes from the literature on socialization and social influence. Socialization is a term used to describe the learning process that takes place when newcomers to an organization learn dominant values, goals, norms and role expectations (Fisher, 1986). Co-workers, and in particular the members of one's primary work group, often play a key role in the socialization process; existing group members are likely to be seen as readily available experts who possess reward power while at the same time being similar to the newcomer (Fisher, 1986; Rakestraw & Weiss, 1981; Weiss & Nowicki, 1981).

Socialization is often viewed in terms of the transmission and assimilation of substantive information regarding such matters as how things are done in a group, how they ideally should be done, and so forth. However, it also is likely that during the socialization process newcomers also learn more subtle aspects of group life, such as the group's affective tone. By seeing that other group members are enthusiastic and excited, for example, a newcomer may come to learn that this is a desired affective response in a group and strive to be similarly positively activated.

Reinforcing the impact of socialization are more general social influence processes whereby individuals may be "infected" by the affect of those around them. Contagion theories of the spread of affect or emotion describe some of these mechanisms which may promote homogeneity in affect within groups.

Group Tasks and Outcomes

Members of groups often perform similar tasks and are exposed to similar kinds of group outcomes. These tasks and outcomes are likely to impact individual affective experience. For example, George (1995) found that receiving contingent rewards from one's supervisor was positively associated with the experience of positive mood states at work among a sample of managers. As another example, performing intrinsically enjoyable work may result in positive affective experience. The fact that group members are exposed to similar kinds of group tasks and outcomes which are likely to influence their affective experience also supports the notion that their affective experiences should be similar, resulting in a group affective tone.

When Group Affective Tone Might Not Exist

While the three complementary perspectives described above lead to the conclusion that group affective tone should exist, it might not always exist, as research has shown (George, 1995). Essentially, homogeneous affective reactions within a group are less likely when the processes described above are constrained in some way or not able to operate. First, under certain conditions, attraction, selection and attrition processes are not able to function to produce similarity within groups. This can occur, for example, when groups are formed with little information about the personalities and other characteristics of group members, such as when military units are formed, when newcomers have little or no choice about group membership (which may be true in lean economic times), and when group membership is constantly changing.

Group affective tone also might not be prevalent when group members do not actively play a role in the socialization process and ongoing social influence in a group is the exception rather than the norm. This might occur, for example, when group members are physically separated from one another.

Finally, relatively homogeneous affective reactions in a group may not be that common when group members perform different kinds of tasks and receive different kinds of outcomes. For example, in an academic department in a university, such as a psychology department or a management department, professors teach different kinds of classes, do different kinds of research, and may be engaged in different kinds of other activities (such as service in collegial organizations and consulting). Faculty members also receive different kinds and levels of outcomes. Some group members are rewarded for their research activities with prestigious journal publications, pay raises and promotions, while others face the disappointment of rejections from journals. In light of their varied activities and outcomes, members of such a group may not be expected to experience similar affective reactions at work.

Ascertaining and Measuring Group Affective Tone

Because group affective tone is defined as relatively homogeneous affective reactions within a group, ascertaining whether it actually exists in any given group revolves around determining if individual affect is homogeneous within the group. This determination can be made through using indices of agreement, such as that described by James, Demaree & Wolf (1984). As George & James (1993) point out, ANOVA-based statistics may not be as appropriate in this context due to their emphasis on between-group differences, which are likely to be affected by restriction of range across groups nested in the same organization or similar kinds of organizations.

Once it has been determined that there is actual agreement in affective reactions within groups, then measurement of group affective tone can proceed as follows. Individual self-reports of affective reactions can be aggregated to the group level of analysis and the mean levels of positive and negative affect within the groups can be used as the measure of group affective tone. Importantly, however, if agreement in affect is not found in one or more groups, then the aggregate scores should not be used, as they are essentially meaningless for groups that do not have an affective tone.

Individual affect can be measured by the use of self-report affect scales such as the PANAS scale (Watson, Clark & Tellegen, 1988) or the JAS (Brief et al., 1988; Burke et al., 1989). Time-frames for these self-report scales should be short-term (e.g. the past week) so as to avoid inadvertently measuring affect as a trait (i.e. positive affectivity and negative affectivity) rather than as a state.

There are alternatives to this measurement route, such as using third party observations of affect. However, research is needed to determine the appropriateness of such measures and the potential for emotional expressions to be deliberately manipulated by group members irrespective of experienced affect (as in the case of an unhappy salesperson who nonetheless smiles and displays positive affect for the benefit of customers).

At this point, it is important to note that whenever group constructs are measured by aggregating individual responses, it is crucial that the group-level construct be theoretically based (George & James, 1993). Group affective tone is a theoretically based construct and in the preceding pages I have described some of its theoretical underpinnings. When, for example, the processes which are theorized to give rise to group affective tone are not allowed to operate in a particular setting, or there is no strong theoretical basis for expecting group affective tone to exist, then aggregation is inappropriate.

POTENTIAL ANTECEDENTS OF GROUP AFFECTIVE TONE

Given that the theorized mechanisms which give rise to group affective tone are allowed to operate, what are the antecedents of group affective tone? Some of the antecedents have already been discussed such as the dispositional composition of the group in terms of the personality traits of positive affectivity and negative affectivity. Here three additional antecedents are discussed; leader affect, key group members, and rewards and punishments.

Leader Affect

George and Brief (1992) reasoned that leader affect is a powerful source of group affective tone. Just as group members experience positive and negative affect at work, so too do group leaders, and it is likely that the affect leaders experience rubs off on their groups in the form of group affective tone. Leaders who feel excited, enthusiastic and energetic themselves are likely to similarly energize their followers, as are leaders who feel distressed and hostile likely to negatively activate their followers.

In order for leader affect to influence group affective tone, however, it may be necessary for group leaders to work side by side with group members and be engaged in similar kinds of tasks. When leaders do not work with group members and perform different functions, their affective experience may have less of a direct effect on the groups they manage (George, 1995).

Key Group Members

In the foregoing discussion and in preliminary studies of group affective tone, it has been implicitly assumed that each member of a group contributes similarly to the group's affective tone. However, it may be the case that in some groups, there are key group members who are decisive in setting the affective tone of the group as a whole. Just as a group's leader may have a powerful influence on group affective tone, so too may very influential group members be a potent source of group affective tone, especially in groups that do not have formal leaders, such as self-managed work teams. Thus, the affective states experienced by key group members may play an important role in the etiology of group affective tone.

Rewards and Punishments

At the individual level, positive affect and negative affect are associated not only with different personality traits but also with different kinds of events (Clark & Watson, 1988). Analyses of these events, as well as discussions of the physiological structure of the central nervous system, suggest that positive and negative affect have their origins in different systems of the brain which are differentially responsive to various kinds of stimuli (Clark & Watson, 1988; Gray, 1971, 1981, 1987; Tellegen, 1985). For example, the work of Gray (1987) and others suggests that the behavioral activation system in the brain is responsible for positive affect and positive affect which is experienced when signals of reward are detected by this system (Larsen & Katelaar, 1991). Similarly, the behavioral inhibition system is responsible for negative affect which is experienced when signals of punishment are detected by this system. As Larsen & Katelaar indicate (1991, p. 135):

> When exposed to signals of reward, one experiences positive affect, and when exposed to signals of punishment, one experiences negative affect.

Rewards and punishments are one of the primary means through which behavior is controlled and managed in groups and organizations, whether they be intrinsic or extrinsic rewards, just or unjust punishments. To the extent that members of a work group are exposed to similar levels and kinds of rewards and punishments, then the rewards and punishments experienced should help to determine the positive and negative affective tones of the groups, respectively.

Summary

These are just a few of the potential antecedents of group affective tone. Due to the paucity of research in this area, this discussion of potential antecedents (like much of the other material in this chapter) is necessarily tentative and pending further research. Moreover, in order to discover additional causes of group affective tone, qualitative research may be warranted which focuses on studying the affective experience of ongoing groups over time.

POTENTIAL CONSEQUENCES OF GROUP AFFECTIVE TONE

Group affective tone has the potential to impact a wide variety of group and organizational outcomes. Here a sampling of some of these potential consequences is provided. More specifically, the potential effects of group affective tone on team mental models, decision-making, prosocial behavior, withdrawal behaviors and group member well-being are discussed. It should be emphasized at the outset that, given the lack of empirical research on many of the relationships discussed, they are necessarily tentative and are provided in the spirit of interesting links for future research to focus on.

Team Mental Models

Klimoski & Mohammed (1994) use the term "team mental model" to capture the shared cognitive structures that groups use to represent and make sense of knowledge and information. Group members collectively make sense of the issues and situations which confront them through these cognitive structures. These cognitive structures are collective as opposed to individual in that they are shared by group members. However, they reside in the minds of individual group members and, similar to work on individual cognition, are thought to be category-based (like schemas). Team mental models capture how a group, as a group, categorizes and makes sense of phenomena. As Klimoski & Mohammed point out, "group-mind" kinds of constructs akin to what these authors describe as team mental models have been variously labeled and described by authors in a variety of areas, including human resources and organizational behavior (e.g. Cannon-Bowers & Salas, 1990; Innami, 1992; Walsh & Fahey, 1986; Weick & Roberts, 1993). What these various writings have in common is a focus on how groups collectively make sense of the situations and issues confronting them through the use of shared cognitive structures.

At the individual level of analysis, a substantial body of literature attests to the interdependence of affect and cognition (Clark & Fiske, 1982; Clark & Isen, 1982). The positive and negative affective states of individuals have been shown to have far-reaching effects on their cognitive processes, just as cognitive processes can help to determine affective states (Lazarus, 1982, 1984). Consistent with the relative independence of positive and negative affect (Watson & Tellegen, 1985), positive and negative affect do not tend to have parallel or symmetrical influences on cognition (Isen & Baron, 1991). For example, while positive affect tends to facilitate the recall of positive material from memory, negative affect does not always result in more negative material being recalled (Blaney, 1986; Isen, 1985).

While team mental models focus on collective cognitive structures, they are "housed" in individuals. Individual cognitive structures play a key role in their development (Damon, 1991; Resnick, 1991). As Klimoski & Mohammed (1994, p. 404) indicate, "We will only come to understand the notion of team mental models if we first focus on individual cognitive processes". In one sense, the team mental model construct can be seen as the "cognitive analogue" of group affective tone. Both are shared and collective properties of groups which have their roots in individual level processes and experiences that come to be relatively homogeneous within a group and thus group-level constructs.

The nature of these two group constructs, and the highly interdependent nature of affect and cognition at the individual level of analysis, suggest that group affective tone and team mental models might have reciprocal influences on each other. On the one hand, it is likely that group affective tone impacts the cognitive structures and processes by which group members make sense of situations and issues. For example, it has been found that when individuals are in positive affective states, they tend to make more connections and integrations of divergent stimulus materials (Isen & Daubman, 1984; Isen, Daubman & Nowicki, 1987; Isen et al., 1985). Essentially, it appears that experiencing positive affect results in people perceiving more interrelatedness among stimuli and using broader, more inclusive categories (Isen & Daubman, 1984; Isen, Daubman & Nowicki, 1987). More specifically, Isen & Daubman (1984) found that individuals in positive affective states exhibited greater categorization breadth than a control group; by categorization breadth what is meant, for example, is the likelihood of seeing a stimulus as belonging to a certain category or of seeing two stimuli as being similar (Sinclair, 1988).

Murray et al. (1990) extended this work and proposed that positive affective states might promote cognitive flexibility, such that individuals in positive affective states might be more flexible in their categorizations. Results of three laboratory studies they conducted demonstrated that individuals in positive moods created and used both more narrow *and* more inclusive categories (i.e. they were more flexible in approaching categorization tasks). As Isen & Baron (1991, p. 21) suggest

> Persons who are feeling happy are more cognitively flexible—more able to make associations, to see dimensions, and to see potential relations among stimuli—than are persons in a neutral state.

It is important to keep in mind that the research discussed above pertains to the individual level of analysis. However, it is interesting to explore how these individual-level findings may play out at the group level of analysis. First, if individuals in a group all tend to experience positive affective states at work (i.e. the group has a high positive affective tone), then as individuals they may tend to be more cognitively flexible. Second, through social influence and other processes in a group, individual cognitive flexibility may be reinforced and strengthened. Third, as a result of these individual and group level processes the group as a whole may be more cognitively flexible, which will be reflected in its shared mental models. This may result, for example, in a group with a high positive affective tone being more creative, because one of the hallmarks of creativity is making connections between things that on the surface are dissimilar and combining ideas and concepts in unique ways. Obviously, whether or not these conjectures are valid is an empirical question. However, this is one example of the ways in which group affective tone may influence team mental models.

It also is likely that team mental models impact group affective tone. A group whose mental model emphasizes defensiveness and protection from threatening competitors, for example, might be more likely to have a high negative affective tone categorized by hostility and anger.

Group Decision-making

To the extent that group affective tone influences team mental models, it is likely that group decision-making will be affected. While there have been few direct tests of the team mental model construct and analogous concepts, theory and indirect evidence suggest that team mental models play an important role in group decision-making (Klimoski & Mohammed, 1994). It has been proposed that team mental models impact aspects of group decision-making ranging from problem definition, speed and flexibility, alternative evaluation, and choice to implementation (e.g. Innami, 1992; Klimoski & Mohammed, 1994; Walsh & Fahey, 1986; Walsh, Henderson & Deighton, 1988). For example, a group with a mental model which emphasizes threat and which has a high negative affective tone (which mutually reinforce and affect each other) may tend to be more rigid when making decisions (Staw, Sandelands & Dutton, 1981). To the extent that the proposed reciprocal relationship between group affective tone and team mental models is confirmed by research, the nature and outcomes of group decision-making are likely to be a result of the interaction of group affective tone and team mental models.

Prosocial Behavior

George (1990) reasoned that group affective tone would influence the extent to which a group performed prosocial behaviors. Her reasoning was relatively straightforward: the more favorable the affective tone of a group, the more likely the group is to engage in prosocial behavior because the work setting will be attractive to group members and will foster positive behaviors. As expected, she found negative affective tone to be negatively related to prosocial behavior performed by a group. However, contrary to expectations, group positive affective tone was not significantly associated with prosocial behavior. This may have been due to the fact that the form of prosocial behavior investigated was role-prescribed, that is, customer service behavior. George (1990) suggested that group positive affective tone might still be related to prosocial behavior but this helping behavior might be more oriented toward other group members rather than customers. However, in another retail setting, George (1995) found that positive affective tone was significantly and positively related to helping behavior directed at customers or customer service behavior. Clearly, more research is needed to understand the implications of group affective tone for role-prescribed and extra-role forms of prosocial behavior directed at both other group members and people outside the group such as customers, clients, supervisors and other members of an organization.

Withdrawal Behaviors

Group affective tone also is likely to influence withdrawal behaviors such as absenteeism and turnover, to the extent that members of a group have discretion over these behaviors. By discretion, I mean that they can be absent without excessive penalties and can voluntarily quit their jobs due to the presence of viable alternative employment options. Put simply, it is likely to be enjoyable to be working in a group with a high positive affective tone. Group members are more likely to be nice to each other in such a group, will be more likely to laugh and display other signs of positive feelings, and will be pleasant to be around (George & Brief, 1992). Conversely, it is likely to be unpleasant to work in a group with a high negative affective tone. Being surrounded by others who are feeling bad and have a negative outlook (even when your own feelings are similarly negative) is likely to be distasteful when such collective negative feelings are chronic and do not seem to improve over time. Consistent with this reasoning, at the individual level of analysis, it has been suggested that people consciously strive to maintain positive feelings or affective states and change or improve negative feelings or affective states (e.g. Clark & Isen, 1982; Morris & Reilly, 1987; Thayer, Newman & McClain, 1994). Absence and turnover may occur at the individual level of analysis as a result of these processes. At the group level of analysis, to the extent that the members of a group experience similar kinds and levels of affect at work (i.e. the group has an affective tone), this affective tone, as a collective construct, might impact group absence and turnover rates. Preliminary research is consistent with these proposed effects of group affective tone on withdrawal. For example, George (1990) found positive affective tone to be negatively related to group absence rates and negative affective tone to be positively related to group absence rates. More indirect support is provided by George & Bettenhausen (1990) who found leader positive mood to be negatively related to group turnover rates.

Group Member Well-being

The final potential consequence of group affective tone, group member well-being, is rather different from the other consequences discussed above, for several reasons. First, the group affective tone construct, in a sense, captures the overall collective well-being levels of groups. Second, group member well-being is more of an individual-level potential consequence than the other potential consequences considered. And third, it is almost too much of an intuitive, "common-sense" kind of argument to propose that group member well-being will be enhanced by a high positive affective tone and detracted from by a high negative affective tone. However, group member well-being is also an important potential consequence of group affective tone for future research to focus on.

CONCLUSIONS

Probably more so than some of the other chapters in this handbook, the ideas, proposed relationships, and findings reported in this chapter are quite tentative due to the fact that group affective tone has only recently been studied and discussed in the literature. This chapter was written not only to be a guide to existing theory and research but also (and perhaps more importantly) to stimulate future interest and research on group affective tone. Groups and teams are important building blocks of almost all organizations (Cummings, 1981; Hackman & Morris, 1975). Just as it is important to understand how groups "think" (Klimoski & Mohammed, 1994), it is important to understand how they feel—such feelings are likely to have wide-ranging effects on the functioning of work groups, their members and the organization as a whole.

REFERENCES

Argyle, M. & Little, B.R. (1972). Do personality traits apply to social behavior? *Journal for the Theory of Social Behaviour*, **2**, 1–35.

Blaney, P.H. (1986). Affect and memory: a review. *Psychological Bulletin*, **99**, 229–246.

Bowers, K.S. (1973). Situationism in psychology: an analysis and critique. *Psychological Review*, **30**, 307–336.

Brief, A.P., Burke, M.J., George, J.M., Robinson, D. & Webster, J. (1988). Should negative affectivity remain an unmeasured variable in the study of job stress? *Journal of Applied Psychology*, **73**, 193–198.

Bryne, D., Griffitt, W. & Stefaniak, D. (1967). Attraction and similarity of personality characteristics. *Journal of Personality and Social Psychology*, **5**, 82–90.

Burke, M.J., Brief, A.P., George, J.M., Roberson, L. & Webster, J. (1989). Measuring affect at work: confirmatory analyses of competing mood structure with conceptual linkage to cortical regulatory systems. *Journal of Personality and Social Psychology*, **57**, 1091–1102.

Cannon-Bowers, J.A. & Salas, E. (1990). Cognitive psychology and team training: shared mental models in complex systems. *Human Factors Bulletin*, **33**, 1–4.

Carson, R.C. (1989). Personality. *Annual Review of Psychology*, **40**, 227–248.

Church, A.T. & Burke, P.J. (1994). Exploratory and confirmatory tests of the Big Five and Tellegen's three- and four-dimensional models. *Journal of Personality and Social Psychology*, **66**, 93–114.

Clark, M.S. & Fiske, J.T. (eds) (1982). *Affect and Cognition*. Hillsdale, NJ: Erlbaum.

Clark, M.S. & Isen, A.M. (1982). Toward understanding the relationship between feeling states and social behavior. In A.H. Hastorf & A.H. Isen (eds), *Cognitive Social Psychology*. New York: Elsevier Science, pp. 73–108.

Clark, L.A. & Watson, D. (1988). Mood and the mundane: relations between daily life events and self-reported mood, *Journal of Personality and Social Psychology*, **54**, 296–308.

Costa, P.T. & McCrae, R.R. (1980). Influence of extraversion and neuroticism on subjective well-being: happy and unhappy people. *Journal of Personality and Social Psychology*, **38**, 668–678.

Cummings, T. (1981). Designing effective work groups. In P.C. Nystrom & W.H. Starbuck (eds), *Handbook of Organizational Design*, Vol. 2. Oxford: Oxford University Press, pp. 250–271.

Damon, W. (1991). Problems of direction in socially shared cognition. In L.B. Resnick, J.M. Levine & S.D. Teasley (eds), *Perspectives on Socially Shared Cognition*. Washington, D.C.: American Psychological Association, pp. 384–397.

Digman, J.M. (1990). Personality structure: emergence of the five-factor model. *Annual Review of Psychology*, **41**, 417–440.

Endler, N.S. (1975). The case for person–situation interactions. *Canadian Psychological Review*, **16**, 12–21.

Fisher, C.D. (1986). Organizational socialization: an integrative review. In K.M. Rowland & G.R. Ferris (eds), *Research in Personnel and Human Resources Management*, Vol. 4. Greenwich, CT: JAI Press, pp. 101–145.

George, J.M. (1989). Mood and absence. *Journal of Applied Psychology*, **74**, 317–324.

George, J.M. (1990). Personality, affect, and behavior in groups. *Journal of Applied Psychology*, **75**, 107–166.

George, J.M. (1991a). Time structure and purpose as a mediator of work–life linkages, *Journal of Applied Social Psychology*, **21**, 296–314.

George, J.M. (1991b). State or trait: effects of positive mood on prosocial behaviors at work. *Journal of Applied Psychology*, **76**, 299–307.

George, J.M. (1992). The role of personality in organizational life: issues and evidence. *Journal of Management*, **18**, 185–213.

George, J.M. (1995). Leader positive mood and group performance: the case of customer service. *Journal of Applied Social Psychology*, **25**, 778–794.

George, J.M. & Bettenhausen, K. (1990). Understanding prosocial behavior, sales performance, and turnover: a group level analysis in a service context. *Journal of Applied Psychology*, **75**, 698–709.

George, J.M. & Brief, A.P. (1992). Feeling good—doing good: a conceptual analysis of the mood at work–organizational spontaneity relationship. *Psychological Bulletin*, **112**, 310–329.

George, J.M. & James, L.R. (1993). Personality, affect, and behavior in groups revisited: comment on aggregation, levels of analysis, and a recent application of within and between analysis. *Journal of Applied Psychology*, **78**, 798–804.

George, J.M. & James, L.R. (1994). Levels issues in theory development. *Academy of Management Review*, **19**, 636–640.

George, J.M., Reed, T.F., Ballard, K.A., Colin, J. & Fielding, J. (1993). Contact with AIDS patients as a source of work-related distress: effects of organizational and social support. *Academy of Management Journal*, **36**, 157–171.

Gray, J.A. (1971). The psychophysiological basis of introversion–extraversion. *Behavior Research and Therapy*, **8**, 249–266.

Gray, J.A. (1981). A critique of Eysenck's theory of personality. In H.J. Eysenck (ed.), *A Model for Personality*. New York: Springer, pp. 246–276.

Gray, J.A. (1987). Perspectives on anxiety and impulsivity: a commentary. *Journal of Research in Personality*, **21**, 493–509.

Griffitt, W. (1966). Interpersonal attraction as a function of self-concept and personality similarity–dissimilarity. *Journal of Personality and Social Psychology*, **4**, 581–584.

Hackman, J.R. & Morris, C.G. (1975). Group tasks, group interaction process, and group performance effectiveness: a review and proposed integration. In L. Berkowitz (ed.), *Advances in Experimental Social Psychology*, Vol. 8. New York: Academic Press, pp. 45–99.

Holland, J.L. (1985). *Making Vocational Choices: A Theory of Careers*. Englewood Cliffs, NJ: Prentice-Hall.

Innami, I. (1992). Determinants of the quality of group decisions and the effect of the consensual conflict resolution. *Academy of Management Best Papers Proceedings*, 217–221.

Isen, A.M. (1985). Asymmetry of happiness and sadness in effects on memory in normal college students: comments on Hasher, Rose, Zacks, Sanft, and Doren. *Journal of Experimental Psychology: General*, **114**, 388–391.

Isen, A.M. & Baron, R.A. (1991). Positive affect as a factor in organizational behavior. In L.L. Cummings & B.M. Staw (eds), *Research in Organizational Behavior*, Vol. 13. Greenwich, CT: JAI Press, pp. 1–53.

Isen, A.M. & Daubman, K.A. (1984). The influence of affect on categorization. *Journal of Personality and Social Psychology*, **47**, 1206–1217.

Isen, A.M., Daubman, K.A. and Nowicki, G.P. (1987). Positive affect facilitates creative problem solving. *Journal of Personality and Social Psychology*, **52**, 1122–1131.

Isen, A.M., Johnson, M.M.S., Mertz, E. & Robinson, G.F. (1985). The influence of positive affect on the unusualness of word associationa. *Journal of Personality and Social Psychology*, **48**, 1413–1426.

James, L.R., Demaree, R.G. & Wolf, G. (1984). Estimating within-group interrater reliability with and without response bias. *Journal of Applied Psychology*, **69**, 85–98.

Klimoski, R. & Mohammed, S. (1994). Team mental model: construct or metaphor? *Journal of Management*, **20**, 403–437.

Larsen, R.J. & Katelaar, T. (1991). Personality and susceptibility to positive and negative emotional states. *Journal of Personality and Social Psychology*, **61**, 132–140.

Lazarus, R.S. (1982). Thoughts on the relations between emotion and cognition. *American Psychologist*, **37**, 1019–1024.

Lazarus, R.S. (1984). On the primacy of cognition. *American Psychologist*, **39**, 124–129.

McCrae, R.R. (1989). Why I advocate the five-factor model: joint factor analyses on the NEO-PI with other instruments. In D.M. Buss & N. Cantor (eds), *Personality Psychology: Recent Trends and Emerging Directions*. New York: Springer-Verlag, pp. 237–245.

Meyer, G.J. & Shack, J.R. (1989). Structural convergence of mood and personality: evidence for old and new directions. *Journal of Personality and Social Psychology*, **57**, 691–706.

Mischel, W. (1968). *Personality and assessment*. New York: Wiley.

Mischel, W. (1973). Toward a cognitive social learning reconceptualization of personality. *Psychological Review*, **80**, 252–283.

Mobley, W.H. (1982). *Employee turnover in organizations*. Reading, MA: Addison-Wesley.

Morris, W.N. & Reilly, N.P. (1987). Toward the self-regulation of mood: theory and research. *Motivation and Emotion*, **11**, 215–249.

Murray, N., Sujan, H., Hirt, E.R. & Sujan, M. (1990). The influence of mood on categorization: a cognitive flexibility interpretation. *Journal of Personality and Social Psychology*, **59**, 411–425.

Norman, W.T. (1963). Toward an adequate taxonomy of personality attributes: replicated factor structure in peer nomination personality ratings. *Journal of Abnormal and Social Psychology*, **66**, 574–583.

Pervin, L.A. & Lewis, M. (1978). Overview of the internal–external issue. In L.A. Pervin

& M. Lewis (eds), *Perspectives in Interactional Psychology*. New York: Plenum, pp. 1–22.

Rakestraw, T.L. & Weiss, H.M. (1981). The interaction of social influences and task experience on goals, performance, and performance satisfaction. *Organizational Behavior and Human Performance*, **27**, 326–344.

Resnick, L.B. (1991). Shared cognitions: thinking as social practice. In L.B. Resnick, J.M. Levine & S.D. Teasley (eds), *Perspectives on Socially Shared Cognition*. Washington, D.C.: American Psychological Association, pp. 1–20.

Schneider, B. (1987). The people make the place. *Personnel Psychology*, **28**, 447–479.

Sinclair, R.C. (1988). Mood, categorization breadth, and performance appraisal: the effects of order of information acquisition and affective state on halo, accuracy, informational retrieval, and evaluations. *Organizational Behavior and Human Decision Processes*, **42**, 22–46.

Staw, B.M., Sandelands, L.E. & Dutton, J.E. (1981). Threat-rigidity effects in organizational behavior: a multilevel analysis. *Administrative Science Quarterly*, **26**, 501–524.

Tellegen, A. (1985). Structures of mood and personality and their relevance to assessing anxiety, with an emphasis on self-report. In A.H. Tuma & J.D. Maser (eds), *Anxiety and the Anxiety Disorders*. Hillsdale, NJ: Erlbaum, pp. 681–706.

Thayer, R.E., Newman, J.R. & McClain, T.M. (1994) Self-regulation of mood: strategies for changing a bad mood, raising energy, and reducing tension. *Journal of Personality and Social Psychology*, **67**, 910–925.

Tom, V.R. (1971). The role of personality and organizational images in the recruiting process. *Organizational Behavior and Human Performance*, **61**, 573–592.

Walsh, J.P. & Fahey, L. (1986). The role of negotiated belief structures in strategy making. *Journal of Management*, **12**, 325–338.

Walsh, J.P., Henderson, C.M. & Deighton, J. (1988). Negotiated belief structures and decision performance: an empirical investigation. *Organizational Behavior and Human Decision Processes*, **42**, 194–216.

Watson, D. & Clark, L.A. (1984). Negative affectivity: the disposition to experience aversive emotional states. *Psychological Bulletin*, **98**, 219–235.

Watson, D., Clark, L.A. & Tellegen, A. (1988). Development and validation of brief measures of positive and negative affect: the PANAS scales. *Journal of Personality and Social Psychology*, **54**, 1063–1070.

Watson, D. & Pennebaker, J.W. (1989). Health complaints, stress and distress: exploring the central role of negative affectivity. *Psychological Review*, **96**, 234–254.

Watson, D. & Tellegen, A. (1985). Toward a consensual structure of mood. *Psychological Bulletin*, **103**, 193–210.

Weick, K.E. & Roberts, K.H. (1993). Collective mind in organizations: heedful interrelating on flight decks. *Administrative Science Quarterly*, **38**, 357–381.

Weiss, H.M. & Nowicki, C.E. (1981). Social influences on task satisfaction: model competence and observer field dependence. *Organizational Behavior and Human Decision Processes*, **27**, 345–366.

Zautra, A.J. (1983). Social resources and the quality of life. *American Journal of Community Psychology*, **11**, 275–290.

Chapter 5

Group Task Structure, Processes and Outcome

Franziska Tschan
and
Mario von Cranach
Institute of Psychology, University of Bern, Switzerland

Abstract

There is widespread agreement that task characteristics are very important for group processes and outcomes. Yet, the influence of specific task characteristics is all too often neglected in small group research. Most task classifications concern the task *in toto*, classifying it, for instance, in terms of complexity, divisibility, involvement of manual operations vs. conceptual work, etc. While such classifications represent an important starting point, they do not specify what exactly has to be done with regard to which (sub-)goal at what time (or in what sequence) has to be attained. The functionality of many group and individual behaviors can only be judged, however, if these requirements are known. It is therefore proposed to describe tasks in more detail, specifying: (a) their hierarchical requirements in terms of goals and sub-goals at different levels; (b) their sequential requirements in terms of restrictions imposed on the sequence in which certain sub-tasks should be dealt with; and (c) with regard to the cyclical nature of information processing (orienting, planning, executing, evaluating) with regard to each sub-goal. Such a specific task analysis, for which action regulation theories are a good basis, allows judgement of single behaviors with regard to their relationship to task requirements at a much higher level of specificity than classifications which only describe the task as a whole. As behaviors are described in terms of the task-requirements they are related to, such a classification also allows description of tasks and behaviors in corresponding terms. Especially where tasks are difficult and task requirements not obvious, the group has to develop a common understanding of the task and its requirements. The necessity for more research on this problem is underscored. Communication is discussed as the most important means to achieve a common understanding and to regulate group behavior. Its functionality should be different at different levels of task requirements, as communication is very difficult—and may even be disrupting—at very low levels of regulation ("automated behaviors", which do occur in groups as well as individuals) as well as on the level of "intuitive" strategies. It is outlined that group processes must be in accordance to the task demands of different levels, ranging from a very general level of structuring of the process over logical sequences of problem-solving steps to task-adequate verbal communication cycles at all goal levels. The higher performance of groups with a high amount of "ideal communication cycles"—(sub-)goal-related cycles of orientation/planning/action, and evaluation—which we found in our research is shown to exemplify the fruitfulness of this approach. Finally, we discuss how the structure of the group itself—role structure as well as sub-group formation for dealing with sub-tasks in smaller units—has to conform to task requirements and how failures to achieve this correspondence may impair group performance.

INTRODUCTION

What factors should one expect to influence the successful performance of a group when success is assessed in terms of "originality"—defined as "the degree to which the ideas and/or mode of presentation of a product are fresh and unusual as opposed to obvious and mundane" (Hackman, Jones & McGrath, 1967, p. 384)? Would not most people expect originality to be highly dependent on the group members' individual creativity, combined with a style of interaction that allows each member to develop and voice their ideas, as, for instance, prescribed by the rules of brainstorming? In other words, would not many of us expect characteristics of the *group* to be mainly responsible for an outcome such as originality?

In light of these considerations, it is interesting that Hackman (1968) and, in a replication and extension, Kent & McGrath (1969) found the characteristics of the *task* to account for much more variance in "originality" than *group* characteristics. In their study, three different types of tasks were examined that all yield a written product (production, discussion, and problem-solving). Most of the variance (87.9%) in their study was explained by *task* characteristics, but only 3.4% by *group* characteristics.

Originality was not the only outcome found that varies more with task than with group characteristics: a similar pattern has been found for action orientation, optimism and issue involvement (taking point of view regarding goal, values, procedures) (Hackman, Jones & McGrath, 1967; Hackman, 1968; Kent & McGrath, 1969; Hackman & Vidmar, 1970; Morris, 1966; Kabanoff & O'Brien, 1979).

This is not to say that group characteristics are unimportant. However, such findings suggest that certain tasks "allow" groups to come up with uncommon, original outcomes, while others make it more difficult to be original. Analogous to "powerful" vs. "weak" situations in the person–situation debate (cf. Mischel, 1977) we might talk of "strong" vs. "weak" tasks in terms of the influence of task vs. group characteristics. This becomes clearer when we look at the examples given for some of the tasks used in the Kent & McGrath (1969) study. An example for their production task is "Write a story about this inkblot" whereas one of the problem-solving tasks reported is "How could you safely change a tyre on a busy expressway at night". With this description of the task in mind, one can easily explain the differences in originality as a result of the task assignment, because it might be easier to come up with uncommon ideas for an inkblot than for changing a tyre.

Although task influences in principle are widely acknowledged in small group research and even more so in research about work teams (Goodman, 1990; Ilgen et al., 1993), in much research we find those influences are underestimated and not studied systematically.

In this chapter we stress the importance of task characteristics and their influence on group processes and outcomes. We emphasize the need to use a general theory of tasks for studying processes and outcomes of groups and work teams, and we propose that action regulation theories may be a fruitful way to describe behaviour requirements of group tasks as well as actual group behaviour in the same terms, thus allowing an assessment of compatibility of group behaviour with task requirements. We then discuss how different tasks influence: (a) to what extent a group can establish a common understanding or representation of a task; (b) how task goals influence the direction in which the group moves and how goals influence group performance; we propose (c) that group processes, in order to lead to a successful product, need to be structured in a way that is compatible with task demands; and (d) the same holds for group structures, which also need to be compatible with task requirements enable good performance.

Because task influences affect groups in many ways, this chapter cannot be comprehensive. Specifically, we do not focus on the motivational properties of tasks that lead to various job design propositions (see Chapter   in this book). We also do not discuss specific, task-related organizations of work groups such as autonomous work groups, because this is done in chapter   and chapter

SELECTING A WAY TO DESCRIBE TASKS

The acknowledgment of the impact of tasks on group processes and outcomes has led to several task classifications for group tasks (e.g. Steiner, 1972; Hackman, 1968; Shaw, 1976; McGrath, 1984). Task types have been classified along dimensions, for example in Shaw's empirical classification along the dimensions *difficulty* (easy vs. difficult tasks), solution *multiplicity* (number of correct solutions), *intrinsic interest* (motivating potential of the task), *cooperation requirements*, *intellectual–manipulative requirements* (ratio of mental to motor requirements), and population *familiarity*. Steiner (1972) distinguishes *unitary* and *divisible* tasks. Unitary tasks, which require a joint product for the group as outcome, are further distinguished into disjunctive tasks (a single member can solve the task for the group), conjunctive tasks (each group member must solve the task) additive tasks (the contribution of the group members are added for the outcome), and discretionary tasks (the group has the latitude to choose its own process). McGrath (1984) developed a circumplex model of group tasks, claiming that it can classify types of tasks in an exhaustive and mutually exclusive way. It combines the dimensions conflict vs. cooperation, and conceptual (intellectual) vs. behavioural (actional) tasks with four general types of tasks. Each of these is further divided into two sub-types, so the complete circumplex model contains eight different types of tasks. *Generate* contains (1) generating plasn or (2) ideas; *choose* can mean (3) choose the correct answer or (4) decide issues along preferences; *negotiate* includes (5) resolving conflict of viewpoints or (6) conflict of motive-interest and *execute* is further divided into (7) competition and (8) the performance of psycho-motor tasks.

These task classification schemes have been both very influential and useful in small group research. Interestingly, however, they are not very much taken up in research about teams in organizations. Although in this research the importance of tasks is stressed as well, these classifications are not often reported as used or regarded as useful for research on work teams (Guzzo & Shea, 1992; Hackman, 1990a; Hackman & Oldham, 1980). One of the reasons for this seems to be that such clear-cut distinctions can only be made for strongly controlled and short-term laboratory tasks. In contrast, the task of a real work group is likely to contain several sub-tasks, each representing a different type of Steiner's or McGrath's dimensions (Goodman, 1990). A decision-making team, for example, may be confronted with problems that represent several of McGrath's task types of generate, choose, and negotiate—all in one meeting. It seems, therefore, that for the investigation of "real" groups, task classifications used in laboratory research have a limited usefulness.

Wood (1986) stresses the need for a general theory of tasks and proposes to describe tasks in terms of a combination of behavioural and objective task requirements (Hackman, 1968). Wood's model is based on Naylor, Pritchard & Ilgen's theory of behaviour in organizations (1980). In their terminology, acts (as the basic units of behaviour) result in *products*, and those are the starting point of task analysis, Wood (1986) assesses task requirements in terms of (a) the behavioural acts that must be performed in order to attain the product, and (b) the informational cues that must be attended to for successful performance. Based on these considerations, Wood developed a framework to assess *task complexity* as one part of a theory of tasks. He distinguishes three facets of complexity. *Component complexity* is described in terms of how many different acts a given product requires, how many informational cues are needed for each act and the number of sub-acts required for each act. *Coordinative complexity* refers to the coordinative requirements that are inherent in the task. It is important to note that it does *not* refer to coordinating people, but to coordinating acts. Coordinative complexity is high to the extent that the task requires timing or sequencing of subjects. The third aspect, *dynamic complexity*, describes the need to adapt to changes in the cause–effect or means–end hierarchy of the task. Dynamic complexity is high to the extent that, during task performance, changes in the environment occur which alter the way a task has to be conceptualized. Wood's system enables a calculation of the overall complexity of a task, and thus comparisons of different tasks in terms of their complexity level (see also Dörner, 1989).

THE NEED FOR MORE SPECIFIC DESCRIPTIONS OF TASKS IN HIERARCHICAL AND SEQUENTIAL TERMS

Whatever distinguishes the task classifications described so far, they all have one element in common: they describe tasks in global terms, e.g. divisibility or complexity. While it is interesting and fruitful to use such classifications for investigating which type of group (in terms of group composition, style of behaviour such as interruptions, etc.) does well with what type of tasks, these classifications do not enable one to specify what behaviours may be necessary, helpful or inhibiting at what point in time. A conclusion like, "The group could not finish the task in time, because they failed to realize that their solution was based on assumption X, that turned out to be wrong, but this was not checked until the very end of the session..." cannot be drawn based on the task analysis made possible by these approaches. As a consequence, such classifications leave us astonishingly ignorant about what *exactly* went wrong or well in the time-course to a group's action.

In order to answer such questions, we have to ask, "What has to be done, when?" This implies that the task can be described in terms of the goals and subgoals that need to be reached. Thus, for example, a task like "preparing dinner" might involve frying steaks, boiling vegetables, preparing the salad, serving the food, etc. The various tasks can further be broken down into sub-tasks (e.g. putting oil into a pan, heating it, putting the steaks in the pan, salting the meat, etc.). In addition, there are certain requirements with regard to sequence. It would not be wise to fry the steaks before starting to peel the potatoes because the potatoes take much longer, etc. Of course, tasks differ with regard to the strictness of sequential requirements: some are prescribed quite strictly, some leave quite a few options, but normally there are at least some sequential requirements that have to be met.

Thus, we must not only ask about general classes of behaviour favourable for successful group action, such as "not interrupting others". It may, indeed, be quite functional to interrupt others in order to avoid hasty action without sufficient exploration of the problem and its different facets. We therefore have to ask what different kinds of behaviours are required, what steps a group has to perform, and in what sequence they have to perform them, if a group is to be successful.

Most existing task classifications are limited in this respect, although Wood's approach certainly represents a major step in this direction. There are, however, approaches which concentrate on hierarchical and sequential analyses of action requirements. These are usually described as theories of action regulation (von Cranach et al., 1982; Frese & Zapf, 1994; Hacker, 1986; Volpert, 1984). They specify regulatory processes necessary in goal-directed behaviour, such as decomposing high-level goals (preparing meals in a restaurant) into lower level sub-goals; constantly checking to what extent they are fulfilled; taking action as a result of these checks; keeping to a sequence of orientation, planning, deciding, acting and controlling each (sub-)action; and choosing the correct (or, if there are several ways to proceed, a feasible) sequence in which the various sub-goals should be worked on. The basic idea has been described in terms of the famous TOTE (test–operate–test–exit)-unit (Miller, Galanter & Pribram, 1960). Taken up and refined by European psychologists (especially Hacker, 1985; Volpert, 1987; von Cranach et al., 1982; Frese & Zapf, 1994), this approach has been applied to individual behaviour and extended to group behaviour by von Cranach and his co-workers (von Cranach, Ochsenbein & Valach, 1986; von Cranach et al., 1989; von Cranach (in press); Tschan, 1995). Since in these approaches tasks are described in terms of goals and subgoals, task requirements and (individual or group) behaviour can be described in the same terms.

Action theories are both more global and more specific than most of the group task classifications. They are more global in that they deal with goal-directed behaviour in general. They are more specific in their description of the regulatory processes in task fulfilment. They are similar to Naylor, Pritchard's and Ilgen (1980) as well as Woods' (1986) approach of tasks via products, in that products can be described as goals. They are different to those approaches, in that they distinguish between different hierarchical levels of an action and propose specific characteristics of those levels.

Action theories define an action as behaviour that is related to a goal. Most tasks can be described in terms of goals to be accomplished, "deciding about next year's budget", to "landing planes safely" and "mining coal". Such tasks are then analysed with respect to their (a) hierarchical and (b) sequential requirements as well as with respect to (c) cyclical process requirements (Frese & Zapf, 1994; von Cranach, in press).

1. The *hierarchical* organization of a task is given by the goals, sub-goals and sub-sub-goals that have to be accomplished in order to achieve the main goal or product. Sub-goals have to be identified that invariably have to be fulfilled in order to achieve the main goal. "Invariably" is important here, because most tasks contain degrees of freedom over how to perform them: some sub-goals can be left out, changed or added, and the main goal can still be achieved.

    Different regulatory mechanisms are postulated at different levels of the goal hierarchy. More abstract and general goals require conscious attention (cf. Shiffrin & Schneider's "controlled" mode) while lower level goals may (given sufficient practice) become "automatized" (cf. Shiffrin & Schneider's "automatic" mode: Shiffrin & Schneider, 1977; Schneider & Shiffrin, 1977). Hacker (1986) speaks of an "intellectual level" which involves the conscious development of plans, based on rather extensive orientation about the task and the prevailing conditions, and a "sensorimotor level" of regulation which involves highly automatized patterns of movement. In addition, he postulates a medium level that has been called the "level of flexible action pattern" by Frese & Zapf (1994) and Semmer & Frese (1985; cf. also Rasmussen's, 1987, distinction between knowledge-based, rule-based, and skill-based behaviour). This "medium" level involves the triggering of behavioural schemata (e.g. "shift gear" in driving) on the basis of the identification of appropriate environmental cues and the application of well established if–then rules (Rasmussen's "rule-based behaviour"). While there are classifications assuming four (Semmer & Frese, 1985) or five (Oesterreich, 1981) levels, the three-level classification by Hacker is the most widely acknowledged (see also von Cranach et al., 1982). In all cases, however, the basic idea is the same, involving consciously controlled, slow processes at higher levels, and more automatic, not consciously controlled, and fast processes at lower levels of action regulation.

2. The second characteristic of tasks refers to their *sequential* requirements. In the dinner example, for instance, there is a clear sequential requirement in that the salad needs to be washed before it is seasoned and served. Again, some of the sequential requirement may be invariant (e.g. washing before eating), while others can be changed (e.g. seasoning before or after serving). Thus, as for hierarchical requirements, tasks contain more or fewer degrees of freedom for the sequence that has to be followed in completing the various subtasks.

3. Actions can also be described as *cyclical regulation processes*. For each (sub-)task, actors have to orientate, to generate or choose goals, to develop plans, to decide on a course of action, to execute the behaviour, and to assess how far the goal has been reached (feedback). A complete action cycle contains preparatory as well as evaluative information processing, and execution of behaviour. The concept of different levels of regulation combined with the elements of action processes allows description of regulation requirements of tasks, and allows us to identify and classify errors (Frese & Zapf, 1994), as well as regulation obstacles (Semmer, 1984).

THE GROUP AS AN ACTING SYSTEM

A group cannot act except through its individual members who are the basic acting units. However, the group has to go beyond individual acts; it has to coordinate its actions towards a common goal, and in this sense, the group can be regarded as an acting unit, or an acting system, in its own right (von Cranach, Ochsenbein & Valach, 1986; Larson & Christensen, 1993). Group action is, therefore, a two-level process where individuals have to meet the requirements of their individual sub-tasks in such a way that the group as whole meets the requirements of the task as a whole.

Of course, most groups are, in turn, parts of larger systems. Therefore, more than two levels have to be considered when analysing, for instance, group action in organizations (cf. von Cranach, in press, Tschan, 1990; Tschan & von Cranach, 1990). This however will not be pursued here.

To achieve a common product, for most tasks, the group has to develop a common understanding of the task, to develop goals, to structure the processes, and to establish a group structure that helps rather than hinders task completion. Unless a group has established routines for the interpretation of tasks and situations and the behaviours that each group member has to fulfil (as described, for instance, by von Cranach, Ochsenbein & Valach, 1986 or by Gersick & Hackman, 1990) it is evident that communication among groups members is vital. The function that communication fulfils in the regulation of group action may be seen as analogous to the function that conscious thinking fulfils for individual action regulation processes (von Cranach, Ochsenbein & Valach, 1986).

ESTABLISHING A COMMON UNDERSTANDING OF THE TASK

Probably the first challenge for groups trying to complete a task is to establish a common concept of this task. If this is not achieved, different individual concepts are likely to generate confusion and conflict. if groups have a common redefinition of the task (Hackman & Morris, 1975; Hackman, 1990b) as well as of how to proceed, process losses may be minimized and group performance may be enhanced, as is suggested by research that provides groups with rules about how to proceed (Erffmeier & Lane, 1984; Firestien, 1990; Ganster, Williams & Poppler, 1991).

The development of a common concept of the task implies that task demands are interpreted in equal (or, at least, reasonably similar) terms; there is agreement at least about the general way of proceeding; the most important and likely difficulties are being anticipated. In other words, a "mental model" of the task has to be built up. Hacker and his group (e.g. Hacker & Clauss, 1976) have shown that individuals with a better mental model (they speak of a system of "operative images" to emphasize that it must contain not only declarative but also procedural knowledge) have a wider range of anticipation, know more about possible obstacles, machine failures and action errors, as well as ways to correct them. This enables them to perform better without necessarily spending more effort because their work behaviour is more economical. In the same vein, a group has to develop its "mental model" of the task which, however, has to contain an additional element, which is coordination requirements. Of course, building up such a mental model can be done in a very limited way in advance; feedback from (group) action is usually needed to clarify misunderstandings, correct errors and acquire an understanding of what can reasonably be expected of the other group members. To the extent that this happens, communication requirements decrease, and routines are developed on a group level (Gersick & Hackman, 1990).

This is not to say, of course, that diversity is, by definition, a disadvantage. Having multiple views on a task can result in a broader and more thorough understanding of the problem (Lord, 1976), and not allowing dissenting views may be very detrimental, as in group-think (Janis, 1972). On the other hand, at least to some degree a common problem definition is necessary to be able to develop common action plans and finally show coordinated action (Larson & Christensen, 1993; Moreland & Levine, 1992; von Cranach, Ochsenbein & Valach, 1986; Wilson & Canter, 1993). Time is likely to be of crucial importance here: just as individual action seems to profit from a "deliberative" state of mind, where one is open to a diversity of informational cues—*before*, but an "implemental" state of mind—which "protects" the decision from being constantly changed on the basis of new information—*after* a decision is taken, group action may also profit from diversity in the beginning, but from a restriction of diversity once a course of action has been started (Beckmann & Gollwitzer, 1987).

Tasks differ in the extent to which they will be perceived similarly by all group members, and thus in the likelihood of a common understanding and conceptualization. Some tasks rank high in population familiarity (Shaw, 1976), that is, there exists a widely shared social representation for them (Thommen, Amman & von Cranach, 1988). In this case, the task is likely to be perceived in a more similar way by all group members and, therefore, establishing a common understanding of the task and the action it requires should be relatively easy (Hackman, Brousseau & Weiss, 1976; Hackman & Morris, 1975) and quick (Moreland & Levine, 1992).

One can also expect that for problems that are not very complex and have either few or obvious sequential requirements, it should be easier to establish a common understanding of the tasks. In this case, this may happen more implicitly. Also, it can lead to a definite solution early in the group's work, whereas more complex problems may require recurrent phases of problem-definition (Badke-Schaub, 1993; Mintzberg, Raisinghani & Theoret, 1976).

Of course, familiarity and complexity of a task are not constant; they change with experience. Thus, Kanki & Foushee (1989) showed that aircraft crews that have flown together perform better in a flight-simulator task than crews that are unfamiliar with each other, even though the former were more tired. As expertise of the individual members was constant in their study (all crew members were experts on how to fly an airplane), it is likely, as the authors state, that at least part of this effect is due to the development of group specific procedures on the basis of common experience. This should reduce explicit coordination requirements, and thus reduce the effects of fatigue.

The performance strategies chosen depend on how the task is redefined (Hacker, Freedman & Gorman, 1990), and problematic redefinition can have quite disastrous consequences (Janis, 1972). Establishing a common understanding of the task is, therefore, a crucial step in successful performance.

REGULATING THE ACTION PROCESS ON DIFFERENT LEVELS

Distinguishing between different hierarchical levels of action regulation implies that at higher levels information processing is more conscious and elaborate, while at lower levels it is more automatic. Also, at lower levels, orientation and feedback often are confined to intermittent checks rather than continuous vigilance, with sub-actions in between these checks running smoothly "on their own" once they are triggered, and so long as no serious deviation requires "reinstallation" of controlled regulation modes.

While in the beginning, most tasks require regulation at high levels, tasks differ in how much they can be routinized and "delegated" to lower levels with practice (cf. Frese & Zapf, 1994). There are indications that this way of thinking can be applied to group action as well (Gersick & Hackman, 1990).

Higher levels of regulation imply that it is easier to verbalize what one is planning and doing. This, in turn, implies that it should be easier for a group to communicate about tasks that require much conscious regulation, as has been pointed out by von Cranach, Ochsenbein & Valach (1986). Indeed, for complex tasks, a higher rate of communication has been found to be positively related to group performance (Foushee, 1984; Williges, Johnston & Briggs, 1966), whereas for less complex tasks, communication does not seem to enhance performance (Lanzetta & Roby, 1956, 1960; Mueller, 1992).

It is important to emphasize, however, that it is not the complexity of the task *per se* that determines the possibility and fruitfulness of verbal communication. Highly skilled performance, even in originally very complex tasks, often is characterized by a declining ability to verbalize one's own action regulation processes. Indeed, highly skilled experts tend to resort to "intuitive" strategies which they describe in words like "playing it by ear", "having a feeling for it", etc. (cf. Hacker & Skell, 1993). Communicating about this seems to require a vocabulary on its own. And, indeed, long-standing groups tend to develop their own "vocabulary" (which is not only verbal but also contains many signs and symbols) (Meissner, 1976). These "languages" tend to show characteristics of "restricted" codes in that communication presupposes that the receiver knows the background and context of what is being communicated. This may partly explain the advantage of a flight crew that has flown together in comparison with a crew which is newly composed, as shown by Kanki & Foushee (1989). In line with this reasoning, Mueller (1992) reports that the amount of verbal communication is negatively related to performance for a task that required groups to coordinate movements—something where verbalization and coordination are extremely difficult.

It follows that it often is not a wise strategy to have the group as a whole work on tasks for which highly skilled—and hard to verbalize—procedures exist in individuals or sub-groups. Anyone who has tried to formulate a letter or any other text jointly in a group knows that in most cases this is a very difficult thing to do. It is much easier if the group agrees on the basic content, and one person writes a draft, which subsequently may be revised by others.

Such an analysis of action regulation requirements highlights an inappropriate assumption in much of the literature on groups: that "the group" is working on a task. In reality, however, "the" group does not necessarily work *as a whole* on each sub-task—and in many cases, it should not! Many sub-tasks might better be delegated to individuals, dyads, etc.

Questions such as:

- To what extent does a task require regulation on high levels—and thus requires the group, most likely, to communicate about:
- To what extent does the task involve highly skilled components over which the group has no command and which therefore should be delegated to individuals or sub-groups? Or:
- How necessary is it to acquire this type of skilled regulation *on the group level* which may imply the need for a specific, group-related training phase?

are important both for the analysis and the training of group performance, and the action regulation approach may be fruitful for this, especially if the originally approach which is oriented towards the individual is extended to the group level (cf. von Cranach, Ochsenbein & Valach, 1986).

THE IMPORTANCE OF GOALS

Task groups have one or several goals to fulfil. They are expected to show coordinated action towards a final state. In definitions of task groups, the notion of goal-relatedness often is explicitly included (von Cranach, Ochsenbein & Valach, 1986; Hackman, 1990), and goal fulfilment is the main constituting factor of task-force groups, the existence of which is justified by specific goals (McGrath, 1984; Ilgen et al., 1993). In groups as multilevel systems, the concordance of individual and group goals also must be considered. If individual and group goals differ too much, group performance as well as individual satisfaction may suffer (Hackman & Oldham, 1980). Indeed, goals have an impact on groups in several respects. They can build identify, guide behaviour, increase motivation and influence the development of long-term strategies.

When group members "identify" with the goal of the group (Hackman, 1990a), this can have consequences for group identification, as postulated by Social Identity Theory (Tajfel & Turner, 1979) such as in-group favouritism and derogation of outgroups. Identifying with the goal(s) of a group may be part of group members' roles and have persuasive influence on their attitudes, as shown, for instance, in Lieberman's study of men who became shop stewards or foremen and changed their attitudes according to their new roles (Lieberman, 1956). In extreme and unstructured situations, developing and following concrete goals seems to enhance the chance of survival. Air force crews going down in enemy territory that succeeded in establishing common goals have been captured less often than groups that failed to establish a goal (Torrance, 1954a). Torrance concludes that the structuring effect of goals helped the group in an otherwise ambiguous situation, and establishing goals also seemed to enhance staying power. Conversely, a group may fall apart when it loses its goal, as shown in Festinger, Reider & Schachter's case study about a cult that lost the goal of surviving the end of the world (Festinger, Reider & Schachter, 1956).

As a representation of a state which is to be achieved, goals are *standards* against which feedback about the current state, the effect of past actions and new developments can be judged. Goals therefore have an important guiding function, and they can reduce uncertainty and confusion, be that about what should be done (content goals) or when and how fast it should be done (time related goals, i.e. time limits). Clear goals should therefore enhance the coordination of actions. It is plausible to expect that goals will fulfil this function better, the more concrete they are.

With regard to *motivation*, the mere fact of setting goals has been shown to enhance performance of individuals, provided the goals conform to certain conditions. The most important of these are that goals should be concrete and challenging but attainable (Bandura, 1989; Locke, Shaw, Sari & Latham, 1981; Hacker, 1983). Studies of groups and simulated organizations show that systems react similarly to goal-setting (Smith, Locke & Barry, 1990; Pritchard et al., 1989; Weingart, 1992; Weingart & Weldon, 1991). Groups with concrete and challenging goals show a higher work rate and work harder (Weingart & Weldon, 1991; Weingart, 1992). Set or perceived time limits in teams also seem to be a powerful organizing force (Gersick, 1989; Hackman, 1990a).

However, goals do not only have an impact on immediate group processes. Goal-setting also seems to have *long-term consequences* for the later behaviour of a group. Thus, research by Weldon, Jehn & Pradhan (1992) and Weingart & Weldon (1991) suggests that groups with challenging goals are more likely to develop effective strategies which, however, may not pay off immediately but can be regarded as an investment, because they enhance performance in later sessions (the development of strategies is also one of the mechanisms that Locke & Latham, 1990, mention as being responsible for the effects of goal-setting). In a similar vein, goal-setting may induce groups to develop specific ways of dealing with tasks which may then be retained even under new circumstances. Thus, groups working under high time pressure in their first session tend to develop a high working pace which is upheld in later sessions, even if time pressure is removed (Kelly & McGrath, 1985; Kelly, Fotoran & McGrath, 1990).

As with individuals, goals must be judged by the group to be attainable in order to increase motivation and performance. For groups, however, this implies an additional aspect: not only must the goal be attainable in principle but the conditions must allow the group members to coordinate their efforts effectively, if necessary for task fulfilment. If the group members are hindered in generating and coordinating an action plan, goal-setting is not likely to be effective, as shown by Larson & Schaumann (1993).

Since we have argued that tasks can be described in terms of goals and sub-goals, the emphasis on goals is another way of repeating our emphasis on more detailed analyses of tasks in group research. Except in research which is specifically devoted to the investigation of goals, however, questions such as how concrete, challenging and attainable the goals are, are seldom prominent in small group research.

STRUCTURING THE PROCESS ACCORDING TO TASK DEMANDS

Studies examining the relationship between group processes all propose a certain degree of structuring of group processes, to improve group performance. Structuring the group process means that the group follows a regular or organized pattern of behaviour, rather than being chaotic and unpredictable. This pattern can be given to the group or emerge spontaneously.

An unstructured and chaotic group would suffer large process losses (Steiner, 1972), and would perform well below its potential. Given the hierarchical and sequential organization of tasks, one can assume that structuring processes in ways compatible with hierarchical and sequential task requirements (von Cranach, Ochsenbein & Valach, 1986) would lead to higher group performance. The more strict the requirements of a task, the closer would be the relationship between process characteristics and performance.

In what terms should this structuring be conceived and described? Even though various authors differ with regard to terminology and the exact number of requirements specified, there seems to be little disagreement that goal-directed behaviour typically requires at least a minimal amount of the following:

- Exploring and understanding the task and the situation in which it has to be fulfilled (task orientation).
- Deciding on goals.
- Developing and selecting strategies (planning).
- Executing behaviour.
- Evaluating the result.

(cf. Miller, Galanter & Pribram, 1960; Frese & Zapf, 1994; Hacker, 1985)

Of course, in many cases these processes do not have to be very elaborate. Orientation may be quick if the situation is familiar; goals may be accepted as given; strategies may be recalled rather than developed; parts of execution may be highly automatized; and evaluation may be reduced to a quick check if the results conforms to a familiar "gestalt". Nevertheless, at least in some very basic form, all these functions must be fulfilled if goal directed behaviour is to be carried out successfully.

Many approaches which deal with the structuring of group behaviour deal with one, several, or all of these functions. Some emphasize phases over time; some sequences of steps, some the importance of certain of these functions; and some cyclical processes specifically related to task requirements at different goal-levels.

General Phases Over Time

In their well-known studies of problem-solving groups, Bales and his co-workers (Bales, 1950; Bales & Strodtbeck, 1951) rated group communication with regard to its functionality. They found that higher percentages of exploration or orientation in the first phase, evaluation in the middle phase and control in the third phase of a group's work were typical.[1] Note that these phases are specified with regard to their distribution over time (which should be approximately equal), but are not specified with regard to the task at hand. Indeed, they are often perceived as generally occurring in problem-solving groups (Bales, 1950; McGrath, 1984) and thus are basically conceived of as typical for the task type problem-solving tasks. However, a second requirement was specified, in order for these phases to occur: The problem-solving tasks had to be "fully fledged". This means that "... functional problems of orientation, evaluation and control are each to a major degree unsolved at the beginning of observation ..." (Bales & Strodtbeck, 1951, p. 487). In other words, the problem as a whole must be unresolved at the beginning of the group's work. If the group has had some experience with the problem before working together, fewer orientation activities are expected to occur; then, the task is "truncated" instead of "fully fledged" and there is no need for the three phases to occur.

The model has found empirical support. Thus, Landsberger (1955) found that groups working on a problem-solving task which distinctly followed this predicted structure, performed well. Talland (1955) did not confirm this in therapy groups, but their tasks have quite different requirements to the problem-solving tasks used in Bales' studies.

Thus, while there is some support for the utility of Bale's three-phase model the phases are rather general descriptions of group processes for the broad class of problem-solving tasks and do not further specify task-specific requirements. Nevertheless, they certainly do represent a major breakthrough for task-related thinking in small group research.

---

[1] It should be noted that Bales terminology differs from that used here. By "evaluation", Bales refers to the evaluation of plans which we—in accordance with many others—simply call planning. What he calls, "control", however, we refer to as, "evaluation" because here the outcome of an action is being evaluated with respect to the goal (the standard) adopted.

General "Logical Sequences"

For certain tasks, there seem to be clear steps to be taken, as well as a logical *sequence* of these steps. The general hypothesis of many studies is that groups that follow sequential task-requirements better show higher performance. These approaches are similar to the "phases" model in that they stay on a rather general level, referring to the task as a whole, not to its specific elements in terms of subtasks. They also resemble the phases model in that they postulate a rather strict (albeit very general) linear sequence which has to be followed, with each step occurring once. A final similarity is that these models also refer to the class of problem-solving tasks. The main difference to the proposed "phases" is that these models do not necessarily make assumptions about the distribution over time. All that is required is that the steps are there and in the right order.

The various models differ, ranging from five steps (Dewey, 1933) to the proposition of two major processes, e.g. developing a problem space and searching for possible solutions (Newell & Simon, 1972). Research on these models tends to follow one of two lines: one is to compare different prescribed formats, and the other is to examine whether groups without a preassigned format spontaneously follow the proposed sequential requirements. In general, findings support such models in a "weak" form. Thus, different assigned formats (e.g. a different number of steps or different sequences) (Brilhart & Jochem, 1964; Erffmeyer & Lane, 1984; Eils & John, 1980) do not necessarily lead to differences in performance. This does not mean, however, that format does not matter. Rather, there are various but not unlimited sequences that are appropriate for the task at hand. Studies which do not use preassigned formats show that groups in general do not follow the *sequential pattern* of problem-solving steps proposed by the models (Poole, 1983; Poole & Roth, 1989). Also, no particular sequential pattern has been found to be related to performance (Hirokawa 1983, 1985, 1988, 1990). However, while sequence did not prove to be especially important, groups that failed to perform a necessary step altogether did show lower performance. The one finding that seems to emerge is that groups which show more orientation and problem definition activities in the beginning show higher performance, compared to groups that immediately start generating solutions—a phenomenon that is often found for individuals as well as for groups (Hoffman & Maier, 1967; Janis & Mann, 1977).

It seems that for problem-solving tasks, groups have to work through the different steps of problem-solving, although there are degrees of freedom in terms of the sequential pattern to follow. Hirokawa (1990) and Poole & Roth (1980) therefore propose a task-contingency model of problem-solving steps in contrast to a "one best way of step sequences". In this model, the main problem-solving steps have to be present for high performance, but a strong sequential requirement is not proposed. It seems from this research that proposed sequential requirements for problem-solving tasks are not without merit but are too rigorous for the problems they describe.

However, the absence of co-variation of more specific stages of problem-solving with performance could also be attributed to differences in dynamic task requirements, as proposed by Wood (1986) and examined in groups, for example, by Badke-Schaub (1993). If a task has high dynamic properties, that is if the group works in a changing and dynamic environment, some of the problem-solving steps need to be repeated during the course of action in order to fulfil the dynamic requirements of the task. Thus, decisions already taken may be reconsidered in light of "new evidence" such as changing conditions or incompatibility with decisions taken later. Mintzberg, Raisinghani & Theoret (1976) studied decision-making processes in organizations and found that organizations recycle steps in problem-solving and decision-making, thus satisfying dynamic task or environmental demands. In a similar vein, Tschan (1990) found that decisions already taken were reconsidered repeatedly. Some of these reconsiderations were provoked by new partners in the environment of the organization, others followed changes in personnel within the organization, while still others were triggered by social conflicts within the organization.

In sum, it seems that a sequential model of problem-solving can be upheld only a molar level of abstraction. Groups are likely to perform better if they engage in diagnosis or orientation activities early in the process (Landsberger, 1955; Hirokawa, 1990) than if they immediately jump into solution generation, and certain steps do have to be gone through if the group is to be successful. Apart from these rather general requirements, however, there seem to be many different strategies that can be followed successfully.

That it seems to be more difficult to specify sequential task-requirements than many of these models plausibly suggest may be related to the fact that the tasks being studied all can be solved verbally. In this case, steps that are not successful can quite easily be reversed. This is, of course, quite different when we are dealing with tasks where physical changes are involved. In these cases, reversibility is often quite limited. It may well be that tasks involving physical activities are more affected by sequential stages of task performance than those involving verbal activities.

Differential Importance of Specific Steps

Models which emphasize the necessity of certain steps start with the task and what is logically required in order to fulfil it. Beyond the logical requirement, however, certain steps may be more important, not because there is a stronger necessity for them but because there is a stronger tendency for groups (and individuals) to neglect them. Since it is a frequently observed phenomenon that people come up with solutions before they have thoroughly understood the problem and planned their steps, preparatory steps of task fulfilment are likely candidates for aspects that should be emphasized. In line with this, it has been often assumed that groups perform better to the extent that they plan extensively. While this has, indeed, been found, it does not seem to be true under all circumstances but depends on task complexity. Hackman, Brousseau & Weiss (1976) and Larson & Schaumann (1993) showed that more planning enhanced group performance only for tasks that are complex enough to require planning, whereas planning inhibited performance or was of no influence on performance for very simple tasks. The same relationship seems to hold for individuals as well (Earley & Perry, 1987).

While the mere fact of planning seems to influence performance in complex tasks, one would also expect the *quality* of planning to be important. Weingart (1992) assessed the quality of planning processes in groups that assembled structures. She found that planning quality varied with task demands and goal-setting, but there was no relationship between high quality planning and performance. In contrast, Smith, Locke & Barry (1990) did find time spent in *high quality* planning to be positively related to performance. Again, task complexity seemed to be responsible for this finding. The task used by Weingart did not require high quality planning at group level, whereas Smith et al. worked with an organizational simulation involving a complex task.

We have mentioned that research on "logical sequences" has established a trend that early engagement in orientation and problem definition is helpful. Findings from studies that examine planning are consistent with this but they reveal an important prerequisite: the task has to be complex enough to require extended preparatory activities.

Cycles of Information Processing Related to Specific Goals at Various Levels

The approaches presented so far tend to deal with the task *in toto*, and thus in a very global way. However, the processes involved—orientating, adopting goals, developing plans, executing and evaluating behaviour—may refer to acts or sub-acts at very different hierarchical levels. Preparing a meal involves high-level ("strategic") aspects such as deciding about serving meat, fish, a vegetarian meal, etc. but also low-level aspects such as deciding how small the onions should be cut, cutting them and evaluating the result. Planning each little step in advance would be quite uneconomical and lead to very rigid and inflexible plans, so action theorists emphasize that the importance of breaking down tasks into sub-tasks and those into sub-sub tasks etc. *as they are dealt with* (von Cranach et al., 1982; Volpert, 1987). It follows that orderly sequences of orientating/planning, executing and evaluating can be expected to occur (if they occur at all) mainly with regard to the specific (sub-)task at hand. In contrast to a phase model, which postulates that "orientation" is something that only happens in the beginning, this reasoning would lead to quite a different expectation. Many cycles of preparation (i.e. orientating and planning), execution and evaluation should be expected, each being related to a sub-goal.

This does not necessarily contradict the expectation that there should be more orientation/planning in the beginning, and more evaluation towards the end of task completion (provided, of course, that the task has a minimum amount of complexity). Some basic orientation about the task as a whole may be necessary in the beginning, and some strategic decisions (fish or meat?) have to be taken early. Also, many sub-tasks have to evaluated not only with regard to whether they are completed correctly (did we boil as many potatoes as we had planned?) but also with regard to whether they do, indeed, fulfil the function they have for the task as a whole (did we calculate enough potatoes per person?), and these latter aspects often can only be judged towards the end (there may be too few potatoes but since there are so many vegetables this does not matter too much). Therefore, it still makes sense to expect more orientating/planning in the beginning and more evaluation towards the end of the task as a whole. However—and this is the difference from general phase or sequence models—these would be expected to relate to high-level goals, whereas many little cycles of orientating/planning, execution and evaluation would be expected to occur with regard to lower level goals throughout the process.

Thus, cycles of preparatory and evaluative steps are related to task requirements in a more specific way. Rather than considering only the task as a whole and its global characteristics (e.g. complexity), it is postulated that such cycles should be compatible with the hierarchical structure of the task and therefore have to be investigated with regard to specific goals or sub-goals.

Tschan (1995) has done this type of analysis using a task that required building a roller-coaster type construction out of plastic pieces. The task had a strong manual component involving low-level goals. For these, orientation and planning may involve considering what parts can be stuck together to make a good support, and evaluation would imply checking if the support is high enough, stable enough, etc. On the other hand, the task also had strategic requirements such as deciding on the general shape of the structure, building a loop (which is difficult to build but yields points in the experiment) vs. having a slow and gradual decline (which is easier to build but does not earn as many points). The tasks were broken down hierarchically, leading to sub-goals that had to be fulfilled at various levels of the goal hierarchy. Analysing communication segments (segments of related communication units as defined by Futoran, Kelly & McGrath, 1989), Tschan defined an "ideal" communication cycle as consisting of a preparatory and evaluative component within one segment, which are related to the same (sub-)goal. She hypothesized that the proportion of ideal cycles would be positively correlated with performance. This hypothesis was confirmed with triads working on the problem (Tschan, 1995). It has also been replicated for dyads (Jaeggi, 1994). This indicates that some of the difficulties of empirically establishing general phases may be due to their general nature, whereas a certain regularity of preparatory and evaluative information processing is useful if these are related to more specific task requirements.

The approach, presented earlier, for describing tasks in terms of hierarchical structure, seems to be a promising way for analysing these specific requirements. One might conclude that it is the combination of sequential and hierarchical aspects that made this possible, or, to put is another way, that sequential requirements can be understood only with reference to hierarchical requirements.

GROUP STRUCTURE AND TASK DEMANDS

Group Size

There is a large body of literature assessing the relationship between different aspects of group structure and performance. Group size is one of the most obvious of those factors. While there may be an upper limit for effective group functioning regardless of the specific tasks at hand, the task again plays an important role. If, for instance, a task has a single solution that is obvious as soon as it is communicated, larger groups tend to perform better, due to the simple fact that the probability is enhanced that there is at least one group member who knows the answer. On conjunctive tasks where performance depends on the weakest member, large groups should perform worse. However, Frank & Anderson (1971) found that for conjunctive tasks, performance remains stable in groups ranging from three to eight members. Bray, Kerr & Atkin (1978) proposed the concept of "functional group size" to explain these results. They argued that groups regulate their group size by adjusting their participation patterns. If a group has too many members for the task at hand, the number of non-participative members increases and the active members form a smaller subgroup which largely takes over the functions of the group. Group size therefore needs to be assessed also by means of active, not just present, members (Littlepage, 1991). Manning theories state that a given task requires a given number of group members to work on it so that, for a given task, groups can be overstaffed or understaffed. Too few as well as too many group members are found to impair performance (Perkins, 1982). Group members in overstaffed groups feel less involved in the group and the task (Wicker et al., 1976), so the likelihood of processes like social loafing is enhanced.

Role Structure

Compared to individuals, groups and teams have the advantage of being able to divide the work, and to combine specialized individual efforts. Many groups have a pre-assigned role structure and, where this is not the case, such a structure tends to develop quite quickly (Katz & Kahn, 1978). For many, the development of such a structure is regarded as a defining element of groups (cf. Brown, 1988).

Roles, too, should be analysed with regard to their functionality for the tasks a group has to carry out. von Cranach, Ochsenbein & Vallach (1986) emphasize that for formalized tasks, the task structure tends to be imposed on the group and determines the role structure to a very large extent. They illustrate this with the example of a sailing crew. In sailing, the skipper as the highest-ranking member sets the main goals (what course the boat has to take, change of direction). The helmsman, next in the hierarchy, coordinates the action of a turn (a sub-goal of changing direction) and gives the specific commands (e.g. "ship ready for turn"). The sailors carry out the concrete steps of the commands. In this example, the task is "mirrored" in the formal role structure.

Highly formalized roles may, however, become dysfunctional if they are not adapted to a given task. Lanzetta & Roby (1956) imposed structures on groups that made it more or less difficult to exchange information between group members. When confronted with a task which is high in information demands, all groups have a higher rate of errors than usual, but this effect is much stronger for groups whose structure is unfavourable for information exchange. This example highlights the problem that perfect adaptation to a certain task or class of tasks may have "costs" in terms of flexibility, at least if the structure becomes rigid. The development of "informal" group structures may counter these rigid formal structures and thus be regarded as a means to adapt better to task demands than the formal group structure allows.

All through this chapter we have argued that it is not enough to analyse tasks according to their general structure but that task requirements should be analysed in a rather specific way. A recent study from our laboratory (Jaeggi, 1994; cf. Tschan, Jaeggi & von Cranach, 1994) illustrates this point. One member of each dyad that was to perform the "roller-coaster assembly-task" (Tschan, 1995) was trained in how to use the various pieces that were provided. Thus, one member of each dyad might be considered an "expert", and this should predispose him/her for a leading role. Note, however, that the training referred to the functions of the various pieces, that is, it concentrated on low-level task requirements but did not involve training in the more strategic aspects, e.g. the optimal shape of the structure as a whole. It turned out that the dyads where one member had been trained performed worse than those without any training. In the training conditions, it was quite obvious that the "experts" extended their "expertise" to the task as a whole and assumed a leading role that was not confined to their actual area of expertise. It is tempting to speculate that people in leading roles easily get tempted to "stretch their role" and extend it to areas where they are not experts. Certainly everyday experience would support this speculation, but further research is needed.

Once established, group structures tend to remain relatively stable across situations. The advantage is obvious: the group does not have to constantly renegotiate its division of labour, roles are clear, power-struggles may be reduced—in other words, process losses are minimized. As mentioned above, however, the disadvantage of established group structures increases with the likelihood of new and unfamiliar tasks, the demands of which do not correspond to the structure of the group (Gersick & Hackman, 1990). Thus, if standing cockpit crews were given a problem-solving task which bore no relationship to their usual tasks of flying, failure to accept the correct answer was more likely if the correct answer was given by the lowest-ranking member. This effect was found to a lesser degree if the crews were new (Torrance, 1954b). Experienced groups therefore seem to establish permanent structures that are more likely to be projected on a new task. If task and group structure are not compatible, as in Torrance's research, performance is impaired.

Again, of course, such an effect is not likely to last very long but may be countered by informal processes as the group gains experience with new and changing task conditions. This is exemplified by research on cockpit crews. It is well known that status differences between pilot and co-pilot can be quite dysfunctional. Co-pilots tend to hold back information; pilots tend to ignore warnings of co-pilots (Retzlaff & Gibertini, 1987). Research by Kanki & Foushee (1989) has shown such role differences to be less prominent and dysfunctional for crews that had previously flown together than for newly composed crews. Thus, task-related adaptation processes in groups that stay together for a longer period of time than the usual laboratory groups should be kept in mind and deserve more attention in research.

CONCLUSIONS

Tasks have a major impact on group processes and performance. Most researchers would agree with this statement, yet many studies in small group research do not go beyond very global analyses of the tasks involved, describing them in very general terms rather than analysing task demands in detail. As Ilgen et al. (1993) remark, tasks have been included in much of small group and team research only as a means of standardizing situations but have received too little attention in their own right. We have tried to show how pervasive the influence of task characteristics can be. Depending on these characteristics, it can be easy or difficult to establish a common representation of the task, the range of behaviours may be more or less limited, there may be more or less stringent demands on planning, on keeping to a given sequence, on flexibly adjusting the size of the "functional group", etc. We have proposed that a generic approach of analysing tasks in terms of their sequential and hierarchical components, as proposed by action regulation theories, can be fruitful for getting a clearer picture of the specific task demands that have to be met, the most convincing example of this usefulness being that cycles of preparatory and evaluative communication can be shown to enhance performance when analysed with regard to specific sub-goals, while they have been quite difficult to establish with regard to the task as a whole.

We believe that analysing tasks in this way can be very helpful in determining what structure(s) might be optimal for what kind of tasks, in devising training, in analysing failures, etc. Basically, we have emphasized: (a) that the nature of tasks is important for understanding group performance; (b) that tasks should be analysed not only in general terms but with regard to their requirements *in detail*;

and (c) that action regulation approaches can be useful in this. Of course, new developments may lead to better and more refined methods than this approach can offer so far and, therefore, our third point may be true for quite a limited time only. We are firmly convinced, however, that the first two points should be on the agenda for group research for quite some time.

ACKNOWLEDGEMENTS

We thank Peter Beck, Marianne Gertsch, Heiner Dunckel, and especially Norbert Semmer for helpful comments on earlier drafts of this paper.

LITERATURE

Badke-Schaub, P. (1993). *Gruppen und komplexe Probleme. Strategien von Kleingruppen bei der Bearbeitung einer simulierten AIDS-Ausbreitung.* Frankfurt a.M.: Lang.
Bales, R.F. & Strodtbeck, F.L. (1951). Phases in group problem-solving. *The Journal of Abnormal and Social Psychology,* **46,** 485–495.
Bales, R.F. (1950). *Interaction Process Analysis. A method for the study of small groups.* Cambridge, MA: Addison-Wesley.
Bandura, A. (1989). Self-Regulation of motivation and action through internal standards and goal systems. In L.A. Pervin (ed.), *Goal Concepts in Personality and Social Psychology.* Hillsdale, NJ: Erlbaum.
Beckmann, J. & Gollwitzer, P.M. (1987). Deliberative versus implemental states of mind: the issue of impartiality in predecisional and postdecisional information processing. *Social Cognition* (Special issue—Cognition and Action) **5,** 259–279.
Bray, R.M., Kerr, N.L. & Atkin, R.S. (1978). Effects of group size, problem difficulty, and sex on group performance and member reactions. *Journal of Personality and Social Psychology,* **36,** 1224–1240.
Brilhart, J.K. & Jochem, L.M. (1964). Effects of different patterns on outcomes of problem-solving discussion. *Journal of Applied Psychology,* **48,** 175–179.
Brown, R. (1988). *Group processes, Dynamics Within and Between Groups.* Oxford: Blackwell.
Cranach, M. von. (in press). Towards a theory of the acting group. To appear in E. Witte & J.H. Davis (eds), *Understanding Group Behavior: Small Group Processes and Interpersonal Relations.* Hillsdale, NJ: Erlbaum.
Dewey, J. (1933). *How We Think.* Boston: D.C. Heath.
Dörner, D. (1989). *Die Logik des Misslingens. Strategisches Denken in komplexen Situationen.* Hamburg: Rowohlt.
Earley, P.C. & Perry, B.C. (1987). Work plan availability and performance: an assessment of task strategy priming on subsequent task completion. *Organizational Behavior and Human Decision Processes,* **39,** 279–302.
Eils, L.C. & John, R.S. (1980). A criterion validation of multiattribute utility analysis and group communication strategy. *Organizational Behavior and Human Decision Processes,* **25,** 268–288.
Erffmeyer, R.C. & Lane, I.M. (1984). Quality and acceptance of an evaluative task: the effects of four group decision-making formats. *Group and Organization Studies,* **9,** 509–529.
Festinger, L., Rieder, H.W. & Schachter, S. (1956). *When Prophecy Fails. A Social and Psychological Study of a Modern Group that Predicted the Destruction of the World.* New York: Harper & Row.

Firestien, R.L. (1990). Effects of creative problem solving training on communication behaviors in small groups. *Small Group Research*, **21**(4), 507–521.
Foushee, M.C. (1984). Dyads and triads at 35000 feet. Factors affecting group process and aircrew performance. *American Psychologist*, **39**, 885–893.
Frank, F. & Anderson, L.R. (1971). Effects of task and group size upon group productivity and member satisfaction. *Sociometry*, **34**, 135–149.
Frese, M. & Zapf, D. (1994). Action as the core of work psychology: a German approach. In H.C. Triandis, M.D. Dunnette & L.M. Hough (eds), *Handbood of Industrial and Organization Psychology*, Vol. 4, 2nd Edn. Palo Alto: CA Consulting Psychologists Press, pp. 271–340.
Futoran, G.C., Kelly, J.R. & McGrath, J.E. (1989). TEMPO: a time-based system for analysis or group interaction processes. *Basic and Applied Social Psychology*, **10**, 211–232.
Ganster, D.C., Williams, S. & Poppler, P. (1991). Does training in problem solving improve the quality of group decisions? *Journal of Applied Psychology*, **76**(3), 479–483.
Gersick, C.J. & Hackman, J.R. (1990). Habitual routines in task-performing groups. *Organizational Behavior and Human Decision Processes*, **47**, 65–97.
Gersick, C.J.G. (1989). Marking time: predictable transitions in task groups. *Academy of Management Journal*, **32**, 274–309.
Goodman, P. (1990). Impact of task and technology on group performance. In P. Goodman (ed.), *Designing Effective Work Groups*. San Francisco, CA: Jossey-Bass, pp. 120–167.
Guzzo, R.A. & Shea, G.P. (1992). Group performance and intergroup relations in organizations. In M.D. Dunette & L.M. Hough (eds), *Handbook of Industrial and Organization Psychology*, Vol. 3. Palo Alto, CA: Consulting Psychologists Press, pp. 269–313.
Hacker, K.I., Freedman, E.G. & Gormann, M.W. (1990). The emergence of task representation in small-group simulations of scientific reasoning. *Journal of Social Behavior and Personality*, **5**, 175–186.
Hacker, W. & Clauss, A. (1976). Kognitive Operationen, inneres Modell und Leistung bei Montagetätigkeiten. In W. Hacker (ed.), *Psychische Regulation von Arbeitstätigkeiten*. Berlin: VEB, pp. 88–102.
Hacker, W. & Skell, W. (1993). *Lernen in der Arbeit*. Berlin: Bundesinsitut für Berufsbildung.
Hacker, W. (1983). Ziele—eine vergessene psychologische Schluesselvariable? Zur antriebsregulatorischen Potenz von Taetigkeitsinhalten. *Psychologie für die Praxis*, **2**, 5–26.
Hacker, W. (1985). Activity: a fruitful concept in industrial Psychology. In M. Frese & J. Sabini (eds), *Goal Directed Behavior*. Hillsdale, NJ: Erlbaum, pp. 262–285.
Hacker, W. (1986). *Arbeitspsychologie, Psychische Regualtion von Arbeitstaetigkeiten*. Berlin (DDR): Deutscher Verlag der Wissenschaften.
Hackman, J.R. & Oldham, G.R. (1980). *Work Redesign*. Reading, MA: Addison-Wesley.
Hackman, J.R. & Vidmar, N. (1970). Effects of size and task type on group performance and member reactions. *Sociometry*, **33**, 37–54.
Hackman, J.R. (1968). Effects of task characteristics on group products. *Journal of Experimental Social Psychology*, **4**, 162–187.
Hackman, J.R. (ed.) (1990a). *Groups That Work (and Those That Don't). Creating Conditions for Effective Teawork*. San Francisco: Jossey Bass.
Hackman, J.R. (1990b). Creating more effective work groups in organizations. In J.R. Hackman (ed.), *Groups That Work (and Those That Don't). Creating Conditions for Effective Teamwork*. San Francisco, CA: Jossey-Bass, pp. 479–504.
Hackman, J.R., Jones, L.E. & McGrath, J.E. (1967). A set of dimensions for describing the general properties of group-generated written passages. *Psychological Bulletin*, **67**, 379–390.
Hackman, R.J. & Morris, C.G. (1975). Group tasks, group interaction process, and group performance effectiveness: a review and proposed integration. In: L. Berkowitz (ed.),

Advances in Experimantal Social Psychology, Vol. 8. New York: Academic Press, pp. 47-97.
Hackman, R.J., Brousseau, K.R. & Weiss, J.A. (1976). The interaction of task design and group performance strategies in determining group effectiveness. *Organizational Behavior and Human Performance*, **16**, 350-365.
Hirokawa, R.Y. (1983). Group communication and problem-solving effectiveness: an investigation of group phases. *Human Communication Resarch*, **9**, 291-305.
Hirokawa, R.Y. (1985). Discussion procedures and decision-making performance. A test of a functional perspective. *Human Communication Research*, **12**, 203-224.
Hirokawa, R.Y. (1988). Group communication and decision-making performance. A continued test of the functional perspective. *Human Communication Research*, **14**, 487-515.
Hirokawa, R.Y. (1990). The role of communication in group decision-making efficacy: a task-contingency perspective. *Small Group Research*, **21**, 190-204.
Hoffman, L.R. & Maier, N.R.F. (1967). Valence in the adoption of solutions by problem-solving groups: II Quality and acceptance as goals of leaders and members. *Journal of Personality and Social Psychology*, **6**, 175-182.
Ilgen, D.R., Major, D.A., Hollenbeck, J.R. & Sego, D.J. (1993). Team research in the 1990s. In M.M. Chemers & R. Ayman (eds), *Leadership Theory and Research. Perspectives and Directions*. San Diego: Academic Press, pp. 245-270.
Jaeggi, C. (1994). Rollen im dvadischen Handeln (roles in dyadic actions). Unpublished master's thesis. University of Bern: Psychologisches Institut.
Janis, I.L. (1972). *Victims of Groupthink*. Boston: Houghton Mifflin.
Janis, I.L. & Mann, L. (1977). *Decison Making*. New York: Free Press.
Kabanoff, B. & O'Brien, G.E. (1979). The effects of task type and cooperation upon group products and performance. *Organizational Behavior and Human Performance*, **23**, 163-181.
Kanki, B.G. & Foushee, H.C. (1989). Communication as group process mediator of aircrew performance. *Aviation, Space and Environmental Medicine*, **4**, 402-410.
Katz, D. & Kahn, R.L. (1978). *The Social Psychology of Organizations*, 2nd Edn. New York: Wiley.
Kelly, J.R. & McGrath, J.E. (1985). Effects of time limits and task types on task performance and interaction of four-person groups. *Journal of Personality and Social Psychology*, **42**, 248-264.
Kelly, J.R., Futoran, G.C. & McGrath, J.E. (1990). Capacity and capability. Seven studies of entrainment of task performance rates. *Small Group Research*, **21**, 283-314.
Kent, R.N. & McGrath, J.E. (1969). Task and group characteristics as factors influencing group performance. *Journal of Experimental Social Psychology*, **5**, 429-440.
Landsberger, H.A. (1955). Interaction process analysis of the mediation of labor-management disputes. *Journal of Abnormal and Social Psychology*, **51**, 552-228.
Lanzetta, J.T. & Roby, T.B. (1956). Effects of work-group structure and certain task variables on group performance. *Journal of Abnormal and Social Psychology*, **53**, 307-314.
Lanzetta, J.T. & Roby, T.B. (1960). The relationship between certain group process variables and group problem solving efficiency. *The Journal of Social Psychology*, **52**, 135-148.
Larson, J.R. & Christensen, C. (1993). Group as problem-solving units: towards a new meaning of social cognition. *British Journal of Social Psychology*, **32**, 5-30.
Larson, J.R. & Schaumann, L.J. (1993). Group goals, group coordination, and group member motivation. *Human Performance*, **6**, 49-69.
Liebermann, S. (1956). The effects of changes in role on the attitudes of role occupants. *Human Relations*, **9**, 383-402.
Littlepage, G.E. (1991). Effects of group size and task characteristics on group performance: a test of Steiner's model. *Personalitiy and Social Psychology Bulletin*, **17**, 449-456.

Locke, E.A. & Latham, G.P. (1990). *A Theory of Goal Setting and Task Performance*. Englewood Cliffs, NJ: Prentice-Hall.

Locke, E.A., Shaw, K.N., Sarri, L.M. & Latham, G.P. (1981). Goal setting and task performance: 1969–1980. *Psychological Bulletin*, **90**, 125–152.

Lord, R.G. (1976). Group performance as a function of leadership behavior and task structure: toward an explanatory theory. *organizational Behavior and Human Performance*, **17**, 76–96.

McGrath, J.E. (1984). *Groups, Interaction and Performance*. Englewood Cliffs, NJ: Prentice-Hall.

Meissner, M. (1976). The language of work. In R. Dubin (ed.), *Handbook of Work, Organization, and Society*. Chicago: Rand McNally, pp. 205–280.

Miller, G.A., Galanter, E. & Pribram, K.H. (1960). *Plans and the Structure of Behavior*, New York: Holt.

Mintzberg, H., Raisinghani, D. & Theoret, A. (1976). The structure of "unstructured" decision processes. *Administrative Science Quarterly*, **21**, 246–275.

Mischel, W. (1977). The interaction of person and situation. In D. Magnusson & N.S. Endler (eds), *Personality at the Crossroads*. Hillsdale NJ: Lawrence Erlbaum, pp. 333–352.

Moreland, R.L. & Levine, J.M. (1992). Problem identification by groups. In S. Worchel, W. Wood & J.A. Simpson (eds), *Group Process and Productivity*. Newbury Park: Sage, pp. 17–47.

Morris, C.G. (1966). Task effects on group interaction. *Journal of Personality and Social Psychology*, **4**, 545–554.

Mueller, G.F. (1992). Psychological and communicational influences on coordination effectiveness. *Basic and Applied Social Psychology*, **13**(3), 337–350.

Naylor, J.C., Pritchard, R.D. & Ilgen, D.R. (1980). *A Theory of Behavior in Organizations*. New York: Academic Press.

Newell, A. & Simon, H-A. (1972). *Human Problem Solving*. Englewood Cliffs NJ: Prentice-Hall.

Oesterreich, R. (1981). *Handlungsregulation und Kontrolle (Action Regulation and Control)*. München: Urban & Schwarzenberg.

Perkins, D.v. (1982). Individual differences in the performance of a behavior setting: an experimental evaluation of Barker's manning theory. *American Journal of Community Psychology*, **10**, 617–634.

Poole, M.S. (1983). Decision development in small groups II: a study of multiple sequences in decision making. *Communication Monographs*, **50**, 206–232.

Poole, M.S. & Roth, J. (1989). Decision development in small groups V. Test of a contingency model. *Human Communication Research*, **15**, 549–589.

Pritchard, R.D., Jones, S.D., Roth, Ph.L., Stuebing, K.K. & Ekeberg, S.E. (1989). The evaluation of an integrated approach to measuring organizational productivity. *Personnel Psychology*, **42**, 69–115.

Rasmussen, J. (1987). Cognitive control and human error mechanisms. In J. Rasmussen, K. Duncan & J. Leplat (eds), *New Technology and Human Error*. Chichalter: Wiley, pp. 53–61.

Retzlaff, R.D. & Gibertini, M. (1987). Air Force pilot personality: Hard data on the "right stuff". *Multivariate Behavioral Research*, **22**, 383–399.

Schneider, W. & Shiffrin, R.M. (1977). Controlled and automatic human information processing. I. Detection, search, and attention. *Psychological Revies*, **84**, 1–66.

Semmer, N. & Frese, M. (1985). Action theory in clinical psychology. In M. Frese & J. Sabini (eds), *Goal Directed Behavior*. Hillsdale, NJ: Erlbaum, pp. 296–310.

Semmer, N. (1984). *Stressbezogene Tätigkeitsanalyse. Psychologische Untersuchungen zur Analyse von Stress am Arbeitsplatz*. Weinheim and Basel: Beltz.

Shaw, M.E. (1976). *Group Dynamics. The Psychology of Small Group Behavior*. New York: McGraw-Hill.

Shiffrin, R.M. & Schneider, W. (1977). Controlled and automatic human information processing. II. Perceptual learning, automatic attending and a general theory. *Psychological Review*, **84**, 127–190.

Smith, K.G. Locke, E.A. & Barry, D. (1990). Goal setting, planning, and organizational performance: an experimental stimulation. *Organizational Behavior and Human Decision Processes*, **46**, 118–134.

Steiner, I.D. (1972). *Group Processes and Productivity*. New York: Academic Press.

Tajfel, H. & Turner, J.C. (1979). An integrative theory of intergroup conflict. In W.G. Austin & S. Worchel (eds), *The Social Psychology Intergroup Relations*. Monterey, CA: Brooks.

Talland, G.A. (1955). Task and interaction process: some characteristics of therapeutic group discussion. *Journal of Abnormal and Social Psychology*, **50**, 105–109.

Thommen, B., Amman, R. & von Cranach, M. (1988). *Handlungsorganisation durch soziale Repraesentation*. Bern: Huber.

Torrance, E.P. (1954a). The benhavior of small groups under the stress conditions of "survival". *American Sociological Review*, **19**, 751–755.

Torrance, E.P. (1954b). Some consequences of power differences on decision making in permanent and temporary three-man groups. *Research Studies, State College of Washington*, **22**, 130–140.

Tschan, F. (1990). Organisationen als sich zielgerichtet verhaltende Systeme. Entwicklung eines theoriegeleiteten Beschreibungssystems im Rahmen einer Fallstudie. Unpublished dissertation, University of Bern: Psychologisches Institut.

Tschan, F. (1995, in press). Communication enhances small group performance if it conforms to task requirements. The concept of "ideal communication cycles". *Basic and Applied Social Psychology*, **17**.

Tschan, F., Jaeggi, C. & von Cranach, M. (1994). Kommunikationszyklen und Leistung in Kleingruppen. Paper presented at the 39th Kongress der Deutschen Gesellschaft für Psychologie, 25–29 September, Hamburg.

Tschan, F. & von Cranach, M. (1990). Zielgerichtetes Verhalten sozialer Systeme als mehrstufiger Prozess. In R. Fisch & M. Boos (eds), *Vom Umgang mit Komplexität in Organisationen. Konzepte—Fallbeispiele-Strategien*. Konstanz: Universitätsverlag.

Volpert, W. (1984). *Handlungsstrukturanalyse als Beitrag zur Qualifikationsforschung*. Kön: Pahl Rugenstein.

Volpert, W. (1987). Psychische Regulation von Arbeitstätigkeiten. In U. Kleinbeck & J. Rutenfranz (eds), *Arbeitspsychologie*. (Enzyklopädie der Psychologie, Themenbereich D, Serie II, Band 1, pp. 1–42). Göttingen: Hogrefe.

von Cranach, M., Kalbermatten, U., Intermühle, K. & Gugler, B. (1982). *Goal-directed Action*. London: Academic Press.

von Cranach, M., Ochsenbein, G. & Valach, L. (1986). The group as a self-active system: outline of a theory of group action. *European Journal of Social Psychology*, **16**, 193–229.

von Cranach, M., Ochsenbein, G., Tschan, F. & Kohler, H. (1989). Untersuchungen zum Handeln sozialer Systeme, Bericht ueber ein Froschungsprogramm. *Schweizerische Zeitschrift für Psychologie*, **46**, 213–226.

Weingart, L. & Weldon, E. (1991). Processes that mediate the relationship between a group goal and group member performance. *Human Performance*, **4**, 33–54.

Weingart, L. (1992). Impact of group goals, task component complexity, effort, and planning on group performance. *Jopurnal of Applied Psychology*, **77**, 682–693.

Weldon, E., Jehn, K.A. & Pradhan, P. (1991). Processes that mediate the ralationship between a group goal and improved group perpormance. *Journal of Personality and Social Psychology*, **61**, 555–569.

Wicker, A.W., Kirmeyer, S.L., Hanson, L. & Alexander, D. (1976). Effects of manning levels on subjective experiences, performance, and verbal interaction in groups. *Organizational Behavior and Human Performance*, **17**, 251–274.

Williges, R.C., Johnston, W.A. & Briggs, G.E. (1966). Role of verbal communication in teamwork. *Journal of Applied Psychology*, **50**, 473–478.

Wilson, M. & Canter, D. (1993). Shared concepts in group decision making: a model for decisions based on qualitative data. *British Journal of Social Psychology*, **32**, 159–172.

Wood, R.E. (1986). Task complexity: definition of the construct. *Organizational Behavior and Human Decision Processes*, **37**, 60–82.

Section III

Group Processes

Chapter 6

Making Work Groups More Effective: the Value of Minority Dissent

Charlan Nemeth
and
Pamela Owens
University of California, Berkeley, USA

Abstract

Most treatises on the current business climate talk of "revolution" and, increasingly, stress the need for adaptation and innovation. As a result, a number of corporations have tried to instil a corporate culture that values innovation. This generally consists of expectations (norms) that are shared by the majority, by higher as well as lower status persons. While the value and the power of such norms are not at issue, the present article contends that such mechanisms actually constrain thought and may inadvertently produce conformist rather than innovative thought and may lead to poorer quality decision-making. Rather, we contend that innovation and high quality decision-making may be better served by exposure to minority views, by the harnessing of dissent and conflict. A number of studies, mostly experimental, permit us to argue that minority dissent stimulates: (a) the search for more information; (b) the consideration of the information from more perspectives; and (c) on balance, aids the quality of performance, decision-making and even creativity. Thus, we note and even emphasize the positive aspects of conflict and of exposure to minority views.

In most considerations of conflict or disagreement in working groups, the negative consequences are apparent. People dislike disagreement; it makes them uncomfortable (Nemeth & Staw, 1989). Conflict may cause people to decrease their own effort or participation, to feel less satisfaction with the group and to experience increased hostility between co-workers (see generally Levine & Moreland, 1990). To the extent that conflict also lowers cohesion (Jackson, 1992), it is also likely to lessen satisfaction with co-workers (Bass & Barrett, 1981) and lessen the likelihood of remaining in the group (Levine & Moreland, 1990).

But there is another side to the issue of conflict and disagreement. One possibility is that the opposing view, while promoting conflict, may be correct. As Oscar Wilde reminded us:

> We dislike arguments of any kind; they are always vulgar and often convincing.

Another possibility is that conflict and disagreement promote divergent thinking, a consideration of multiple viewpoints and, in the process, provide contributions to the quality of decision-making and performance.

In this chapter we will consider varying theories about how to improve organizational performance, decision-making and innovation. Recognizing the importance of "corporate culture" in achieving these aims, our position is that, while even the most enlightened set of norms, rules and procedures can achieve coordination, high morale and cohesion, they also tend to produce uniformity. They tend not to promote flexibility and innovation. By contrast, there is a powerful and often untapped resource that has repeatedly been found to stimulate better decision-making, better performance and more creativity. That resource is dissent and, properly harnessed, it can be invaluable to an organization.

CORPORATE CULTURE

In most recent treatises on the business world, particularly in the USA, there is talk of "revolution", not just one but several. Stewart (1993) suggests four: "globalization of markets, the spread of information technology and computer networks, the dismantling of hierarchy, (and) . . . an information age economy". One consequence of these particular revolutions is that knowledge and communication are now the sources of wealth, rather than natural resources and physical labor. Another is that businesses need "quick responses to changing circumstances" (Stewart, 1993, p. 72). More than ever before, the emphasis is on adaptation and innovation—and the utilization of human resources. The model is one of a "more flexible organization adaptable to change, with relatively few levels of formal hierarchy and loose boundaries among functions and units, sensitive and responsive to the environment". (Kanter, Stein & Jick, 1992, p. 3).

For many observers and researchers of organizations, one of the keys to adaptation and especially innovation is "corporate culture". Schein (1989) refers to it as the *"real key* to creativity" (p. 73, our emphasis). Variously defined, corporate culture involves "the underlying assumptions about the goals of the organization and what has been learned through the company's successes and failures" (Schein, 1989, p. 73). O'Reilly (1989) likens it to the social psychological concept of norms, the "shared expectations" about what is appropriate and what is not.

Most researchers and many businesses have touted the power of such "corporate culture" and have credited it with the successes (or failures) of major business ventures. As illustrations, 3M's success in developing new products has long been credited to a corporate culture that favors innovation. Allen Jacobsen, the CEO at 3M, advises giving people "responsibility for their own destinies and encourage them to take risks" (Labich, 1988). The NUMMI plant at Fremont, CA, a joint venture between Toyota and GM, has double the productivity of any other GM plant. Its success is usually credited to a Japanese style of management—a "culture" where the assembly line workers "maintain their machines, ensure the quality of their work and improve the production process" (Kraar, 1989). Failures, too, are credited to the culture. Smith Kline's CEO, Henry Wendt, wanted to "create a new culture", implicating the company's prior success as part of the problem, one which led to complacency.

While these global visions coupled with shared expectations about goals, attitudes and behaviors are undoubtedly important, most researchers have also recognized that these expectations or norms need to be "shared" by people at *all* levels of the organization. Often, there is a discrepancy between the stated goals or "vision" of the company from the CEO and another, much more cynical version, of life at the mid- or lower-management levels. A speech about the value of dissent from the CEO may not be an expression of "shared expectations" at lower levels if every expression of dissent is punished. Thus, many researchers have argued that you need not only have shared expectations (i.e. consensus) but also careful monitoring and a consistent reinforcement of these expectations through rewards and punishments.

The Power of Norms

Social psychologists have long recognized the power of shared expectations for effecting certain behavioral outcomes. And, importantly, it appears that they are more potent than tangible rewards or punishments (see generally Asch, 1955; Allen, 1965; Aronson, 1995). Such norms can become so habitual, so recognizable, so familiar, that they are adhered to without question. As examples, when you go to the cinema, you go to the end of the line to buy your tickets; when in a crowded elevator, you avoid eye contact; when listening to a symphony, you do not clap between movements.

One of the powers of such "shared expectations" or norms is that they are not only expectations; they are demands. They not only dictate what is "appropriate" but what is even considered "true", "normal" or "healthy". Consider the implications of a stranger staring at you from a distance of 18 inches. He had better be your ophthamologist. Otherwise, is this "normal" or even "mentally healthy"?

As the preceding would suggest, one of the best ways to recognize that a norm exists is to violate that norm. In the USA, the appropriate distance for a stranger is approximately 4 feet. Thus, the stranger referenced above, by standing 18 inches away, is likely to see us recede, look away or show signs of discomfort, even anger (Altman & Vinsel, 1978). Similarly, if the norm is for the head seat to be reserved for the leader or a high status person, it would be inappropriate for a lower status person to take the head seat at a rectangular table; that person is likely to see frowns or indications of disapproval.

The Perils of Norms and of Majorities

Much as the above suggests, norms can be a powerful mechanism for achieving desired behaviors and rendering them uniform. Further, norms operate as a very effective control mechanism. Not only do people adhere to the norms but they enforce them. The person jumping the queue at a cinema may be subject to outbursts from people who are not only adhering to the norm by taking their turn but are also enforcing the norm.

Such enforcements have been found to lower the quality of decision-making. In his study of cabinet level decision-making, Janis (1982) reports that people enforced favored proposals, e.g. those wanted by the President, and specifically punished the expression of dissent or the offering of alternatives. One should "get behind the president". Not only did some members actively discourage dissent, others monitored themselves and avoided expressing their doubts or suggestions (see, generally, Janis, 1982).

Majorities pose a different kind of problem, precisely because people assume that truth lies in numbers. Further, people are motivated to assume that the majority is correct since this would warrant movement to the majority position (Asch, 1955; Deutsch & Gerard, 1955). They would prefer being a member of a majority than remaining a "deviate", that is, maintaining a minority position. They fear disapproval and rejection.

The problem is that such fear of rejection is not illusory. Deviates, i.e. those who maintain a minority position, have been found to be the target of communication aimed at changing their position and, if these attempts are unsuccessful, the deviate is rejected (Schachter, 1959).

As indicated earlier, this power of the majority to gain adoption of its position can have perils. The majority may be wrong, a situation depicted in the hundreds of studies on conformity where individuals were found to move to the majority's position even when it was in error (see generally Allen, 1965). Further, there is evidence that the majority exerts approximately equal influence whether it is right or wrong (Nemeth & Wachtler, 1983).

Similar findings come from research on status. Persons of higher status or credibility are more effective in gaining adoption of their position than are persons of lower status or lacking in credibility (Hovland & Weiss, 1951). And higher status does not carry with it a guarantee of correctness. Consider the work by Torrance (1954) on aircraft bomber crews in solving the horse trader problem. It is as follows:

A man buys a horse for $60, sells it for $70, buys it back again for $80 and sells it again for $90. How much profit did he make? (Maier & Salem, 1952).

Most people cannot solve this problem correctly. Three different answers tend to be given ($0, $10, $20). The answer is $20. One would expect that, if one member of a group knew the correct answer, the group would adopt that correct answer. Optimally, one would expect 100% of the groups to get the correct answer if one of the members of each group knew it. Torrance's research shows that it depends on *who* knows the correct answer. If it is the pilot (highest status), 96% of the group adopted the correct answer; if it was the tailgunner (lowest status), only 63% of the groups adopted it. In other words, adoption of the correct position was a direct function of the status of the person holding that position.

Separating the Tasks: When the Solution is Known

It is clear that norms, majorities and higher status people can all form a "corporate culture" supporting a given set of attitudes and behaviors. As findings from numerous studies attest, this can be a highly effective mechanism for gaining desired behavior. However, the question is whether or not that set of norms, that "corporate culture", is in fact the clearly correct prescription. If one is dealing with productivity, for example, and the task is quite simple or well learned, a norm or goal of high productivity could well be effective in gaining the desired behavior.

A number of theories and data underscore the effectiveness of goals. Group goals have been found to improve group performance (Yukl & Latham, 1976), especially when performance feedback is available (Zander, 1971). The theory of goal-setting further argues that specific goals are better than general goals and research has generally confirmed that setting goals leads to more effort, which improves performance (Hall & Hall, 1976; Hall & Foster, 1977). In general, the prescription is to have clear but difficult concrete goals with contingent rewards (see generally Zander, 1977). This may be one reason why 3M, rather than just valuing innovation in the abstract, decided that 25% of its annual sales should come from products developed within the past 5 years and why NUMMI, in wanting to break down status barriers, had management and workers wear similar uniforms.

Goals and norms appear to be powerful mechanisms for improving productivity, an outcome that Blake & Mouton (1981) regard as the most important concern in the industrial setting. Yet even they recognize that norms, with their ability to improve productivity and reduce absenteeism, also give rise to a strain to uniformity. And, as we will see, uniformity is what hampers the quality of decision-making and the finding of new solutions. It hinders the flexibility, adaptability to change and willingness to take risks that are the desired traits of many companies of the 1990s.

QUALITY OF DECISION-MAKING VS. CREATIVITY

As we try to understand how an enlightened culture can promote quality of decision-making and creativity, we need to distinguish between these laudable goals. Good decision-making involves an adequate survey of information without biased processing, a consideration of this information from multiple perspectives, an examination of the costs and risks of each alternative as well as monitoring and contingency plans (Janis, 1982). Creativity is more elusive, involving uniqueness or originality, but also providing solutions that are appropriate to the problem. It seems to require variability, even "blind" variability (Campbell, 1969), but it also includes "processes more complex and more mysteriously rational than this ordinary routine of variability will explain" (Royce, 1896).

One of the major problems with group decision making is that people "strain towards uniformity" (Janis, 1982). As we noted briefly in our discussion of conformity and norms, people want to agree. They assume that truth lies in numbers and, furthermore, they are motivated to agree with the majority. They fear the disapproval and possible rejection that emanates from maintaining a minority view (Asch, 1955; Deutsch & Gerard, 1955; Schachter, 1959). Even when a majority is not apparent, people search for agreement. In Janis' work on major cabinet-level policy decisions, the major culprit for the poor decision-making that led to fiascos, e.g. the Bay of Pigs, was this "groupthink," this strain to uniformity.

The decision to back the invasion of Cuba by a brigade of Cuban exiles was clearly a fiasco. The cabinet level members assumed that Castro's army was so weak, so low in morale and so under-equipped that such an invasion not only would be successful but that it would inspire an uprising by the Cuban people. On the contrary, this brigade was surrounded within hours and the USA was publicly embarrassed. Even the contingency plan to escape to the Escambray Mountains proved to be unfeasible. It required an escape route of hundreds of miles through treacherous swamp, a fact that could easily have been discerned by consulting an atlas.

Often, people assume that stupid decisions are made by stupid people. This was certainly not the case with this group. In fact, they could be considered the "best and the brightest". The problem was with the process. Consider the members. Among others, they included Dean Rusk, who was recruited from his position as head of the Rockefeller Foundation, Robert NcNamara, former president of Ford Motor, Co., leading intellectuals such as McGeorge Bundy and Arthur Schlesinger, Robert Kennedy, three Joint Chiefs of Staff, etc. Thus we can see that, even a decision to hire the brightest individuals, while it has merit, does not ensure that such individuals with make intelligent decisions, especially in groups. The problem appears to be this "strain to uniformity", a tendency that appears endemic to groups that are highly cohesive and have a strong directive leader (Janis, 1982; Tetlock et al., 1992).

The fact that people want to agree is not something that is easily changed. However, its deleterious consequences in terms of decision-making can be countered by the expression of dissent. In Janis' (1982) examples of cabinet level "fiascos", there is clear evidence that dissent was discouraged and even avoided by the dissenters themselves. Open straw votes were taken which raised the likelihood of conformity. Some individuals, e.g. Robert Kennedy, actively discouraged the expression of dissent, arguing that ". . . the President has made his mind up. Don't push it any further". Schlesinger (1972), who opposed the invasion, was quoted later:

> In the months after the Bay of Pigs I bitterly reproached myself for having kept so silent during those crucial discussions . . . though my feelings of guilt were tempered by the knowledge that a course of objection would have accomplished little save to gain me a name as a nuisance (Janis, 1982, p. 39).

Such active suppression of the expression of alternative views is one of the negative consequences of this strain to uniformity. As a result, researchers, e.g. Janis, have argued for mechanisms that increases the likelihood that dissent will be expressed. Some of those "antidotes" include the presence of a devil's advocate, the usage of outside experts, and a "second chance" meeting where members are encouraged to express residual doubts and rethink the entire issue (Janis, 1982, pp. 269–271).

Business organizations have attempted similar remedies. Cosier (1981), for example, reports on the effectiveness of devil's advocate and dialectic inquiry as techniques for formalizing dissent in decision-making. The dialectic inquiry method involves presenting a plan with its underlying assumptions and then subsequently presenting a counterplan based on different and often opposing assumptions. In the final stage, a debate ensues with the intent of gauging the reasonableness of the assumptions and recommendations in order to arrive at the best decision (Stone, Sivitanides & Magro, 1994).

The devil's advocate is similar in that the plan is presented along with its underlying assumptions. However, an individual is specifically charged with exposing the problems and the hidden or erroneous assumptions. Available evidence suggests that the devil's advocate leads to better decisions than dialectic inquiry or methods that exclude formalized dissent (Cosier, 1981).

Brainstorming is another technique whose aim is to increase the number of options that are expressed. In brainstorming, the individuals are instructed to generate as many ideas as possible, to build upon other's ideas whenever possible and to refrain from criticizing any other members's ideas (Osborn, 1957). The claim was that "the average person can think up twice as many ideas when working with a group than when working alone" (Osborn, 1957, p. 229).

Research shows that brainstorming groups are superior compared with other groups, i.e. those not given brainstorming instructions. However, the research is mixed. If the efforts of individuals working in isolation are pooled, they are superior in terms of producing more unique and high quality ideas relative to brainstorming groups (Dunnette, Campbell & Jaastad, 1963). However, brainstorming groups have been found to be superior to solitary individuals, although still not at the level of the combined abilities of the members (Taylor, Berry & Block, 1958). Further, there appears to be some value in this instructional method of brainstorming in that asking people to suspend judgment has been found to increase the number of alternatives generated, though not the quality (Levy, 1968; Manski & Davis, 1968).

The Positive Aspects of Conflict

As much of the preceding literature suggests, there is an increasing recognition that the expression of alternative views is an essential ingredient to good group decision-making. Such expressions of dissent clearly invoke conflict, a result that many researchers want to reduce or "resolve". Of interest is that, for years, the main journal for negotiation research was called the *Journal of Conflict Resolution*.

Other inquiries have recognized the value of conflict. Guetzkow & Gyr (1954), for example, recognize the potential value of conflict but make an important distinction between substantive conflict and affective conflict. The former is more intellectual in origin and is rooted in the substance of the task, whereas the latter, which is personal in origin, derives from the emotional aspects of the group's interpersonal relations. Guetzkow & Gyr's research found that successful conferences were marked by substantive conflict, whereas unsuccessful ones were marked by affective conflict.

Another area where the value of differing views and its attendant conflict is underscored is in the research on heterogeneity of groups. Demographic diversity, for example, has been found to increase conflict, reduce cohesion and complicate internal communications (Dougherty, 1987; Kiesler, 1978; Shaw, 1971; Pfeffer & O'Reilly, 1987) and yet there is a fairly strong relationship between various forms of heterogeneity and performance and quality of decision-making (Hoffman, 1959; Hoffman & Maier, 1961; May, 1994). Bantel & Jackson (1989), for example, found that heterogeneity of age, tenure and educational background was linked to innovation among top management.

Perhaps the value of dissent is best summarized by Hackman's (1987) question, "why do groups plagued with conflict and dissension sometimes perform better than those with an abundance of warmth and mutual respect among members?" (p. 320).

Empirical Evidence for the Value of Minority Dissent

Over the past decade, there has been a considerable amount of research in the social psychological arena on the value of exposure to minority dissent (see generally Nemeth, 1986; Nemeth & Rogers, 1995). Its value must be seen in the context of numerous studies which show that groups are usually "less than the sum" of their individuals. In performance, groups perform somewhat above the average individual and somewhat below the "best" individual (McGrath, 1984). Group decision-making is often defective and the major culprits appear to be social embarrassment and conformity pressures, which stifle the generation and expression of divergent views, of alternative solutions. And when it comes to creativity, most believe it is best left to the individual and considerable research shows that individuals generate more creative ideas than do groups (see generally McGrath, 1984).

There is also reason to believe that groups *can* be better than the sum of their individuals. Hackman & Morris (1975), for example, have shown that specific instructions, e.g. telling group members to develop a strategy, can be effective. The recent social psychological research on minority dissent, however, does not stem from a concentration on instruction or training but from a recognition of the "natural" and powerful processes that are unleashed by disagreement or dissent.

The major premise behind this work is that dissent stimulates cognitive effort but the form of that effort is very different, depending on whether the source of that dissent is a majority or minority (Nemeth, 1976, 1986). Specifically, Nemeth predicts that both majorities and minorities induce more cognitive thought. However, majorities induce convergent thinking and a focus on the issue from their perspective. By contrast, minorities stimulate cognitive activity that is divergent in form. Individuals exposed to minority dissent consider the issue from multiple perspectives, one of which is that posed by the minority (De Dreu & de Vries, 1995; Martin & Noyes, 1995; Nemeth & Rogers, 1995).

The reasons for these predictions are complex but, briefly, majorities who offer a differing viewpoint induce a great deal of stress. Such stress is likely to cause a focus of attention (Yerkes-Dodson, 1908; Easterbrook, 1959). Why such focus is on the perspective posed by the majority is because majorities are assumed to be correct and, further, people are motivated to assume that. Thus, people try to ascertain the truth or falsity of the majority position and often convince themselves of its truth, thus permitting movement to the majority position.

By contrast, minorities are initially derided and assumed to be incorrect. With consistency on the part of the minority, however, individuals come to reappraise the situation. They make a more thorough, broad-ranging analysis of the stimulus or issue, one that is motivated not so much by being accepted as by being correct. On balance, such divergent thought is hypothesized to aid the quality of judgments, decisions and performance.

The research to date supports such contentions. In an early study (Nemeth & Kwan, 1987), for example, individuals were shown a series of letter strings, e.g. tDAMop. When asked to name the first 3 letter word they noticed (under short exposures), people named "DAM", the word formed by the 3 capital letters. After 5 such slides, they were given feedback as to the answers of the 4 members of their group. In the majority condition, feedback indicated that *all 3* of the other individuals first noticed the word formed by the backward sequencing of the capital letters (e.g. MAD). In the minority condition, the feedback indicated that *one* of the other individuals first noticed the word formed by the backward sequencing of capital letters. Individuals were then shown 10 letter strings and were asked to write down all the words they could form from the sequence of letters.

It is clear that you can form words using a forward sequence of letters (e.g. mop, top, tam), a backward sequence of letters (e.g. mat, pot, pad) or a mixed sequence (e.g. map, mod, opt). Findings showed that individuals exposed to majority dissent excelled in the usage of backward sequencing. They found significantly more words using a backward sequencing than did a control group (that is, those not exposed to dissent), but this was at the expense of finding words using forward or mixed sequencing. Thus, their overall performance was comparable to the control group. By contrast, those exposed to minority dissent found significantly more words than did those exposed to the majority or the control individuals, and they did so by utilizing all three strategies. As predicted, those exposed to majority disagreement showed convergent thinking from the perspective posed by the majority. They utilized backward sequencing in their attempt to solve the problem. By contrast, those exposed to the minority dissent manifested divergent thought; they utilized all strategies (forward, backward and mixed) in the service of better performance.

By switching the task to one that favors convergent thought, Nemeth, Mosier & Chiles (1992) were able to underscore these cognitive processes that are stimulated by majority vs. minority dissent. Here the majority should have the advantage, provided their perspective is appropriate to the task.

Very few tasks are aided by convergent thought (that is, from a single perspective) but one is the Stroop task (Stroop, 1935). For this task, individuals are shown the name of a color in an ink of a different color and are asked to read the color of ink). As an example, the word "blue" written in red ink should be read as "red". For this task, it is helpful to ignore the name of the word; in other words, convergent thought from the perspective of *ink* is adaptive; convergent thought from the perspective of the *name* of the word is maladaptive.

Given the prediction that majorities induce convergent thought from the perspective they pose, Nemeth, Mosier & Chiles (1992) predicted that a majority focus on "ink" should aid performance while a majority focus on "name" of color should impede performance. To test such hypotheses, they showed individuals (in groups of 4) a series of slides in which they were asked to name the first color they noticed. Each slide consisted of two words. One was centrally positioned and was the name of a color printed in ink of the same color (e.g. the word "blue" in blue ink). The other word was positioned much lower and was the name of a different color printed in an ink of still a different color (e.g. the word "red" in yellow ink).

When asked the first color they noticed, people reported "blue". After 3 such slides, they were then given feedback that 3 of the others (majority condition) or 1 of the others (minority condition) consistently noticed a different color. Depending on the condition, this color was either the *name* of the second word (red) or the color of *ink* of the second word (yellow). They were then asked to do the Stroop test, which consisted of reading aloud the ink color of a series of words in which the name of the color was different than the ink in which it was printed.

Results indicated that individuals performed better on the Stroop test when exposed to a majority who had concentrated on *"ink"*. Individuals could read the ink colors more quickly and with fewer errors. They performed poorest on this test when exposed to a majority who concentrated on *"name"*. Here, speed was the slowest and errors the highest. Those exposed to a minority who focused on "ink" or "name" fell in between the two majority conditions. Presumably because they engaged in divergent thinking, a consideration of both name and ink, their performance was in between and not significantly different from the control group.

Thus, again, there is evidence that majorities induce cognitive thought from the perspective they pose. In most situations, this convergent thought would be maladaptive, as a consideration of various strategies or positions is conducive to good performance or decision-making. It is only when the majority perspective is the correct one, appropriate to the task, that the convergent thought induced by majorities can be helpful.

This stimulation of divergent thought is only one contribution of minority dissent. Other studies show that minorities also stimulate the search for and the recall of, information. In one study, minority dissent was found to improve the recall of information (Nemeth et al., 1990). Perhaps even more importantly, another study has shown that minority dissent increased the desire for more information. Furthermore, this search for additional information is relatively unbiased. Individuals search for information on *both* sides of the issue (Nemeth & Rogers, 1996).

This latter finding is relatively important in that there is evidence that people favor information that is consistent with their own position and may even actively avoid information that opposes their position (Frey, 1982). Thus, people are often biased in their information search and, to the extent that minority dissent stimulates an unbiased search for more information, it is likely to improve the quality of decision-making.

IMPROVING OUTCOMES BY MINORITY DISSENT

Consistent with the predictions that minority dissent stimulated divergent thought which, on balance, serves performance and decision-making, is research showing better outcomes as a result of exposure to minority dissent. Atsumi & Burnstein (1992), for example, studied majority vs. minority dissent in an air traffic controller situation. The task involved viewing a matrix showing landing patterns of 100 possible positions with either a plane in that slot or not, and then determining whether another plane could be permitted to enter the landing pattern. Simulating the stress facing these people, subjects had only 2 seconds to view the matrix. Results showed that the majority lowered acuity while the minority, even when incorrect, raised acuity.

Another study (Nemeth & Wachtler, 1983) used an embedded figures task. Those exposed to a disagreeing majority chose the majority solution. However, those faced with a disagreeing minority detected novel solutions—those not suggested by the minority or ones that would have been detected alone. And they were correct.

Still another positive outcome is the raised creativity found by exposure to minority ideas. Creativity, as noted earlier, is quite different from good decision-making. One of its defining elements is uniqueness of thought and expression. In studying this aspect, Nemeth & Kwan (1985) exposed individuals to either a majority or minority view that consistently maintained that blue slides were "green". Subsequent to this situation, they were asked to give word associations to "blue" and to "green" seven times. Those associations were then compared with the published list of frequency of associations (Postman & Keppel, 1970). As an example, a common or conventional association to the word "blue" might be "sky". A less common or more unique association might be "jazz".

Findings showed that individuals exposed to minority dissent gave more original associations to these words than did individuals exposed to majority dissent or to no dissent (the controls). By contrast, individuals exposed to majority dissent gave even less original (more conventional) associations to the words "blue" and "green" than did control individuals.

Orchestrating the Quality of Decision-making and Innovation

Many companies have come to recognize the importance of flexibility and adaptation in the current business climate. As a result, they have attempted to create corporate climates that value innovation. While the valuing of innovation is an important aspect, the achievement of originality and high quality decision-making is not so easily achieved.

Desiring to be creative does not ensure it. In fact, there are reasons to assume that high motivation may actually impede the process. Stress, as noted previously, often leads to a narrow focus of thought, characterized by convergent thought (Easterbrook, 1959) when, in fact, one needs divergent thought for creativity (Guilford, 1950). Such stress and strong motivation can also lessen the playfulness that often characterizes creative thought (Barron, 1955, 1968).

Rewards may not be the answer either, depending on how they are used. For years, there has been a recognition that creativity is served by *intrinsic* motivation (Deci, 1975), the pursuit of the issue for reasons intrinsic to the task, such as curiosity or the "love of it". External rewards can often serve to diminish this intrinsic motivation and, with it, creative thought (Amabile, 1983, 1988).

Quality of decision-making is a somewhat different issue, in that one wants to ensure that people search for available information in a relatively unbiased way and consider alternatives prior to making a decision—and even then, to reconsider the chosen alternative relative to other possibilities. The primary difficulty is that people are not motivated to seriously search for information or to consider alternatives when they believe that they hold the correct answer. And they are very likely to hold such a belief if it is shared by others (a majority) and if it is shared by persons of higher status (e.g. management). Thus, a strong corporate culture may in fact have unintended consequences that thwart good decision-making.

The beauty of the work on minority dissent is that it suggests that one does not always have to know the correct answer and then find effective ways of implementing it. People can find the correct answer for themselves if they learn to search for information and to think about that information in divergent ways. The motivation to do this does not appear to be promoted by a goal or a desire to consider multiple perspectives. Good intentions are hindered by tendencies to search for and think about information in ways that fit our preconceived ideas (see generally Markus & Zajonc, 1985; Taylor & Fiske, 1975).

Instead, we have found that dissenting minority views stimulate information search and thought processes that are divergent in form. People search for information in an unbiased way; they consider multiple perspectives; they utilize multiple strategies in the service of performance. Importantly, the effects of exposure to minority dissent do not depend on the correctness of their position. It is not because they might hold the truth or even a partial truth. It is because they maintain a dissenting view and, by casting doubt on the position held by the majority, they stimulate those individuals to engage in precisely the kinds of thought processes that, on balance, serve decision-making and creativity. In fact, minority dissent appears superior to instruction—and that is assuming that we knew what to teach or instruct people and that we had the power and resources to motivate them.

In contrast to such contributions of minority dissent, we have seen the deleterious effects of majority views. Not only do they encourage adoption of the majority position but they constrain thought to the perspective posed by the majority. People are less likely to search for information and such search is often biased; they tend not to consider alternatives and, in the process, the value of their decisions or judgments is dependent on the truth and the appropriateness of the majority view.

While we do not intend to make minority dissent a panacea for all that ails work groups or business organizations, we note the value—and even the economy in cost and knowledge—that minority dissent provides. Rather than continually striving to reduce conflict on the assumption that harmony and comfort are the only desirable goals, perhaps one needs to recognize the value of certain types of conflict for the stimulation of divergent thought and creativity. And, in the process, we may learn to heed the words of US Senator Fulbright, who advised that "we should welcome and not fear the voices of dissent" (Fulbright, 1964).

ACKNOWLEDGMENTS

We wish to express our appreciation to the Center for Research in Management (now named the Institute of Management, Innovation and Organization) and to the Institute for Industrial Relations at the University of California, Berkeley, for their generous support.

REFERENCES

Allen, V.L. (1965). Situational factors in conformity. In L. Berkowitz (ed.), *Advances in Experimental Social Psychology*. New York: Academic Press, pp. 133–175.

Altman, I. & Vinsel, A.M. (1978). Personal space: an analysis of E.T. Hall's proxemics framework. In I. Altman & J. Wohlwill (eds), *Human Behaviour and The Environment*. New York: Plenum.

Amabile, T.M. (1983). *The Social Psychology of Creativity*. New York: Springer-Verlag.

Amabile, T.M. (1988). A model of creativity and innovation in organizations. *Research in Organization Behavior*, **10**, 123–167.

Aronson, E. (1995). *The Social Animal*. New York: W.H. Freeman.

Asch, S. (1955). Opinions and social pressure. *Scientific American*, **193**, 31–35.

Atsumi, T. & Burnstein, E. (1992). How is Minority Influence Different from Majority Influence and What Does It Have to do with Awareness of Being Influenced? Unpublished Manuscript. University of Michigan.

Bantel, K.A. & Jackson, S.E. (1989). Top management and innovation in banking: does the composition of the top team make a difference? *Strategic Management Journal*, **10** (Special Issue), 107–124.

Barron, F. (1955). The disposition toward originality. *Journal of Abnormal and Social Psychology*, **51**, 478–485.

Barron, F. (1968). *Creativity and Personal Freedom*. New York: Van Nostrand.

Bass, B.M. & Barrett, G.V. (1981). *People, Work, and Organizations*. Boston: Allyn & Bacon.

Blake, R.R. & Mouton, J.S. (1981). *Productivity: The Human Side*. New York: Amacom.

Campbell, D.T. (1969). Variation and selective retention in sociocultural evolution. *General Systems: Yearbook of the Society for General Systems Research*, **16**, 69–85.

Cosier, R.A. (1981). Further thoughts on dialectic inquiry in strategic planning: rejoinder to Mitroff and Mason. *Academy of Managements Review*, **6**, 653–654.

Deci, E.L. (1975). *Intrinsic Motivation*. New York: Plenum.

de Dreu, C.K.W. & de Vries, N.K. (1995). Differential processing and attitude change following majority versus minority arguments. To appear in C.J. Nemeth (ed.), *British Journal of Social Psychology*, Special Issue on Minority Influence, in press.

Deutsch, M. & Gerard, H.B. (1955). A study of normative and informational social influences upon individual judgment. *Journal of Abnormal and Social Psychology*, **51**, 629–636.

Dougherty, D. (1987). New Products in Old Organizations: The Myth of the Better Mousetrap in Search of the Beaten Path. PhD dissertation, Sloan School of Management, M.I.T.

Dunnette, M.D., Campbell, J.P. & Jaastad, K. (1963). The effects of group participation on brainstorming effectiveness for two industrial samples. *Journal of Applied Psychology*, **47**, 30–37.

Easterbrook, J.A. (1959). The effect of emotion on the utilization and the organization of behavior. *Psychological Review*, **66**, 183–201.

Frey, D. (1982). Different levels of cognitive dissonance, information seeking, and information avoidance. *Journal of Personality and Social Psychology*, **43**, 1175–1183.

Fulbright, J.W. (1964). Speech to the United States Senate, March 27.

Guetzkow, H. & Gyr, J. (1954). An analysis of conflict in decision making groups. *Human Relations*, **7**, 367–382.

Guilford, J.P. (1950). Creativity. *American Psychologist*, **14**, 469–479.

Hackman, J.R. (1987). The design of work teams. In J.W. Lorsch (ed.), *Handbook of Organizational Behavior*. Englewood Cliffs, NJ: Prentice-Hall.

Hackman, J.R. & Morris, C.G. (1975). Group tasks, group interaction process, and group performance effectiveness: a review and proposed integration. In L. Berkowitz (ed.), *Advances in Experimental Social Psychology*, Vol. 9. New York: Academic Press, pp. 35–99.

Hall, D.F. & Foster, L.W. (1977). A psychological success cycle and goal setting: goals, performance and attitudes. *Academy of Management Journal*, **2**, 282–290.

Holl, D.F. & Hall, F.S. (1976). The relationship between goals, performance, success, self-image, and involvement under different organizational climates. *Journal of Vocational Behavior*, **9**, 267–278.

Hoffman, L.R. (1959). Homogeneity of member personality and its effect on group problem-solving. *Journal of Abnormal Psychology*, **58**, 27–32.

Hoffman, L.R. & Maier, N.R.F. (1961). Quality and acceptance of problem solutions by members of homogeneous and heterogeneous groups. *Journal of Abnormal and Social Psychology*, **62**(2), 401–407.

Hovland, C. & Weiss, W. (1951). The influence of source credibility on communication effectiveness. *Public Opinion Quarterly*, **15**, 635–650.

Jackson, S.E. (1992). Team composition in organizational settings: issues in managing a diverse work force. In S. Worchel, W. Wood & J. Simpson (eds), *Group Process and Productivity*. Beverly Hills, CA: Sage.

Janis, I.L. (1982). *Groupthink: Psychological Studies of Policy Decisions and Fiascos*. Boston: Houghton Mifflin.

Kanter, R.M., Stein, B.A. & Jick, T.D. (1992). *The Challenge of Organizational Change*. New York: Free Press.

Keisler, S.B. (1978). *Interpersonal Processes in Groups and Organizations*. Arlington Heights, IL: AHM Publishing.

Kraar, L. (1989). Japan's gung-ho US car plants. *Fortune*, **119**(3), 98–108.

Labich, K. (1988). The innovators. *Fortune*, **117**(12), 50–64.

Levine, J.M. & Moreland, R.L. (1990). Progress in small group research. *Annual Review of Psychology*, **9**, 72–78.

Levy, L.H. (1968). Originality as a role-defined behavior. *Journal of Personality and Social Psychology*, **9**, 72–78.

Maier, N.R.F. & Solem, A.R. (1952). The contribution of a discussion leader to the quality of group thinking: the effective use of minority opinion. *Human Relations*, **5**, 277–288.

Manski, M.E. & Davis, G.A. (1968). Effects of simple instructional biases upon performance in the unusual uses test. *Journal of General Psychology*, **78**, 25–33.

Markus, H. & Zajonc, R.B. (1985). The cognitive perspective in social psychology. In G. Lindzey and J.E. Aronson (eds), *The Handbook of Social Psychology*. Reading, MA: Addison-Wesley, pp. 137–230.

Martin, R. & Noyes, C. (1995). Minority influence and argument generation. To appear in C.J. Nemeth (ed.), *British Journal of Social Psychology*, Special Issue on Minority Influence, in press.

May, K. (1994). Understanding the Differential Effects of Demographic- and Ability-based Diversity on the Processes and Performance of Decision-making Teams. Doctoral thesis, University of California, Berkeley.

McGrath, J.E. (1984). *Groups: Interaction and Performance*. Englewood Cliffs, NJ: Prentice-Hall.

Nemeth, C.J. (1976). A camparison between conformity and minority influence. Invited address, International Cargress of Psychology, Paris, France.
Nemeth, C. (1986). Differential contributions of majority and minority influence. *Psychological Review*, **93**, 23–32.
Nemeth, C. & Kwan, J. (1985). Originality of work associations as a function of majority vs. minority influence processes. *Social Psychology Quarterly*, **48**, 277–282.
Nemeth, C. & Kwan, J. (1987). Minority influence, divergent thinking and the detection of correct solutions. *Journal of Applied Social Psychology*, **9**, 788–799.
Nemeth, C., Mayseless, O., Sherman, J. & Brown, Y. (1990). Exposure to dissent and recall of information. *Journal of Personality and Social Psychology*, **58**, 429–437.
Nemeth, C., Mosier, K. & Chiles, C. (1992). When convergent thought improves performance: majority vs. minority influence. *Personality and Social Psychology Bulletin*, **81**, 139–144.
Nemeth, C. & Rogers, J. (1996). Dissent and the search for information. *British Journal of Social Psychology*, in press.
Nemeth, C. & Staw, B.M. (1989). The tradeoffs of social control and innovation in groups and organizations. In L. Berkowitz (ed.), *Advances in Experimental and Social Psychology*, Vol. 22. San Diego, CA: Academic Press, pp. 175–210.
Nemeth, C. & Wachtler, J. (1983). Creative problem solving as a result of majority v. minority influence. *European Journal of Social Psychology*, **13**, 45–55.
O'Reilly, C. (1989). Corporations, culture, and commitment: motivation and social control in organizations. *California Management Review*, **Summer**, 9–25.
Osborn, A.F. (1957). *Applied Imagination*. New York: Scribners.
Pfeffer, J. & O'Reilly, C. (1987). Hospital demography and turnover among nurses. *Industrial Relations*, **26**, 158–173.
Postman, L. & Keppel, G. (1970). *Norms of Word Association*. New York: Academic Press.
Royce, J. (1896). The psychology of invention. *Psychological Review*, **5**, 111–143.
Schachter, S. (1959). *The Psychology of Affiliation*. Stanford: Stanford University Press.
Schein, E.H. (1989). Corporate culture is the real key to creativity. *Business Month*, **May**, 73–75.
Schlesinger, A.M. Jr. (1972). *A Thousand Days*. Boston: Houghton Mifflin (1965). Cited by I.L. Janis in *Victims of Groupthink*. Boston: Houghton Mifflin, p. 40.
Shaw, M.E. (1971). *Group Dynamics: The Psychology of Small Group Behavior*. New York: McGraw-Hill.
Stewart, T.A. (1993). Welcome to the revolution. *Businessweek*, December 13.
Stone, D.N., Sivitanides, M.P. & Magro, A.P. (1994). Formalized dissent and cognitive complexity in group processes and performance. *Decision Sciences*, **25**, 243–261.
Stroop, R.J. (1935). Studies of interference in serial verbal reactions. *Journal of Experimental Psychology*, **18**, 643–662.
Taylor, D.W., Berry, P.C. & Block, C.H. (1958). Does group participation when using brainstorming facilitate or inhibit creative thinking? *Administrative Science Quarterly*, **3**, 23–47.
Taylor, S.E. & Fiske, S.T. (1975). Point of view and perceptions of causality. *Journal of personality and Social Psychology*, **32**, 439–445.
Tetlock, P.E., Peterson, R.S., McGuire, C., Change, S. & Feld, P. (1992). Assessing political group dynamics: a test of the groupthink model. *Journal of Personality and Social Psychology*, **63**, 403–425.
Torrance, E.P. (1954). Some consequences of power differences on decision making in permanent and temporary three-man groups. *Research Studies, State College of Washington*, **22**, 130–140.
Yerkes, R.M. & Dodson, J.D. (1908). The relation of strength of stimulus to rapidity of habit formation. *Journal of Comparative Neurological Psychology*, **18**, 459–482.

Yukl, G.A. & Latham, G.P. (1976). Interrelationships among employee participation, individual differences, goal difficulty, goal acceptance, instrumentality and performance. *Personnel Psychology*, **26**, 221–231.

Zander, A.W. (1971). *Motives and Goals in Groups*. New York: Academic Press.

Zander, A.W. (1977). *Groups at Work*. San Francisco: Jossey-Bass.

Chapter 7

Unconscious Phenomena in Work Groups

Mark Stein
The Tavistock Institute*, London, UK

Abstract

The increasing awareness of the importance of groups in the workplace has prompted a renewed interest in the more subtle, irrational and often unconscious facets of group functioning. This chapter uses a psychodynamic framework to examine such phenomena. At the centre of this framework lies the notion that unconscious phenomena are governed by emotions that may easily subvert rational task activity. Several different types of phenomena are examined. First, certain features of the work and environment of the group may give rise to anxieties which are too painful to bear. Such anxieties may therefore operate at an unconscious level and lead to defensive responses in the group and the organization. Second, certain aspects pertaining to individuals or groups may be experienced by them as too uncomfortable and may thus be split off and projected into other individuals or groups; the mechanisms of "splitting" and "projective identification" are employed here. Third, there are circumstances in which the group maintains an unconscious, shared "basic assumption" which inhibits it from pursuing its task. Fourth, the largely unexplored but important issue of envy is examined. Unconscious envy is understood to explain phenomena where individuals in groups appear to be thwarting the development or blocking the contribution of other members, managers or consultants associated with the group. This is followed by a description of ways in which unconscious phenomena may be learnt about. Finally, practical interventions with work groups using

---

* Address for correspondence: Human Resource Management, South Bank Business School, South Bank University, 103 Borough Road, London SEI OAA.

Handbook of Work Group Psychology. Edited by M.A. West.
© 1996 John Wiley & Sons Ltd.

psychodynamic concepts are explored. It is concluded that psychodynamic research is of considerable value in helping us understand the more difficult and intractable aspects of group functioning. It also provides practical opportunities for exploring and trying to deal with some of the issues raised.

INTRODUCTION

Few scholars and researchers today expect organizations and their constituent work groups to act entirely rationally. In contrast with the hegemony of the scientific management view of Taylor, Gilbreth & Urwick earlier this century, there has been of late an increased emphasis on the role of the irrational and of emotions in the workplace. Peters & Waterman (1982), for example, speak of the passion for work, Moss Kanter (1983) of empowerment, and Hochschild (1983) of emotional labour in the workplace.

One set of concepts which provide a particularly valuable framework for understanding the emotions and the irrational is that deriving from the psychodynamic tradition. At the core of these concepts lies the notion that certain aspects of the functioning of work groups and their members operate at an unconscious level. Such a view postulates that these phenomena are not easily accessible to the conscious minds of individual members of a group. In some cases such phenomena may be shared by all group members and the notion of a "group unconscious" may be referred to. Such unconscious phenomena—thoughts, feelings, mechanisms and processes—may in some circumstances become accessible to consciousness, but frequently with considerable struggle, and even then often only temporarily and partially.

Central to this view is Bion's (1961) notion that such unconscious phenomena in a group may run counter to and undermine the rational pursuit of its task. The group functions as if it is working on its task, but factors which group members are largely unaware of prevent it from actually doing so. Bion's view suggests that the concept of the unconscious may help us to understand the irrationality of work groups that most of us have at some point had some experience of. Our own involvement in the group may make it difficult to recognize what is going on, and it often requires an outsider with a more neutral position to make sense of what is happening. Exploring and understanding these unconscious phenomena may help to unburden the group and enable it engage more effectively with its task and progress with its work.

This chapter describes the main concepts used by researchers in the exploration of unconscious phenomena within work groups. It examines the notions of the individual and group unconscious, defences against anxiety, splitting and projective identification, the basic assumptions, transference and envy. Each concept is illustrated by examples from the literature or from the author's own research. This is followed by an examination of a variety of methods and opportunities that have been developed to foster learning about such phenomena.

After this several different types of practical application and intervention in work groups are explored.

KEY PSYCHODYNAMIC CONCEPTS IN THEORY AND PRACTICE

The Individual and Group Unconscious

When defining the unconscious, Freud (1915, in 1984) introduced the following distinction. Certain contents of the mind, while not currently in consciousness, are in principle easily capable of entering consciousness. To take a simple example, while I may not currently be thinking what my own name is, this can easily be brought to mind. These types of thoughts constitute the preconscious mind. However, there exist other mental contents which are currently actively denied access to consciousness, and may be brought into consciousness only with difficulty; these constitute the unconscious mind.

Despite many developments in psycho-analytic thinking, Freud's theory of the unconscious continues to provide us with a sound basis for the study of these phenomena (see Isaacs, 1948; Hinshelwood, 1989). Freud, and Bion after him, extended the notion of the individual unconscious by postulating that there are unconscious thoughts pertaining to the group, as well as those that belong to the individual. Group unconscious phenomena are simply those that individuals in a group have in common that exist within their individual minds.

A person who joins a group, therefore, enters it with his or her own individual unconscious mind. Several people entering a group are likely to have unconscious minds which have both different properties as well as certain aspects in common. The hypothesis of the group unconscious suggests that in most circumstances there is a tendency for certain of the common aspects to increase and be fostered by the individual members' experience in the group. These common unconscious thoughts are the "group unconscious", and may contribute to the distorting of the external reality that the group inhabits.

Halton (1994) provides a useful example of the group unconscious in a medical setting. The staff group of a hospital unit designated for closure employed a consultant and mounted a major campaign to keep the unit open. The campaign helped the staff to maintain a strong feeling that closure was unthinkable. Yet, the evidence increasingly suggested that closure was unavoidable. During one meeting with the consultant, the discussion strayed onto the apparently irrelevant topic of the merits of euthanasia. The consultant understood this to be a reference to an unconscious feeling in the staff group that—in the current circumstances—it may be a relief to face the inevitability of the death of the unit. The consultant believed that, despite their difficulty in consciously recognizing the inevitability of closure, the group was unconsciously aware that this was now unavoidable. The consultant made an interpretation along these lines which, following the initial reaction of shock, later enabled the group to face the reality of closure and begin planning for the future of the patients.

One of the features of the psychodynamic view is that certain individuals are understood to take on the role of expressing different aspects of the group's unconscious thoughts. One example may be when a group member expresses anger towards a manager over some time, without apparent response of any kind from others. There may of course be several reasons why group members do not voice their opinions, including their lack of power or their position in a particular interest group. However, if the group allows this voicing of anger to go on unabated, the psychodynamic view would suggest that this may be an expression of certain feelings of the group and not just of the individual. Horwitz (1985) refers to this as "the use of a member as spokesman" (1985, p. 29). Becoming aware of the way it allows an individual member to express its views and feelings may enable the group to take more responsibility for itself and proceed with the pursuit of its task.

Defences Against Anxiety

A major constituent part of the group unconscious are the anxieties that group members are unable to bear and therefore block from entering into consciousness. Researchers who have experience of psychodynamic work with groups have found that the emotion of anxiety is of considerable importance in determining the nature of the group, and, by extension, the organization. They believe that the anxiety of individuals is always present in differing shapes and degrees in groups within organizations. The types of anxiety experienced in a workplace are likely to be related to the nature of the work undertaken and the environment in which it is undertaken. Further, a great deal about the nature of the group and the organization, including its structure, may be shaped by the need to avoid the experience of these anxieties. These authors thus spoke of defences, and defensive systems, which the organization and its constituent groups unconsciously construct to attempt to avoid these experiences. In reviewing her many years of organizational and group work, Menzies Lyth (1989), who, alongside Elliott Jaques, played a pivotal role in developing this point of view, commented: "... in all situations where I have worked, *anxiety* has been a central issue: how *anxiety*, its experience and expression and the related defences, adaptations and sublimations are a major factor in determining personal and institutional behaviour". (1989, Preface, p. viii; my italics)

In her now classic study of hospitals, Menzies Lyth (1959, in 1988) argued that work with ill, vulnerable and sometimes dying patients was associated with degrees of anxiety that had major consequences for the work group and the organization. For example, by a process of unconscious collusion the nursing task was often designed to preclude individual nurses from relating too closely to individual patients. This included an over-emphasis on checklists and ritual activity in preference for more substantial and considered work in pursuit of the task. It also included job designs which ensured that nurses would be moved from ward to ward or even hospital to hospital. Instead of finding some way of helping nurses manage the considerable anxieties of their jobs, this was seen by Menzies Lyth as a type of collusion that avoided the issue and thereby contradicted the nursing task at hand. While it may be predicted that such anxieties are likely to be of concern in the health sector, other researchers have found similar phenomena in other sectors. Hirschhorn's (1988) study of the NASA programme, for example, revealed evidence of the operation of anxieties and their consequences for the organization (see also Colman & Bexton, 1975; Colman & Geller, 1985).

Splitting and Projective Identification

Central means of unconscious defending against anxiety involve the mechanisms of splitting and projective identification. These concepts were developed by Melanie Klein (1946, in 1975) and build on Freud's (1915, in 1984) idea of projection. Although developed initially in relation to the functioning of the individual, these concepts may also be applied to group functioning.

These phenomena involve experiences, feelings, qualities or attributes pertaining to the group being unconsciously experienced as threatening. When these become too threatening, the group may psychologically split them off and thereby get rid of them by projecting or lodging them in another individual or group. Any awareness in the minds of group members that these aspects belong to them is therefore generally consigned to their unconscious; in their conscious minds, these are solely the property of the other person or group.

Two distinct types of aspects may be subject to splitting and projective identification. First, aspects that the group experiences as especially "bad" may be split off because members find them too painful to deal with in themselves. As the recipient group or individual is now felt to contain these bad aspects, they may be experienced as detestable, and deserving of derision. Not infrequently this may be a manager whose every statement and action is understood only in terms of giving expression to his or her malign influence on the group. The difficulty here is not only that the group is unable to work effectively with this manager, but also that it is unable to acknowledge which of its own shortcomings it has projected into him or her. It is therefore unable to examine these issues and develop its work and the capacity of its members.

Second, aspects of the group that members find especially "good" may be split off and projected. In this case the splitting enables the group unconsciously to keep these good aspects separate and safe from their own bad aspects by lodging the good aspects in another individual or group. The recipient is then experienced by the group in an idealized way. Situations where the group is unquestioningly respectful of someone they regard as a hero, a genius or an invincible leader, are those in which this kind of splitting, projective identification and idealization are understood to have taken place. Attending a group meeting with a respected and famous person and feeling unable to make any contribution is a typical example of this. Here the good aspects of the group which have been split off remain unavailable to it. The result is a significant loss of capacity in the group.

The projection of parts of the group, whether good or bad, creates a relationship of identification with the recipient (hence, projective identification). This means that splitting and projective identification do not enable the group to get rid of that which is split off in any effective way; instead, by shifting the issue to a group or individual recipient the group unconsciously identifies with that recipient, and this contributes to a seemingly endless unfruitful relationship with this recipient. This identification thus involves a considerable lack of clarity of boundary between the group and the other.

Jaques' (1955) account provides a good example of group splitting and projective identification in the workplace. The evidence on board ship, as Jaques understood it, suggests that the crew may unconsciously lodge their bad qualities in the first officer of the ship. By making the first officer responsible for much that goes wrong, including that for which he is not responsible, the crew are able to unburden themselves of their own anxieties and responsibilities. It also then enables them unconsciously to lodge their good aspects with the ship's captain, so that he becomes an idealized, protective figure.

The use of unconscious projective identification may also be illustrated by research undertaken by the author in a learning event (or group relations) event setting. The purpose of the learning event (expanded later in greater detail in the section "Learning about Psychodynamic Phenomena") is to provide an opportunity for members to explore their relatedness to other members of the group, and its connections with their work and lives outside the group, in the service of learning. This particular group met once a week for one-and-a-half hours over ten weeks and meetings were attended by the author as a participant observer.

One of the major features of this group was the considerable conflict that developed between one member (John) and the remaining five. There was a strong feeling in the group that John was difficult to deal with and inhibited the development of the group. Group members explained this by saying that John had personal difficulties which were making his role in the group problematic.

Progress on the task of the group was limited by a series of circular discussions. John would make a sequence of comments which were felt to be unhelpful and undermining of the group. For example, he would generalize about group members, suggesting that they faced identical difficulties and shared the same feelings. Members responded to this by suggesting that it was insensitive and denied the differences between them. This was often followed by attempts to stop John, which appeared to have the opposite consequence of providing him with further opportunity to continue with these comments. Finally, some members would formulate explanations of why John behaved as he did. These speculations were of four kinds: that John's difficulties resulted from his being the oldest, that he was physically unwell, that he was unemployed, and that he was lonely. These in turn led to further of John's comments, made in an even more persistent style than before.

Participant observation in the group setting, together with follow-up interviews and a respondent validation exercise with group members revealed that while John was consciously believed to embody the features attributed to him, the evidence indicated that members themselves had strong concerns about these four issues in relation to themselves.

For example, it emerged that one member was a geriatrician working with the very elderly and disabled, who was acutely aware both of the suffering of his patients and of his own age, being second oldest to John in the group. Another member was a bereavement counsellor for whom illness and death were both of particular personal and professional concern.

Further, group members were worried about their own progress in their work settings and about the possibility of becoming unemployed. The geriatrician was worried that, with further cuts in the health services, his job might be at risk. Another was an employee in an auction and valuation company whose success depended on other companies being declared bankrupt; he was acutely aware that their success hinged on a situation in which others became unemployed, and was also concerned that fewer bankruptcies might make his own job vulnerable. Another group member was an employee development manager who had chosen to attend the group because he felt he needed to explore his concerns about his job and progress at work. Yet these issues were never examined in the group meetings. The follow-up interviews and respondent validation exercise revealed considerable evidence that members were projecting unwanted aspects of themselves—such as their fears of illness, death, and unemployment—onto John.

Establishing that these projective mechanisms were operating in the group does not imply that all the members' views about John's characteristics were false; some of them may have been accurate. However, what it does suggest is that group members' projections into John enabled them to avoid examining these very same concerns in themselves because they were then psychologically lodged with him rather than themselves. This thereby helped them avoid the task of the group, which was to examine their own relatedness to the group and their work, and which therefore should have involved these very issues.

Splitting and projective identification may also operate in work settings, as is exemplified by the author's research in the European marine industry (Dyer-Smith & Stein, 1993). It was found that seafarers have particularly strong feelings about the start of journeys at sea, often also the time when a new work team is created. The task of the previous crew is to hand over all relevant information to the new crew, especially about ongoing operational problems on which the safety of all may depend. Not only do these hand-overs frequently fail to occur, but the previous crew are often to be found going down the gangplank apparently rushing to get off as the new crew are embarking. The evidence suggests that in this action the despair and loneliness of the previous crew is projected into the new crew. Such an unfortunate start to a journey seems to contribute to a sense of despair in the new crew, which then reduces their capacity to work effectively. This in turn appears to be one of the contributing factors in the malaise in the European shipping industry, for which there is considerable other evidence (see Dyer-Smith & Stein, 1993).

The Basic Assumptions

An alternative way of conceptualizing the phenomena described above was provided when Bion (1961) introduced the notion of the "basic assumption". Bion suggested that shared, unconsciously held assumptions may prevent a group from engaging in effective task activity, and these he called "basic assumptions". As they are unconsciously held, they are not generally acknowledged as such by members of the group, but may be inferred from their speech and behaviour. What is essential here is the role of the emotions in the constitution of the basic assumption group; in particular, the group's experience of certain feelings, and their desire to avoid experiencing other feelings, leads to the holding of basic assumptions. The emotion that needs to be avoided, according to Bion's original formulation, is that of anxiety; basic assumptions therefore are essentially the group's unconscious thoughts that constitute its defence against anxiety.

Bion described three sorts of basic assumptions. First, there is the basic assumption of *dependence*, in which the group operates with the assumption that one of its members is able to look after and satisfy its needs, and that other group members therefore need to do very little other than allow this member to act on behalf of, and for, them. There is no sense, therefore, in which such a group would be inclined to meet for the purposes of doing work, or to achieve something through scientific endeavour, which is associated with too much anxiety and is anathema to it.

The second type of basic assumption is that of *pairing*, which occurs when a group shares the unconscious belief that two members of the group will join together, or may have already joined together, to produce a leader. As in the dependent group, the notion of a leader acting for and saving the group is central; in contrast with the dependent group, however, the leader is not present but "unborn"; in the unconscious of the group he or she is the "child" of the couple who make up the "pair". As a consequence the pairing group is permeated with an air of hopefulness and expectation, with the sense of Messianic anticipation of the arrival of the new leader. This hope must always remain unfulfilled because, in principle, the unborn leader's task to save the group from its difficulties can never be achieved.

The third basic assumption is one in which there is an unconscious shared belief that the group has met either to fight an external enemy or to run away from it. This, the *fight–flight* group, is therefore unable to do any effective work, because the compulsion to "deal" with the enemy by fight-or-flight is overwhelming. It should be noted here that Bion does not imply that fighting or fleeing are in principle in contradiction with the notion of task; clearly, in circumstances such as war these might constitute the task at a particular moment in time. His point, however, concerns the use of fight-or-flight as a method of evading a proper consideration of the task, which he sees as particularly damaging.

Before moving on to the next section, several points need to be noted. First, Bion made it clear that any group of individuals may at one time manifest the characteristics of one sort of group (e.g. of the basic assumption of dependence) and then shortly after of another sort (e.g. of the fight–flight basic assumption group). Fluctuations can and do occur within the same group of people.

Second, Bion's concept of basic assumption activity hinges on the concepts of group splitting and projective identification, and is an extension and more specific application of these ideas. In particular, the dependent group is one in which members' capacities are split off and projected into an individual or another group, thus depleting the group itself of resources; in the pairing group such splitting and projective identification occurs in relation to a couple; and the fight–flight group is the classic example of the splitting and projection of bad aspects into another.

The Transference

A work group may have unconscious thoughts and feelings about an individual with whom it works, such as a director, manager or consultant. When these feelings and thoughts are transferred from other past or present relationships in the experience of the group, they are understood to be "transference" phenomena. For example, research in educational settings by Salzberger-Wittenberg, Henry & Osborne (1983, pp. 32–33) suggests that school children in the classroom are likely to transfer feelings from their relationships with their parents onto the teacher.

In the relationship between consultants and work groups, recognizing such phenomena may be critical if an effective working relationship is to be established. In some cases such phenomena may correspond with an accurate perception of the consultant and his/her role, while in others it may not.

Envy

The ideas explored above all hinge on concepts that were initially examined in the psychodynamic study of individuals by Klein, Bion and their colleagues. However, an examination of this literature on individuals reveals a somewhat surprising finding: one of its central concepts is largely unrepresented in the psychodynamic study of groups and organizations, and this is the concept of envy.

For example, the concept is not listed in the index of Colman & Bexton's (1975) *Group Relations Reader 1*, which contains the most comprehensive collection published in the field prior to the 1980s, and neither is it listed in the index in de Board's (1978) otherwise useful book *The Psycho-Analysis of Organisations*.

This is particularly surprising in the light of the quintessential role envy has played in the psychodynamic perspective on individuals over the past four decades (see Hinshelwood, 1989). Why then has envy played a relatively minor role in the psychodynamic studies of groups and organizations? One reason is that the most important and innovative contributions to the field were written prior to Klein's development of the envy notion in 1957 and its publication in her book, *Envy and Gratitude* (1957, in 1975). In particular, the defences against anxiety perspective was formulated and published by Jaques in 1955. Klein formulated and published the concepts of splitting and projective identification in 1946 (see Klein, 1975) without reference to the notion of envy. Further, the papers that introduced the concept of the basic assumption—which constitute Bion's book *Experiences in Groups* (1961)—were all first published between 1943 and 1952. All these concepts were elaborated prior to Klein's *Envy and Gratitude*, published in 1957, and formulated largely in exclusion of the envy concept.

The question, of course, is to what extent envy is relevant to groups and organizations. *Prima facie* it appears that, if envy is an emotion of some importance in the life of the individual, there is little reason to believe it would be any less important in his or her experiences in groups and organizations. Indeed, the ambitions, power struggles and rivalries that are familiar in most work organizations would suggest that envy is equally important there.

What then is meant by "envy"? How may it be applied to the psychodynamic understanding of work groups? A dictionary definition suggests two main components to the concept. First, envy involves the relation to another who is perceived to have good fortune or to be in some way better off than oneself. Second, envy involves feelings of ill-will or "mortification" towards that other. The psychodynamic concept of envy builds on these two aspects by adding the following components. Third, the ill-will manifests in an unconscious attack on the envied other; in some cases an attack may be made in external reality as well. Fourth, among the unconscious motives in such an envious attack are likely to be the desire to exert control over the other and the desire to prevent the other from exercising authority or power or simply enjoying their good fortune. Fifth, psychodynamic research suggests that such envious feelings are experienced most powerfully in relation to those on whom one is dependent. Relationships are of course often characterized by a two-way interdependence, but the psychodynamic view is that envy is likely to be evoked specifically by the dependence on the other, regardless of whatever dependence the other may have on oneself. Sixth, such unconscious attacks on those on whom one is dependent destroy one's capacity to be helped by or learn from the other. In a group setting the object of such attacks may well be an individual who is particularly skilled, a leader, manager or consultant to the group. This destruction of capacity is one reason why the psychodynamic concept of envy is particularly relevant to work groups. Seventh, as with the psychodynamic concepts described earlier, envy may in some circumstances be understood to be operating not just between individuals in a group, but between the group and an individual or another group.

Despite the relative dearth of studies of envy in work groups, there have been some studies in this area. An early contribution was made by Bion in his neglected *Attention and Interpretation* (1970, in 1977). Here he makes the distinction between the "symbiotic" relationship, capable of both hostility and benevolence and which is able to grow and develop, and the "parasitic" relationship, unable to grow and characterized by a predominance of envy. A more recent contribution was made by Kreeger (1992), who proposed the notion that certain group phenomena may be explained by the group's need to pre-empt envy that they would find painful. The concept has also received further attention in more recently edited volumes, such as Colman & Geller (1985), and Obholzer & Roberts (1994), but it is notable that this has occurred several decades after the envy concept was formulated, and then only within limited areas of the literature.

Research by the author (Stein, 1995) found evidence for envy in work groups in both organizational and experimental settings. One example is from customer service teams in a large organization in the transport sector. These teams comprised of voluntary members and managers and were modelled on quality circle principles. Their task was to explore ideas and make proposals for changes which would promote better customer service. After a promising start, the teams entered a phase of acrimonious and angry interchange between managers and employee members. Finally the teams broke down.

The fight between the managers and employee members could be partly explained as a power struggle between two structurally opposed interest groups. However, this does not explain the extent of the hatred and what appeared to be a degree of purposeful destructiveness that emerged in the teams. A supplementary explanation which hinges on the notion of envy may be offered. This suggests that being put together to work "as equals" evoked considerable envy between the employees and managers in the teams. The employees envied the formal authority of the managers and used the teams to attack them. On the other hand, managers within and outside of the teams envied the new and alternative authority the teams had and did what they could to thwart them. Ultimately, the teams approximated a "parasitic group" (Bion, 1977, Part 4, p. 78). "In the parasitic relationship", Bion suggests, "the product of the association is something that destroys both parties to the association" (ibid). Further, it is a manifestation of a "setting dominated by envy. Envy begets envy, and this self-perpetuating emotion finally destroys host and parasite alike. The envy cannot be satisfactorily ascribed to one party or another; in fact it is a function of the relationship" (ibid.). As may be expected, the acrimony within the teams eventually led to their breakdown.

LEARNING ABOUT PSYCHODYNAMIC PHENOMENA

Those who have used and developed psychodynamic concepts have also developed methods for learning to apply them. These methods invariably involve participation in temporary groups that are usually attended as part of a "group relations event" or "learning event", held over a period of a week or two. The principal aim of these is to facilitate learning about the personal, group and institutional relationships that develop within and between groups, including those facets of these relationships that are unconscious. The emphasis is more on learning rather than training because of the difficulty of training candidates to deal with psychodynamic issues, intractable as they sometimes are.

The classic and most enduring of these has been the two-week conference of "Authority, Leadership and Organization" held annually in Leicester, UK, under the auspices of the Tavistock Institute and the Tavistock Clinic Foundation. Its design has been developed and modified over its 40-year history, and includes small study groups, large study groups, intergroup events and institutional events. Candidates who have attended a conference as members may apply to join the training group in later events.

A second model has been developed by Bridger, a founder member of the Tavistock Institute, and is run annually in the UK or France. This is the "double-task" model, which proposes that those attending such events should focus on two distinct tasks: an "external" task selected by the group itself for the achievement of a specific purpose; and a second task of examining the relations and processes—including those that are unconscious—which impinge on this.

Similar such events are now held throughout the world. The main sponsoring organization in the USA is the A. K. Rice Institute, named after one the principal architects of the Leicester conference. Variations on the Leicester conference are run in the UK by the Tavistock Institute, the Tavistock Clinic, the Grubb Institute, the Bayswater Institute and OPUS. They are also run by a variety of organizations in France, Switzerland, Germany, India, Australia and Israel.

TYPES OF PRACTICAL APPLICATION AND INTERVENTION

We now move to examine types of practical application and intervention using the psychodynamic approach and how these may be applied to work groups. Psychodynamic understanding has been used in many and varied ways in work groups, and there is no definitive way of categorizing these. The situation is complicated by the fact that it is often used in tandem with a variety of different research, diagnostic and intervention methods that derive from other traditions.

Despite this some typical forms of practical application and intervention may be isolated, and these are elaborated here. The types which will be described here are psychodynamic consulting to teams and in-house group relations events. These methods may be used by consultants working on their own, in pairs, or, in the case of larger interventions, by several consultants trained in the same method. These various types of practical application and intervention are explored below and examples given.

Psychodynamic Consulting to Teams

There are two main circumstances in which a consultant working psychodynamically may be brought in to work with a team or group in an organization. The first is where the team is stuck, unable to proceed with its task and work effectively together. There may be a perception in the team that the main problem concerns the relationships in the team; some of us will be aware of situations in which the acrimony and rivalry between team members is all too obvious. Alternatively the situation may be considerably more opaque than this, with a feeling among team members that something is blocking the team, but with little idea of what it may be. Whether the problem is clearly to do with relationships or not, a psychodynamic consultant may provide useful insights which will help the group to develop. Invariably an agreement will be made with the team that the consultant may attend team meetings and comment on the process he/she observes. Much of the work of the Tavistock Clinic Consultancy Service is of this type (see Obholzer & Roberts, 1994).

The second type of circumstance in which someone will consult to a team is when it needs to deal with a specific practical issue or set of issues. It may need help defining its strategic direction, reorganizing a work force, dealing with imminent closures, etc. In these circumstances the consultant will often agree an intervention design with the team, play an active role in leading the intervention, and consult to the process at the same time. It is this last aspect of consulting to the process by making interpretations about the dynamics that is the distinctively psychodynamic component of the intervention. Much of the work of the Tavistock Institute is of this type (see Miller, 1993).

One example of this is from work undertaken by the author and two colleagues with the senior management team of a manufacturing plant. The company manufactured an obsolescent product in a shrinking market that could only last a few more decades at most; the technology of its plant would make a shift to manufacturing different product very difficult. Its best hope of survival was to become considerably more efficient by radically reorganizing its work along flexible manufacturing and teamwork principles.

Over several months the consultant group undertook a variety of activities which assisted the team in developing the company's vision for the future, and a method of implementation that would lead to its realization. Some of this inevitably included planning for redundancies. During this time, however, data emerged which suggested significant tensions within the senior team that were blocking its work. In one off-site meeting there was considerable discussion in the team about difficulties in the workforce, especially concerning the issue of the redundancies. The consultants interpreted that this also appeared to refer to unacknowledged difficulties within the team, which had been present but not spoken about in earlier meetings.

This was followed by an acknowledgement by various members that there were indeed tensions that had not been spoken about. One member who had been especially quiet began speaking about his own fear of redundancy, and told the group how this fear had been inhibiting his work in the team. He expressed considerable relief that he could now talk about this issue openly. Evidence from later meetings suggested that he and others were able to play a much stronger role in the team following this intervention.

In-house Group Relations Events

A second way in which psychodynamic ideas are employed in work groups is by running group relations events within the organization. Behind such an intervention lies the ambition to influence the entire culture of the organization. Membership in the group events is voluntary, and they are usually run in combination with a range of other intervention techniques.

One example of this type of intervention is that described by Miller (1993) within a manufacturing firm called Omicron. The background to the intervention was the takeover of Omicron by a larger company and the removal of its sales function into the bigger organization. The consultant group's initial research and diagnosis suggested that understanding and negotiating boundaries in the organization was of considerable concern. This led to the proposal that a group relations event for all managers be held. The event was successful enough to prompt the managers to take over and continue running a large group meeting based on group relations principles for several years following it. A survey following the event and the programme of which it was a part indicated that half the respondents found it useful, and that there was a general perception that communication had improved. It also emerged that a number of problem-solving groups were formed as a direct result of it. Ironically, however, it does appear that Omicron became too powerful in relation to the larger organization, and this caused certain problems later.

CONCLUSION

In conclusion, psychodynamic research makes a contribution that is especially helpful in explaining some of the more difficult and intractable features of work groups. It suggests that the problems facing work groups are compounded by certain phenomena which involve mental contents that are unavailable for conscious consideration and exploration, and that by remaining unconscious are likely to exert a damaging influence on the group's capacity to pursue its task.

The anxieties characteristic of a particular work group are one such phenomenon. While the group may have some awareness of certain of its anxieties, other anxieties may be too difficult to bear and may therefore operate at a more insidious, unconscious level. In such cases psychodynamic researchers have found that both the group's culture and its structure may embody features which enable it to defend against these anxieties, but in their defensiveness simultaneously diminish its likelihood of achieving its objectives.

Another phenomenon occurs when individuals or groups split off and project unwanted aspects of themselves into other individuals or groups. Such splitting and projective identification may enable the group to avoid dealing with its task because its members remain unaware that they have lodged aspects of themselves in other individuals or groups. In some cases group members may split off and project into one of its members, a manager, or a consultant, who is blamed for having all the difficulties and for blocking the achievement of the group's task.

Splitting and projective identification are also involved when group members maintain a shared basic assumption that remains unconscious and unexpressed. One type of basic assumption is that of "fight–flight", which involves holding an unconscious assumption that the task of the group is to fight or flee from an individual or group. In a second type the leadership qualities of members are projected into one individual (the dependency basic assumption), allowing members to absolve themselves of any of their own responsibility for leadership. In a third type, group members may project their leadership qualities into a couple, enabling them to believe that the couple will produce the solution to all their problems (the pairing basic assumption).

Then there is the relatively unexplored but important phenomenon of envy in groups. While members may be conscious of some of their envy, it is the unconscious aspects of their envy that are critical. In particular, the not uncommon phenomenon of group members thwarting the development and skills of certain of its members, or of consultants or managers that work with it, may be explained by unconscious envy of those others. Such envy is sometimes too painful to recognize, deal with or modify. It is particularly unfortunate that this thwarting activity may continue even when there is considerable cost to the group as a whole.

Finally, the evidence of unconscious phenomena should remind us that, while critical to the functioning of organizations, work groups do not constitute a cure for all manner of problems. Indeed, it suggests that such groups inevitably embody a variety of difficulties, and that these may benefit from clarification and exploration. In such cases an understanding of these phenomena may help us to promote more effective membership and leadership in work groups.

REFERENCES

Bion, W.R. (1961). *Experiences in Groups and Other Papers*. London: Tavistock.
Bion, W.R. (1977). *Seven Servants*. New York: Jason Aronson, Inc.
Colman, A.D. & Bexton, W.H. (eds) (1975). *Group Relations Reader 1*. Washington, D.C.: A.K. Rice Institute.
Colman, A.D. & Geller, M.H. (eds) (1985). *Group Relations Reader 2*. Washington, D.C.: A.K. Rice Institute.
De Board, R. (1978). *The Psychoanalysis of Organisations*. London: Tavistock.
Dyer-Smith, M.B.A. & Stein, M. (1993). Human Resourcing in the European Marine Industry, *European Review of Applied Psychology*, **43**(1), pp. 5–10.
Freud, S. (1984). *11. On Metapsychology. The Theory of Psychoanalysis*. Harmondsworth: Penguin.
Halton, W. (1994). Some unconscious aspects of organisational life: contributions from psycho-analysis. In A. Obholzer & V.Z. Roberts (eds), *The Unconscious at Work: Individual and Organisational Stress in the Human Services*. London: Routledge, pp. 11–18.
Hinshelwood, R.D. (1989). *A Dictionary of Kleinian Thought*. London: Free Association Books.
Hirschhorn, L. (1988). *The Workplace Within: Psychodynamics of Organisational Life*. Massachusetts: MIT Press.
Hochschild, A.R. (1983). *The Managed Heart: Commercialization of Human Feeling*. Berkeley: University of California Press.
Horwitz, L. (1985). Projective Identification in Dyads and Groups. In A.D. Colman & M.H. Geller (eds), *Group Relations Reader 2*. Washington, D.C.: A.K. Rice Institute.
Isaacs, S. (1948). On the Nature and Function of Phantasy. *International Journal of Psychoanalysis*, **29**, 73–97.
Jaques, E. (1955). Social systems as defence against persecutory and depressive anxiety. *Human Relations*, **20**, 478–498.
Klein, M. (1975). *Envy and Gratitude, and Other Works*. London: The Hogarth Press Ltd and the Institute of Psycho-Analysis.
Kreeger, L. (1992). Envy pre-emption in small and large groups. *Group Analysis*, **25**, 391–412.
Menzies Lyth, I. (1988). *Containing Anxiety in Institutions*. London: Free Association Books.
Menzies Lyth, I. (1989). *The Dynamics of the Social*. London: Free Association Books.
Miller, E.J. (1993). *From Dependency to Autonomy: Studies in Organisation and Change*. London: Free Association Books.
Moss Kanter, R. (1983). *The Change Masters*. London: Unwin.
Obholzer, A. & Roberts, V.Z. (1994). *The Unconscious at Work: Individual and Organisational Stress in the Human Services*. London: Routledge.
Peters, T.J. & Waterman, R.H. Jr (1982). *In Search of Excellence*. London: Harper & Row.
Salzberger-Wittenberg, I., Henry, G. & Osborne, E. (1983). *The Emotional Experience of Learning and Teaching*. London: Routledge.
Stein, M. (1995). *Envy and Related Unconscious Phenomena in Groups within Organisations*. Unpublished PhD thesis, Brunel University.

Chapter 8

Interaction and Decision-making in Project Teams

Marjolein van Offenbeek
Rijksuniversiteit Groningen, Groningen, The Netherlands and
Paul Koopman
Vrije Universiteit, Amsterdam, The Netherlands

Abstract

This chapter is concerned with the interaction and decision-making in project teams, whose task is often unstructured. Moreover, project teams function within an organizational context, meaning that effectiveness will often encompass reconciling seemingly incompatible goals and conflicting interests within certain time–money boundaries. Therefore, cognitions and power are important determinants as well as outcomes of the group process. The central aim is to show how psychological knowledge about cognitive and political group processes can be applied to this field, leading to models and guidelines that enlarge the behavioural capabilities of the team. Examples are largely drawn from case studies in the field of technological process innovation, but could as well involve tasks such as product innovation and strategy development. The chapter is built around a contingency model. The effectiveness of the decisions a project team makes about their management approach is contingent upon the critical aspects of their task in its context. According to the model, contingency factors give rise to five types of risk: functional uncertainty, conflict potential, technical uncertainty, resistance potential and material resources. Three levels of project management are distinguished; these concern respectively the nature of the innovation process, the structuring of the process and the interaction during the process. For each level we not only describe which project management choices are possible, but we also discuss in which way these choices can be matched with the five types of risk. Special attention is given to four important functions of interaction for innovative project teams: exchanging information, learning, motivating and negotiating. In the concluding section the limitations as well as the value of a contingency approach are discussed. From a practitioner's point of view, contingency models can help project teams to adopt an interpretation mode in which they interpret their context in an active way and experience it as analysable. In so far as innovation encompasses changes in the social or organizational structure, the project team realises innovation by (accommodating) social interaction processes. These considerations result in some recommendations for further research.

INTRODUCTION

There are two reasons for concentrating on the management of innovative project teams. First, change is an essential feature of organizing (Argyris & Schön, 1978; Frank & Brownell, 1989; Rockart & Short, 1989). Nowadays, one can expect to find one or more project teams operating in every organization. It is also not unusual to encounter "supraprojects" consisting of several parallel projects, and series of (partly overlapping) projects. Mintzberg (1979) introduced the concept of the "adhocracy" structure: an organisational structure that is built upon multidisciplinary *ad hoc* workgroups or project teams. Rightly, he called this one of the structures of the future. Adhocracies use project teams to respond to clients who confront them with unique problems or to meet the organization's strategic needs for innovation. In such organizations, innovation and teamwork are crucial elements. There is another development that requires project teams: the emergence of network organizations and interorganizational collectives within which two or more organizations share resources to attain specific goals (van Gils, 1993; van de Ven, Emmett & Koenig, 1974). An interorganizational network may, for example, set up an electronic data interchange project to create a computer-based network that will sustain a regular information flow among the organizations involved. In such a situation, members from the different organizations may work together in project teams. In this way the participation of the various parties can be ensured.

The second reason for concentrating on project teams is the recognition that the tasks and composition of innovative project teams differ greatly from regular work groups in organizations. The latter have traditionally been studied the most (Payne & Cooper, 1981; Goodman, 1986; Hackman, 1992; Guzzo & Shea, 1992). Although a substantial part of the knowledge obtained in these studies may be applied to the functioning of project teams, the management of this category of work groups poses special questions. Project teams have to perform tasks that demand the awareness and use of specific psychological models and knowledge. Hackman & Morris (1975) pointed out that groups rarely discuss what approach they should adopt in tackling a decision-making task, but that when they do, they tend to perform better: discussion about the approach has to be treated as a separate task if it is to be taken seriously.

The distinguishing nature of project teams is a result of the unique cognitive and political aspects of their task and composition. Usually the tasks of project teams are non-routine. In terms of Perrow's (1970) technology variables this means that the stimuli (demands, signals) on which a project team has to act will often present a new problem that is not immediately analysable. Moreover, project teams are often created when input from different specialisms is needed to perform the task. This heightens the complexity of decision-making and interaction—the interfaces among different fields of expertise must be managed and differences in professional views and jargon bridged. In order for the project team to effectively manage non-routine processes and multidisciplinary inputs, knowledge is needed of the way in which teams interpret the task in its context and of the way in which they communicate and collectively assemble, process and apply information. This suggests a cognitive perspective in which typical social psychological knowledge can be applied.

However, project teams also function within an organizational context, indeed they exist because of the organizational context. This context is political in nature. Even in stable and harmonious circumstances, organizations consist of (groups of) people with differing ideas, motives and backgrounds, which may at any time give rise to conflicting forces within organizations. When the outcome of the innovation process has valued consequences for different intra- or interorganizational groups, the task of the project team is also political. Many innovations require the active participation of different groups with different interests in the process. Consequently, a political perspective is essential to understand the functioning of project teams. In this respect organizational psychology can offer important insights.

In this chapter we will concentrate on how project teams can manage decision-making and interaction within the innovation process. We will in particular discuss how project teams can manage the cognitive and political aspects of their tasks, by presenting a framework within which the (management) approach a team adopts can be described and the character of their task in its context can be diagnosed. Regular diagnosis of the contextualized characteristics should help project teams in choosing an effective management approach. We will end this chapter by discussing the applicability of such a contingency framework to the management of project teams.

THEORETICAL BACKGROUND

In the organizational literature, universal models have been replaced by contextual or contingency models. Structural contingency theories are based on the assumption that the effectiveness of an organization is dependent on the congruence or "goodness of fit" between its social structure and its context (Mintzberg,

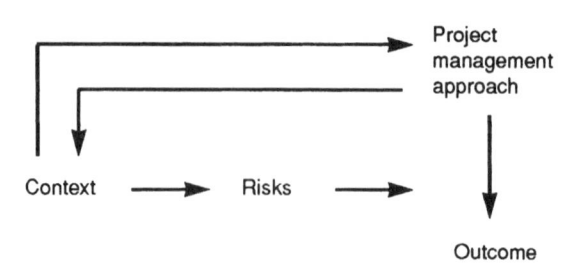

Figure 8.1 A contingency framework

1979). As Galbraith (1973: 2) stated, "There is no one best way to organize and any way of organizing is not equally effective". In most of these contingency theories a management view is taken, meaning that the dependent variable is the effectiveness of the organization. Likewise, contingency approaches have also been applied in research into motivation, leadership style, decision-making and innovation (e.g. Latham, 1974; Vroom & Yetton, 1973; Hackman & Lawler, 1971; Fiedler, 1978; Heller et al., 1988; Koopman, 1988). In many contingency models of decision-making, the context is characterized by a political and a cognitive dimension (Thompson & Tuden, 1959; Axelsson & Rosenberg, 1979; McMillan, 1980; Koopman, 1992; Grandori, 1984). The analysis of Hickson et al. (1986) of 150 strategic decisions in 30 organizations yielded a classification of three decision types: vortex (highly complex and highly political); tractable (complex, but less political); and familiar (less complex, but more political than the tractable ones). Decisions low on complexity and political import were not found, most likely because all decision processes were strategic ones.

In innovation research, the complicated task of developing information systems for work organizations also gave rise to the development of a number of contingency models (e.g. Naumann, Davis & McKeen, 1980; McFarlan, 1981; Shomenta et al., 1983; Burns & Dennis, 1985; Weitzel & Kerschberg, 1989). The premises underlying these models is that for effective performance the management (approach) of a project team should be directed at controlling the risks that are connected with the team's task and its context (Figure 8.1). The majority of these models only recognize cognitive risks, but some of them distinguish both cognitive and political risks (e.g. Schonberger, 1980; Episkopou & Wood-Harper, 1986). Sometimes situations will occur that are relatively simple. In these instances, because the risks are low, the project team can succesfully apply principles of technical rationality (see example 1), meaning that to a large extent the innovation process can be seen beforehand as a closed system of cause–effect relationships that will lead to desired outcomes (Thompson, 1967).

Example 1: An Interim Planning System for Sales
A project team developed an information system for a decentralized sales unit. The project team consisted of an information analyst, two computer programmers, the planner of the sales unit and, on an *ad hoc* basis, his colleague from the central planning department. The system was intended to support the existing sales fore-

casts planning process and to forward the forecasted figures to the systems at headquarters. The system had to make use of the sales information from the order processing system with which it had to be connected. The system was to be used directly by only one person, the decentral planner. His colleague was an indirect user: he needed the decentral forecasted figures in a standardized format. Both were used to working with information systems and the content of their tasks would not change. They would use the system for 10–20% of their working time. They agreed about the overall goals of the project, differing only on some minor issues. The system would not support complex or new tasks, because it had to be an interim system and would be replaced after a few years. The information analyst was quite experienced. Moreover, the team could use existing planning systems in two other decentralized units as examples. One of the computer programmers had been involved in the development of one of these systems. This project team conducted an information analysis, after which the interim system was developed and implemented in 8 months.

In circumstances like these, the project team can easily identify the most economic management approach. But most often project teams operate in a context characterized by uncertainly, heterogeneity of goals and organizational conservatism (see Example 2). The project team cannot be sure of either the inputs or the desired outputs of the innovation process and has to deal with political influences. In that case technical rationality will have to be replaced by organizational (Thompson, 1967) and political rationality (Pfeffer, 1981).

Example 2: Innovation in a Municipal Register Office
An on-line information system with a central database and a connection to the national register network was being developed for the municipal register office of a big city. The system would support all the mutations in the Register of Population as well as the supply of management, external and lateral information. At the same time the city council had ordered for lower cost of labour and for decentralization of the registry to 16 district offices.

The project team had the task of physically implementing the information system (which was largely being developed outside the organization); describing the procedure for the administrative organization of the registry; redesigning its work organization; communicating with the personnel of the registry about the changes and designing and coordinating the training of the registry's personnel.

In accomplishing its task the team had to meet the sometimes conflicting demands of different parties in and outside the organization. On top of that, some of these demands, like the legislation of the national government, were subject to change during the innovation process. Many of these changes had consequences for the design of the information system. Every time the system design changed, this led to changes in, consecutively, the administrative procedures, the user manual and the training course material. At the end of the process more than 2000 requests for change had been registered.

The project team itself consisted of employees of the organization and external consultants. Because of their different backgrounds, they had to get used to each other's working style. To the surprise of the consultants, using formal planning methods was not very important to their clients; discussions were not necessarily closed after a decision had been taken and the communication climate was much more open than they were used to in other organizations. In charge of the project team was one of the four directors. He had a formal mandate for the project, but the distribution of responsibilities between him and the managing director remained unclear. The linking pin between this intra-organizational project team and the automation project outside the organization was the busy head of the registry's automation department, who had quite different opinions than the other members of the team. It can be concluded that the context of their task was highly uncertain and political.

If a project team is faced with risks to their effective functioning, as in Example 2, their management approach should be directed to the control of these risks. A review of existing literature on social and organizational aspects of project management and information system development, as well as the analysis of seven technological innovation projects (see Box 1) has led to the formulation of a contingency framework (Van Offenbeek, 1993), which we will outline below. The framework is composed of, on the one hand, contingency factors associated with five types of risks (see below) and, on the other hand, management approach characteristics that can be matched with these risks, at a strategic (see section on "Choices at the Strategic Level"), tactical (see section on "Choices at the Tactical Level") and operational level (see section on "Choices at the Operational

---

Box 8.1   Risk profile and amount of control measures taken in ten episodes of ISD

The study was undertaken to preliminary test the contingency framework introduced in this chapter. Case material consisted of analyses of seven information system development (ISD) processes, that could be divided into five successful episodes and five episodes that were considered failures. In each site data from interviews with project team members and other key actors and project documents were used to retrospectively analyse the contingency and approach factors. About six months later questionnaires were completed to evaluate the outcome of the process. The table offers a quite simplified representation of the results of the study: the risks and the amounts of control measures taken are both indicated by being either low, moderate or high. However, it can be seen that neither the risks (taken separately or together) nor the amount of control measures (taken separately or together) could explain subsequent failure or success, but the fit between risks and specific control measures taken could. These results give some evidence for the application of contingency theory to the management of project teams.

Case	Risk 1	Approach	Risk 2	Approach	Risk 3	Approach	Risk 4	Approach
Success								
a	Low	Low	Low	Low	Low	Low	Low	Low
b	Moderate	Moderate	High	High	Moderate	High	High	High
c	Moderate	High	Low	Low	Low	Moderate	Low	Moderate
d	Moderate	Moderate	High	High	Moderate	High	Moderate	Moderate
e	Low	High	Moderate	High	Low	Moderate	Moderate	Moderate
Failure								
f	Moderate	Moderate	Moderate	Low	Low	Moderate	Moderate	Low
g	Moderate	Moderate	Moderate	Low	Moderate	Moderate	Moderate	Low
h	High	Moderate	High	Low	High	Moderate	Moderate	Low
i	Moderate	High	High	Low	Moderate	Low	High	Low
j	Moderate	Low	Low	Low	Low	Low	Low	Low

Level"). These levels refer to the management of respectively the nature of the project, the structuring of the project, and the interaction in the project. In a later section we will give some more thought to the functions of the interaction processes which project teams engage in.

CONTINGENCY FACTORS AFFECTING PROJECT EFFECTIVENESS

We distinguish four types of substantial risks. These have been derived from the four interdependent domains of the organization as defined by Leavitt (1965): tasks, structure, technology and people. According to his balance model, any organizational change will to a greater or lesser extent cause changes in all

Table 8.1 Contextual factors determining the five risk types

Risk 1: functional uncertainty	Risk 3: technical uncertainty

Existing situation (problem system)
  Complexity of tasks
  Stability of tasks
  Acquaintance with tasks
	Existing situation (problem system)
	  Complexity of technology
	  Newness of technology

Change situation
  Acquaintance with problem(s)
  Acquaintance with goal(s)/needs/criteria
  Amount of change in businessprocess
  Experience with innovation-type
	Change situation
	  Acquaintance with software environment
	  Complexity of technological innovation
	  Quality and commitment of technical experts

Risk 2: conflict potential	Risk 4: resistance potential

Pluriformity of problem system
  Number of groups involved
  Heterogeneity of interests, ideas, semantics
  Extensiveness of innovation (people, time)
	Changeability of problem system
	  Change potential of workers (management)
	  Willingness to change by workers (management)

Desired homogeneity
  Needed integration among groups
  Dependency on third parties, other projects
	Desired change
	  Quantitative impact on work organisation
	  Qualitative impact on work organisation

	Risk 5: material conditions
	  Importance for organisation
	  Time pressure
	  Budget
	  Human, machine and computer resources

domains. Technological innovation may be primarily directed towards the technological domain, but some change will occur in every domain. Therefore each domain can cause a risk to the effectiveness of the innovation process, that is the adoption of the innovation by the organization. Furthermore, the material conditions define the degrees of freedom the project team has in matching the other four risk-types with their approach. Table 8.1 shows the factors constituting these risks.

Contingency factors in the task domain determine what we have come to call *functional uncertainty*: the risk that the project team chooses a wrong solution or solves the wrong problem. Take, for instance, the risk that a company develops a new product for which there turns out to be no market. Or imagine a project in which an advanced communication system is developed to ameliorate pool cooperation among police departments, when the reason for their defective cooperation has to be sought in the competitive, almost hostile climate. The seriousness of this risk is determined by characteristics of the task domain in the existing situation and of the (expected) changes in this domain. High complexity, low stability of the tasks and maybe even unacquaintedness of the members of the problem system with the tasks at which the innovation is directed will heighten the functional uncertainty with which the project team is confronted. So will obscurity of the problem(s), unknown goal(s) or needs, and the absence of criteria against which the solution will be judged. Two other factors that will increase functional uncertainty are when extensive changes in the task system are foreseen and when the organizational members have little experience with the intended kind of innovation.

Contingency factors in the stucture domain determine the *conflict-potential*: the risk that incompatible needs and interests will block the innovation. Conflict potential is determined by the pluriformity of the stakeholders within the problem system compared with the extent to which a uniform solution is desired. This risk-type is heightened when more parties are involved whose ideas, language and/or interests are heterogeneous or even conflicting and when the scope of the innovation process (in terms of people and money) is large. Furthermore, risk is heightened when the need for integration among these parties is high and when the project is dependent on third parties or on the results or progress of other projects.

Technical uncertainty is the risk that the solution the project team will conceptualize cannot be realized. In technological innovation projects, this risk is greater to the extent that the existing technology is complex and new; that technical experts are unacquainted with the software environment; complexity of the technological innovation is high; and the quality and commitment of the technical experts is low.

Resistance potential is the risk that organizational members will be dissatisfied with the solution, because they feel the quality of their working life will be decreased. The height of this risk is determined by the willingness to change of the organizational members concerned, compared with characteristics of the wanted change. The risk is heightened when the workers (and management) have a low willingness to change and when the qualitative and quantitative impact on the work organization is high.

Material resources is the risk that the innovation will be aborted prematurely because of a lack of resources in terms of budget; human, machine and computer resources; and time pressure. Insufficient material resources will have a limiting influence on the degree of freedom the project team has in matching its approach with the former four (substantive) risks.

In this section we have determined critical factors, which create five types of risk for project effectiveness (Table 8.1). In the next section we will define three project management levels (Table 8.2) and describe the choice parameters available at each level (Table 8.3). For each of these levels we will next address the way in which the risks types can be controlled by the project team, as the management choices the project team makes on each of these levels should be contingent upon critical aspects of their task in its context.

THREE LEVELS OF PROJECT MANAGEMENT DECISIONS

The management choices that can be made by project teams can be divided into three types: strategic, tactical and operational (Table 8.2). Consideration of these choices provides insight respectively into the nature of the innovation process, the structuring of the process and interactions during the process.

At a *strategic* level, the project team has to establish which parts of the organization (in the case of process innovation) or to which parts of the potential output of the organization (in the case of product innovation) the work of the team is directed. In terms of systems theory we would call this the definition of the "problem system" (Checkland, 1981). The problem system is that part of reality at which the innovation is directed. Using this terminology, the project itself can be seen as the "problem-solving system".

Moreover, when considering innovation as organizing (Weick, 1979), the project can be seen as a temporary organization with certain explicit or implicit goals. These determine the orientation of the problem-solving system. Defining the problem system and developing an orientation within

Table 8.2 Three levels of project management decisions

Level	Determines	Decisions about
Strategic	Nature of innovation task	Definition of problem system Orientation of problem-solving system
Tactical	Structuring of innovation task	Differentiation of innovation process Coordination of innovation process
Operational	Performance of innovation task	Interaction during innovation process

the problem-solving system we call the strategic level of the functioning of the project.

At the *tactical* level, the activites of the project need to be structured. This encompasses not only differentiating the project activities, but also coordinating them. The differentiation and coordination of the project activities can be seen as the tactics of project management.

The third level of management choices is concerned with the *operational* activities: managing the actual performance of the innovation task and monitoring these work processes. Innovation is a continuous process that evolves on the interface between the existing organization(s) and the project. From a social psychological point of view, this process can be seen as consisting of the participation of people in the innovation and the interaction among them. From a management point of view, effectiveness of innovation is defined by two criteria: quality of the innovation (cognitive criterion) and acceptance of the innovation by the problem system (political criterion) (e.g. Ives and Olson, 1984). Also, when we look to the individual level, both knowledge and motivation seem necessary for enhanced performance (Arnold, Cooper & Robertson, 1995). The enhancement of both quality and acceptance leads to four functions of interaction processes among organizational groups in innovation processes: exchanging information, collective learning, negotiating and motivating.

Below we describe the choices available at each of the three levels (see Table 8.3). The management choices made at each level will not be entirely independent.

Choices at the Strategic Level

Defining the Problem System

In defining the problem system, the project team establishes, on the one hand, the functional domain and, on the other hand, the social domain of the project. The functional domain defines what project team members see as the organizational functions or activities the innovation is directed at. Their definition of the social domain delineates the organizational and/or other groups at which the innovation is directed and thereby limits the stakeholders (customers, suppliers, competitors and regulatory bodies) the project team has to deal with. The social domain can be compared with Thompson's (1967) task environment. Often the social and the functional domain will co-vary but, as Example 3 shows, this is not necessarily the case.

Example 3: A Pilot Project
In a service organization with 30 branches, an information system was developed to automate the administrative functions of which the primary process consisted (functional domain). The innovation process was directed at developing such an information system for only one of the branches (social domain). After the system was developed, implemented and adopted in this branch, a new project was started to

diffuse the system to the other branches (broadening the social domain, while the functional domain is being kept constant).

In most cases, widening the social domain will heighten the risks involved in the project. However, if the functional goals cannot be achieved without the political or cognitive support of others, a higher risk will have to be accepted by the project team. It can help to enlist external advisers to the project team to legitimate the functional goals of the project team by means of their expertise or by means of objective data sampled by them (Koopman & Pool, 1991). Also, consultants can sometimes give useful pointers about the strategic and tactical manoeuvring in the power constellation. Expertise and political skills are two important sources of power (Mintzberg, 1983). In one case, the fact that management hired expensive consultants to support the innovation was seen by the employees as a token of the comittment of the management and motivated them to give the project their full support (Van Offenbeek, 1993). Another way of strengthening one's own position is by seeking support at higher levels in the organization or support from external parties who can put pressure on the organization. Politically, if one's own power is sufficient, then the participation of more parties only generates more risks (Bacharach & Lawler, 1980). Each party that is given access to the team may make additional demands.

Choosing an Orientation for the Problem-solving System

The orientation of the project team also encompasses a functional and a social component. The functional orientation defines the extent to which the project team is directed towards diagnosing and analysing the problem system, or towards the development of a solution for a given need or problem.

When the needs are known it is quickest to start looking for a ready-made solution or, if not available, start working towards a customized solution. Also, an acute situation, which demands a quick reaction, provides little opportunity for diagnosing the problem system. However, in studying strategic decisions in a high-velocity environment, Eisenhard (1989) found that in fast decision-making processes (which were more effective) more information was used and more alternatives were considered than in slow ones. A problem-oriented approach has the advantage that a thorough analysis of the problem and the elaboration of alternatives is beneficial to the quality of the solution (Schwenk, 1988). An advantage of an open-mined problem diagnosis is that the risk of solving the wrong problem is greatly reduced. Most of the time a project team working on a certain task will alternate between a problem- and a solution-oriented approach. However, it is an important strategic choice whether the emphasis is on a problem- or solution-orientation.

The social orientation determines the extent to which the project team is directed towards social-organizational as opposed to technical-administrative issues within the problem system. This will influence which criteria are assigned most weight in the decision-making process (Hartwig, 1978; Vroom & Jago,

1988). Above, we have defined effectiveness of the innovation process by two criteria: quality and acceptance. Moreover, in most cases the project team should keep the costs of innovation within certain limits. Sometimes these three criteria are contradictory with one another. In these instances they should be kept in balance. When one of the criteria becomes dominant, this can create substantive problems for meeting the other criteria (Janis, 1989).

Important in this respect is the perception of the risks faced by the project team. In the case of a high resistance potential a social–organizational orientation seems to be a necessary condition for adoption of the innovation, because the innovation has an impact on the work organization. While cases with a moderate or high resistance potential were not successful when a technical administrative approach was taken, in two cases where the conflict potential and resistance potential were low, a technical–administrative approach proved successful (Van Offenbeek, 1993). Sometimes, however, the managers of the problem system think it attractive to define the problem as technical–economical in nature, precisely because this affects the entire subsequent approach. They may hope to avoid a political tug-of-war about the issue. This often happens in automation projects (Child, 1987).

In technological innovation projects, Blackler & Brown (1986) distinguish two archetypal approaches which differ in their functional and social orientation. A Model I approach stresses tasks and technology, is solution- and technical-administrative-oriented, and is based on a "top down" approach to work systems control; for instance, people are seen as a costly resource to be reduced if possible and planning objectives are tightly prescribed: while a Model II approach stresses organizational structure and members and is problem-oriented; here, because people are costly they should be more fully utilized, and general policy formation replaces tight planning. Nonetheless, in the 1980s, Blackler & Brown often found a third approach, which they have called a Model-Zero approach: management in charge of the project avoided the strategic choices and followed a muddling-through approach by reacting to *ad hoc* events and taking *ad hoc* decisions. The same conclusion can be drawn from the case studies by Vijlbrief, Algera & Koopman (1986).

Choices made at the strategic level should be the prime responsibility of the management of the problem system who have assigned the project team their task (Koopman & Pool, 1990). The strategic choices determine the possible effects the innovation will have in the problem system. For workers and their organizations it is never easy to pave new directions. This is because people have basic limitations of being able to handle complexity, of (unconsciously) adapting to gradually changing conditions, of conforming to group and organizational norms, and of focusing on repetitive activities (van de Ven, 1986). In a muddling-through approach where strategic choices are avoided, the *status quo* is taken for granted anyhow, making substantial innovation impossible. Blackler (1990) has concluded: "The management of the details of choices concerning particular projects is less important than management of their formative context ... which shapes the organizational choices that are made".

It is also important for the project team that these choices are made explicitly and on the basis of sound arguments, because these choices have a major impact on project team functioning. If not, problems may arise because of different interpretations of the team's task among team members and/or between the team and the management of the problem system. By choosing the project definition, the team determines to a certain extent the contingency factors and thereby the risk profile. For instance, when material resources (risk 5) are insufficient (so a match between context and approach cannot be realized) risk reduction must be accomplished by redefinition of the problem system. In that way a more efficient approach becomes feasible.

Choices at the Tactical Level

Differentiating Project Activities

The differentiation concerns the decomposition of the problem-solving system in parallel and succeeding activities. The innovation can be broken down into activities, which can be separated in terms of time and/or people who perform them.

Grouping of activities in time results in project phases. The number of phases and the extent to which these phases are clearly separated determines the *linearity* of the process. A linear approach is characterized by a large measure of phasing and specialization, whereby iterations among successive activities are hindered by the establishment of so called milestones (Keller, 1990). When more activities are placed within one phase, feedback (or iteration) among them becomes easier. In this case the approach becomes a more iterative one (Davis & Olson, 1985). For example, a process in which "defining problem", "diagnosing problem", "designing solution", "testing solution" and "implementing solution" are clearly separated activities in time is more linear than a process in which only "diagnosis", "design" and "implementation" phases are distinguished.

Besides, it is possible that the task of the project team does not consist of one innovation but of a series of consecutive innovations. This choice concerns the *magnitude of the steps taken*. In this case the project team passes more times through the phases constituting the innovation process: e.g., "diagnosis", "design", "implementation", "evaluation" and "further diagnosis", "further design", "further implementation". In extreme terms, the choice is between making an entirely new design to replace the problem situation (an integral or revolutionary process) or advancing in little steps (a step-by-step or evolutionary process). Furthermore, the decision about and the implementation of the changes can be more or less incremental. In Example 4 the innovative steps are small. Another choice might have been to make an integral analysis of and design for all the business logistic functions.

Example 4: Logistical Innovation in a Corrugated Cardboard Factory
As a first step, the project team identifies the problem areas in business logistics.

Subsequently, in a global analysis, an assessment is made of the domain in which the best gain can be made. This is the domain within which they start to work. So the first subproject of the team is to plan the dispatch of cardboard products in a more efficient way by combining the shipments of two production plants. When this innovation is implemented and evaluated, the team goes on with the diagnosis of the paper supply, another part of business logistics.

When we look to the *parallellization of activities*, we can see to what extent the problem-solving system is broken down into activities which are performed are performed simultaneously but relatively independently from each other. For example, during the diagnosis phase different members of the project team might analyse different parts of the logistic functions as preliminary work before the team makes an integral analysis. Or, workers are being sent on a course to learn to use new equipment while the equipment is simultaneously being installed at their workplaces.

In the case of high functional uncertainty the project team can stimulate learning processes by choosing an iterative process model, thereby facilitating the necessary feedback-loops (Algera, Koopman & Vijlbrief, 1989). Projects with a high resistance potential require a "step-by-step" approach, because this provides for the necessary recovery points for the organization and makes sure the innovation process does not surpass the comprehension of organizational members. In cases of high technical uncertainty, the diagnostic activities of the problem and the design and realization of a solution should be clearly separated, while within the design and realization of the solution, iterations are needed.

Coordinating Project Activities

The project team is responsible for the coordination of the different activities of the problem-solving system. Mintzberg (1979) describes five coordinating mechanisms within organizations. These coordinating mechanisms can also be found in projects, which can be seen as a temporary organizational form (Heemstra, 1990; Nadler, Hackman & Lawler, 1979):

- Mutual adjustment—Two or more people communicate informally (between themselves) to coordinate their work, as when members of a team meet together in a space agency to design a new rocket component.
- Direct supervision—One person gives direct orders to others and so coordinates their work, as when a team leader tells different members to perform specific activities in the innovation process.
- Standardization of skills—Persons are trained in a certain way so that they coordinate automatically, as when two team members with the same technical background understand each other with a few words.
- Standardization of outputs—One person specifies the general outputs of the work of another, as when management tells the project team to develop a solution for their problem that meets certain criteria.

- Standardization of work processes—The general work procedures are being designed beforehand to ensure that these are all coordinated. In projects, standardization of work processes can be achieved by the definition of standards for documentation and reporting and by choosing known methods and techniques, as when a team of information system developers decides to adopt a certain method for information analysis. To a certain extent, work processes can also be standardized by methods for project management or for problem-solving. See, for example, Flood & Jackson (1991), who describe various problem-solving approaches.

Standardization of work processes is the most formal mechanism. Mutual adjustment and direct supervision, while being the least formal coordinating mechanisms, can be given a more or less formal character. With regard to mutual adjustment, this coordinating mechanism becomes more formal when occurence of the communication is planned. For example, a project team can schedule their meetings and set an agenda for them. The formality of direct supervision is dependent on whether the leader of a project team is formally appointed with formal responsibilities and authority. The most informal direct supervision is the emergence of an informal leader. Research results indicate that line manages should hold project management responsibility (Clegg & Symon, 1989; Vaas, 1989).

In cases of high conflict potential, formal coordination mechanisms are necessary to unequivocally take and record decisions and communicate them to the grass-roots and others involved (Van Offenbeek, 1993). An advantage of a formalized coordination approach, with precise rules and procedures, is that it is clear to everyone where they stand (Koopman, 1992). Wissema, Messer & Wijers (1988), who analysed seven innovation processes, reported that creating clarity about the approach can prevent resistance. However, if people expect unwanted changes, formalized procedures can be the first step towards postponement, perhaps with the hope that the whole project will be abandoned (Koopman & Pool, 1991). In cases of high technical uncertainty, coordination within the problem-solving system among different specialists should consist of formal as well as informal mechanisms (McFarlan, 1981).

Choices at the Operational Level

Interaction

Interaction is necessary to process information and create commitment. Both activities are necessary for innovation. In the literature on decision-making, a lot of attention has been given to the participation of workers in all kinds of managerial decision-making (e.g. Ashmos, McDaniel & Duchon, 1990; Koopman & Wierdsma, 1988; Heller et al., 1988; IDE, 1993). In the field of automation, much research has been concerned with the participation of users in the design process, which was historically dominated by automation experts (e.g. Mumford, 1983; Koopman & Algera, 1990; Cressey, 1989).

However, it has been shown more than once that participation is not effective—in terms of higher performance, quality and/or satisfaction of participants—in all circumstances (Locke & Schweiger, 1979; Vroom & Jago, 1988; Heller et al., 1988; Algera & Koopman, 1989; Ives & Olson, 1984). Lack of consistent results probably means that various forms of participation (e.g. more or less formalized, more or less intense, direct or indirect) are effective in some contexts but not in others. Contextual factors include the issue at stake and the national culture. As a motivational technique, for instance, participation in decision-making seems to have a differential effect across national cultures (Erez, 1992). Erez found that participation in goal-setting to create acceptance of those goals was needed more in Israel than in the USA. In addition, participation is unlikely to be effective if potential participants do not share the dominant actors' objectives; if they do not want to take responsibility for helping to make decisions; if they distrust the dominant actors; or if time pressure and the dispersion of participants make it impractical to consult with individuals or hold group meetings. Group forms of participation are unlikely to be effective unless the leader of the group has sufficient skill in managing conflict, facilitating constructive problem-solving, and dealing with common process problems that occur in groups (Yukl, 1994).

In short, contextual factors must be taken into account and a one-dimensional high–low concept of participation is too simple. So we need a multi-dimensional model that enables us to describe and analyse the interactions of which the participation consists. Ashmos, McDaniel & Duchon (1990) formulated a participation model to describe participation in decision-making processes. Van

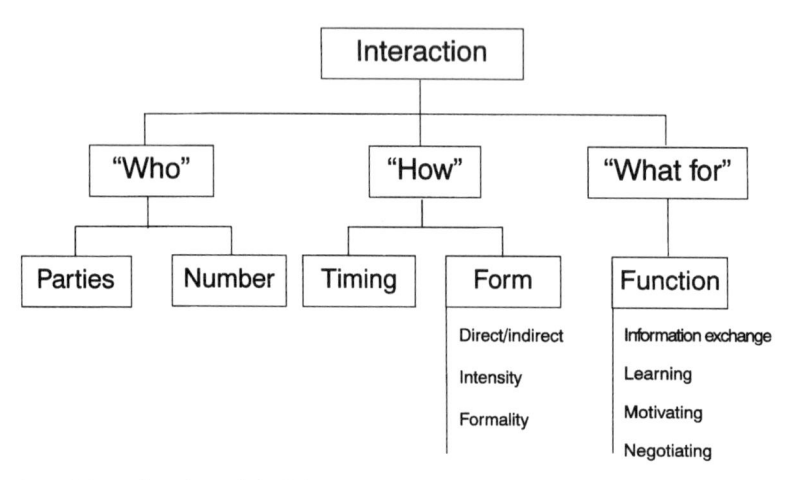

Figure 8.2 Hierarchical model of dimensions of interaction. Adapted from Ashmos et al. (1990)

Offenbeek (1993) adjusted it to a model to describe interaction activities in innovation processes (Figure 8.2).

First, the project team should establish *who* should be involved actively in the innovation process: what *number* of people has to interact together given the circumstances and the function of interaction? The next dimension is formed by the *parties* who have to interact. Not only interaction among these parties, but also interaction within individual groups can be described. The outcome of the interaction is not only dependent on who has to interact with whom but also on *how* the interaction takes place. The *timing of the interaction* determines during which phases the interaction takes place. It follows from the previous section that the choice for structuring the innovation process in phases is an arbitrary one. The *form* of interaction can be described by the formality of the interaction (Ashmos, McDaniel & Duchon, 1990), by its intensity (Vroom & Jago, 1988) or by the extent to which it is direct or indirect (Blackler & Brown, 1986). An example of direct interaction would be discussions among project team members. The interaction between two groups would be indirect when at least one of them is represented by others, for example by a regulatory body.

The last, and by no means the least, important dimension is the *function of interaction*. In the literature on organizational innovation, four important functions of or perspectives on interaction can be distinguished: exchanging information (Ashmos, McDaniel & Duchon, 1990; Markus, 1983; Ives & Olson, 1984); collective learning (Markus, 1983; Ciborra & Lanzara, 1989); motivating (Kotter & Schlesinger, 1979; Markus, 1983; Ives & Olson, 1984); and negotiating (Vaas, 1988; Blackler, 1990). Sometimes interaction activities will be directed towards

Table 8.3 Choices for the project team

Level	Decision	Choices
Strategic	Definition of problem system	Functional domain Social domain
	Orientation of problem-solving system	Problem-oriented Solution-oriented Technical–administrative Social–organisational
Tactical	Differentiation of innovation process	Linearity of activities Magnitude of (innovation) steps Parallellisation of activities
	Coordination of innovation process	Mutual adjustment Direct supervision Standardisation of skills, Work processes and output
Operational	Interaction during innovation process	who: number, parties How: timing, form Function: exchanging information, motivating, learning and negotiating

different functions at the same time, and sometimes the functions will concern interaction activities that are clearly separated in time and place. It is important that these functions are taken into consideration, as the effectiveness of the choices on the other dimensions of interaction will be dependent on the function of interaction (Van Offenbeek, 1993).

The management choices we discussed in this section are summarized in Table 8.3. In the next section we will take a closer look at the functions of interaction.

FOUR FUNCTIONS OF INTERACTION IN INNOVATIVE PROJECTS

Exchanging Information

French & Bell (1990) state that it is necessary to involve anyone who is part of the problem system or can make a contribution to solving the problem. The exchange of information serves purposes such as achieving a better analysis of problem, accessing the latest knowledge and experience, and a better assessment of the usefulness of potential solutions (Kanter, 1983). So, achieving a high quality solution requires exchange of information. Information exchanges lead to a more complete and accurate specification of the needs of the different parties, to interventions and solutions that fit the characteristics of the organization, and to realistic expectations (Ives & Olson, 1984).

In cases of high functional uncertainly, the project team does not have all the relevant information and so information exchange among problem systems and the project team needs to be facilitated (Vroom & Jago, 1988; van Oostrum & Rabbie, 1988). This interaction should be initiated by the project team at an early stage, because then its information-processing capacity will be highest (Ashmos, McDaniel & Duchon, 1990; McFarlan, 1981; Davis & Olson, 1985; Cressey, 1989). Resistance partly has a cognitive base, in the sense that uncertainty heightens resistance. In this respect, in cases of high resistance potential the managers of the problem system should keep all groups involved informed during the process.

Learning

In innovative environments, learning will be needed to achieve project goals. The learning function of interaction differs from the "exchange of information" function in the sense that subsequent behaviour has to be changed. In most innovation projects, individual learning alone will not be sufficient. The problem system and/or problem-solving system as a whole will have to learn, i.e. change its behaviour. For collective learning, interaction among groups and individuals involved is needed (Argyris, 1992; Swieringa & Wierdsma, 1992). Organizational or collective learning is a prerequisite for the development and adoption of complex innovations. Ciborra & Lanzara (1989) and Goedvolk & Smeets (1991) have argued that the innovative potential of technical systems will only be realized if organizational learning is stimulated. This is because, first, technical systems cannot be fully designed at the outset and they are often re-invented by their users; and second, new systems lead to unexpected consequences, some of which may be creative. Of course, the extent to which learning is necessary and the type of learning can differ.

Swieringa & Wierdsma (1992) distinguish three levels of learning, based on the extent and permanence of resulting changes. According to their terminology, single-loop learning is the changing of rules of what we can do, and brings improvement. Double-loop learning also changes the shared insights, the things we know and understand, and leads to more fundamental innovation. Triple-loop learning is radical in nature; it concerns the changing of the commonly shared principles on which the organization is built, of how the organizational members perceive themselves, and this leads to organizational development.

Information exchange alone will not be sufficient to control high functional uncertainty. Second- and/or third-order learning processes will have to take place. In cases of high conflict potential, rational exchange of information will not meet the needs of the project as interests and definitions of reality differ among the groups involved. The way of being, values and norms will be questioned (Hirschheim & Klein, 1989), requiring double-loop learning to occur (Argyris & Schön, 1978; Argyris, 1992). In circumstances characterized by high functional uncertainty and high conflict potential, Bouwen & Fry (1991) found a learning-confrontation approach, in which learning and negotiating are combined, to be successful. As to technical uncertainty, first-order learning will be required whenever the project members have little experience with the technology and methods, or have to improve their skills, and second-order learning will be required when given methods or techniques are insufficient.

Motivating

Interaction is sometimes critical in establishing a high level of acceptance (Erez, Earley & Hulin, 1985). It is important that the people who are involved in the project are committed to attain the goals of the innovation process. We can distinguish between the motivation of people in the problem system and in the problem-solving system. From a managment point of view it is important that project members should become "owners" of the problem-solving system; irrational fears and organizational conservatism should be reduced and goals established and accepted (Ives & Olson, 1984). Acceptance and commitment to the goals are enhanced by participation in goal-setting (Locke & Latham, 1990b).

When we describe the motivation of those involved in an innovation process,

process-oriented motivation theories offer more support than those that are mostly based on reinforcement or oriented on the content of motivation. In the former, the central questions are how behaviour is initiated, how it gets direction and in which way it is continued or changed (Thierry, 1991). Strict behaviouristic reinforcement theories have been criticized for their "black-box" approach to human behaviour. They ignore the obvious influence of cognitive factors (Bandura, 1986). In content-oriented theories, motivation is seen as a product of innate human needs. Arnold, Cooper & Robertson (1995) maintain that accounts of motivation based on needs have only very limited value. Their theoretical base is doubtful, and they offer no clear guidance about how to motivate individuals.

The process-oriented motivation theory that has received the most empirical support is goal-setting (Miner, 1992). It is based on the premise that intentions shape actions. A goal is defined as that which we intend to do at a given time in the future. People are motivated to deliver high work performance when a difficult, precisely formulated goal is set that is accepted by them, and when they receive feedback regularly about their progress towards attainment of the goal (Locke & Latham, 1990a,b).

Motivating activities in project teams would be creating clarity about goals; selling these goals to project members or letting those involved set their own goals; and giving feedback about project as well as individual performance. Many studies have found that feedback is a necessary condition for goal-setting (Kanfer, 1992). This proposition has received much empirical support (see Tubbs, 1986), including that derived from field studies of groups (Arnold, Cooper & Robertson, 1995). However, goal-setting theory has not been properly tested in situations where there are conflicting goals (Austin & Bobko, 1985). When commonly accepted goals in terms of desired outcomes are lacking, the common formulation of process goals will offer better perspectives (Latham, personal communication). An example of a process goal could be the way in which groups decide to try to work together towards a solution. Also, it is suggested that goal-setting may not be helpful in conditions where novelty surrounds the task, and various strategies are available to tackle the situation (Early, Conolly & Ekegren, 1989). In a meta-analysis, Wood et al. (1987) assessed the effect of task complexity. They found that goal-setting effects were weakest for the most complex tasks (business game simulations, scientific and engineering work). Likewise, the findings of Kanfer & Ackerman (1989) indicate that interventions designed to engage motivational processes, like goal-setting, may impede task-learning when presented prior to an understanding of what the task is about. In these instances, cognitive resources necessary for task understanding are diverted towards self-regulatory activities (e.g. self-evaluation). When learning is necessary in the innovation process, people should not be fired up to achieve specific goals: it is probably better to find ways of aiding learning, not performance. This is consistent with Farr, Hofman & Ringenbach (1993), who argue that people with a learning goal orientation, whose main objective is to increase their level of competence on a given task, are in the long run more likely to produce high levels of performance and competence than those who define goals in terms of demonstrating their level of task performance.

Other complementary activities to motivate people are the stimulation of self-efficacy, that is, perceptions of one's ability to achieve the goal (Bandura, 1990), the use of modelling behaviour (Bandura, 1977; House, 1988), team-building and rewarding performance. The last motivating activity is a regulating mechanism in many theories (Thierry, 1991). However, on the whole it seems that factors intrinsic to the work (challenge, autonomy) are more important in fostering commitment than extrinsic factors such as pay and working conditions (Arnold, Cooper & Robertson, 1995). Behavioural change may be brought about very effectively without the use of incentives (Duff et al., 1994). Pritchard et al. (1988) used a mixture of goal-setting, feedback and incentives in group settings. They felt that incentives added little to the improvements brought about by feedback and goal-setting. Social learning theory suggests that internal factors such as expectancies about the eventual consequences of behaviour have a role in controlling it (Bandura, 1977). Also, positive feedback could be implicitly rewarding by heightening factors like self-esteem and job satisfaction.

These findings somewhat limit the effect we may expect of motivating team members by involving them in goal-setting in innovation projects with high functional and/or technical uncertainty. One of the dangers of applying "goal-setting" is that issues on which no goals are formulated get neglected. This may be dangerous in innovative situations with high functional uncertainty. Nevertheless, in cases of high resistance potential, the managers of the problem system may use goal-setting theory to motivate the members of the problem system. Maybe more attention should be given to the emotional aspects of resistance (Carnall, 1990). The experiences of Korteweg (1988) with innovations in the printing trade pointed in this direction: room should be created to discuss fears explicitly, canalize dissatisfactions and mourn about possible personal losses. Personal attention for people may generate willingness to cooperate, even when the solution chosen might turn out to be less than ideal for them. If the innovation process encompasses collective learning processes, learning goals will function better than performance goals. A conflict seems to require the setting of process goals.

Negotiating

Innovation often involves discussion between groups which have different opinions about where the innovation process should lead (conflict potential). Mastenbroek (1982) described the political dimension of interaction as fighting–negotiating–cooperating. Interaction can facilitate processes of negotiation and the exertion of influence. An innovation process involves cooperative relations, but will, in the case of high conflict potential, also have political components. When more parties with different interests interact, the amount of interdependence defines the position the parties will be inclined to take on this dimension.

When the parties are insufficiently interweaved into one shared identity with explicitly shared interests and goals, the interaction cannot consist of cooperation only. Some (Moscovici & Mugny, 1983; Moscovici, 1985) have found that minorities need to disagree consistently with the majority, including on issues other than the one at stake, if they are to exert influence. Minorities do not exert influence by being liked or being reasonable, but by being perceived as consistent, independent and confident, This need not be detrimental to the project effectiveness. As Nemeth (1986, and this volume) concluded, groups exposed to minority viewpoints are more original, use a greater variety of strategies to detect novel solutions, and detect correct solutions. Likewise, the results of Vroom & Jago (1988), Heller et al. (1988) and van Oostrum & Rabbie (1988) show that the creation of constructive conflicts leads to better decision-making and does not magnify the differences in opinion. In cases of conflicting interests, it is important to keep problems manifest and discussable. Especially under circumstances where there is no superordinate power centre that can stimulate cooperative behaviour, it is useful to have set rules, common goals and intervention strategies to prevent escalation. When risks of fighting become too high, reducing the interdependence, where possible, is a good approach. This will require redefinition of the problem system at the strategic level in order to reduce the conflict potential.

In innovation processes with a high conflict potential, integrative bargaining is better than distributive bargaining. In the latter, the parties assume that there is a fixed amount of reward available, so that one party's gain is another's loss, while integrative bargaining involves an attempt to increase the size of the overall reward available to both sides. Win–win outcomes, where all parties gain, often depend on the parties having complementary priorities so that each can make concessions over issues where their subjective loss is smaller than the corresponding gain experienced by another negotiator (Pruitt & Rubin, 1986). Solving conflicts by consensus seems to result in higher long-term effectiveness than solving them by settling for a compromise (Olson, 1990; Barrett & Cooperrider, 1990).

As a consequence, room must be created for negotiation (Mastenbroek, 1982). Negotiation will benefit from being closely monitored by a higher, neutral power centre (Vroom & Yetton, 1973; Mastenbroek, 1982). Alternatively, a third party can be appointed (Ross, 1990) to mediate the negotiation process.

BEYOND CONTINGENCY MODELS

We have argued in this chapter that contingency models are better than universal models for explaining the effectiveness of project teams' management approaches. But still, a contingency framework such as that presented here is limited in its applicability. First, the theoretical distinction between context and approach is an arbitrary one. Only in a specific process can we tell which factors are endogenous (changeable by project team members) and which are exogenous. Second, the extent to which context factors constitute risks is to a large extent a matter of local perceptions (Nijhof, 1990). Therefore the risk profile can only be estimated locally. It cannot be decided beforehand that building a system for 10 people will always constitute a low risk, and building a system for 150 people a high risk. Many contingency factors have to be taken into account, so a project team has to assess how the relevant factors will interact and to what extent this constitutes a risk.

Daft & Weick's (1984) model suggests that contingency models can have practical value. Their model is based on the finding that managers can vary in their beliefs about the environment and in their intrusiveness into and active search of the environment. In the same way, project teams can be categorized according to their interpretation modes, i.e. the process through which information about the context and task is given meaning and an approach is chosen. Figure 8.3 depicts four categories of interpretation behaviour, based on the two dimensions. It follows that a contingency model can help project teams (a) to interpret the context in an active way, and (b) to experience the context as analysable (interpretation mode 4).

First, a contingency model can tell them which contextual factors will give rise to which risks, although the assessment of these risks cannot be quantified in advance by giving objective, absolute scales to compute them. The project team members will have to interpret the situation in an active way: how can we define, influence, interpret a part of reality in such a way that it becomes manageable? In line with our arguments put forward earlier, our hypothesis would be that passive

ASSUMPTIONS ABOUT ENVIRONMENT	1. Muddling through	2. Experimental matching of context and approach
Unanalyzable	Undirected viewing: constrained interpretations nonroutine, informal data hunch, rumor, change, opportunities	Enacting: experimentation, testing, coercion, invent environment learn by doing
	3. Standard method with options	4. Project diagnosis and definition
Analyzable	Conditioned viewing: interprets within traditional boundaries, passive detection, routine, formal data	Discovering: formal search, questioning, surveys, data gathering, active detection
	Passive	Active

PROJECT TEAMS INTRUSIVENESS

Figure 8.3 Project teams interpretation modes in management approach formation. Adapted from Daft & Weick (1984)

interpretation (modes 1 and 3) is not feasible, where the objective is some form of innovation (as stated previously, the choices at the strategic level, definition and orientation, are decisive for the possible outcomes of the innovation process). Second, contingency guidelines may help the project team to choose a suitable approach. In relation to this, Van Offenbeek (1993) found that the risk profile sometimes changes substantially during the process. Project teams will have to rediagnose the contingency factors and if necessary adapt their management approach at regular intervals, as well as in cases of sudden critical changes in the context.

However, the issues raised here should be examined further in future research. This will be especially interesting with regard to the interaction among participants in innovative projects. We have said that, from a psychological point of view, the actual performance of the innovation task (Table 8.2) consists of social interaction (in contrast with work activities like designing, computing, building). This is important because it is through interaction that organizational structure and thereby organizational reality are created (e.g. Giddens, 1982). The existing structure constrains interaction by its rules and resource allocation and, because of this, innovation is difficult to accomplish. At the same time, social interaction becomes translated into significant structures when participants use interpretative schemes to make sense of what they say and do (Weick & Browning, 1986). These structures both enable and constrain subsequent interaction and interpretation. In so far as innovation encompasses changes in the social or organizational structure, innovation is realized by social interaction. Laboratory studies and experimental field studies of interaction in simple work settings are not sufficient to capture these processes. They should be complemented wit more intensive case studies of the functioning of project teams, although these alone will not lead to results that are generally applicable (Weick, 1979).

REFERENCES

Algera, J.A. & Koopman, P.L. (1989). Coping with new technology: central issues in perspective. *Applied Psychology: An International Review*, **38**, 1.

Algera, J.A., Koopman, P.L. & Vijlbrief, H.P.J. (1989). Management strategies in introducing computer-based information systems. *Applied Psychology: An International Review*, **38**, 1.

Argyris, C. (1992). *On Organisational Learning*. Cambridge, MA: Blackwell.

Argyris, C. & Schön, D.A. (1978). *Organisational Learning: A Theory of Action Perspective*. Reading, MA: Addison-Wesley.

Arnold, J., Cooper, C.L. & Robertson, I.T. (1995). *Work Psychology: Understanding Human Behaviour in the Work Place*. London: Pitman.

Ashmos, D.P., McDaniel, R.R. & Duchon, D. (1990). Differences in perception of strategic decision-making processes: the case of physicians and administrators. *Journal of Applied Behavioral Science*, **26**(2), 201–218.

Axelson, R. & Rosenberg, L. (1979). Decision-making and organizational turbulence. *Acta Sociologica*, **22**, 45–62.

Bacharach, S.B. & Lawler, E.J. (1980). *Power and Politics in Organizations*. San Francisco: Jossey-Bass.

Bandura, A. (1977). *Social-Learning Theory*. Englewood Cliffs, NJ: Prentice-Hall.
Bandura, A. (1986). *Social Foundations of Thought and Action: A Social Cognitive Theory*. Englewood Cliffs, NJ: Prentice-Hall.
Bandura, A. (1990). Perceived self-efficacy in the exercise of personal agency. *Applied Sports Psychology*, **2**, 128–163.
Barrett, F.J. & Cooperrider, D.L. (1990). Generative metaphor intervention: a new approach for working with systems divided by conflict and caught in defensive perception. *Journal of Applied Behavioral Science*, **26**(2), 219–239.
Blackler, F.H.M. (1990). Technological choice and organisational cultures; applying Unger's theory of social reconstruction. Paper for the Siofok Workshop "Technological Change Process and its Impact on Work", Hungary.
Blackler, F.H.M. & Brown, C. (1986). Alternative models to guide the design and introduction of the new information technologies into work organisations. *Journal of Occupational Psychology*, **59**, 287–313.
Bouwen, R. & Fry, R. (1991). Organisational innovation and learning: four patterns of dialogue between the dominant logic and the new logic. *International Studies in Management and Organisation*, **21**(4), 37–51.
Burns, R.N. & Dennis, A.R. (1985). Selecting the appropriate application. *Data Base*, **Fall**, 19–23.
Carnall, C.A. (1990). *Managing Change in Organizations*. New York: Prentice-Hall.
Checkland, P. (1981). *Systems Thinking, Systems Practice*. Chichester: Wiley.
Child, J. (1987). Managerial strategies, new technology, and the labor process. In: J.M. Pennings & A. Buitendam (eds), *New Technology as Organisational Innovation: The Development and Diffusion of Microelectronics*. Cambridge, MA: Ballinger, pp. 87–115.
Ciborra, C.U. & Lanzara, G.F. (1989). Designing networks in action; formative contexts and post-modern system development. Paper presented at the 6th Network Workshop Telematics and Work, Bad Homburg, April 13–15.
Clegg, C. & Symon, G. (1989). *A Review of Human-centred Manufacturing Technology and a Framework for its Design and Evaluation*. Memo No. 1036, Sheffield University.
Cressey, P. (1989). *Trends in Employee Participation and New Technology*. University of Glasgow: Working Paper.
Daft, R.L. & Weick, K.E. (1984). Toward a model of organisations as interpretation systems. *Academy of Management Review*, **9**(2), 284–295.
Davis, G.B. & Olson, M.H. (1985). *Management Information Systems: Conceptual Foundations and Development*. New York: McGraw-Hill.
Duff, A.R., Robertson, I.T., Phillips, R.A. & Cooper, M.D. (1994). Improving safety by the modification of behaviour. *Construction Management and Economics*, **12**, 67–78.
Earley, P.C., Conolly, T. & Ekegren, G. (1989). Goals, Strategy development and task performance: some limits on the efficacy of goal-setting. *Journal of Applied Psychology*, **74**, 24–33.
Eisenhardt, K.M. (1989). Making fast strategic decisions in high-velocity environments. *Academy of Management Journal*, **32**, 543–576.
Episkopou, D.M. & Wood-Harper, A.T. (1986). Towards a framework to choose appropriate IS approaches. *The Computer Jounral*, **29**(3), 222–228.
Erez, M. (1992). Work motivation from a cross-cultural perspective. *Proceedings of the XIth International Congress IACCP*, July 14–18, Liege, Belgium.
Erez, M., Earley, P.C. & Hulin, C.L. (1985). The impact of participation on goal acceptance and performance: a two-step model. *Academy of Management Journal*, **28**, 50–66.
Farr, J.L., Hofman, D.A. & Ringenbach, K.L. (1993). Goal orientation and action control theory: implications for industrial and organizational psychology. In: I.T. Robertson & C.L. Cooper (eds), *International Review of Industrial and Organizational Psychology*, Vol. 8. Wiley: Chichester.

Fiedler, F.E. (1978). The contingency model and the dynamics of the leadership process. In L. Berkowitz (ed.), *Advances in Experimental Social Psychology*, Part II. New York: Academic Press.
Flood, R.L. & Jackson, M.C. (1991). *Creative Problem-solving: Total Systems Intervention.* Chichester: Wiley.
Frank, A. & Brownell, J. (1989). *Orangisational Communication and Behavior.* New York/London: Holt, Rinehart & Winston.
French, W.L. & Bell, C.H. (1990). *Organisation Development: Behavioral Science Interventions for Organisation Improvement.* Englewood Cliffs, NJ: Prentice-Hall.
Galbraith, J.R. (1973). *Designing Complex Organizations.* Reading, MA: Addison-Wesley.
Giddens, A. (1982). Action, Structure, Power. In A. Giddens (ed.), *Profiles and Critiques in Social Theory.* London: MacMillan, pp. 28–39.
Gils, M.R. van (1993). Interorganisationele netwerken. In P.J.D. Drenth, H. Thierry & C.J. de Wolf (eds), *Nieuw Handboek Arbeids- and Organisatie-psychologie.* Deventer: Van Loghum Slaterus, pp. 4.4.1–4.4.42.
Goedvolk, J.G. & Smeets, J.J. (1991). Computers en evolutie, een nieuwe basis voor systeemontwerp. *Informatie*, **33**(1), 1–64.
Goodman, P.S. (1986). *Designing Effective Work Groups.* San Fransisco: Jossey-Bass.
Grandori, A. (1984). A prescriptive contingency view of organisational decision-making. *Administrative Science Quarterly*, **29**, 192–209.
Guzzo, G.A. & Shea, G.P. (1992). Group performance and intergroup relations in organisations. In M.D. Dunnette & L.M. Hough (eds), *Handbook of Industrial and Organizational Psychology*, Vol. 3. Palo Alto, CA: Consulting Psychologists' Press.
Hackman, J.R. (1992). Group influences on individuals and organisations. In M.D. Dunnette & L.M. Hough (eds), *Handbook of Industrial and Organizational Psychology*, Vol. 3. Palo Alto, CA: Consulting Psychologists' Press.
Hackman, J.R. & Lawler, E.E. (1971). Employee reactions to job characteristics. *Journal of Applied Psychology Monograph*, **55**, 259–286.
Hackman, J.R. & Morris, C. (1975). Group tasks, group interaction processes and group performance effectiveness: a review and proposed integration. In L. Berkowitz (ed.), *Advances in Experimental Social Psychology*, Vol. 8. London: Academic Press.
Hartwig, R. (1978). Rationality and the problems of administrative theory. *Public Administration*, **5**, 159–179.
Heemitra, F.J. (1990). Software outwikkleing beheersen en onzekerheid. *Informatie*, **32**, 192–200.
Heller, F.A., Drenth, P.J.D., Koopman, P.L. & Rus, V. (1988). *Decisions in Organisations: A Three-country Comparative Study.* London: Sage.
Hickson, D.J., Butler, R.J., Cray, D., Mallory, G.R. & Wilson, D.C. (1986). *Top Decisions: Strategic Decision-making in Organisations.* Oxford: Basil Blackwell.
Hirschheim, R. & Klein, H.K. (1989). Four paradigms of information system development. *Communications of the ACM*, **32**(10), 1199–1216.
House, R.J. (1988). Power and personality. *Research in Organisational Behavior*, **10**, 305–357. Greenwich: JAI Press.
IDE-International Research Group (1993). *Industrial Democracy in Europe Revisited.* Oxford: Oxford University Press.
Ives, B. & Olson, M.H. (1984). User involvement and MIS success; a review of research. *Management Science*, **30**, 586–603.
Janis, I.L. (1989). *Crucial Decisions: Leadership and Policymaking in Crisis Management.* New York: Free Press.
Kanfer, R. (1992). Work motivation: new directions in theory and research. In I.T. Robertson & C.L. Cooper (eds), *International Review of Industrial and Organizational Psychology*, **7**, Chichester: Wiley.

Kanfer, R. & Ackerman, P.L. (1989). Motivation and cognitive abilities: an integrative\aptitude-treatment interaction approach to skill acquisition. *Journal of Applied Psychology*, **74**, 657–690.
Kanter, R.M. (1983). *The Change Masters: Corporate Entrepeneurs at Work*. New York: Simon & Schuster.
Keller, W.J. (1990). *Automatisering: Kunst of Vliegwerk?* Inaugurele rede bij aanvaarding van het hoogleraarschap in de Kwantitatieve Informatica. Amsterdam: Vrije Universiteit.
Kotter, J.P. & Schlesinger, L.A. (1979). Choosing strategies of change. *Harvard Business Review*, **57**, 106–113.
Koopman, P.L. (1988). *Tussen Beheersing en Betrokkenheid: Management als Kunst van het Balanceren*. Alphen a/d Rijn, The Netherlands: Samson.
Koopman, P.L. (1992). Between economic-technical and socio-political rationality: multi-level decision making in a multinational organization. *The Irish Journal of Psychology*, **13**, 32–50.
Koopman, P.L. & Algera, J.A. (1990). Automatisering: sociaal-organisatorische aspecten. In P.J.D. Drenth, H. Thierry & C.J. de Wolf (eds), *Nieuw Handboek Arbeids- and Organisatie-psychologie*. Deventer: Van Loghum Slaterus, pp. 4.12.1–4.12.57.
Koopman, P.L. & Pool, J. (1990). Decision making in organisations. In C.L. Cooper & I.T. Robertson (eds), *International Review of Industrial and Organisational Psychology*, Vol. 5. Chichester: Wiley, pp. 101–148.
Koopman, P.L. & Pool, J. (1991). Management dilemmas in reorganisations. *European Work and Organisational Psychologist*, **1**(4), 225–244.
Koopman, P.L. & Wierdsma, A.F.M. (1988). Participatief management. In P.J.D. Drenth, H. Thierry, P.J. Willems & C.J. de Wolf (eds), *Nieuw Handboek Arbeids- and Organisatie-psychologie*. Deventer: Van Loghum Slaterus, pp. 3.3.1–3.3.34.
Korteweg, S.M. (1988). De procesdimensie bij automatisering. *M & O Tijdschrift voor Organisatie-kunde en Sociaal Beleid*, **42**(2), 75–87.
Latham, G.P. (1974). Assigned versus Participative Goal-setting: A Contingency Approach to Worker Motivation. Doctoral dissertation, University of Ohio: Akron.
Leavitt, H.J. (1965). Applied organisational change in industry: structural, technological and humanistic approaches. In J.G. March (ed.), *Handbook of Organisations*. Chigaco: Rand-McNally, pp. 1144–1170.
Locke, E.A. & Latham, G.P. (1990a). Work motivation: the high performance cycle. In U. Kleinbeck & H. Thierry (eds), *Work Motivation*. Hillsdale, NJ: Erlbaum.
Locke, E.A. & Latham, G.P. (1990b). *A Theory of Goal-setting and Task Performance*. Englewood Cliffs, NJ: Prentice-Hall.
Locke, E.A. & Schweiger, U.M. (1979). Participation in decision-making: one more look. In B. Staw (ed.), *Research in Organisational Behavior*. Greenwich, CT: Jai Press, pp. 265–339.
Markus, M.L. (1983). Power, politics and MIS Implementation. *Communication of the ACM*, **26**, 430–444.
Mastenbroek, W.F.G. (1982). *Conflicthantering en Organisatie-ontwikkeling*. Alphen a/d Rijn, The Netherlands: Samson.
McFarlan, F.W. (1981). Portfolio approach to information systems. *Harvard business review*, **59**(5), 142–150.
McMillan, C.J. (1980). Qualitative models of organizational decision-making. *Journal of General Management*, **5**, 22–39.
Miner, J.B. (1992). *Industrial-Organizational Psychology*. New York: McGraw-Hill.
Mintzberg, H. (1979). *The Structuring of Organisations*. Englewood Cliffs, NJ: Prentice-Hall.
Mintzberg, H. (1983). *Power In and Around Organisations*. Englewood Cliffs, NJ: Prentice-Hall.

Moscovici, S. (1985). Social influence and conformity. In G. Lindzey & E. Aronson (eds), *The Handbook of Social Psychology*. New York: Random House.
Moscovici, S. & Mugny, G. (1983). Minority influence. In P.B. Paulus (ed.), *Basic Group Processes*. New York: Springer-Verlag.
Mumford, E. (1983). *Designing Human Systems for New Technology: The ETHICS Method*. Manchester: Manchester Business School.
Nadler, D.A., Hackman, R.J. & Lawler, E.E. (1979). *Managing Organisational Behavior*. Cambridge: Harvard University Press.
Naumann, J.D., Davis, G.B. & McKeen, J.D. (1980). Determining information requirements: a contingency method for selection of a requirements assurance strategy. *The Journal of Systems and Software*, **1**, 273–281.
Nemeth, C.J. (1986). Differential contributions of majority and minority influence, *Psychological Review*, **93**, 23–32.
Nijhof, H. (1990). *Projectdiagnose*. Afstudeerscriptie, Enschede: Hogeschool Enschede, Management Informatica.
Olson, E.E. (1990). The transcendent function in organisational change. *The Journal of Applied Behavioral Science*, **26**(1), 69–81.
van Oostrum, J. & Rabbie, J.M. (1988). Inspraak en effectiviteit; een contingentiebenadering. *Gedrag en Organisatie*. **1**(2), 55–70.
Payne, R. & Cooper, C.L. (eds) (1981). *Groups at Work*. Chichester: Wiley.
Perrow, C. (1970). *Organisational Analysis: A Sociological View*. London: Wadsworth, Tavistock.
Pfeffer, J. (1981). *Power in Organisations*. Boston: Pitman.
Pritchard. R.D., Jones, S.D., Roth, P.L., Stuebing, K.K. & Ekeberg, S.E. (1988). Effects of group feedback, goal-setting, and incentives on organizational productivity. *Journal of Applied Psychology*, **73**, 337–358.
Pruitt, D.G. & Rubin, J.Z. (1986). *Social Conflict: Escalation, Stalemate and Settlement*. New York: Random House.
Rockart, J.F. & Short, J.E. (1989). IT in the 1990s: Managing Organisational Interdependence. *Sloan Management Review*, **Winter**, 7–17.
Ross, W.H. (1990). An experimental test of motivational and content control on dispute mediation. *The Journal of Applied Behavioral Science*, **26**(1), 111–118.
Shomenta, J., Kamp, G., Hanson, B. & Simpson, B. (1983). The application approach work-sheet: an evaluative tool for matching new development methods with appropriate applications. *MIS Quarterly*, **December**, 1–10.
Schonberger, R.J. (1980). MIS design: a contingency approach. *MIS Quarterly*, **March**, 13–20.
Schwenk, C.R. (1988). *The Essence of Strategic Decision Making*. Massachusetts: D.C. Heath & Co.
Swieringa, J. & Wierdsma, A.F.M. (1992). *Becoming a Learning Organisation*. Wokingham, Berkshire: Addison-Wesley.
Thierry, H. (1991). Motivatie en satisfactie. In P.J.D. Drenth, H. Thierry & C.J. de Wolff, *Nieuw Handboek Arbeids- en Organisatiepsychologie*. Deventer: van Loghum Slaterus.
Thompson, J.D. & Tuden, A. (1959). Strategies, strutures, and processes of organisational decision, In J.D. Thompson, P.B. Hammond, R.W. Hawkes, B.H. Junker & A. Tuden (eds), *Comparative Studies in Administration*. Pittsburgh: Pittsburgh University Press.
Thompson, J.D. (1967). *Organizations in Action*. New York: McGraw-Hill.
Tubbs, M.E. (1986). Goal setting: a meta-analytical examination of the empirical evidence. *Journal of Applied Psychology*, **71**, 474–483.
Vaas, S. (1988). A model approach towards industrial automation. Paper presented at the onconference "Joint design of technology organization and people's growth". Venice, October, 12–14.

Vaas, S. (1988). The myth of technology? A reaction to the human-centred approach by Clegg and Symon. Paper presented at the symposium "Psychology of Work and Organization: Design-oriented Research", at the First European Congress of Pscyhology, Amsterdam, July.

van de Ven, A.H. (1986). Central problems in the management of innovation. *Management Science*, **5**, 590–607.

van de Ven, A.H., Emmett, D.C. & Koenig, R. Jr (1974). Frameworks for interorganisational analysis. *Organisation and Administrative Sciences*, **5**(1), 113–130.

Van Offenbeek, M.A.G. (1993). *Van methode naar scenario's*. Amsterdam: Proefschrift, Vrije Universiteit.

Vroom, V.H. & Jago, A.G. (1988). *The New Leadership: Managing Participation in Organizations*. Englewood Cliffs, NJ: Prentice-Hall.

Vroom, V.H. & Yetton, P. (1973). *Leadership and Decision-making*. Pittsburgh: University of Pittsburgh Press.

Vijlbrief, H.P.J., Algera, J.A. & Koopman, P.L. (1986). Management of automation projects. Second West-European Conference on the Psychology of Work and Organisation, Aachen.

Weick, K.E. (1979). *The Social Psychology of Organizing*. Philippines: Addison-Wesley.

Weick, K.E. & Browning, L.D. (1986). Argument and narration in organizational communication. In J.G. Hunt & J.D. Blair (eds), *Yearly Review of Management of the Journal of Management*, **12**(2), 243–259.

Weitzel, J.R. & Kerschberg, L. (1989). Developing knowledge-based systems: reorganizing the system development life cycle. *Communications of the ACM*, **32**(4), 482–488.

Wissema, J.G., Messer, H.M. & Wijers, G.J. (1988). *Angst voor veranderen? Een mythe*! Assen: Van Gorcum.

Wood, R., Mento, A. & Locke, E. (1987). Task complexity as a moderator of goal effects: A meta-analysis. *Journal of Applied Psychology*, **72**, 416–425.

Yukl, G. (1994). *Leadership in Organizations*. Englewood Cliffs, NJ: Prentice-Hall.

Chapter 9

Group Leadership: a Levels of Analysis Perspective

Francis J. Yammarino
State University of New York, Binghamton, USA

Abstract

Numerous explanations for understanding the nature of leadership in groups are available in the literature. A common feature of these views is that each one is based implicitly on a particular level of analysis. The purpose of this chapter is to clarify and integrate various theories, models, and frameworks of group leadership by explicitly focusing on multiple levels of analysis. A general conceptual approach to levels of analysis is presented that includes two views of both groups and dyads, a special case of groups. For the *group* level, where the entire group or team is of concern, focus can be on whole groups and how groups differ from one another; or on group parts and the interdependent individuals and superior–subordinate dyads which comprise groups. For the *dyad* level, where interpersonal relationships are of concern, focus can be on whole dyads and balanced/equitable superior–subordinate relationships; or on dyad parts and unbalanced/inequitable relationships within superior–subordinate dyads. By considering dyads and groups concurrently, *cross*- or *multi*-level views are plausible. Balanced interpersonal relationships (whole dyads) can evolve into groups (viewed as wholes or parts), so "aggregated" approaches to group leadership can be clarified. Employing this multiple levels of analysis framework, key formulations involving inspirational (transformational, charismatic, visionary), instrumental (transactional, exchange, contingent reward), and informal (emergent, elected, non-appointed) group leadership theories are reviewed and integrated. Implications of the ideas for theoretical development and testing of group leadership theories as well as managerial practice are discussed.

Handbook of Work Group Psychology. Edited by M.A. West.
© 1996 John Wiley & Sons Ltd.

INTRODUCTION

Numerous explanations for understanding the nature of leadership in groups are available in the extant literature (for reviews, see Bass, 1990; Clark & Clark, 1994; Hollander, 1985; Hughes, Ginnett & Curphy, 1993; Yukl, 1994; Yukl & Van Fleet, 1992). Although these approaches are quite different from one another, a common feature is that each view is based implicitly on a particular level of analysis. Even when the focus is limited to *group* leadership, the levels of analysis involved in various approaches may focus on groups *per se*, dyads (a special case of groups), some combination of dyads and groups, and/or different views of dyads and groups. As such, not one but *multiple* levels of analysis are involved.

Purpose

The objective of this chapter is to clarify and integrate various theories, models and frameworks for understanding group leadership by explicitly focusing on multiple levels of analysis. Toward this end, a general conceptual approach to levels of analysis—developed by Dansereau, Alutto & Yammarino (1984)—is presented. Using this framework, two very different levels of analysis views of groups (whole groups and group parts), of dyads (whole dyads and dyad parts), and of multiple-level approaches (whole dyads-to-whole groups and whole dyads-to-group parts) are developed. This explicit levels of analysis framework is then employed to review, clarify and integrate group leadership theories and models. To focus the discussion, key leadership formulations, based on about 7500 studies of leadership (see Bass, 1990), are viewed as *inspirational* (i.e. transformational, charismatic, visionary), *instrumental* (i.e. transactional, exchange, contingent reward and punishment), or *informal* (i.e. emergent, elected, non-appointed) in nature. The combination of this tripartite view of leadership theories *and* multiple levels of analysis permits the specification of a comprehensive framework for synthesizing the group leadership literature.

Definitions and Scope

Prior to developing these ideas, it seems useful to specify some working definitions of key concepts as well as the scope and limits of the current discussion. To begin, there are literally hundreds of definitions of *leadership* available in the literature (Bass, 1990; Yukl, 1994). While these definitions vary considerably, most involve the ability of an individual (e.g. leader, superior, supervisor) to get others (e.g. followers, subordinates, groups) to accomplish things (e.g. goals, tasks, objectives) willingly in a particular situation. For the present purposes, compatible with prior work, this definition can be stated formally as:

> *Leadership* is a set of observable activities that occur in a group comprising a leader and followers who willingly subscribe to a shared purpose and work jointly to accomplish it.

This working definition permits the specification of additional relevant terms and the limits of the present chapter. In particular, the activities are asserted to be "observable", so the functions served by leaders for their followers are not accomplished by means other than the leaders' behavior. As such, substitutes for leadership (e.g. Kerr & Jermier, 1978; Podsakoff & MacKenzie, 1995) or leadership viewed as an illusory, symbolic or romantic phenomenen (e.g. Meindl & Ehrlich, 1987; Meindl, 1995) are excluded from the discussion (cf. Yammarino & Dubinsky, 1992).

Relatedly, the discussion is limited to "group leadership", or simply, *leadership in groups*. As a result, various individual differences views of leadership (e.g. Lord, Foti & DeVader, 1984; Phillips & Lord, 1981; Eden & Leviatan, 1975; see also Kim & Yukl, 1995) as well as collective, systems or organizational views of leadership (e.g. Gomez-Mejia, Tosi & Hinkin, 1987; Hunt & Osborn, 1978; Hunt, 1991; Hunt & Ropo, 1995; Tosi, 1992) are not a focus of the current discussion. This strategy is not meant to imply that these views are unimportant; rather, that they do not involve groups *per se* (see Yammarino & Bass, 1991; Yammarino & Dubinsky, 1992; and Dansereau, Yammarino & Markham, 1995, for a discussion of these views).

The notion of *group* used in this chapter, however, is rather broad-based (see Miller, 1978). It includes all traditional views of groups, whether small groups in laboratory research or groups in organizations and field research. "Teams" also are included in the view of groups here, and the terms "group" and "team" can be used interchangeably in the current presentation. Stated more formally:

> *Groups* are defined as a collective of individuals who are interdependent and interact face-to-face with one another.

A particular interest is in formal work groups comprising subordinates (followers) who report to a common immediate superior or supervisor (leader). An additional concern is:

> *Dyads*, a special case of groups, are defined as two individuals who are interdependent on a one-to-one basis.

In particular, a current focus is on superior–subordinate dyads (leader–followers dyads) both *within* groups and *independent* of their formal work groups (see below).

Overall, while the focus is on "group leadership", two levels of analysis are thus explicitly included—dyads and groups. *Levels of analysis* are the entities or objects of study; they are typically arranged in hierarchical order such that higher levels (e.g. groups) include lower levels (e.g. dyads or individuals), and lower levels are embedded in higher levels (see Dansereau, Alutto & Yammarino, 1984; Miller, 1978; Yammarino, 1995, 1996).

Beyond these single levels (i.e. dyads or groups viewed separately), a key concern is a type of multiple-level view of group leadership. In particular, *cross-level* formulations are those involving relationships among variables that are likely to hold equally well at a number of levels of analysis (e.g. x and y are positively related for both dyads and groups). Formulations of this type are uniquely powerful and parsimonious because the same effect is presumed to be manifested at more than one level of analysis (e.g. $E = mc^2$) (see Dansereau, Alutto & Yammarino, 1984; Yammarino, 1995, 1996). Therefore, some relevant leadership formulations will include both dyads and groups concurrently or simultaneously. With this perspective in mind, it is now possible to consider several levels of analysis views of group leadership, three substantive views of group leadership, and their integration and various implications.

LEVELS OF ANALYSIS VIEWS OF GROUP LEADERSHIP

Wholes and Parts

Dansereau, Alutto & Yammarino (1984) distinguish conceptually between two different views of any level of analysis (also see Lerner, 1963). First, a *whole* view is defined as a focus between entities (e.g. dyads or groups) but not within them; differences between entities are viewed as valid, and differences within entities are viewed as error (random). This can be viewed as a *between*-units case (Yammarino, 1995, 1996). In this instance, members of a unit are homogeneous, the whole unit is of importance, and relationships among members of units with respect to constructs of a theory are positive. Relationships among theoretical constructs are a function of differences between units.

Second, a *parts* view is defined as a focus within entities (e.g. dyads or groups) but not between them; differences within entities are valid, and differences between entities are erroneous. This can be viewed as a *within*-units case or a "frog pond" effect (Yammarino, 1995, 1996). In this instance, members of a unit are heterogeneous, a member's position *relative* to other members is of importance, and relationships among members of units with respect to constructs of a theory are negative. Relationships among theoretical constructs are a function of differences within units.

These two views—wholes and parts—are conceptually different ways to indicate that a particular level of analysis is relevant for understanding constructs and variables of interest. They can be thought of as two different perspectives on a particular level of analysis. As such, parts and wholes can be viewed as alternative "lenses" through which human beings, in dyads or groups, can be observed.

Group Level: Work Groups and Teams

In terms of leadership issues, a *group* (e.g. work group or team) can be viewed as a homogeneous entity (whole) displaying similar superior–subordinate relationships, but these relationships would differ from those in other groups. This view indicates that a superior displays a similar style toward each subordinate within a group; however, superiors' styles differ from one group to another. This notion is illustrated in the left portion of Figure 9.1 in which the circles, representing superiors' (e.g. SUP 1) and subordinates' (e.g. SUB 1) behaviors and perceptions, vary between the groups but are the same within the groups.

Some researchers argue that superior–subordinate (leader–follower) relationships are based on a style displayed by a superior toward an entire group of subordinates (e.g. Kerr & Schriesheim, 1974; Schriesheim & Kerr, 1977). In this work, called the *average leadership style* approach (Dansereau, Alutto & Yammarino, 1984; Dansereau, Yammarino & Markham, 1995; Yammarino, 1995, 1996; Yammarino & Dubinsky, 1992), a superior (leader) has a similar relationship with each subordinate (follower) in a group (team).

Distinct from this case is a group parts view in which superior–subordinate relationships that are managed by a superior differ within a group (parts), and

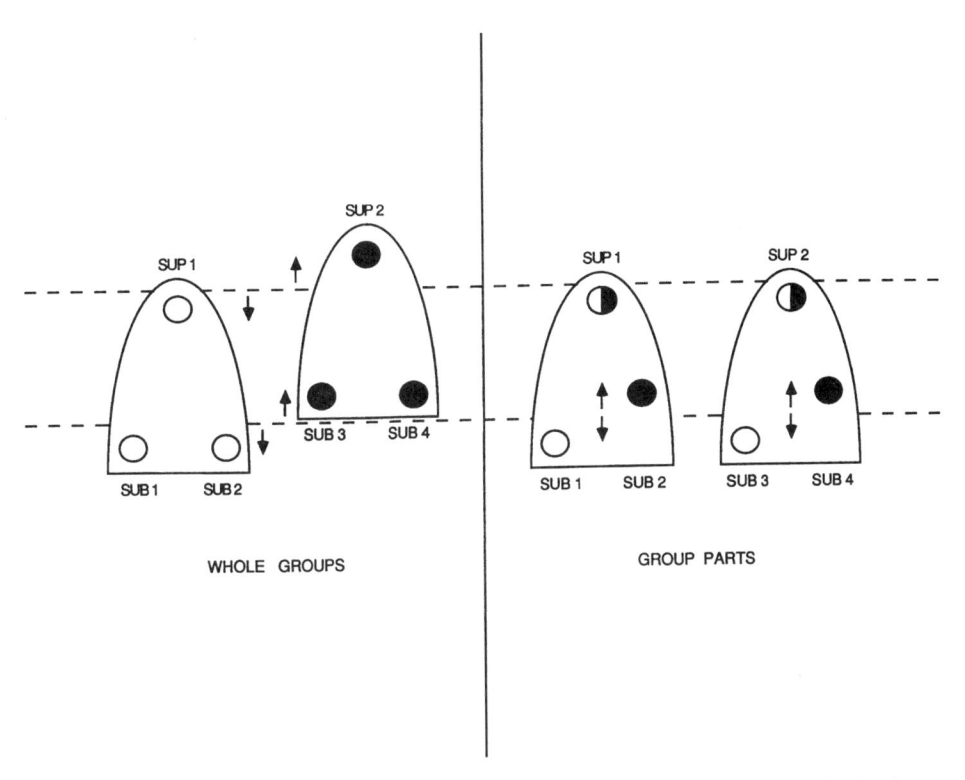

Figure 9.1 Group level of analysis—whole groups and group parts views of leadership

superiors of other groups act similarly. This implies that superiors have relatively similar behavioral repertoires, but that the specific behavior displayed in any situation (group) depends upon the particular superior–subordinate relationship. This view indicates that a superior displays differential styles toward subordinates in a group, and heterogeneity in superiors' styles is also present in other group. Thus, the nature of each relationship in the group differs, and each is managed by the superior relative to the others in the group. This notion is illustrated in the right portion of Figure 9.1, in which the circles, representing superiors' and subordinates' behaviors and perceptions, vary within the groups but are consistent across the groups. As shown in this portion of the figure, each superior has a different relationship with each subordinate (represented by a split circle for the superior and contrasting solid circles for the subordinates).

Other researchers assert that superior–subordinate (leader–follower) relationships occur on a one-to-one basis within a group (team) where the nature of each relationship differs; i.e. the superior (leader) displays a different style toward each subordinate (follower) in the group (see Dansereau, Alutto & Yammarino, 1984; Dansereau, Yammarino & Markham, 1995; Yammarino, 1995, 1996; Yammarino & Dubinsky, 1992, 1994). In this research, called the *vertical dyad linkage/leader–member exchange* approach (e.g. Graen, 1976; Dansereau, Graen & Haga, 1975; Graen, Novak & Sommerkamp, 1982; Graen & Scandura, 1987), the focus is on dyads *within* a group; the relationships are controlled, managed, or influenced by a superior (leader); and superiors are linked more closely with some subordinates/followers (in-group) than with others (out-group)—a relative notion.

Dyad Level: Interpersonal Relationships

Researchers also have focused on superior–subordinate (leader–follower) relationships from a purely dyadic or interpersonal perspective *independent* of groups or teams (Dansereau, Alutto & Yammarino, 1984; Yammarino, 1996; Yammarino & Dubinsky, 1992, 1994; Dansereau, Yammarino & Markham, 1995; Hollander, 1958, 1985). In this work, independent, one-to-one relationships (dyads) are viewed as not influenced by, nor dependent on, group membership of superior (leader) and subordinate (follower). This *independent* dyadic approach, different from the dyads within groups approach discussed above, involves mutual influence of superior (leader) and subordinate (follower) in each dyad. Dyads are not controlled solely by the superior (leader), neither are dyads relatively positioned within a group; dyads are viewed independent of groups.

Continuing with the notion of leadership at a *dyad* level (e.g. interpersonal relationships), whole dyads would refer to a focus on an independent dyad as a homogeneous entity. Some superior–subordinate dyads show stronger relationships than others, and individuals' perceptions or behaviors within a dyad are

GROUP LEADERSHIP

similar to one another. This view indicates that a superior–subordinate relationship is balanced, equitable, or composed of similar individuals (see Yammarino & Dubinsky, 1992, 1994); however, relationships differ from one another. This notion is illustrated in the left portion of Figure 9.2 in which the circles, representing superiors' and subordinates' behaviors and perceptions, vary between the dyads but are the same within the dyads. As shown in this portion of the figure, each superior has an independent relationship (represented by separate rectangles) with each subordinate.

In this case, a superior–subordinate (leader–follower) relationship can be viewed as equitable or balanced (Adams, 1965; Heider, 1958), as composed of similar individuals (Byrne, 1971; Wexley et al., 1980; Hall & Lord, 1995), or drawing on credit balances to induce equity between the individuals involved (Hollander, 1958). Perceived similarity and equity may be more important than actual similarity and equity. These views can be called *balanced interpersonal* relationships (Yammarino & Dubinsky, 1992, 1994). Within each dyad there is superior–subordinate (leader–follower) agreement or consensus.

In contrast, yet also at a dyad level, processes within an independent dyad would be the focus in a dyad parts view. That is, a superior's and subordinate's

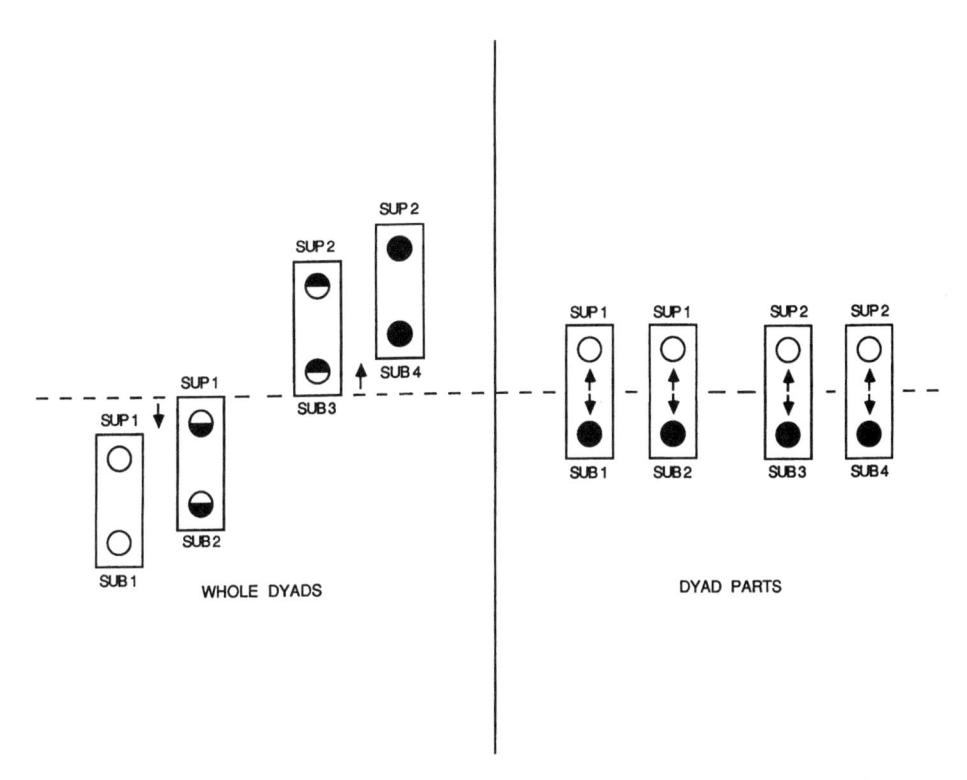

Figure 9.2 Dyad level of analysis—whole dyads and dyad parts views of leadership

perceptions or behaviors differ from one another in a superior–subordinate dyad, and these differences also are present in other superior–subordinate dyads. This view indicates that a superior–subordinate relationship is unbalanced, inequitable, or composed of dissimilar individuals (see Yammarino & Dubinsky, 1992, 1994); and other superior–subordinate relationships also are heterogeneous. This notion is illustrated in the right portion of Figure 9.2 in which the circles, representing superiors' and subordinates' behaviors and perceptions, vary within the dyads but are consistent across the dyads.

In this instance, a superior–subordinate (leader–follower) relationship can be viewed as inequitable or unbalanced (Adams, 1965; Berscheid, 1985), as composed of dissimilar individuals (Berscheid, 1985; Byrne, 1971; Pulakos & Wexley, 1983; Hall & Lord, 1995), or as reflecting status differences and disproportionate credit build-up between the individuals involved (Hollander, 1958). These views can be called *unbalanced interpersonal* relationships (Yammarino & Dubinsky, 1992, 1994). Within each dyad, despite the lack of superior–subordinate (leader–fellower) congruence, the individuals "agree to disagree" and remain connected interpersonally.

Multiple Levels: Cross-Level Views

Assuming only one level of analysis in a theoretical formulation or empirical study, or choosing to focus only on one level without consideration of other levels, can either ignore or mask effects or indicate effects when none exist (Lerner, 1963; Miller, 1978; Yammarino, 1995, 1996). These issues are especially important in areas such as "group leadership" when individuals (leaders and followers) are embedded within larger units such as dyads and groups.

In particular, relationships among leadership constructs may be hypothesized, and/or found empirically, to hold at higher (e.g. group) and lower (e.g. dyad) levels of analysis. These are discussed generally as a homology thesis (Miller, 1978), or empirically, as aggregated or "ecological" effects (Yammarino & Markham, 1992a). Of relevance for the present work, *cross-level* explanations (Miller, 1978; Dansereau, Alutto & Yammarino, 1984; Yammarino, 1995, 1996) specify relationships among theoretical constructs that hold equally well, or are replicated across, higher and lower levels.

Dansereau, Alutto & Yammarino (1984) have extended this work by focusing on multiple levels of analysis simultaneously *and* in conjunction with wholes and parts views of levels. In the realm of "group leadership", two cross-level formulations, cross-level wholes and cross-level parts, are especially relevant.

First, wholes at a lower level can aggregate to wholes at a higher level. Specifically, in terms of leadership issues, balanced interpersonal relationships (whole dyads) can evolve into whole groups. This whole-dyads-to-whole-groups view means that members are homogeneous with respect to the constructs of interest in all dyads and in all group; but dyads and groups differ from one another. In other words, there are between-dyads and between-groups differences, as shown in the left portion of Figure 9.2 *and* the left portion of Figure 9.1—whole groups overlay whole dyads.

This view indicates that within each superior–subordinate (leader–follower) dyad there is agreement or consensus, and the nature of superior–subordinate relationships within a particular group are similar; however, relationships differ from group to group. Whole (between) effects at the dyad level would aggregate to the group level, be homogeneous within a group (team), and superiors' (leaders') styles would vary between groups (wholes) (see Dansereau, Alutto & Yammarino, 1984; Yammarino & Dubinsky, 1992; Yammarino, 1995, 1996).

Second, wholes at a lower level can aggregate to parts at a higher level. Relevant to the leadership realm, balanced interpersonal relationships (whole dyads) can evolve into group parts. This whole-dyads-to-group-parts view means that members are homogeneous in all dyads with respect to the constructs of focus, but in all groups, there is heterogeneity as dyads within the groups differ from one another. In other words, there are between-dyads and within-groups differences, as shown in the left portion of Figure 9.2 *and* the right portion of Figure 9.1—group parts overlay whole dyads.

This view indicates that within each superior–subordinate (leader–follower) dyad there is agreement or consensus, but the nature of superior–subordinate relationships differs within groups. Whole (between) effects at the dyad level would aggregate to the group level, be heterogeneous within a group (team), and a superior (leader) would display different styles within a group relative to different subordinates (parts) (see Dansereau, Alutto & Yammarino, 1984; Yammarino & Dubinsky, 1992; Yammarino, 1995, 1996).

Summary

The levels of analysis views of group leadership discussed in this chapter are summarized in Table 9.1. Six views are identified and defined, and reference to the appropriate figures is indicated. At the group level of analysis, work groups and teams viewed as wholes and parts are specified. At the dyad level of analysis, interpersonal relationships viewed as wholes and parts are presented. In terms of multiple levels of analysis, cross-level whole-dyads-to-whole-groups and whole-dyads-to-group-parts views are specified. This levels of analysis conceptualization of groups/teams and interpersonal relationships can be used to clarify and integrate the literature on group leadership.

SUBSTANTIVE VIEWS OF GROUP LEADERSHIP

Prior to developing this integration, it is useful to briefly develop three key substantive views of group leadership. This tripart classification—instrumental,

Table 9.1 A levels of analysis conceptualization of groups and dyads

Levels of analysis	Members	Variables/constructs	Illustration
Group (Work groups/teams)			
Whole groups	Homogeneous in Groups	Between-groups differences	Figure 1—left portion
Group parts[a]	Heterogeneous in Groups	Within-groups differences	Figure 1—right portion
Dyad (Interpersonal relations)[b]			
Whole dyads	Homogeneous in Dyads	Between-dyads differences	Figure 2—left portion
Dyad parts	Heterogenous in Dyads	Within-dyads differences	Figure 2—right portion
Cross-level (dyads and groups)			
Whole-dyads-to-whole-groups	Homogeneous in dyads *and* homogeneous in groups	Between-dyads *and* between-groups differences	Figure 2—left portion *and* Figure 1—left portion
Whole-dyads-to-group-parts	Homogeneous in dyads *and* heterogeneous in groups	Between-dyads *and* within-groups differences	Figure 2—left portion *and* Figure 1—right portion

[a] Group parts includes "dyads within groups" views in which a superior manages, controls, or influences *all* dyads in a group relative to one another.
[b] Dyad level refers to *independent* dyadic (interpersonal) relationships that are *not* dependent on group membership or superior control; relationships are based on mutual influence.

inspirational, and informal views—is presented as a way to focus the discussion in this chapter and yet capture the breadth and depth of the numerous theories, models and empirical studies of group leadership (see Boss, 1990; Yammarino & Bass, 1991; Yukl, 1994; Clark & Clark, 1994; Hollander, 1985; Hughes, Ginnett & Curphy, 1993; Yukl & Van Fleet, 1992).

Instrumental Views

Instrumental views of group leadership (e.g. Likert, 1961; Fiedler, 1967; House, 1971; Schriesheim & Kerr, 1977; Yukl, 1994) are those approaches that involve a focus on transactions, exchanges and contingent rewards and punishments. These theories, models, and empirical studies tend to describe person- and task-oriented leader behaviors that are instrumental to effective follower/subordinate performance (e.g. goal-setting, coaching and the use of incentives; showing consideration; being participative, empowering and delegative).

Instrumental leaders may attempt to satisfy the current needs of followers by focusing on transactions or exchanges through contingent reward behavior. These leaders recognize follower needs and desires and clarify how those needs and desires will be met in exchange for enactment of the follower's work roles. Because rewards to followers are contingent on performance, performance–outcome expectancies are strengthened. The clarification of task requirements also may contribute to subordinates' confidence that with some degree of effort, they can succeed in accomplishing their assignments. So, effort–performance expectancies are strengthened.

The exchanges or transactions included in instrumental leadership may include both tangible (e.g. pay increases) and intangible (e.g. recognition) commodities. When the rewards are contingent on performance (rather than being non-contingent or punishment-based), effectiveness of individuals and groups is enhanced.

Included under this general classification of instrumental views of group leadership is the following work: Fiedler's contingency theory and cognitive resource theory (e.g. Fiedler, 1967, 1992; Fiedler & Garcia, 1987; Ayman, Chemers & Fiedler, 1995); Ohio State University and University of Michigan approaches (e.g. Stogdill & Coons, 1957; Likert, 1961; Kerr & Schriesheim, 1974; Katz & Kahn, 1978; Schriesheim & Kerr, 1977); social exchange based approaches (e.g. Homans, 1961; Jacobs, 1970; Hollander, 1978, 1985, 1992); Vroom–Yetton participation in decision-making (e.g. Vroom & Yetton, 1973; Vroom & Jago, 1995); path–goal theory (e.g. Evans, 1970; House, 1971, 1995; House & Mitchell, 1974); vertical dyad linkage/leader–member exchange views (e.g. Graen, 1976; Dansereau, Graen & Haga, 1975; Graen & Cashman, 1975; Katerberg & Hom, 1981; Graen & Scandura, 1987; Graen & Uhl-Bien, 1995; Graen, Novak & Sommerkamp, 1982); Podsakoff's contingent reward approach (e.g. Podsakoff & Schriesheim, 1985; Podsakoff & Todor, 1985; Podsakoff, Todor & Skov, 1982; Williams & Podsakoff, 1988); and certain dimensions or aspects of individualized leadership (e.g. Dansereau, Alutto & Yammarino, 1984; Yammarino & Dubinsky, 1992; Dansereau, 1995; Dansereau, Yammarino & Markham, 1995; Dansereau et al., 1995).

Inspirational Views

Inspirational views of group leadership (e.g. Bass, 1985; Burns, 1978; House, 1977; House & Shamir, 1993) are those approaches that involve a focus on transformation, charisma and visioning. These theories, models and empirical studies tend to describe emotional and/or ideological appeals that change individuals' work values to consider not only themselves but also the larger group (e.g. team, organization, society). Typical leader behaviors include providing an inspirational vision, communicating confidence in followers, setting challenging performance expectations, and displaying exemplary actual and symbolic behaviors and actions.

Inspirational leaders attempt to raise the needs of followers and promote the transformation of individuals, groups and organizations. These leaders arouse heightened awareness and interests in the group, increase confidence, and gradually move followers from concerns for existence to concerns for achievement and growth. Inspirational leaders engage in exemplary acts that followers interpret as involving extraordinary abilities, determination and confidence. Such leadership instils intense feelings in followers along with a desire to identify with the leader.

Inspirational leadership can achieve major changes in the attitudes and assumptions of followers and can build commitment for the group's mission. It is generally agreed the inspirational leadership includes behaviors such as identifying and articulating a vision; providing an appropriate role model for others; fostering the acceptance of group goals; setting high performance expectations; providing individualized support to followers; being intellectually challenging and stimulating; recognizing accomplishments of followers; empowering others; and taking great personal risks for the betterment of others.

Included under this general classification of inspirational views of group leadership is the following work: Burns' (1978) and Bass' (1985, 1990) views of transformational leadership (e.g. Avolio & Bass, 1988, 1995; Bass & Avolio, 1993, 1994; Yammarino & Bass, 1990a, 1990b; Waldman, Bass & Yammarino, 1990; Avolio & Yammarino, 1990; Avolio, Yammarino & Bass, 1991; Bass & Yammarino, 1991; Atwater & Yammarino, 1992, 1993; Yammarino, Spangler & Bass, 1993; Yammarino, 1994; Yammarino & Dubinsky, 1994; Yammarino, Dubinsky & Spangler, 1994); House's charismatic view (e.g. House, 1977; House, Spangler & Woycke, 1991; Klein & House, 1995); the notion of superleadership (e.g. Manz & Sims, 1987, 1989; Markham & Markham, 1995); various other charismatic views (e.g. Howell & Frost, 1989; Howell, 1988; Shamir, 1991; Graham, 1991; House & Shamir, 1993); and certain dimensions or aspects of individualized leadership (e.g. Dansereau, Alutto & Yammarino, 1984; Yammarino & Dubinsky, 1992; Dansereau, 1995; Dansereau, Yammarino & Markham, 1995; Dansereau et al., 1995).

Informal Views

Informal views of group leadership (see Hollander, 1985; Bass, 1990; Yukl, 1994) are those approaches that involve a focus on emergent, elected and non-appointed leaders. There theories, models and empirical studies tend to describe individual contributions to group/team goals, work facilitation of others, and offering support, direction and collaboration with co-workers or team members. Leader emergence, in contrast to leadership *per se*, is always a result of social interaction and consensus among members of group (team) that a particular individual, more so than another individual, can "lead" the group to attain group goals (Bass, 1990; Hollander, 1985). In other words, an individual group member becomes elevated to a position of status and leadership.

Informal leaders tend to adapt their style of performance to the needs of the group (team). If they also are elected (i.e. not appointed) leaders, their groups show increased productivity over appointed leaders. Elected and emergent leaders are considered to be more responsive to followers' needs, more interested in the group task, and more competent than appointed leaders. Elected and emergent leaders, as compared to appointed leaders, gain influence over time. Although more is expected of emergent and elected leaders in groups, they are given greater latitude to deviate and act on behalf of group goals.

The vast majority of conceptual and empirical work on informal leadership—whether emergent, elected or non-appointed—has been done by Hollander and his colleagues (see Hollander, 1958, 1978, 1985, 1992, 1993, for extensive reviews and discussion). This research shows that the conforming group member is likely to be elevated to a leadership position—"paying one's dues" results in an ability to redirect the group and make changes in group norms. Other representative views of informal leadership are reviewed thoroughly by Bass (1990), Yukl (1994), Clark & Clark (1994), and Hughes, Ginnett & Curphy (1993).

GROUP LEADERSHIP: COMBINING LEVELS OF ANALYSIS AND SUBSTANTIVE VIEWS

Having developed a multiple-level conceptualization of group leadership *and* three substantive views of group leadership, it is now possible to combine these perspectives and integrate the literature on group leadership. The overall approach is summarized in Table 9.2. Relevant and representative literature for each combination of a substantive view (instrumental, inspirational and informal) *and* a levels of analysis view (group wholes and parts, dyad wholes and parts, cross-level wholes and parts) of group leadership are shown in the table.

The intention is to *hypothesize* an appropriate location in the table classification scheme for various bodies of work. Given the paucity of empirical studies involving levels of analysis and group leadership, the entries in the table are based primarily on theoretical/conceptual work. (Where empirical research directly testing these ideas exists, research will be noted in the text below.) As such, this classification can be viewed as a set of propositions or hypotheses that can be subjected to empirical tests in future work. Alternatively, the integration in the table can be viewed as an attempt to clarify and integrate the literature on group leadership by *explicitly* accounting for levels of analysis in work which has typically ignored or only implied a level or levels of focus. While not comprehensive or a definitive statement, the ideas in Table 9.2 serve as a useful starting point for further theory development and theory testing on group leadership.

Levels of Analysis and Instrumental Leadership

Group Views

Group-level views of instrumental leadership have dominated the study of leadership since its beginning (see Bass, 1990; Yukl, 1994). Virtually all the classical

Table 9.2 A levels of analysis perspective on group leadership

Levels of analysis	Theories and models of leadership		
	Instrumental	Inspirational	Informal
Group level			
Whole groups	Average leadership style (Stogdill & Coons, 1957; Likert, 1961; Kerr & Schriesheim, 1974; Schriesheim & Kerr, 1977; Katz & Kahn, 1978)	Transformational (Bass, 1985, 1990; Burns, 1978; Bass & Avolio, 1993, 1994; Yammarino, Spangler & Bass, 1993; Yammarino, 1994)	Emergent, elected, non-appointed (see Bass, 1990; Yukl, 1994)
	Contingency and cognitive resources (Fiedler, 1967; Fiedler & Garcia, 1987; Ayman, Chemers & Fiedler, 1995)	Charismatic (House, 1977; House, Spangler & Woycke, 1991; House & Shamir, 1993; Howell & Frost, 1989; Howell, 1988; Shamir, 1991; Graham, 1991; Klein & House, 1995)	
	Participation in decision—making (Vroom & Yetton, 1973; Vroom & Jago, 1995)	Superleadership &(Manz & Sims, 1987, 1989; Markham & Markham, 1995).	
Group parts	Vertical dyad linkage/leader–member exchange (Graen, 1976; Dansereau, Graen & Haga, 1975; Graen & Scandura, 1987; Graen, Novak & Sommer Kamp, 1982; Graen & Uhl-Bien, 1995)	Transformational (Bass, 1985, 1990; Avolio & Bass, 1988; Bass & Avolio, 1993, 1994; Graen & Uhl-Bien, 1995)	Emergence (Hollander, 1958, 1978, 1985, 1992, 1993)
		Charismatic (House, 1977; House & Shamir, 1993; Klein & House, 1995)	

Social exchange (Homans, 1961; Jacobs, 1970; Hollander, 1978, 1985, 1992; Yukl, 1994)

Path–goal (Evans, 1970; House, 1971, 1995; House & Mitchell, 1974)

Contingent reward (Podsakoff & Schriesheim, 1985; Podsakoff & Todor, 1985; Podsakoff, Todor & Skov, 1982; Williams & Podsakoff, 1988).

Transformational (Bass, 1985, 1990; Burns, 1978; Bass & Avolio, 1993, 1994; Yammarino, 1994; Avolio & Bass, 1988)

Charismatic (House, 1977; House & Shamir, 1993; Klein & House, 1995)

Individualized leadership (Dansereau, Alulto & Yammarino, 1984; Yammarino & Dubinsky, 1992; Dansereau, 1995; Dansereau et al., 1995)

Emergence (Hollander, 1958, 1978, 1985, 1992, 1993)

Dyad level
Whole dyads

Balanced interpersonal (Adams, 1965; Byrne, 1971; Heider, 1958; Hollander, 1958; Hall & Lord, 1995; Wexley et al., 1980; Yukl, 1994)

Individualized leadership (Dansereau, Alulto & Yammarino, 1984; Yammarino & Dubinsky, 1992; Dansereau, 1995; Dansereau et al., 1995)

Contingency (Ayman, Chemers & Fiedler, 1995) and cognitive resources (Fiedler, 1992)

Contingent reward (Podsakoff & Todor, 1985; Podsakoff, Todor & Skov, 1982)

Table 9.2 (Continued)

Levels of analysis	Theories and models of leadership		
	Instrumental	Inspirational	Informal
Dyad parts	Unbalanced interpersonal (Adams, 1965; Berscheid, 1985; Hollander, 1958; Hall & Lord, 1995; Pulakos & Wexley, 1983; Yammarino & Dubinsky, 1992)	?????	Emergence (Hollander, 1958, 1978, 1985, 1992, 1993
Cross-level Whole-dyads-to-whole-groups	Average leadership style (see Yammarino & Dubinsky, 1992; Yammarino & Bass, 1991; Dansereau, Alulto & Yammarino, 1984)	Transformational (Bass, 1985, 1990; Burns, 1978; Bass & Avolio, 1993, 1994; Avolio & Bass, 1988, 1995; Yukl, 1994) Charismatic (House, 1977; House, Spangler & Woycke, 1991; House & Shamir, 1993; Yukl, 1994) Superleadership (see Markham & Markham 1995)	Emergent, elected, non-appointed (see Bass, 1990; Yukl, 1994)
Whole-dyads-to-group-parts	Vertical dyad linkage/leader–member exchange (see Yammarino & Dubinsky, 1992; Yammarino & Bass, 1991; Dansereau, Alulto & Yammarino, 1984) Contingent reward (Podsakoff & Schriesheim, 1985; Podsakoff & Todor, 1985; Williams & Podsakoff, 1988)	Transformational (Bass, 1985, 1990; Bass & Avolio, 1993, 1994; Avolio & Bass, 1988; Yukl, 1994) Charismatic (House, 1977; House & Shamir, 1993; Yukl, 1994)	Emergence (Hollander, 1958, 1978, 1985, 1992, 1993

and contemporary approaches to instrumental leadership can be conceptualized in terms of a group level of analysis. There is, however, a clear distinction between views of instrumental group leadership that focus on whole groups (differences between groups and leaders) and those views which focus on group parts (differences within groups and leaders).

In terms of *whole groups*, the average leadership style approaches in work from Ohio State University (see Stogdill & Coons, 1957; Kerr & Schriesheim, 1974; Schriesheim & Kerr, 1977) and University of Michigan (see Likert, 1961; Katz & Kahn, 1978) are representative. Whether interest is on consideration and initiating structure or employee-centered and job-oriented behaviors, these approaches focus on the style of the leader displayed toward the group as a whole. That is, different leaders use different leadership styles, and these styles are displayed to the entire group. Thus, the assertion is homogeneity among members in a group and differences between groups. It appears that only two studies have tested this levels of analysis hypothesis *directly*. Yammarino (1990) and Schriesheim, Cogliser & Neider (1995), however, found very limited support for the position. Rather, they determined that relationships among traditional Ohio State measures of leadership and outcomes were based primarily on individual differences of subordinates and not between-groups effects.

Contingency and cognitive resources theories (e.g. Fiedler, 1967, 1992; Fiedler & Garcia, 1987; Ayman, Chemers & Fiedler, 1995), are other approaches that appear to assert differences between groups and leaders. As such, they seem to be based on a whole groups view. Leaders' styles differ (task- or relationship-oriented), situations differ (very favorable to very unfavorable), and group effectiveness differs based on these factors. The leader displays a style toward the group as a whole, the entire group faces the same situation, and effectiveness is typically assessed in terms of group performance. To date, this level of analysis assertion has not been tested *directly*.

Another approach that appears to be based on the whole groups level of analysis is participation in decision-making (e.g. Vroom & Yetton, 1973; Vroom & Jago, 1995). Again, the key issue here appears to be the style displayed by a leader toward the group as a whole. An interesting feature is that leaders apparently are able to switch styles depending on the problem (situation) they face, but the style is exhibited toward the group. For example, with the GII style, the leader shares the problem with the subordinates as a group; they generate and evaluate alternatives together and try to reach a consensus solution. The leader acts like a chairperson and is willing to accept and implement any solution that has support of the entire group. In contrast, but again a style of the leader, with the GI style, the leader shares the problem with one subordinate. They analyze it together and arrive at a mutually satisfactory solution in an atmosphere of free and open exchange of information and ideas. Both the leader and subordinate contribute to the problem solution with the relative contribution being dependent on knowledge not authority. As a third example, with the DI style, the leader delegates the problem to one subordinate and provides the subordinate with relevant information that the leader possesses. The leader gives the subordinate responsibility for solving the problem, and the leader supports any solution generated by the subordinate. While these three styles—GII, GI, and DI—may seem to be based on whole groups, group parts, and whole dyads views, respectively, all actually involve a choice of style by the leader that he/she will manifest to the group as a whole. Future empirical research could explore whether this notion of shifting styles is solely leader-based or involves a shifting of levels of analysis in the model. Vroom & Jago (1995) imply it is the latter, but have not tested the notion *directly*.

In term of *group parts*, the vertical dyad linkage/leader–member exchange (VDL/LMX) approach (e.g. Graen, 1976; Dansereau, Graen & Haga, 1975; Graen & Scandura, 1987; Graen, Novak & Sommerkamp, 1982; Graen & Uhl-Bien, 1995) is representative. While there are some differences between the VDL and recent LMX approaches (see Dansereau, Yammarino & Markham, 1995), they can be viewed similarly for the current purposes. In these cases, dyads within groups, a group parts notion, are the focus. Superior–subordinate relationships occur within a group where the nature of each relationship differs (i.e. in-group versus out-group), relationships are controlled by the superior, and he/she displays a different style toward each subordinate in a group. While various studies claim to examine this levels of analysis issue (e.g. Katerberg & Hom, 1981), a *direct* test of the levels involved in the LMX approach has been conducted by Schriesheim (1995) and his colleagues (Schriesheim, Neider & Scandura, 1994). They generally found support for the position and determined that relationships among traditional LMX measures of leadership and outcomes were based primarily on within-groups differences.

Social exchange or transactional approaches (e.g. Homans, 1961; Jacobs, 1970; Hollander, 1978, 1985, 1992; Yukl, 1994) also appear to assert differences within groups and leaders. As such, they seem to be based on a group parts view. Hollander (1978, 1985) views leadership as the occurrence of mutually satisfying transactions among leaders and followers in a particular situation (e.g. group). His notion of idiosyncracy credit (Hollander, 1958) is exchange-based and is one explanation of the various transactions which occur. Likewise, Yukl (1994), in reviewing this body of work as well as various aspects of power and influence, discusses the reciprocal influence and exchange processes in dyads within groups. In all these cases, differentiated exchange processes in work groups and teams are the focus. However, *direct* empirical tests of this group parts level of analysis assertion are lacking in the literature.

Path–goal theory (e.g. Evans, 1970; House, 1971; House & Mitchell, 1974) also is based on a group parts level of analysis, especially focusing on dyads in groups (House, 1995). Again, the leader has a set of available behavioral styles (participative, directive, supportive, achievement-oriented) that are directed and tailored to different subordinates within a group. Thus, a leader displays differential styles within a group depending on his/her assessment of the subordinates' goals, needs and wants. In an empirical study *directly* examining this levels issue, Yammarino (1995) found strong support for the group parts level of analysis when path–goal styles were considered separately; that is, strong within-groups differences were obtained. However, when styles were related to outcomes, relationships were based primarily on individual differences of subordinates and not within-groups effects.

Another view that suggests a group parts perspective on group leadership is the contingent reward approach (e.g. Podsakoff & Schriesheim, 1985; Podsakoff & Todor, 1985; Podsakoff, Todor & Skov, 1982; Williams & Podsakoff, 1988). Again, within-groups differences (dyads within groups) are implied when performance is contingently reward by leaders in groups. In *direct* tests of this notion, Yammarino & Dubinsky (1994) and Yammarino, Dubinsky & Spangler (1994) found that relationships among contingent reward leadership and outcomes were based on individual differences of subordinates and not within-group effects. In these studies, however, measures of contingent reward leadership different from those proposed by Podsakoff and his colleagues were used.

Dyad Views

Interpersonal relationships independent of group membership—the dyad level of analysis—also have been a focus in the literature on instrumental leadership. As noted above, different from a dyads within groups view, dyadic relationships are determined by mutual influence of superior and subordinate, not solely superior control. At the dyad level, however, there is a clear distinction between views of instrumental leadership that focus on whole dyads (differences between dyads) and those views which focus on dyad parts (differences within dyads).

In terms of *whole dyads*, the balanced interpersonal view (e.g. Adams, 1965; Byrne 1971; Heider, 1958; Hollander, 1958; Hall & Lord, 1995; Wexley et al., 1980; Yukl, 1994) is representative. Whether viewed as balanced or equitable relationships, as composed of similar individuals, or drawing on credit balances to induce equity, the focus is on whole dyads and between-dyads differences. There is homogeneity within dyads. Dansereau, Alutto & Yammarino (1984) and Yammarino & Dubinsky (1992) have provided direct empirical support for the whole dyads view of instrumental leadership using dimensions typically associated with interpersonal relationships.

Building on this prior work, the individualized leadership approach (e.g. Dansereau, 1995; Dansereau, Yammarino & Markham, 1995; Dansereau et al., 1995) asserts a whole dyads view of instrumental leadership. Subordinates are independent of each other as individuals, and leaders link with subordinates on an individual basis. This one-to-one connection of individuals creates a dyadic relationship that differs from dyad to dyad. Leaders provide a sense of self-worth for subordinates as unique individuals independent of other individuals with whom they interact. In exchange, subordinates perform in a way that satisfies the leader. So, leaders and followers link in dyads. Direct empirical support for the individualized leadership view of instrumental leadership based on whole dyads is provided in numerous studies reported by Dansereau, Alutto & Yammarino

(1984), Yammarino & Dubinsky (1992), Dansereau, Yammarino & Markham (1995), and Dansereau et al. (1995).

In recent work, a whole dyads perspective on contingency theory (Ayman, Chemers & Fiedler, 1995) and cognitive resource theory (Fiedler, 1992) has been asserted. Ayman, Chemers & Fiedler (1995) note and provide evidence that a dyadic match of superior and subordinate least preferred co-worker (LPC) styles results in greater effectiveness. Also, Fiedler (1992) states and empirically supports that one situational parameter—interpersonal stress—can alter the utilization of specific cognitive resources. In particular, when interpersonal stress caused by a boss is low, leaders use their intellectual abilities but not their experience; when boss-induced stress is high, leaders use their experience but not their intelligence. The whole dyads view of contingency and cognitive resource theories seems worthy of further empirical study.

Another whole dyads assertion about instrumental leadership appears to have been made in the literature on contingent rewards (e.g. Podsakoff & Todor, 1985; Podsakoff, Todor & Skov, 1982). This view also seems to be implied in several recent views of the literature (e.g. Bass, 1990; Yukl, 1994). Yammarino & Dubinsky (1992) provide some *direct* empirical support for the view of contingent reward leadership and its relationships with various outcomes as based on whole dyads (i.e. differences between dyads).

In terms of *dyad parts*, the unbalanced interpersonal view (e.g. Adams, 1965; Berscheid, 1985; Hollander, 1958; Lord & Hall, 1995; Pulakos & Wexley, 1983) is representative. In this case, independent dyadic (interpersonal) relationships can be viewed as inequitable or unbalanced, as composed of dissimilar individuals, or as reflecting status differences and disproportionate credit build-up between individuals. While a theoretically and conceptually viable alternative, to date the *direct* empirical tests of this dyad parts level of analysis view have not been supportive (e.g. Dansereau, Alutto & Yammarino, 1984; Yammarino & Dubinsky, 1992, 1994; Yammarino, Dubinsky & Spangler, 1994; Dansereau et al., 1995).

Cross-Level Views

Yammarino & Dubinsky (1992) note that the average leadership style approaches (e.g. Ohio State University and University of Michigan) can be viewed as asserting *both* a whole dyads and whole groups view of instrumental leadership (also see Yammarino & Bass, 1991). This *whole-dyads-to-whole-groups* view indicates that within each superior–subordinate dyad there is agreement, dyads within a group are similar, but groups differ from one another (i.e. between-dyads and between-groups differences). To date, these theoretical assertions have not been supported empirically (see Dansereau, Alutto & Yammarino, 1984; Yammarino & Dubinsky, 1992; Schriesheim, Cogliser & Neider, 1995).

Relatedly, Yammarino & Dubinsky (1992) state that the VDL/LMX approaches can be viewed as hypothesizing *both* a whole dyads and group parts view of instrumental leadership (also see Yammarino & Bass, 1991). This *whole-dyads-to-group-parts* view indicates that there is agreement within each superior–subordinate dyad, but superior–subordinate relationships differ within groups (i.e. between-dyads and within-groups differences). To date, this conceptualization has not been supported empirically (see Dansereau, Alutto & Yammarino, 1984; Yammarino & Dubinsky, 1992).

Contingent reward leadership also can be interpreted from a whole-dyads-to-group-parts perspective (see Podsakoff & Schriesheim, 1985; Podsakoff & Todor, 1985; Williams & Podsakoff, 1988). The assertions here would parallel those for the VDL/LMX approaches. The empirical work of Yammarino & Dubinsky (1994) and Yammarino, Dubinsky & Spangler (1994), however, provides no support for this cross-level proposition regarding contingent reward instrumental leadership.

Summary

It is possible to assert the level of analysis associated with various approaches to instrumental leadership. Depending on the particular theory or model of leadership, whole groups or group parts, whole dyads or dyad parts, or cross-level formulations may be involved; and these can be specified based on theory. Much more empirical research the *directly* tests these levels of analysis assertions for instrumental leadership is clearly needed.

Levels of Analysis and Inspirational Leadership

Group Views

More recently, a vast amount of theory and research on group leadership has focused on inspirational leadership (see Bass, 1990; Yukl, 1994). Within this genre, conceptual and empirical work has been dominated by Bass and his colleagues on transformational leadership (e.g. Bass, 1985, 1990; Bass & Avolio, 1993, 1994; Yammarino, Spangler & Bass, 1993; Avolio & Bass, 1988, 1995) and House and his colleagues on charismatic leadership (e.g. House, 1977; House, Spangler & Woycke, 1991; House & Shamir, 1993; Klein & House, 1995). In this and other work on inspirational leadership, there has been a focus on both whole groups and group parts views.

In terms of *whole groups*, where differences between groups and leaders are the focus, there has been considerable interest on transformational (Bass, 1985, 1990; Burns, 1978; Bass & Avolio, 1993, 1994; Yammarino, Spangler & Bass, 1993; Yammarino, 1994) and charismatic (House, 1977; House, Spangler & Woycke, 1991; House & Shamir, 1993; Howell & Frost, 1989; Howell, 1988; Shamir, 1991; Graham, 1991; Klein & House, 1995) leadership as a style displayed toward a group of subordinates or followers as a whole. In very simple terms, leaders can be viewed as transformational or non-transformational (e.g. transactional); charismatic or non-charismatic; personalized or socialized charismatics (the former seeking self-interests, the latter pursuing follower interests). Likewise, based on the work of Manz & Sims (1987, 1989) on superleadership—an analogue to transformational leadership—Markham & Markham (1995) note a focus on whole groups and a style displayed toward the entire group of subordinates; there are, simply, superleaders and non-superleaders (the former develop and empower others to lead themselves; the latter do not).

This theoretical focus on a whole groups view of inspirational leadership, asserting homogeneity among group members and between-groups differences in leader styles and group effectiveness, also has been the subject of some empirical research. In a series of studies, this notion has been tested *directly* by Yammarino & Bass (1990a), Avolio & Yammarino (1990), Avolio, Yammarino & Bass (1991), Yammarino & Dubinsky (1994), and Yammarino, Dubinsky & Spangler (1994). In all this research, the whole groups view of transformational leadership as espoused by Bass and his colleagues was not supported; rather, transformational leadership was based on individual differences in perceptions of subordinates and not between-groups differences.

In terms of *group parts*, where differences within groups and leaders are the focus, transformational (e.g. Bass, 1985, 1990; Avolio & Bass, 1988; Bass & Avolio, 1993, 1994) and charismatic (e.g. House, 1977; House & shamir, 1993; Klein & House, 1995) leadership are again representative. In this case, the primary focus has been on dyads within groups, a group parts view. Again, leader–follower relationships are differentiated within a group and controlled, managed or influenced by transformational or charismatic leaders. Said more positively, transformational and charismatic leaders tailor their style to individual subordinates within a group to recognize individual follower needs and wants. So, what it takes to be seen as inspirational to one subordinate differs from what it takes to be viewed inspirationally by another. Relatedly, Graen & Uhl-Bien (1995) note that high quality dyads in groups that engage in leader–member exchange are actually exchanging "higher order commodities" as in transformational leadership. Rather than rewards for performance (instrumental leadership), inspiration for empowerment (inspirational leadership) is exchanged in the dyads within a group.

Empirical research has been conducted that tests *directly* this theoretical focus on a group parts view of inspirational leadership which asserts heterogeneity among group members and within-group differences in leader styles. The work of Yammarino & Bass (1990), Avolio & Yammarino (1990), Avolio, Yammarino & Bass (1991), Yammarino & Dubinsky (1994), and Yammarino, Dubinsky & Spangler (1994) found support for individual differences in subordinates' perceptions of transformational leadership and not for the group parts view (within-groups differences) of inspirational leadership.

Dyad Views

Inspirational leadership also has been implied to hold at the dyad level of analysis. In this case, independent interpersonal (dyadic) relationships are asserted to be a relevant focus for inspirational leadership that is transformational, charismatic or individualized in nature.

In particular, in terms of *whole dyads*, the transformational (e.g. Bass, 1985, 1990; Burns, 1978; Bass & Avolio, 1993, 1994; Yammarino, 1994; Avolio & Bass, 1988), charismatic (House, 1977; House & Shamir, 1993), and individualized leadership (Dansereau, Alutto & Yammarino, 1984; Yammarino & Dubinsky, 1992; Dansereau, 1995; Dansereau, Yammarino & Markham, 1995; Dansereau et al., 1995) approaches are representative. In all these cases, superior–subordinate dyads not dependent on group membership are of concern. Differences between dyads and agreement within dyads are implied or asserted in discussions of inspirational leadership. While the work on transformational and charismatic leadership clearly plays a role here, certain dimensions of individualized leadership, viewed as commodities of a higher order exchange, also are involved.

There is some empirical research that *directly* tests these assertions and hypotheses about whole dyads and between-dyads effects. In the transformational realm, Yammarino & Dubinsky (1994) and Yammarino, Dubinsky & Spangler (1994) found no support for this level of analysis assertion (i.e. associations among transformational leadership and subordinate outcomes were related based on individual differences). In contrast, empirical research on individualized leadership is much more promising and supportive. Specifically, Dansereau, Alutto & Yammarino (1984), Yammarino & Dubinsky (1992), Yammarino, Dubinsky & Spangler (1994), and Dansereau et al. (1995) all have found considerable evidence in numerous studies for the operation of inspiration-like aspects of individualized leadership at the whole dyads level.

In terms of *dyad parts*, the literature on inspirational leadership is silent. This author was unable to discover a suggestion or implication in the extant literature that inspirational leadership may operate at the dyad parts level of analysis. In fact, in the empirical studies noted above, no evidence was found for within-dyads differences. Apparently, inspirational leadership conceptualized at the dyad level is limited to a whole dyads view.

Cross-Level Views

In the realm of inspirational leadership, some of the literature can be viewed as suggesting a cross-level formulation (see Yammarino & Dubinsky, 1994; Yammarino, Dubinsky & Spangler, 1994). In particular, writings on transformational (e.g. Bass, 1985, 1990; Burns, 1978; Bass & Avolio, 1993, 1994; Avolio & Bass, 1988, 1995; Yukl, 1994), charismatic (e.g. House, 1977; House, Spangler & Woycke, 1991; House & Shamir, 1993; Yukl, 1994), and superleadership (e.g. Markham & Markham, 1995) can be viewed as asserting *both* a whole dyads and a whole groups view of inspirational leadership. This *whole dyads-to-whole groups* view indicates homogeneity in dyads and groups and differences between dyads and groups in terms of inspirational leadership. To date, few empirical studies testing this assertion *directly* have been conducted, and there is no supporting evidence for this cross-level effect (see Yammarino & Dubinsky, 1994; Yammarino, Dubinsky & Spangler, 1994).

In a similar way, related literature can be interpreted as suggesting *both* a whole dyads and group parts view of inspirational leadership. This *whole-dyads-to-group-parts* view seems indicated by various proponents of transformational (e.g. Bass, 1985, 1990; Bass & Avolio, 1993, 1994; Avolio & Bass, 1988) and charismatic (e.g. House, 1977; House & Shamir, 1993) leadership as well as by some reviewers of the literature (e.g. Yukl, 1994). Theoretically, homogeneity in dyads and heterogeneity in groups as well as between-dyads and within-groups differences are asserted. In the empirical studies to date that have tested this notion *directly*, Yammarino & Dubinsky (1994) and Yammarino, Dubinsky & Spangler (1994) found no support for this cross-level effect.

Summary

It is possible to assert the level of analysis associated with various approaches to inspirational leadership. Depending on the theory or model of leadership, whole groups or group parts, whole dyads (but not dyad parts), or cross-level formulations may be involved. Although these can be specified based on theory, much more empirical testing that *directly* examines these levels of analysis assertions for inspirational leadership is clearly warranted.

Levels of Analysis and Informal Leadership

Group Views

Theory and research on instrumental and inspirational leadership tend to focus on appointed leaders in formal positions in groups and organizations. A parallel stream of theory and research has developed that focuses on elected, non-appointed or emergent leaders in groups, whether informal or formal. This realm of informal leadership has been dominated by the conceptual and empirical work of Hollander (1958, 1978, 1985, 1992, 1993) and his colleagues (see also Bass, 1990; Yukl, 1994).

In extensive reviews of this work, Bass (1990) and Yukl (1994) described emergent, elected and non-appointed leaders as exhibiting a style toward a group of followers as a whole. This *whole groups* view is the same notion discussed above in terms of instrumental and inspirational leadership views. Homogeneity among followers in a group and between-groups differences can be asserted.

Clearly, the work of Hollander (1958, 1978, 1985, 1997, 1993) on leader emergence allows for the possibility of a *group parts* level of analysis to be hypothesized. In this case, as noted above for instrumental and inspirational views, the emergent leader displays a differentiated style toward subordinates within a group. Dyads within a group can be identified, and an emergent leader can have closer relationships with some than with others. Heterogeneity among followers in a group and within-groups differences can be asserted.

Dyad Views

The work of Hollander (1958, 1978, 1985, 1992, 1993) also suggests the plausibility of viewing leadership emergence at a dyad level of analysis in terms of *whole dyads* and *dyad parts*. In both cases, leader–follower dyads independent of the group can be identified that are based on mutual influence, mutual control and mutual dependence. In the former case, homogeneity in dyads and between-dyads differences are asserted; in the latter case, heterogeneity in dyads and within-dyads differences are specified. As such, this work is analogous to various instrumental and inspirational views of leadership that focus on the dyad level of analysis.

Cross-Level Views

In the realm of informal leadership, some literature also can be interpreted as suggesting cross-level formulations. In particular, reviews by Bass (1990) and Yukl (1994) of elected, non-appointed, and emergent leaders imply that this work asserts *both* a whole dyads and a whole groups view. This *whole-dyads-to-whole-groups* perspective on informal leadership means that between-dyads and between-groups differences of leaders and followers can be hypothesized. Homogeneity in dyads and groups is plausible. Relatedly, Hollander's (1958, 1978, 1985, 1992, 1993) work on leadership emergence also seems to permit *both* a whole dyads and a group parts view. This *whole-dyads-to-group-parts* perspective on informal leadership indicates that between-dyads and within-groups differences of leaders and followers can be asserted. Homogeneity in dyads and heterogeneity in groups is a possibility. Again, a set of formulations for cross-level effects involving informal leadership seem reasonable and parallels those for instrumental and inspirational leadership.

Summary

It is possible to assert the levels of analysis associated with some approaches to informal leadership. Whole groups and group parts, whole dyads and dyad parts, and cross-level formulations seem to be involved based on various theoretical or conceptual views. Hollander's research is quite suggestive of these effects, but did not explicitly account for levels of analysis in the testing procedures. Unfortunately, no empirical studies were found that tested these levels of analysis assertions *directly*.

GROUP LEADERSHIP: IMPLICATIONS

Taking a levels of analysis perspective on group leadership has permitted the integration of a vast literature on instrumental, inspirational, and informal views of leadership (see Table 9.2). At a minimum, the approach presented in this chapter seems to have some implication for future theory formulation, empirical testing and managerial practice.

Theory Development

In terms of theory formulation, the development and extension of current and future theories and models of instrumental, inspirational and informal group leadership could benefit from an explicit consideration of multiple levels of analysis (e.g. Dansereau, Alutto & Yammarino, 1984; Dansereau, Yammarino & Markham, 1995; Yammarino, 1995, 1996). By "pushing" each theoretical formulation to specifically incorporate levels of analysis, clarification of the theories and models occurs and new propositions and hypotheses for testing are generated (see Dansereau, Yammarino & Markham, 1995). Without a focus of group leadership theory on whole groups and group parts, whole dyads and dyad parts, and cross-level views, researchers do not know *precisely* what entities are involved in theoretical formulations. As such, the formulations lack a specification of boundary conditions and rigorous testing is inhibited. Group leadership theory, variables and relationships cannot be assumed to operate at a particular level of analysis; an explication of the level(s) involved is required for more complete theory development.

This approach also permits the identification of commonalities across theories and models of group leadership. For example, several instrumental, inspirational and informal theories appear to hypothesize whole groups effects. Thus, they share a common feature of a similar level of analysis. Likewise, group parts are proposed to account for several formulations in the instrumental, inspirational and informal leadership realms. Similarly, whole dyads and dyad parts, and whole-dyads-to-whole-groups and whole-dyads-to-group-parts, provide a linking mechanism across group leadership theories that are instrumental, inspirational and informal in nature. This suggests that the various theories and models may have more similarities than differences. If this notion is supported in future empirical research, than it may move the field closer to an integrative and comprehensive theory of group leadership—a unified theory that synthesizes instrumental, inspirational and informal approaches across levels of analysis.

The approach presented in this chapter suggests that different theories and models of group leadership may better explain behavior at various points in the leadership development process. Taking a longitudinal perspective, perhaps individuals' (superiors'/leaders' and subordinates'/followers') behaviors may first be explained by informal theories of group leadership. As their relationships develop, they may be better accounted for by the more formal instrumental explanations. Subsequently, when their behaviors move to yet another realm, inspirational theories of group leadership may permit greater understanding of the actions. In other words, over timeshifting behaviors and the changing nature of relationships in leadership development are explained by informal, instrumental and inspirational theories. Obviously, other scenarios are plausible and should be the subject of future longitudinal research.

Likewise, over time, different levels of analysis may better explain the nature of superior–subordinate or leader–follower relationships and the behaviors involved. From a longitudinal perspective, perhaps relationships start out formally at a group level where a superior displays the same style toward the entire group (whole groups)—all followers are treated the same. Then, over time, stronger relationships develop with some but not all followers, and these relationships are managed by the leader (group parts)—followers are treated differently relative to one another. Relationships may then develop, after another period of time, to the point where they are independent of the group (dyad level of analysis). Superiors and subordinates link independently of the groups, reach agreement or consensus on each of these one-to-one relationships (whole dyads), and some relationships are "rich" while others are "poor." These (whole) dyadic relationships could then serve as the basis for integrating entire groups or teams (whole-dyads-to-whole-groups or whole-dyads-to-group-parts). Clearly, there are other possible scenarios, and these seem worthy of testing in future longitudinal research.

Relatedly, when considering the potential types and wide range of work groups/teams and interpersonal relationships, several substantive processes may be occurring at different levels of analysis at various times. Depending on the particular circumstances, however, the specific emphasis may shift. For example, in times of crises, inspirational leadership that employs a common style toward the entire group as a whole may be required. In less stressful times, differentiated instrumental leadership styles in work groups may be appropriate. Alternatively, leaders may adopt implicit whole group-based instrumental theories to guide their behavior under pressure from the external environment and then relax into inspirational dyadic modes of operation in times of peace. Obviously, these shifting views suggest a dynamic and flexible orientation to group leadership that integrates different levels of analysis and substantive approaches depending on time, work situation, and environment.

In yet another realm, different substantive views of group leadership involving multiple levels of analysis may be required when considering cultural context. The meaning of instrumental, inspirational and informal group leadership may shift as one moves across cultural contexts (see Bass, 1990). Likewise, the meaning of, and what constitutes, a group *per se* may be different in alternative cultural contexts. An implication is that whole groups and group parts perspectives might be differentially appropriate depending on the culture involved. For example, Smith & Noakes (this volume) indicate that teams in collectivist cultures, in contrast to those in individualistic cultures, are more concerned with long-term commitment, more deferent toward authority (e.g. leadership), and more concerned with in-group harmony, but just as competitive with out-groups. This view suggests a strong whole groups perspective on leadership, whether instrumental or inspirational. Clearly, these culture-dependent notions would compound group working relations and leadership in groups that are multi-cultural in nature. Future empirical research is warranted on the relevance of the ideas proposed in the current work for various cultural contexts and multi-cultural groups and on how this approach may apply differentially in these alternative situations.

Group leadership theory development also could benefit from a consideration of other levels of analysis (e.g. those excluded at the outset of this chapter). For example, at a lower (e.g. individual) level of analysis, personality traits and characteristics of leaders and subordinates as well as knowledge, skills and abilities of leaders and followers, should influence the development of comprehensive group leadership theories that are instrumental, inspirational and informal. Likewise, at a higher (e.g. organization, social system) level of analysis, situational context and setting characteristics of organizations as well as the norms, values and culture of the large society need to be examined to formulate more complete theories of instrumental, inspirational and informal group leadership. As such, "group" leadership is not limited to groups and dyads *per se*; rather, a broader focus on *multiple* levels of analysis (individuals, dyads, groups, organizations, social systems) can enhance theory development in this area. This would seem to include drawing on theory and ideas from various disciplines that address issues at these other levels (e.g. physiology, psychology, social psychology, sociology, anthropology and political science).

Theory Testing

After clarifying and formulating theories of group leadership, the research process must move to the realm of testing the propositions and hypotheses which have been generated. If the framework presented in Table 9.2 is viewed as a set of propositions about instrumental, inspirational and informal group leadership *and* levels of analysis, then, through a series of studies, it could be subjected to empirical tests. Since multiple levels of analysis are involved, a data analytic technique that explicitly tests levels of analysis effects is required.

One multiple-level data analytic approach that can be used for testing these levels of analysis conceptualizations about group leadership is *within and between analysis* (WABA) (e.g. Dansereau, Alutto & Yammarino, 1984; Schriesheim, 1995; Schriesheim, Cogliser & Neider, 1995; Schriesheim, Neider & Scandura, 1994; Yammarino, Dubinsky & Hartley, 1987; Yammarino & Naughton, 1988, 1992, 1995; Yammarino & Dubinsky, 1990, 1992, 1994; Yammarino, Dubinsky & Spangler, 1994; Yammarino, 1990, 1994, 1995, 1996; Yammarino & Bass, 1990a, 1990b, 1991; Waldman, Yammarino & Avolio, 1990; Avolio & Yammarino, 1990; Avolio, Yammarino & Bass, 1991; Yammarino & Markham, 1992a, 1992b;

Yammarino & Waldman, 1993; Atwater & Yammarino, 1995; Dansereau et al., 1995; Klein, Dansereau & Hall, 1994; Dansereau, 1995). Although a detailed presentation of these procedures is beyond the scope of this chapter, Dansereau, Alutto & Yammarino (1984), Yammarino (1995, 1996), and Yammarino & Markham (1992a, 1992b) have thoroughly developed and illustrated WABA; and Schriesheim (1995), Schriesheim, Cogliser & Neider (1995), and Schriesheim, Neider & Scandura (1994) have developed and illustrated a multivariate extension to WABA.

In brief, WABA integrates various correlational, regression, ANOVA and ANCOVA procedures to assess both variation and covariation in variables and relationships within and between entities (levels of analysis) and across multiple levels. As such, WABA is ideally suited to test the ideas proposed in this chapter. There are three steps in WABA, regardless of the analytic level of analysis.

First, *each variable* is assessed at a particular level to determine whether the variable varies primarily between, within, or both between and within the units of interest (e.g. groups). Within-and-between etas are used to assess sources of variation, and they are tested with *F*-tests of statistical significance and *E*-tests of practical significance (magnitude of effects). These procedures are called *WABA I*.

Second, *each relationship* (whether bivariate or multivariate) among variables of interest is assessed at a particular level to determine whether the covariation among variables is primarily between, within, both between and within, or neither between nor within the focal units (e.g. groups). Between- and within-cell correlations are used to assess covariation among variables, and their differences are tested with *Z*-tests of statistical significance and *A*-tests of practical significance. Moreover, each between- and within-cell correlation is tested for statistical and practical significance using *t*- and *R*-tests, respectively. These procedures are called *WABA II*.

Third, using the WABA equation, the results of the first two steps are combined to draw an overall conclusion from the data. In particular, within and between *components*, which total to the traditional raw-score or multiple correlation, are examined to draw an inference about the level of analysis at which effects operate.

This three-step procedure can be implemented at the dyad *and* group levels and then used to test cross-level effects. In this way, the comprehensive framework proposed here to integrate instrumental, inspirational and informal theories of group leadership can be tested.

Managerial Practice

The development of an integrative framework of understanding group leadership also suggests some key implications for managerial practice. These implications arise from a focus on *both* substantive views (instrumental, inspirational, informal) *and* levels of analysis (dyads, groups, and cross-level effects).

First, managers need to avoid assuming that there is one best way which works. Multiple levels of analysis highlight the fact that what is a hindrance for the group may be an enhancement for the individual, dyad or organization. For example, satisfaction with a leader may depend on feelings of equality in reference to dyadic relationships and feelings of equity with a larger referent (e.g. work group or team). As another example, components of merit pay as controlled by a leader can be broken into a subordinate's independent contribution, contribution within the group and department, and contribution to the larger organization. Moreover, some issues such as safety may be group-wide affairs so that all leaders must show a concern; others, such as educational opportunities, may be most relevant to certain subsets of personnel or units and the leaders of these. Regardless of the issues involved, multiple levels of analysis are an important concern for practising managers.

Second, in diagnosis of whether ability, training, or motivational increases are needed for productivity improvements, or whether resources and facilities changes are needed, a more sophisticated examination becomes possible for practising managers when analyses can be completed to tease out the relative contributions of the different effects. Thus, multiple levels of analysis issues should be of concern in managerial policy formulation and implementation. Training programs, selection devices, planned change and resource allocation all require an assessment of the levels of analysis involved and the influences of levels on the desired outcome. For example, what is often presumed by management to be an individual- (person-)level policy of rewarding the meritorious employee may actually be a work group-based managerial practice of giving pay raises to meritorious groups.

Third, time and timing of managerial practices are critical and depend on levels of analysis. For example, extended training of individuals in the short run may lead to higher group performance in the long run. The diurnal cycles of individuals may enhance or inhibit the work group. For example, a manager who assigns a tight deadline to a team project may miss the goal because of time constraints on some but not all of the individuals in the group. As such, time dependencies in managerial practice also depend on multiple levels of analysis.

Fourth, managers must be cognizant of the particular dimensions of group leadership in use—instrumental, inspirational, and informal—and their focal level of analysis. For example, if leadership or its outcomes are instituted or manipulated on a group-wide basis, but subordinates perceive these notions on an individualized (dyadic) basis, managerial efforts will fail. For example, fostering subordinate motivation and performance with inspirational leadership may occur on a dyadic basis for each subordinate, while instrumental approaches to enhancing these subordinate efforts may work better on a group basis. If empirically supported, to do otherwise would seemingly be inappropriate and not improve managerial effectiveness. Clearly, other dimensions and aspects of instrumental, inspirational and informal group leadership may operate differently in terms of levels of analysis.

Fifth, the nature of training and development programs, selection devices and team-building efforts should differ based on the theory of group leadership and level of analysis involved. For example, traditional individual-focused training programs may fail to have the desired impact if the content actually involves a group leadership model that operates at the dyad and/or group level of analysis. Rather, dyad- or group-focused training programs need to be developed and delivered to units (e.g. dyads or groups) and not individuals. Likewise, traditional individual-oriented selection systems and instruments will fail to hire the "best" employees if the tasks require individuals to work in dyads or teams. Clearly, these two activities—training and selection—are critical in terms of team-building. Most current approaches to team-building are based on relevant theories and models of *group* leadership. However, members of teams are typically selected and trained as *individuals*. This mismatch of levels of analysis may explain some current failures of team-building efforts. In other words, a *theoretical* level of analysis that is supported by a matching *empirical* level of analysis effect ought to result in a corresponding *managerial practice* level of analysis policy or procedure to ensure effectiveness.

CONCLUSION

The intent of this chapter was to integrate and clarify various theories and models of group leadership by using multiple levels of analysis. Inspirational (transformational, charismatic, visionary), instrumental (transactional, exchange, contingent reward, punishment), and informal (emergent, elected, non-appointed) views of group leadership were explicated using two views of groups (whole groups and group parts), dyads (whole dyads and dyad parts), and cross-level formulations (whole-dyads-to-whole-groups and whole-dyads-to-group-parts). Employing this levels of analysis perspective on group leadership also resulted in several implications for future theory development and theory testing as well as managerial practice. The ideas presented here are offered as one small step toward the development of a comprehensive theory of group leadership.

ACKNOWLEDGEMENTS

I gratefully acknowledge discussions with and suggestions from Bernard Bass, Fred Dansereau, Robert House and Michael West that improved this chapter.

REFERENCES

Adams, J.S. (1965). Inequity in social exchange. In L. Berkowitz (ed.), *Advances in Experimental Social Psychology*, Vol. 2. New York: Academic Press, pp. 266–300.

Atwater, L.E. & Yammarino, F.J. (1992). Does self–other agreement on leadership perceptions moderate the validity of leadership and performance predictions? *Personnel Psychology*, **45**, 141–164.

Atwater, L.E. & Yammarino, F.J. (1993). Personal attributes as predictors of superiors' and subordinates' perceptions of military academy leadership. *Human Relations*, **46**, 645–668.

Atwater, L.E. & Yammarino, F.J. (1995). Bases of power in relation to leader behavior: a field investigation. *Journal of Business and Psychology*, **10**, forthcoming.

Avolio, B.J. & Bass, B.M. (1988). Transformational leadership, charisma and beyond. In J.G. Hunt, H.R. Baliga, H.P. Dachler & C.A. Schriesheim (eds), *Emerging Leadership Vistas*. Lexington, MA: Heath, pp. 29–50.

Avolio, B.J. & Bass, B.M. (1995). Individual consideration viewed at multiple levels of analysis: a multi-level framework for examining the diffusion of transformational leadership. *Leadership Quarterly*, **6**, 199–218.

Avolio, B.J. & Yammarino, F.J. (1990). Operationalizing charismatic leadership using a levels of analysis framework. *Leadership Quarterly*, **1**, 193–208.

Avolio, B.J., Yammarino, F.J. & Bass, B.M. (1991). Identifying common methods variance with data collected from a single source: an unresolved sticky issue. *Journal of Management*, **17**, 571–587.

Ayman, R., Chemers, M.M. & Fiedler, F. (1995). Contingency model of leadership effectiveness: its levels of analysis. *Leadership Quarterly*, **6**, 147–167.

Bass, B.M. (1985). *Leadership and Performance Beyond Expectations*. New York: Free Press.

Bass, B.M. (1990). *Bass & Stogdill's Handbook of Leadership*. New York: Free Press.

Bass, B.M. & Avolio, B.J. (1993). Transformational leadership: a response to critiques. In M.M. Chemers & R. Ayman (eds), *Leadership Theory and Research: Perspectives and Directions*. San Diego: Academic Press, pp. 49–88.

Bass, B.M. & Avolio, B.J. (eds) (1994). *Improving Organizational Effectiveness Through Transformational Leadership*. Thousand Oaks, CA: Sage.

Bass, B.M. & Yammarino, F.J. (1991). Congruence of self and others' leadership ratings of naval officers for understanding successful performance. *Applied Psychology: An International Review*, **40**, 437–454.

Berscheid, E. (1985). Interpersonal attraction. In G. Lindzey & E. Aronson (eds), *Handbook of Social Psychology*. New York: Random House, pp. 413–484.

Burns, J.M. (1978). *Leadership*. New York: Harper & Row.

Byrne, D. (1971). *The Attraction Paradigm*. New York: Academic Press.

Clark, K.E. & Clark, M.B. (1994). *Choosing to Lead*. Charlotte, NC: Leadership Press/ Iron Gate Press.

Dansereau, F. (1995). The dyadic approach to leadership: creating and nurturing this approach under fire. *Leadership Quarterly*, **6**, forthcoming.

Dansereau, F., Alutto, J.A. & Yammarino, F.J. (1984). *Theory Testing in Organizational Behavior: The Variant Approach*. Englewood Cliffs, NJ: Prentice-Hall.

Dansereau, F., Graen, G. & Haga, W. (1975). A vertical dyad linkage approach to leadership within formal organizations: a longitudinal investigation of the role-making process. *Organizational Behavior & Human Performance*, **13**, 46–78.

Dansereau, F., Yammarino, F.J. & Markham, S.E. (1995). Leadership: the multiple-level approaches. *Leadership Quarterly*, **6**, 97–109.

Dansereau, F., Yammarino, F.J., Markham, S.E., Alutto, J.A., Newman, J., Dumas, M., Nachman, S.A., Naughton, T.J., Kim, K., Al-Kelabi, S.A.H., Lee, S. & Keller, T. (1995). Individualized leadership: a new multiple-level approach. *Leadership Quarterly*, **6**, 413–450.

Eden, D. & Leviatan, N. (1975). Implicit leadership theory as a determinant of the factor structure underlying supervisor behavior scales. *Journal of Applied Psychology*, **60**, 736–741.

Evans, M.G. (1970). The effect of supervisory behavior on the path–goal relationship. *Organizational Behavior & Human Performance*, **5**, 277–298.

Fiedler, F.E. (1967). *A Theory of Leadership Effectiveness*. New York: McGraw-Hill.

Fiedler, F.E. (1992). Time-based measures of leadership experience and organizational performance: a review of research and a preliminary model. *Leadership Quarterly*, **3**, 5–23.
Fiedler, F.E. & Garcia, J.E. (1987). *New Approaches to Effective Leadership: Cognitive Resources and Organizational Performance*. New York: Wiley.
Gomez-Mejia, L.R., Tosi, H.L. & Hinkin, T. (1987). Managerial control performance and executive compensation. *Academy of Management Journal*, **30**, 51–70.
Graen, G. (1976). Role-making processes within complex organizations. In M.D. Dunnette (ed.), *Handbook of Industrial and Organizational Psychology*. Chicago: Rand McNally, pp. 1210–1259.
Graen, G. & Cashman, J.F. (1975). A role-making model of leadership in formal organizations: a developmental approach. In J.G. Hunt & L.L. Larson (eds), *Leadership Frontiers*. Kent, OH: Kent State University Press, pp. 154–175.
Graen, G., Novak, M. & Sommerkamp, P. (1982). The effects of leader–member exchange and job design on productivity and satisfaction: testing a dual attachment model. *Organizational Behavior and Human Performance*, **30**, 109–131.
Graen, G. & Scandura, T.A. (1987). Toward a psychology of dyadic organizing. *Research in Organizational Behavior*, **9**, 175–209.
Graen G. & Uhl-Bien, M. (1995). Relationship-based approach to leadership: development of leader–member exchange (LMX) theory of leadership over 25 years: applying a multi-level multi-domain perspective. *Leadership Quarterly*, **6**, 219–247.
Graham, J.W. (1991). Servant–leadership in organizations: inspirational and moral. *Leadership Quarterly*, **2**, 105–119.
Hall, R.J. & Lord, R.G. (1995). Multi-level information-processing explanations of followers' leadership perception. *Leadership Quarterly*, **6**, 265–287.
Heider, F. (1958). *The Psychology of Interpersonal Relations*. New York: Wiley.
Hollander, E.P. (1958). Conformity, status, and idiosyncrasy credit. *Psychological Review*, **65**, 117–127.
Hollander, E.P. (1978). *Leadership Dynamics*. New York: Free Press.
Hollander, E.P. (1958). Leadership and power. In G. Lindsey & E. Aronson (eds), *The handbook of social psychology*, 3rd edn. New York: Random House, pp. 485–537.
Hollander, E.P. (1992). Leadership, followership, self, and others. *Leadership Quarterly*, **3**, 43–54.
Hollander, E.P. (1993). Legitimacy, power, and influence: a perspective on relational features of leadership. In M.M. Chemers & R. Ayman (eds), *Leadership Theory and Research: Perspectives and Directions*. San Diego, CA: Academic Press, pp. 29–47.
Homans, G.H. (1961). *Social Behavior: Its Elementary Forms*. New York: Harcourt, Brace.
House, R.J. (1971). A path–goal theory of leadership effectiveness. *Administrative Science Quarterly*, **16**, 321–338.
House, R.J. (1977). A 1976 theory of charismatic leadership. In J.G. Hunt & L.L. Larson (eds), *Leadership: The Cutting Edge*. Carbondale, IL: Southern Illinois University Press, pp. 194–205.
House, R.J. (1995). Path–goal theory of leadership: lessons, legacy, and a reformulated theory. *Leadership Quarterly*, **6**, forthcoming.
House, R.J. & Mitchell, T.R. (1974). Path–goal theory of leadership. *Journal of Contemporary Business*, **3**, 81–97.
House, R.J. & Shamir, B. (1993). Toward the integration of transformational, charismatic, and visionary theories. In M.M. Chemers & R. Ayman (eds), *Leadership Theory and Research: Perspectives and Directions*. San Diego, CA: Academic Press, pp. 81–107.
House, R.J., Spangler, W.D. & Woycke, J. (1991). Personality and charisma in the US presidency: a psychological theory of leadership effectiveness. *Administrative Science quarterly*, **36**, 364–396.

Howell, J.M. (1988). Two faces of charisma: socialized and personalized leadership in organizations. In J.A. Conger & R.N. Kanungo (eds), *Charismatic Leadership*. San Francisco: Jossey-Bass, pp. 213–236.

Howell, J.M. & Frost, P.J. (1989). A laboratory study of charismatic leadership. *Organizational Behavior and Human Decision Processes*, **43**, 243–269.

Hughes, R.L., Ginnett, R.C. & Curphy, G.J. (1993). *Leadership: Enhancing the Lessons of Experience*. Homewood, IL: Irwin.

Hunt, J.G. (1991). *Leadership: A New Synthesis*. Thousand Oaks, CA: Sage.

Hunt, J.G. & Osborn, R.N. (1978). A multiple approach to leadership for managers. In J. Stinson & P. Hersey (eds), *Leadership for Practitioners*. Athens, OH: Ohio University Center for Leadership Studies, pp. 56–75.

Hunt, J.G. & Ropo, A. (1995). Multi-level leadership: grounded theory and mainstream applications to the case of General Motors. *Leadership Quarterly*, **6**, 479–512.

Jacobs, T.O. (1970). *Leadership and Exchange in Formal Organizations*. Alexandria, VA: Human Resources Research Organization.

Katerberg, R. & Hom, P.W. (1981). Effects of within-group and between-group variation in leadership. *Journal of Applied Psychology*, **66**, 218–223.

Katz, D. & Kahn, R.L. (1978). *The Social Psychology of Organizations*, 2nd edn. New York: Wiley.

Kerr, S. & Jermier, J.M. (1978). Substitutes for leadership: their meaning and measurement. *Organizational Behavior and Human Performance*, **22**, 375–403.

Kerr, S. & Schrieshiem, C.A. (1974). Consideration, initiating structure, and organizational criteria: an update of Korman's 1966 review. *Personnel Psychology*, **27**, 555–568.

Kim, H. & Yukl, G.A. (1995). Relationships of managerial effectiveness and advancement to self-reported and subordinate-reported leadership behaviors from the multiple-linkage model. *Leadership Quarterly*, **6**, 361–377.

Klein, K.J., Dansereau, F. & Hall, R.J. (1994). Levels issues in theory development, data collection, and analysis. *Academy of Management Review*, **19**, 195–229.

Klein, K.J. & House, R.J. (1995). On fire: charismatic leadership and levels of analysis. *Leadership Quarterly*, **6**, 183–198.

Lerner, D. (ed.) (1963). *Parts and Wholes*. New York: Free Press.

Likert, R. (1961). *New Patterns of Management*. New York: McGraw-Hill.

Lord, R.G., Foti, R.J. & DeVader, C.L. (1984). A test of leadership categorization theory: internal structure, information processing and leadership perceptions. *Organizational Behavior and Human Performance*, **34**, 343–378.

Manz, C.C. & Sims, H.P. (1987). Leading workers to lead themselves: the external leadership of self-managing work teams. *Administrative Science Quarterly*, **32**, 106–128.

Manz, C.C. & Sims, H.P. (1989). *Superleadership: Leading Others to Lead Themselves*. Englewood Cliffs, NJ: Prentice-Hall.

Markham, S.E. & Markham, I.S. (1995). Self-management and self-leadership re-examined: a levels of analysis perspective. *Leadership Quarterly*, **6**, 343–359.

Meindl, J.R. (1995). The romance of leadership as a follower-centric theory: a social constructionist approach. *Leadership Quarterly*, **6**, 329–341.

Meindl, J.R. & Ehrlich, S.B. (1987). The romance of leadership and the evaluation of organizational performance. *Academy of Management Journal*, **30**, 91–109.

Miller, J.G. (1978). *Living Systems*. New York: McGraw-Hill.

Phillips, J.S. & Lord, R.G. (1981). Causal attributions and perceptions of leadership. *Organizational Behavior and Human Performance*, **28**, 143–163.

Podsakoff, P.M. & MacKenzie, S.B. (1995). An empirical examination of the effects of substitutes for leadership at the individual-level and group-level of analysis. *Leadership Quarterly*, **6**, 289–328.

Podsakoff, P.M. & Schriesheim, C.A. (1985). *Leader Reward and Punishment Behavior: A Methodological and Substantive Review*. Bloomington, IN: Working Paper, Graduate School of Business, Indiana University.

Podsakoff, P.M. & Todor, W.D. (1985). Relationships between leader reward and punishment behavior and group processes and productivity. *Journal of Management*, **11**, 55–73.

Podsakoff, P.M., Todor, W.D. & Skov, R. (1982). Effects of leader contingent satisfaction. *Academy of Management Journal*, **25**, 810–821.

Pulakos, E.G. & Wexley, K.N. (1983). The relationship among perceptual similarity, sex, and performance ratings in manager–subordinate dyads. *Academy of Management Journal*, **26**, 129–139.

Schriesheim, C.A. (1995). Multivariate and moderated within- and between-entity analysis (WABA) using hierarchical linear multiple regression. *Leadership Quarterly*, **6**, 1–18.

Schriesheim, C.A., Cogliser, C.C. & Neider, L.L. (1995). Is it "trustworthy"? A multiple-levels-of-analysis re-examination of an Ohio State leadership study, with implications for future research. *Leadership Quarterly*, **6**, 111–145.

Schriesheim, C.A. & Kerr, S. (1977). Theories and measures of leadership: a critical appraisal of current and future directions. In J.G. Hunt & L.L. Larson (eds), *Leadership: The Cutting Edge*. Carbondale, IL: Southern Illinois University Press, pp. 9–45.

Schriesheim, C.A., Neider, L.L. & Scandura, T.A. (1994). A within- and between-groups analysis of leader–member exchange as a correlate of delegation and as a moderator of delegation relationships with performance and satisfaction. Manuscript submitted for review.

Shamir, B. (1991). The charismatic relationship: alternative explanations and predictions. *Leadership Quarterly*. **2**, 81–104.

Stogdill, R.M. & Coons, A.E. (1957). *Leader Behavior: Its Description and Measurement*. Columbus, OH: Ohio State University, Bureau of Business Research.

Tosi, H.L. (1992). *The Environment/Organization/Person Contingency Model: A Meso Approach to the Study of Organization*. Greenwich, CT: JAI Press.

Vroom, V.H. & Jago, A.G. (1995). Situation effects and levels of analysis in the study of leader participation. *Leadership Quarterly*, **6**, 169–181.

Vroom, V.H. & Yetton, P.W. (1973). *Leadership and Decision Making*. Pittsburgh, PA: University of Pittsburgh Press.

Waldman, D.A., Bass, B.M. & Yammarino, F.J. (1990). Adding to contingent reward behavior: the augmenting effect of charismatic leadership. *Group and Organization Studies*, **15**, 381–394.

Waldman, D.A., Yammarino, F.J. & Avolio, B.J. (1990). A levels of analysis investigation of training needs. *Personnel Psychology*, **43**, 811–835.

Wexley, K.N., Alexander, R.A., Greenwalt, J.P. & Couch, M.A. (1980). Attitudinal congruence and similarity as related to interpersonal evaluations in manager–subordinate dyads. *Academy of Management Journal*, **23**, 320–330.

Williams, M.L. & Podsakoff, P.M. (1988). A meta-analysis of attitudinal and behavioral correlates of leader reward and punishment behaviors. In D.F. Ray (ed.), *Proceedings of the Southern Management Meetings*, pp. 161–163.

Yammarino, F.J. (1990). Individual- and group-directed leader behavior descriptions. *Educational and Psychological Measurement*, **50**, 739–759.

Yammarino, F.J. (1994). Indirect leadership: transformational leadership at a distance. In B.M. Bass & B.J. Avolio (eds), *Improving Organizational Effectiveness Through Transformational Leadership*. Thousand Oaks, CA: Sage, pp. 26–47.

Yammarino, F.J. (1995). The varient/WABA approach for multi-level theory testing. *Advances in Research Methods and Analyses for Organizational Studies*, **1**, forthcoming.

Yammarino, F.J. (1996). A conceptual-empirical approach for testing meso and multi-level theories. In H.L. Tosi (ed.), *Extensions of the Environment/Organization/Person Model* (forthcoming). Greenwich, CT: JAI Press.

Yammarino, F.J. & Bass, B.M. (1990a). Transformational leadership and multiple levels of analysis. *Human Relations*, **43**, 975–995.
Yammarino, F.J. & Bass, B.M. (1990b). Long-term forecasting of transformational leadership and its effects among naval officers. In K.E. Clark & M.B. Clark (eds), *Measures of Leadership*. West Orange, NJ: Leadership Library of America, pp. 151–169.
Yammarino, F.J. & Bass, B.M. (1991). Person and situation views of leadership: a multiple levels of analysis approach. *Leadership Quarterly*, **2**, 121–139.
Yammarino, F.J. & Dubinsky, A.J. (1990). Salesperson performance and managerially controllable factors: an investigation of individual and work group effects. *Journal of Management*, **16**, 87–106.
Yammarino, F.J. & Dubinsky, A.J. (1992). Superior–subordinate relationships: a multiple levels of analysis approach. *Human Relations*, **45**, 575–600.
Yammarino, F.J. & Dubinsky, A.J. (1994). Transformational leadership theory: using levels of analysis to determine boundary conditions. *Personnel Psychology*, **47**, 787–811.
Yammarino, F.J., Dubinsky, A.J. & Hartley, S.W. (1987). An approach for assessing individual versus group effects in performance evaluations. *Journal of Occupational Psychology*, **60**, 157–167.
Yammarino, F.J., Dubinsky, A.J. & Spangler, W.D. (1994). Transformational and contingent reward leadership: individual-, dyad-, and group-level effects. Manuscript submitted for review.
Yammarino, F.J. & Markham, S.E. (1992a). On the application of within and between and analysis: are absence and affect really group-based phenomena? *Journal of Applied Psychology*, **77**, 168–176.
Yammarino, F.J. & Markham, S.E. (1992b). Correction to Yammarino and Markham. *Journal of Applied Psychology*, **77**, 426.
Yammarino, F.J. & Naughton, T.J. (1988). Time spent communicating: a multiple levels of analysis approach. *Human Relations*, **41**, 655–676.
Yammarino, F.J. & Naughton, T.J. (1992). Individualized and group-based views of participation in decision-making. *Group and Organization Management*, **17**, 398–413.
Yammarino, F.J. & Naughton, T.J. (1995). A multiple-level examination of job activities and employee outcomes. *Journal of Business and Psychology*, **10**, forthcoming.
Yammarino, F.J., Spangler, W.D. & Bass, B.M. (1993). Transformational leadership and performance: a longitudinal investigation. *Leadership Quarterly*, **4**, 81–102.
Yammarino, F.J. & Waldman, D.A. (1993). Performance in relation to job skill importance: a consideration of rater source. *Journal of Applied Psychology*, **78**, 242–249.
Yukl, G.A. (1994). *Leadership in Organization*. Englewood Cliffs, NJ: Prentice-Hall.
Yukl, G.A. & Van Fleet, D.D. (1992). Theory and research on leadership in organizations. In M.D. Dunnette & L.M. Hough (eds), *Handbook of Industrial and Organizational Psychology*, Vol. 3. Palo Alto, CA: Consulting Psychologists Press, pp. 147–198.

Chapter 10

Autonomous Work Groups and Quality Circles

John L. Cordery
Department of Organisational & Labour Studies,
The University of Western Australia

Abstract

This chapter reviews the literature dealing with two of the most common organizational manifestations of teamwork, namely quality circles and autonomous work groups. Quality circles are small volunteer groups of employees, generally from the same work area, who meet regularly to participate in the process of identifying work-related problems and generating ideas for solutions or improvements. They are termed parallel participation structures, as they operate to the side of the main authority structure of an organization, and must rely on management acceptance and support for their existence and if their ideas are to be implemented. Their efficacy, in terms of the performance and the satisfaction of members, is founded on the opportunity for participation in problem-solving and decision-making afforded to circle members. Research suggests that many quality circles have a limited life span of effectiveness, largely as a result of declining motivation of circle members and the difficulties in managing the boundaries between the group and the formal organization. Management surveys suggest that the incidence of quality circles has been overtaken in many settings by autonomous work groups. These are permanent groups of employees, frequently at shop floor level, who collectively exercise a substantial degree of operational responsibility in relation to the performance of some natural unit of work. Studies reviewed here indicate that autonomous work groups are associated with increased employee job satisfaction, although their impact on other work attitudes is far less consistent. Performance effects are also found to be modest and variable, leading to speculation that contingency factors are operating. Future research, it is suggested, will need to focus mainly on autonomous work groups. In particular, there is a need to understand more about how such work groups function internally, and to investigate cognitive explanations for their impact on work performance and employee psychological well-being.

INTRODUCTION

The past decade has seen a substantial resurgence of management interest in team-based work organization, as organizations search for increased productivity and competitiveness (Walton, 1985; Bettenhausen, 1991; Lawler, Mohrman & Ledford, 1992; Sundstrom, De Meuse & Futrell, 1990). Whilst teams may take many different forms and exist for many different purposes (Hackman, 1990), a great deal of attention has focused on two particular structural manifestations of the team concept, namely quality circles and autonomous work groups. These two organizational forms have now become so common as to almost constitute a defining characteristic of contemporary management practice. As Osterman (1994) notes:

> A new conventional wisdom has emerged concerning work organization in the United States... that gains in productivity depend on adopting new models of work organization, models that entail internal labor market (ILM) innovations such as broad job definitions and the use of teams, employee problem-solving groups and quality circles (p. 173).

This popularity is confirmed in the results of periodic surveys of management practice. Lawler, Mohrman & Ledford (1992) found that 47% of Fortune 1000 companies in the USA had installed autonomous or self-managing teams, while 66% reported that they had quality circles in operation. Osterman's (1994) survey of over 600 leading US enterprises found that self-directed teams (autonomous work groups) were present in 54% of firms. This made it easily the most widespread "flexible work practice" overall, although quality circles still featured strongly (40%). Macduffie (1995) reports on the findings of a 1989–1990 survey of 62 automotive plants in which it was reported that, on average, 32% of employees within plants were members of employee involvement or quality circle groups, whilst 22.4% of the workforce on average were members of work teams (in which a degree of self-management is implied). In plants characterized as flexible production plants, the incidence increased to 77% and 70% of employees respectively. Research in other countries has yielded a similar body of evidence (Storey, 1993; Callus et al., 1991).

The impression gained from such surveys of contemporary practice is that quality circles have passed a peak in popularity, featuring less and less as stand-alone interventions and more as components of broader total quality management approaches, whilst autonomous work groups are very much in the ascendancy. To understand the reasons why, it is necessary first to describe the essential features of each structural form, and to examine the research into their efficacy.

QUALITY CIRCLES

Quality circles are "small groups of employees who get together regularly to identify and generate solutions for problems which they encounter in their work situation" (Mohrman & Lawler, 1989: 258). Membership is voluntary, and meetings usually take place in working hours, and on a weekly basis at least (Griffin, 1988; Sheffield, Godkin & Drapeau, 1993). Quality circles have their origin in participative management techniques developed within Japanese industry and "exported" to the rest of the world, as organizations sought to borrow ingredients thought to be responsible for Japan's rapid post-war industrial growth and success (Goldstein, 1985; Griffin, 1988; Hill, 1991).

Quality circles (QCs) are parallel participation structures (Mohrman & Lawler, 1989), as are many other team structures such as task forces. They run alongside the regular formal authority structure of the organization, providing employees with the opportunity to participate in organizational problem-solving, dealing with issues and problems that the mainstream organization is not well equipped to handle (Lawler & Mohrman, 1987). This may be because management lacks sufficient operational knowledge to develop problem solutions, or because operational pressures prevent problem solutions being developed directly as the need arises. The parallel arrangement is not permanent, and it can only exist with the cooperation and approval of management. No formal authority is vested in the QC, and it must seek to have its ideas and solutions accepted by management by virtue of the quality of the solution forwarded and supporting argument.

From the earliest reports of their implementation within US industry in the early 1970s (e.g. Dewar, 1980), the QC movement boomed throughout the 1980s, with reports of benefits covering a wide range of individual and organizational outcomes. Over and above any evidence of direct outcome benefits, Mohrman & Lawler (1989) offer the following reasons for the widespread managerial appeal of QCs. First, they are easily packaged and marketed by organizational consultants. Second, management feels that it can readily control the degree of employee involvement. It is possible to start small, to readily control their incidence (where they exist and who takes part) as well as their use of resources. Failure, or unintended consequences, can be readily managed without major organizational disruption. Third, managers perceive QCs as posing no significant threat to the existing configuration of authority. QC output can be simply ignored, if needs be.

Quality Circle Effectiveness

Essentially, arguments as to QC efficacy centre on the proposed impact of employee participation in decision-making on work attitudes such as job satisfaction and organizational commitment, and on the impact of the adoption of analytical problem-solving techniques on performance.

Steel & Lloyd (1988) have conceptualized these arguments in the form of a model which proposes that the participative nature of QCs creates improved organizational climate, intragroup cooperation and trust, leading to more positive work attitudes, less withdrawal from work and a lower incidence of industrial conflict. Tackling problems in a systematic and analytic fashion provides opportunities for improved motivation through role clarification, improved control over work system variances, and the opportunity to develop increased competence through learning. Ultimately this is reflected in system and job performance.

The research testing such claims has been patchy at best, with the early literature being dominated by simple case study reporting within the popular management press and very few failures documented (Wayne, Griffin & Bateman, 1986). Feeling that this possibly had led to a positive findings bias in reporting of QC outcomes, Barrick & Alexander (1987) reviewed 33 published studies on QCs up to 1985. They concluded that there was no evidence of positive findings bias. However, they noted a strong preference in the US literature for examining human relations and quality of work life outcomes, in contrast to productivity, efficiency and "sweating labour" outcomes (Kano, 1993), which had been the traditional concerns of Japanese management.

In the earliest of the few systematic evaluations of QCs, Marks et al. (1986) compared the behaviour and attitudes of 46 QC participants with the same number of non-participants over a 2-year period. They found little effect of QC membership on employee quality of work life, and only modest effects on performance and absenteeism.

A contingency perspective on this problem is adopted by Brockner & Hess (1986). They found that employee self-esteem was higher for QCs judged as successful in terms of having generated at least two problem solutions which had been accepted and acted on by management. However, it is difficult to assess whether or not such differences were accounted for by selection effects, whether self-esteem led to the success of the QC, or *vice versa*.

In a quasi-experimental longitudinal study of employees from a US Airforce installation, Steel & Lloyd (1988) found only weak support for the impact of the QC intervention on a range of cognitive, affective and behavioural indicators.

Perhaps the most thorough and widely cited evaluation of the impact of QCs is that of Griffin (1988). Using two comparable manufacturing plants, the author tracked the operation, performance and work attitudes of QCs and their members from one plant, comparing the results to those obtained from matched employees in the second plant. Four waves of data were gathered (baseline, followed by three post-intervention collection points) the latest being 36 months after the intervention. The result clearly showed that individual work attitudes, performance and turnover intentions improved in the experimental condition up to the 18-month mark, then declined to original levels.

In a quasi-experimental longitudinal study, Adam (1991) found no differences in work attitudes between quality circle and control groups over time, though there were performance improvements. He also found that initially high levels of QC membership tended to drop off, stabilizing after 6 months.

The limited cycle of success described by Griffin (1988) has been termed the "honeymoon" effect (Lawler & Mohrman, 1987) and it appears consistently in performance outcome evaluations. Shenkar, Hattem & Globerson (1992) carried out a cost–benefit study over a 4-year period of 15 QCs randomly selected from a much larger pool operating within a large manufacturing organization. They found that the program was effectively self-financing over the 4 years, although labour savings achieved peaked at about year 2, again showing a rapid decline thereafter.

The obvious performance effectiveness (even if temporary) of QCs helps to further account for their popularity. Barrick & Alexander (1992) report the results of utility analyses demonstrating performance improvements of over $60 000 from five QCs within the first year of operation.

QCs thus do not appear to offer in themselves much scope for employees to transform their quality of working life. The pattern of employee influence over work-related issues and the day-to-day experience of work is changed little, if at all (Head et al., 1986), and the desire for further participation appears unaffected by this particular involvement strategy, at least in the short term (Liverpool, 1990; Bruning & Liverpool, 1993). Buch & Spangler (1990) report that QC members were more likely to be promoted than non-QC members, though the reasons for this are not made clear.

Factors Influencing Quality Circle Success

Mohrman & Lawler (1989) identify the following threats to the successful operation of circles. First, circles encounter difficulties gaining access to scarce resources (time, money, management attention). Second, negotiating the boundaries between the two organizational structures (formal vs. parallel) poses challenges for both communication and influence. Third, employees may need additional knowledge and skill (technical and managerial) in order to effectively operate in a circle and this may strain existing human resource policies and practices (e.g. reward systems).

Hill (1991) reports the following difficulties with QC operation. First, there is a set of operational problems. These include the inherent problem of separating the problem-solving from the actual implementation of the solution, the restricted range of circle focus (generally only within members' immediate familiar work area), the fact that circles soon run out of readily solvable "simple" problems and lack of ability or skill of members. Second, he argues that circles are frequently blighted and fail to survive because of unfavourable employee attitudes stemming from a poor organizational climate characterized by low trust (Bramel & Friend, 1987).

Wood, Hull & Azumi (1983) argue that two preconditions are necessary for QC success from a member point of view, namely the belief by employees that their support and involvement will benefit themselves as well as the organization (an instrumental orientation); and that participants are well trained in problem-solving techniques and group skills.

Fabi (1992) has identified the following factors as being associated with QC success in the literature. Management commitment and support appears essential, followed by the involvement and support of employees and their unions. Interestingly, Drago (1987) has argued that unionization both creates a positive environmental support for circles and is adversely affected by their introduction. In many instances, the failure of middle and senior management to support circles through acting on suggestions, or providing support in the form of resources and encouragement, has constrained circle life and effectiveness. The training of members and leaders, organizational and financial stability (many fail due to takeovers, business collapses, etc), personal characteristics of the facilitator (authoritarian vs. participative style), and member characteristics (interested, available, experienced, instrumental view) and other factors.

Tang, Tollison & Whiteside (1987) examined numbers of participants in QCs, meeting attendance, completed projects and speed of decision-making within 47 QCs from a single structures fabrication and assembly plant, as a function of whether or not the QC was "self-initiated" (where the QCs and their activities were initiated by the workers themselves) as opposed to "management-initiated". They found that attendance motivation and overall membership was greater in self-initiated QCs. However, management-initiated QCs appeared to show greater output and to deal with problems more rapidly.

Quality Circles as Proto-autonomous Work Groups

Lawler & Mohrman (1985, 1987) characterize parallel structures in general, and quality circles in particular, as an important first step in the development of high employee involvement management practices such as autonomous work groups. It is suggested that the QC may be useful in establishing the credibility of participative processes in organizations, establishing the necessary foundation of employee problem-solving and group process skills before organizations develop more inclusive and delegated models of decision-making, such as those provided by autonomous work groups.

However, it is noted that QCs rarely develop naturally into autonomous work groups, largely because of the challenge that this poses to existing management philosophy and practice. QCs operate comfortably within existing structural arrangements and may thereby provide a comfortable means for management to appear as if it is engaging in high employee involvement whilst at the same time retaining overall control. This would appear to be a particularly safe strategy, given the evidence of the limited time-span of effectiveness of such organizational forms.

It may be that QCs do provide the opportunity for subsequent transition to more participative team structures, such as autonomous work groups. However, the literature does not abound with evidence that QCs naturally evolve into such participative structures. In fact there is a risk that, over time, QC experience may lead to disillusionment on the part of management and employees with involvement strategies in general.

AUTONOMOUS WORK GROUPS

An autonomous work group is a formally constituted permanent team of employees who interact directly to perform a relatively complete set of interdependent tasks (such as assembling a whole product or providing a complete service), whilst exercising a high level of collective discretion over matters to do with the performance of work (Cohen & Ledford, 1994). In addition, group members typically possess broad overlapping sets of skills, sometimes called multiskilling (Cordery, 1995). Other terms frequently used to describe this form of work organization include self-managing, self-directed, self-regulating, semi-autonomous, self-governing or empowered teams (Carnall, 1982; Cohen & Ledford, 1994; Pearce & Ravlin, 1987; Wall et al., 1986; Wellins, Byham & Wilson, 1991).

In essence, autonomous work groups vary on two main design dimensions: the extent to which managerial authority is delegated (autonomy), and the degree of intragroup task specialization (multiskilling).

The Nature and Extent of Team Autonomy

The authority to make decisions (formally or informally) is an important variable in the design of all work groups although, by definition, critical to autonomous group working (Sundstrom, DeMeuse & Futrell, 1990).

The type of decisions potentially delegated to autonomous work groups are listed in Table 10.1.

Susman (1979) groups these into three categories of work group autonomy. First, there are "decisions of self-regulation"—those decisions directly associated with the effective day-to-day regulation of the work process itself, such as quality assurance, equipment maintenance, resource allocation and production scheduling. Second, there are "decisions of independence"—decisions reflecting a group's capacity to operate independently of technological and organizational constraints, such as determining where, when and in what order work will be performed and determining the overall strategic direction of work. Finally, there are "decisions of self-governance", concerning the internal governance of the group, such as those to do with group membership, how meetings are conducted, who becomes the leader, how members are to be disciplined, etc.

These distinctions are reflected in a measure of the degree of work group autonomy developed by Breaugh and colleagues (Breaugh, 1985, 1989; Breaugh & Becker, 1987), incorporating three factors: method autonomy, scheduling autonomy and criteria autonomy. Method autonomy deals with discretion the group has in the choice of procedures and techniques they use in carrying out

Table 10.1 Typical responsibilities of autonomous work groups

Area of Responsibility

1. Housekeeping
2. Training other group members
3. Basic maintenance and fault rectification
4. Scheduling production flows
5. Quality auditing
6. Continuous improvement
7. Dealing direct with suppliers
8. Dealing direct with customers
9. Recruiting new group members
10. Organizing leave
11. Appointing team leaders
12. Ordering new equipment
13. Designing plant layout
14. Budgeting
15. Product modification and development
16. Member performance appraisal
17. Disciplining group members
18. Making compensation decisions

Adapted from Wellins, Byham & Wilson (1991).

their work; scheduling autonomy deal with decisions to do with the sequencing of work; whilst criteria autonomy describes the extent to which the basis for evaluating work performance is determined by a work group. Brady, Judd & Javian (1990) failed to replicate this factor structure using the same instrument, finding instead a single factor (see also measures developed by Little, 1988, and Gulowsen, 1972).

Flexibility and Multiskilling

The other main design feature of autonomous work groups is that they contain employees whose skills overlap and who interpret their task requirements in terms of a broad responsibility to maintain and improve on work system performance (Walton, 1985). Such employees are sometimes referred to as being multiskilled (Cordery, 1995), because they possess a broad repertoire of skills which they may match to the varying demands of the work situation. This may take the form of rotation through distinct positions within the group (Blumberg, 1980), or may involve expanding or enlarging the range of tasks performed in the course of daily employment. Multiskilling may be viewed as a process occurring in three major dimensions, one of which encapsulates the autonomy/responsibility variable. First, there is horizontal skilling. This is the extent to which tasks are learned which are part of traditionally occupational or job families. For example, a mill operator in a mine may learn how to drive a truck and to carry out laboratory and stores work, or a clerk may learn word processing and record-keeping skills. Depth skilling refers to the extent to which skills are developed which are traditionally associated with different job titles, but within the same occupational or skill group. For example, a mechanical tradesperson may learn to work with equipment of increasing complexity (e.g. advanced hydraulics). Finally, vertical skilling refers to the extent to which elements of the supervisory role are learned. Autonomous work groups tend to be characterized by medium to high degrees of vertical and horizontal multi-skilling, and low levels of depth multiskilling (see Table 10.2).

Rationale Underlying Autonomous Work Group Effectiveness

It is possible to identify a range of reasons why autonomous work groups might be held to be effective organizational forms, and why they might contribute an employee's quality of working life.

The earliest advocates of autonomous work groups were the proponents of the socio-technical systems perspective (Trist & Bamforth, 1951; Rice, 1958; Miller, 1959; Herbst, 1962; Trist et al., 1963; Bucklow, 1966; Cooper & Foster, 1971; Kelly, 1978). Socio-technical systems theorists broadly hold that autonomous work groups frequently provide a structure through which the demands of "tech-

Table 10.2 Examples of work group types with differing degrees of autonomy and horizontal task overlap

Task overlap	Autonomy		
	Little or no autonomy	Moderate	High
Complete	Multiskilled, "manager-led" teams	Autonomous work groups with control over work procedures	Autonomous work groups with control over goals
Partial	Production team with overlapping inspection tasks and no discretion-setting capabilities	Quality circle teams with overlap in problem-solving skills	New product/process implementation team with overlap in knowledge of new product/process
Low	Product design team with functional objectives provided and specialized skill membership	Airplane crews	Customer-based product design team with specialized skill membership

Adapted from Majchrzak & Gasser (1992).

nical" systems and "social" systems are most readily balanced or "jointly optimized" (Pasmore, 1988). The key to improved "technical" system performance lies in the direct control by teams of work system "key variances" (variations from an optimum operating state to which the work system as a whole is sensitive) as close as possible to the source of that variation. In this way, autonomous work designs (both individual and group) are held to be an effective structural response to conditions of environmental and production uncertainty, such as that arising from technical complexity (Susman, 1979; Susman & Chase, 1986; Walton & Susman, 1987; Wall & Jackson, 1995). For example, advanced manufacturing technology (AMT), as with conventional forms of automation, supports accurate, high-speed machine operation, lowered labour costs, consistent product quality as well as higher output, but with the additional advantages of better machine utilization and greater flexibility in responding to market requirements (Wall & Davids, 1992). However, capital cost and reliability problems associated with AMT, combined with the speed with which such systems drive production, typically require frequent and rapid human intervention if the costs of deviations from ideal operating states are to are to be contained.

In addition to providing improved performance through more rapid decision-making, it has been argued that autonomous work designs also create shifts in the nature of knowledge and skill for employees, which in turn are reflected in improved employee and system performance. The empirical evidence for this mechanism is not strong, though the argument is compelling (Wall & Jackson, 1995). Wall, Jackson & Davids (1992) have argued that AMT operators in high control work designs learn to see the "bigger picture", developing tacit skill and increased knowledge of how the technology really functions. Evidence for this comes in the form of delayed performance effects for work redesign involving giving operators broad responsibility for fault diagnosis and repair and other aspects of work system management. Having learned more about how the system operates and developed skills in regulating its functioning, operators are then in a better position to exercise effective (and proactive) control. In this view, the work design both creates the opportunity to learn a new skill, as well as the opportunity to apply that skill to the advantage of the system (Blumberg & Pringle, 1982).

There is also some evidence that the opportunity to learn and apply a new skill has a powerful impact on employee quality of work life outcomes. Research by O'Brien (1983, 1986) and others (e.g. Warr, 1990) has shown that perceived skill utilization (the opportunity a job affords to learn and apply meaningful skill) is powerfully linked to job satisfaction. It is also noticeable that measures of decision latitude, a key construct within the demands–constraints model of job-related well-being (Karasek, 1979; Karasek & Theorell, 1990) include items dealing with skill utilization in addition to those dealing with control (Wall et al., 1995). Opportunity to control and opportunity to learn are obviously related. Cordery, Sevastos & Parker (1992) have found that work group autonomy, measured using Little's (1988) scale, and job complexity (assessed in terms of the number of distinct tasks performed during work) are causally related to perceived opportunities for skill utilization. In turn, it was found that skill utilization was the most powerful predictor of both intrinsic job satisfaction (+) and job-related depression (−). However, they are certainly not one and the same thing. In the model proposed by Cordery, Sevastos & Parker (1992), skill utilization mediates between control opportunities and job-related affective well-being.

Another cognitive perspective on the performance effectiveness of autonomous work groups centres on the role of perceived self-competence and self-efficacy beliefs in effecting job performance (Bandura, 1986; Wood & Bandura, 1989). Research into self-efficacy has confirmed the existence of a mutually reinforcing relationship between perceived control over environmental conditions surrounding task performance and perceived self-competence (Williams & Lillibridge, 1992). Furthermore:

> ... perceptions that the environment is controllable may lead people to exercise their personal efficacy strongly, while perceptions that the environment is uncontrollable may lead people to exercise their personal efficacy weakly (Williams & Lillibridge, 1992, p. 158)

Whilst this author is not aware of any empirical research which directly tests the notion that autonomous work groups lead to enhanced performance via improved self-efficacy beliefs, this would certainly appear to be a mechanism worthy of further investigation. Certainly, this view underlies the theory of the external leadership of autonomous work groups developed by Manz & Sims, and latterly extended into a general theory of leadership for high performance, or "superleadership" (Manz & Sims, 1980, 1987, 1991). In this perspective, effective leader behaviour is described as those actions which develop "follower" perceived self-competence along with feelings of personal control and which are designed to model and encourage self-reinforcement, self-observation/evaluation, self-expectation, self-goal-setting, and self-criticism.

One of the general arguments forwarded in favour of team structures more generally, and one which applies to autonomous work groups as well as quality circles, concerns the synergistic effects of group problem-solving in a work context (Cohen, 1991). Group decision-making within a climate of trust and openness that may develop within autonomous work groups can increase the pool of information and expertise available to solve frequently occurring operational problems. This group participation may lead to heightened creativity and innovation (Anderson & West, 1994).

There are further explanations for the possible benefits of autonomous group working which arise from need satisfaction theories of motivation. Job characteristics theorists (e.g. Hackman & Lawler, 1971; Hackman & Oldham, 1976) have identified a number of core job features (autonomy, feedback, task significance, task identity and skill variety) which are held to contribute to intrinsic or higher order need satisfaction, and thence to a variety of outcomes such as reduced absenteeism, increased intrinsic work motivation and high quality work performance. Hackman & Oldham (1980) have suggested that the potential for enhancing such job characteristics is often greater in group-based work designs than within individual job designs.

Socio-technical systems theory has also identified a similar set of work design characteristics (Rousseau, 1978) whose presence is often enhanced with the introduction of autonomous work groups, and which are seen as satisfying important "human" or "social" needs. Cherns (1976, p. 791) lists these as:

1. The need for the content of a job to be reasonably demanding of the worker in terms other than sheer endurance, and yet to provide a minimum of variety (not necessarily novelty);
2. The need to be able to learn on the job and go on learning (... neither too much nor too little);
3. The need for some minimal area of decision-making that the individual can call his own;
4. The need for some minimal degree of social support and recognition in the workplace;
5. The need for the individual to be able to relate what he does and what he produces to his social life; and
6. The need to feel that the job leads to some sort of desirable future (not necessarily promotion).

Autonomous Work Groups, Performance and Productivity

The research findings on the individual and organizational performance effectiveness of autonomous work groups are somewhat surprising in the face of so many different theoretical arguments indicating potential positive performance benefits. Studies and reviews conducted over several decades indicate generally only modest improvements in productivity and performance quality can be expected (Beekun, 1989; Cohen & Ledford, 1994; Goodman, Devadas & Hughson, 1988; Guzzo, Jette & Katzell, 1985; Pasmore et al., 1982; Pearson, 1992; Wall et al., 1986). It is worth noting, however, that in a recent field study Campion, Medsker & Higgs (1993) found that of all work group characteristics, self-management and participation at the group level were among the strongest predictors (though the effects were still "modest") of productivity as well as managers' judgements of work group effectiveness. It should be noted that in many cases, indirect savings in labour costs may be responsible for productivity increases (Cordery, Mueller & Smith, 1991). Research also tends to show that autonomous work groups are not consistently associated with improvements in motivation, absenteeism, safety or labour turnover (Goodman, Devadas & Hughson, 1988; Cohen & Ledford, 1994).

Autonomous Work Groups and Work Attitudes

Work redesign involving the introduction of autonomous work groups has been shown in the majority of cases to contribute to enhanced employee job satisfaction and positive work attitudes (Wall et al., 1986; Cordery, Mueller & Smith, 1991; Campion, Medsker & Higgs, 1993; Cohen & Ledford, 1994), although these and other studies have failed consistently to find a predicted impact on job-related mental health (Sonnentag, this volume) and on organizational commitment.

The variable findings in relation to organizational commitment are interesting, since autonomous work groups are at the core of so-called "commitment" strategies advocated by human resource management theorists (Walton, 1985; Beaumont, 1992). Part of the reason for these findings may lie in the measurement and conceptualization of organizational commitment. Recent research has tended to separate organizational commitment as a construct into "continuance" and "affective" commitment (Somers, 1993). It may be the case that group work redesign has a differential impact on these two dimensions. Or it may also be that team members shift the focus of their loyalties from the organization to the team (Klein, 1991). Recent research helps to support this view. Hodson et al. (1993) used ethnographic research techniques to examine published case studies of autonomous group working and found evidence that workers experience increased feelings of group cohesiveness and solidarity under this form of work organization. Interestingly, the researchers had hypothesized that increased group control might reduce feelings of team solidarity once the focus of conflict had been moved from the traditional "us vs. them" of the vertical supervisory relationship.

A recent study by Barker (1993) sheds further light on this particular outcome of autonomous group working. This study examined how the nature of control shifts within an organization as a result of the introduction of autonomous teams. Barker hypothesizes that self-managing teams develop powerful internal systems of values and norms which act as a form of concertive control over member behaviour. This "negotiated consensus" concerning team and organizational values is, he argued, a far more potent and unavoidable influence on worker behaviour than prior systems of technological and bureaucratic control.

> Peer management increases the total amount of control in a concertive system through two important dynamics. The first is that concertive workers have created this system through their own shared value consensus, which they enforce on each other.... The second reason for the increased power of concertive control is that the way it becomes manifest is less apparent than bureaucratic control.... Concertive control is much more subtle than a supervisor telling a group of workers what to do (Barker, 1993, pp. 433-434).

Contingency Variables and Autonomous Work Group Outcomes

Oldham & Hackman (1980) have referred to the often unconvincing findings in the work redesign literature generally as the "small change and vanishing effects" phenomenon. One obvious explanation for this involves the operation of contingency factors (Wall & Jackson, 1995). The most frequently discussed of these concerns individual differences. Growth-need strength is a moderator within the Job Characteristics Model of motivation (Hackman & Oldham, 1976), as is context satisfaction and employee knowledge and ability. Pearce & Ravlin (1987) argue strongly that employees need to see autonomy as a desirable outcome before autonomous work groups can be considered as a work design option. Similar values and expectations would appear to be relevant to the learning that is also a feature of multiskilling development within autonomous work groups (Cordery et al., 1993). Stevens & Campion (1994) identify goal setting, performance management, planning and task coordination as necessary knowledge, skills and abilities for members of autonomous work groups, and it has been suggested that the requirements of autonomous group working are so different to those of traditional work designs that members need to be specifically selected for their capacity to operate effectively within such working arrangements (Neuman, 1991).

The next, and possibly most important, group of contingency factors relates to the degree of uncertainty or variability arising out of the work context (Pearce & Ravlin, 1987; Wall & Jackson, 1995). It seems reasonable to suggest that the strategy of increasing group control in conditions where there is little inherent variability in work processes (and therefore few significant work-related decisions to be made) is unlikely to have a direct impact on performance or on opportunities to learn and apply new skills.

Thus, in work situations where the technology is simple, predictable in its operation and relatively unchanging, the direct performance gains from autonomous work design could also be expected to be small. It is worth pointing out, however, that such conditions rarely apply within modern manufacturing settings, particularly since the rapid influx of computer-controlled advanced manufacturing systems (Wall & Jackson, 1995).

Another contributor to work uncertainty is task or technical interdependence (Kiggundu, 1983). Sequential and reciprocal forms of interdependence (Thompson, 1967) would appear to generate decision-making requirements associated with the coordination of work flows which may benefit from collective forms of control. Pearce & Ravlin (1987) argue that there must be some logical or natural interdependence of tasks which means that organization of work at a group level is desirable. That is, the management of interdependence must itself be a source of performance variances such that it makes sense to locate those variances within a single team boundary.

Klein (1991) suggests that it is important to take into account the interaction between autonomous working arrangements and process control systems, such as "just-in-time". Tightly coupled systems, for example, may actually reduce autonomy, in relation to decisions about pace and work methods. On the other hand, it may be possible to develop collective autonomy over task design as opposed to task execution decisions.

Finally, where the product/market is characterized by turbulence or rapid change and/or where organization–environment linkages are critical (e.g. service organizations), again uncertainty is created, and autonomous work groups may be a desirable option. Cohen (1991), for example, has suggested that autonomous work groups are not appropriate for groups which do not have product or market linkages to internal or external clients.

Another important set of contextual variables which impinge on the performance effectiveness of autonomous work groups relates to the attitudes and behaviours of supervisors and management (Oldham & Hackman, 1980). Autonomy is a feature of work which can vary directly as a function of the exercise of first-level supervisory control (Cordery & Wall, 1985; Clegg, 1984). Managers and supervisors who may have been comfortable with the limited devolution of authority implied by QCs, may feel threatened by the additional formal delegation of responsibility and authority implied by autonomous work groups (Kerr, Hill & Broedling, 1986; Manz, Keating & Donnellon, 1990; Carnall, 1982) and respond in ways inappropriate to the successful maintenance of group autonomy.

Denison (1982) compared plants designed according to socio-technical systems principles, and which operated autonomous work groups, with traditionally organized plants. He found that whilst workers in the socio-technical plants perceived higher levels of control over decisions than their counterparts in the traditional plants, there was not a perception of a more democratic distribution of control. Workers and supervisors in these plants actually attributed higher levels of influence and control to middle and senior managers than in the traditional plants. He offers the explanation that whilst management delegated control over aspects of the immediate work environment to work teams, they still tended to retain control over what were seen as more important elements, such as budgets, planning decisions, etc. Manz (1992) points out that autonomy is inevitably constrained in this way, and that, whilst it is often called self-management, autonomous group working frequently operates as a system of management control in which employees are allowed discretion over how to complete a task, but not over what must be done.

Carnall (1982) suggests that the design of autonomous work groups is a matter of striking a balance such that there is sufficient autonomy to have an effect, but not so much that the groups become too independent within the overall organization. Generally speaking, the effective exercise of self-management at the group level (in addition to the developmental aspects addressed by Manz and colleagues) requires considerate, participative supervision, an absence of close monitoring, along with effective boundary management (Cordery & Wall, 1985; Cummings, 1978).

A final set of contingency factors relate to human resource management policies and practices. For example, team performance-based and individual skill-based approaches to pay (Lawler, 1990), collective approaches to performance appraisal (Saavedra & Kwun, 1993), and an emphasis on cross-functional training systems are frequently associated with such flexible work organization approaches (Osterman, 1994). Osterman (1994) also found that firms adopting autonomous work groups tended to accord human resource management issues a high level of importance.

DIRECTIONS FOR FUTURE RESEARCH

It is apparent from the preceding review that research into QCs is declining along with their popularity as an organizational intervention, and that much more academic and practitioner interest is being expressed in autonomous work groups. Furthermore, the findings in relation to quality circles appear relatively clear and unambiguous. Research into autonomous work groups, however, represents a much more fertile ground, and these opportunities are now discussed.

First, there is a need for empirical research which examines the impact of contingency factors on the effectiveness and quality of work life outcomes of autonomous group working. The zealous advocacy of self-managing teams in the popular management press runs counter to research evidence as to their modest performance effectiveness, and there is a strong sense of organizational fashion and prescription about their widespread adoption (Yorks & Whitsett, 1985; Guest, 1992). Whilst it makes sense to believe that autonomous work designs are an effective structural response to conditions characterized by uncertainty (production process, technological and environmental), there may be conditions where autonomous work groups are less effective than other forms of work organization (e.g. job rotation or individual job designs).

The role of individual differences has to date only been weakly explored in relation to autonomous work groups. There is a need to expand the range of individual difference variables traditionally studied in the context of job design theory (Hulin & Blood, 1968; Hackman & Oldham, 1980) to include such variables as perceived self-competence and self-efficacy. Do prior perceptions of self-competence affect the willingness of employees to take on added responsibilities, and does the experience of autonomous group working enhance personal feelings of efficacy and competence over time? Furthermore, is there a useful distinction to be made between individual and collective efficacy beliefs, such as group potency beliefs (Guzzo et al., 1993) in predicting performance and development within autonomous work groups. Can the same modelling techniques used in self-efficacy research be used to facilitate the development of autonomous work groups ? Finally, what is the role of social orientation of group members (e.g. individualist vs. collectivist, autonomous vs. relational) in predicting attitudinal and behavioural outcomes of autonomous work groups (Brown et al., 1992)?

In addressing the context of autonomous work groups, a more sustained effort needs to be directed towards explaining the lack of positive findings in relation to absenteeism, turnover and occupational health and safety. This points to a need to examine the nature and functioning of autonomous work groups using perspectives other than the traditional need-satisfaction and socio-technical systems job design frameworks. Wall & Jackson (1995) have pointed to the potential significance of learning and knowledge as a first-level outcome or mediating variable within job design theory, but research has yet to directly test this proposition. Recently, much research has focused on the impact of control within demanding work contexts on performance and well-being (see Sonnentag, this volume). Karasek (1979) and Karasek & Theorell (1990) have postulated that jobs which are high on both control opportunities and demands or challenges lead to positive mental health outcomes for employees. Karasek's theoretical framework would appear to be applicable to the context of autonomous group working, yet no research has examined this to date. One avenue of investigation suggested by the demand–constraints model relates to the extent of multiskilling within autonomous work groups. At what point does the requirement to master and apply an increasing range of skills in the face of increasing production uncertainty generate excessive cognitive demands?

It is also worth investigating how autonomous work designs interact with other management systems, for example goal-setting. The literature on individual goal-setting (Locke & Latham, 1990) suggests that clear difficult goals enhance performance, but that this is less so for complex tasks, where guidance and support to facilitate task strategy development becomes necessary. The literature on managing autonomous work groups suggests that group goal-setting generally assists in the development of self-regulatory capacity (Cordery & Wall, 1985; Manz & Sims, 1991). Research is needed to examine the impact of goal-setting within autonomous work groups on performance and members' perceptions of control as potentially moderated by the complexity of the tasks being performed.

Finally, it is apparent that we still know very little about social processes which occur within autonomous work groups. Barker's (1993) paper helped to highlight some of the potential pathologies of group process to which autonomous work groups are prey. Autonomous work groups are groups, after all, and as a result are just as liable to suffer from "groupthink" (Manz & Sims, 1982) and process losses as other groups. Research is needed which examines how decisions are made within autonomous work groups, how internal leadership is exercised, and how conflict is regulated. The development of trust and commitment within such teams and its relationship to organizational attachment and attitudes to management would also be a fruitful area of future research.

In conclusion, the advocacy of autonomous work groups as a high performance work design strategy appears to be out of proportion to our detailed knowledge of their efficacy and operation. It is to be hoped that their popularity will provide opportunity and motivation for researchers to address the many important theoretical issues raised above.

REFERENCES

Adam, E.E. (1991). Quality circle performance. *Journal of Management*, **17**(1), 25–39.
Anderson, N.R. & West, M.A. (1994). *The Team Climate Inventory: Manual and User's Guide*. Windsor, Berks: ASE Press.
Bandura, A. (1986). *Social Foundations of Thought and Action: A Social Cognitive Theory*. Englewood Cliffs, NJ: Prentice-Hall.
Barker, J.R. (1993). Tightening the iron cage: concertive control in self-managing teams. *Administrative Science Quarterly*, **38**, 408–437.

Barrick, M.R. & Alexander, R.A. (1987). A review of quality circle efficacy and the existence of positive findings bias. *Personnel Psychology*, **40**, 579–592.

Barrick, M.R. & Alexander, R.A. (1992). Estimating the benefits of a quality circle intervention. *Journal of Organizational Behavior*, **13**, 73–80.

Beaumont, P.B. (1992). The US human resource management literature: a review. In G. Salaman (ed.), *Human Resource Strategies*. London: Sage, pp. 20–36.

Beekun, R.I. (1989). Assessing the effectiveness of sociotechnical interventions: antidote or fad? *Human Relations*, **42**(10), 877–897.

Bettenhausen, K.L. (1991). Five years of groups research: what we have learned and what needs to be addressed. *Journal of Management*, **17**(2), 345–381.

Blumberg, M. & Pringle, C.D. (1982). The missing opportunity in organizational research: some implications for a theory of work performance. *Academy of Management Review*, **7**(4), 560–569.

Blumberg, M. (1980). Job switching in autonomous work groups: an exploratory study in a Pennsylvania coal mine. *Academy of Management Journal*, **23**, 287–306.

Brady, G.F., Judd, B.B. & Javian, S. (1990). The dimensionality of work autonomy revisited. *Human Relations*, **43**(12), 1219–1228.

Bramel, D. & Friend, R. (1987). The work group and its vicissitudes in social and industrial psychology. *Journal of Applied Behavioral Science*, **23**(2), 233–253.

Breaugh, J.A. (1985). The measurement of work group autonomy. *Human Relations*, **38**, 551–570.

Breaugh, J.A. (1989). The work autonomy scales: additional validity evidence. *Human Relations*, **42**(11), 1033–1056.

Breaugh, J.A. & Becker, A.S. (1987). Further examination of the work autonomy scales: three studies. *Human Relations*, **40**, 381–400.

Brockner, J. & Hess, T. (1986). Self-esteem and task performance in quality circles. *Academy of Management Journal*, **29**(3), 617–623.

Brown, R., Hinkle, S., Ely, P.G., Fox-Cardamone, L., Maras, P. & Taylor, L.A. (1992). Recognising group diversity: individualist–collectivist and autonomous–relational social orientations and their implications for intergroup processes. *British Journal of Social Psychology*, **31**, 327–342.

Bruning, N.S. & Liverpool, P.R. (1993). Membership in quality circles and participation in decision making. *Journal of Applied Behavioral Science*, **29**(1), 76–95.

Buch, K. & Spangler, R. (1990). The effects of quality circles on performance and promotions. *Human Relations*, **43**, 573–582.

Bucklow, M. (1966). A new role for the work group. *Administrative Science Quarterly*, **11**(1), 72–74.

Callus, R., Moorehead, A., Cully, M. & Buchanan, J. (1991). *Industrial Relations at Work*. Canberra: Australian Government Publishing Service.

Campion, M., Medsker, G.J. & Higgs, A.C. (1993). Relations between work group characteristics and effectiveness: implications for designing effective work groups. *Personnel Psychology*, **46**, 823–847.

Carnall, C.A. (1982). Semi-autonomous work groups and the social structure of the organisation. *Journal of Management Studies*, **19**(3), 277–294.

Cherns, A.B. (1976). Behavioural science engagements: taxonomy and dynamics. *Human Relations*, **29**, 783–792.

Clegg, C.W. (1984). The derivation of job designs. *Journal of Occupational Behaviour*, **5**, 131–146.

Cohen, S. (1991). *Teams and teamwork: Future directions* (CEO Publication No. G91-9 (194)). Center for Effective Organizations, School of Business Administration, University of Southern California.

Cohen, S.G. & Ledford, S.G. (1994). The effectiveness of self-managing teams: a quasi-experiment. *Human Relations*, **47**(1), 13–43.

Cooper, R. & Foster, M. (1971). Sociotechnical systems. *American Psychologist*, **26**, 467–474.

Cordery, J.L. (1995). Autonomous work groups. In N. Nicholson (ed.), *The Blackwell Dictionary of Organizational Behaviour*. Oxford: Blackwell.

Cordery, J.L. & Wall, T.D. (1985). Work design and supervisory practice: a model. *Human Relations*, **38**(5), 425–441.

Cordery, J.L., Sevastos, P., Mueller, W.S. & Parker, S. (1993). Correlates of beliefs towards functional flexibility within a white collar public sector organization. *Human Relations*, **46**, 705–723.

Cordery, J.L., Mueller, W.S. & Smith, L.M. (1991). Attitudinal and behavioural outcomes of autonomous group working: a longitudinal field study. *Academy of Management Journal*, **34**, 464–476.

Cordery, J.L., Sevastos, P.P. & Parker, S. (1992). Job design, skill utilization and psychological well-being at work: preliminary test of a model. Paper presented at XXV International Congress of Psychology Brussels, July.

Cummings, T.G. (1978). Self-regulating work groups: a sociotechnical synthesis. *Academy of Management Review*, **3**, 625–634.

Denison, D.R. (1982). Sociotechnical design and self-managing work groups: the impact of control. *Journal of Occupational Behaviour*, **3**, 297–314.

Dewar, D.L. (1980). *The Quality Circle Guide to Employee Participation*. Englewood Cliffs, NJ: Prentice-Hall.

Drago, R. (1987). Circles and unions. *The Quality Circles Journal*, **10**(2), 26–29.

Fabi, B. (1992). Contingency factors in quality circles: a review of empirical evidence. *International Journal of Quality and Reliability Management*, **9**(2), 18–33.

Goldstein, S.G. (1985). Organizational dualism and quality circles. *Academy of Management Review*, **10**, 504–517.

Goodman, P.S., Devadas, R. & Hughson, T.G. (1988). Groups and productivity: analyzing the effectiveness of self-managing teams. In J.P. Campbell, R.J. Campbell & Associates (eds), *Productivity in Organizations*. San Francisco: Jossey-Bass, pp. 295–327.

Griffin, R. (1988). Consequences of quality circles in an industrial setting: a longitudinal assessment. *Academy of Management Journal*, **31**(2), 338–358.

Guest, D.E. (1992). Right enough to be dangerously wrong: an analysis of the "In Search of Excellence" phenomenon. In G. Salaman (ed.), *Human Resource Strategies*. London: Sage, pp. 5–19.

Gulowsen, J.A. (1972). A measure of work group autonomy. In L.E. Davis & J.C. Taylor (eds), *Design of Jobs*. Harmondsworth: Penguin, pp. 374–390.

Guzzo, R.A., Jette, R.D. & Katzell, R.A. (1985). The effects of psychologically based intervention programs on worker productivity: a meta-analysis. *Personnel Psychology*, **38**, 275–291.

Guzzo, R.A., Yosst, P.R., Campbell, R.J. & Shea, G.P. (1993). Potency in groups: articulating a construct. *British Journal of Social Psychology*, **32**, 87–106.

Hackman, R.J. (ed.) (1990). *Groups That Work (and Those That Don't)*. San Francisco: Jossey-Bass.

Hackman, J.R. & Lawler, E.E. (1971). Employee reactions to job characteristics. *Journal of Applied Psychology*, **55**, 259–286.

Hackman, J.R. & Oldham, G.R. (1976). Motivation through the design of work: test of a theory. *Organizational Behavior and Human Performance*, **16**, 250–279.

Hackman, J.R. & Oldham, G.R. (1980). *Work Redesign*. Reading, MA: Addison-Wesley.

Head, T.C., Molleston, J.L., Sorenson, P.F. & Gargano, J. (1986). The impact of implementing a quality circles intervention on employee task perception. *Group & Organizational Studies*, **11**(4), 360–373.

Herbst, P.G. (1962). *Autonomous Group Functioning*. London: Tavistock.

Hill, S. (1991). Why quality circles failed but total quality management might succeed. *British Journal of Industrial Relations*, **29**, 541–568.

Hodson, R., Welsh, S., Rieble, S., Jamison, C.S. & Creighton, S. (1993). Is worker solidarity undermined by autonomy and participation? Patterns from the ethnographic literature. *American Sociological Review*, **58**(June), 398–416.

Hulin, C.L. & Blood, M.R. (1986). Job enlargement, individual differences and work resources. *Psychological Bulletin*, **69**, 41–55.

Kano, N. (1993). A perspective on quality activities in American firms. *California Management Review*, **Spring**, 12–31.

Karasek, R. (1979). Job Demands, job decision latitude and mental strain. *Administrative Science Quarterly*, **24**, 285–308.

Karasek, R. & Theorell, T. (1990). *Healthy Work: Stress, Productivity and the Reconstruction of Working Life*. New York: Basic Books.

Kelly, J. (1978). A reappraisal of sociotechnical systems theory. *Human Relations*, **31**, 1069–1099.

Kerr, S., Hill, K.D. & Broedling, L. (1986). The first-line supervisor: phasing out or here to stay? *Academy of Management Review*, **11**(1), 103–117.

Kiggundu, M.V. (1983). Task interdependence and job design: test of a theory. *Organizational Behavior and Human Performance*, **31**, 145–172.

Klein, J.A. (1991). A re-examination of autonomy in light of new manufacturing practices. *Human Relations*, **44**, 21–38.

Lawler, E.E. (1990). The new plant revolution revisited. *Organization Dynamics*, **19**(2), 5–14.

Lawler, E.E., Mohrman, S.A. & Ledford, G.E. (1992). *Employee Involvement and Total Quality Management: Practices and Results in Fortune 1000 Companies*. San Francisco: Jossey-Bass.

Lawler, E.E. & Mohrman, S.A. (1985). Quality circles after the fad. *Harvard Business Review*, **63**, 65–71.

Lawler, E.E. & Mohrman, S.A. (1987). Quality circles: after the honeymoon. *Organizational Dynamics*, **15**, 42–54.

Little, L. (1988). The Group Participation Index: a measure of work group autonomy. *Asia Pacific Human Resource Management*, **26**, 23–36.

Liverpool, P.R. (1990). Employee participation in decision-making: an analysis of perceptions of members and non-members of quality circles. *Journal of Business and Psychology*, **4**(4), 411–422.

Locke, E.A. & Latham, G.P. (1990). *A Theory of Goal Setting and Task Performance*. Englewood Cliffs, NJ: Prentice-Hall.

Macduffie, J.P. (1995). Human resource bundles and manufacturing performance: organizational logic and flexible manufacturing systems in the world auto industy. *Industrial and Labour Relations Review*, **48**(2), 197–221.

Majchrzak, A. & Gasser, L. (1992). Towards a conceptual framework for specifying manufacturing workgroups congruent with technological change. *International Journal of Computer Integrated Manufacturing*, **5**(2), 119–131.

Manz, C.C. (1992). Self-leading work teams: moving beyond self-management myths. *Human Relations*, **45**(11), 1119–1140.

Manz, C.C. & Sims, H.P. (1980). Self management as a substitute for leadership: a social learning perspective. *Academy of Management Review*, **5**(3), 361–367.

Manz, C.C. & Sims, H.P. (1982). The potential for "groupthink" in autonomous work groups. *Human Relations*, **35**(9), 773–784.

Manz, C.C. & Sims, H.P. (1987). Leading workers to lead themselves: the external leadership of self-managing teams. *Administrative Science Quarterly*, **32**, 106–128.

Manz, C.C. & Sims, H.P. (1991). Superleadership: beyond the myth of heroic leadership. *Organizational Dynamics*, **19**(4), 18–35.

Manz, C.C., Keating, D.E. & Donnellon (1990). Preparing for an organizational change to employee self-management: the managerial transition. *Organizational Dynamics*, **19**(2), 15–26.

Marks, M.L., Mirvis, P.H., Hackett, E.J. & O'Grady, J.F. (1986). Employee participation in a quality circle program: impact on quality of work life, productivity and absenteeism. *Journal of Applied Psychology*, **71**, 61–69.

Miller, E.J. (1959). Technology, territory and time: the internal differentiation of complex production systems. *Human Relations*, **12**, 243–272.
Mohrman, S. & Lawler, E.E. (1989). Parallel participation structures. *Public Affairs Quarterly*, **Summer**, 255–272.
Neuman, G.A. (1991). Autonomous work group selection. *Journal of Business and Psychology*, **6**(2), 283–291.
O'Brien, G.E. (1983). Skill utilization, skill variety and the job characteristics model. *Australian Journal of Psychology*, **35**(3), 461–468.
O'Brien, G.E. (1986). *The Psychology of Work and Unemployment*. Chichester: Wiley.
Oldham, G.R. & Hackman, J.R. (1980). Work design in the organizational context. *Research in Organizational Behavior*, **2**, 247–278.
Osterman, P. (1994). How common is workplace transformation and who adopts it? *Industrial and Labour Relations Review*, **47**(2), 173–188.
Pasmore, W., Francis, C., Haldeman, J. & Shani, A. (1982). Sociotechnical systems: a North American reflection on empirical studies of the Seventies. *Human Relations*, **35**, 1179–1204.
Pasmore, W.A. (1988). *Designing Effective Organizations: The Sociotechnical Systems Perspective*. New York: Wiley.
Pearce, J.A. & Ravlin, E.C. (1987). The design and activation of self-regulating work groups. *Human Relations*, **40**(11), 751–782.
Pearson, C.A.L. (1992). Autonomous workgroups: an evaluation at an industrial site. *Human Relations*, **45**, 905–936.
Rousseau, D.M. (1978). Technological differences in job characteristics, employee satisfaction and motivation: a synthesis of job design research and sociotechnical systems theory. *Organizational Behavior and Human Performance*, **19**, 18–42.
Rice, A.K. (1958). *Productivity and Social Organisation: The Ahmedabad Experiment*. London: Tavistock.
Saavedra, R. & Kwun, S.K. (1993). Peer evaluation in self-managing work groups. *Journal of Applied Psychology*, **78**(3), 450–462.
Sheffield, D.T., Godkin, L. & Drapeau, R. (1993). An industry-specific study of factors contributing to the maintenance and longevity of quality circles. *British Journal of Management*, **4**, 47–55.
Shenkar, O., Hattem, E. & Globerson, S. (1992). Cost–benefit analysis of quality circles: a case study. *Human Systems Management*, **11**, 35–40.
Steel, R.P. & Lloyd, R.F. (1988). Cognitive, affective and behavioral outcomes of participation in quality circles: conceptual and empirical findings. *Journal of Applied Behavioral Science*, **24**(1), 1–17.
Stevens, M.J. & Campion, M.A. (1994). The knowledge, skill, and ability requirements for teamwork: implications for human resource management. *Journal of Management*, **20**(2), 503–530.
Storey, J. (1993). The take-up of human resource management by mainstream companies: key lessons from research. *International Journal of Human Resource Management*, **4**, 529–553.
Somers, M.J. (1993). A test of the relationship between affective and continuance commitment using non-recursive models. *Journal of Occupational and Organizational Psychology*, **66**, 185–192.
Sundstrom, E., De Meuse, K.P. & Futrell, D. (1990). Work teams. *American Psychologist*, **45**(2), 120–133.
Susman, G.I. (1979). *Autonomy at Work: A Sociotechnical Analysis of Participative Management*. New York: Praeger.
Susman, G.I. & Chase, R. (1986). A sociotechnical systems analysis of the integrated factory. *Journal of Applied Behavioral Science*, **22**, 257–270.
Tang, T.L., Tollison, P.S. & Whiteside, H.D. (1987). The effect of quality circle initiiation

on motivation to attend quality circle meetings and on task performance. *Personnel Psychology*, **40**, 799–814.

Thompson, J. (1967). *Organizations in Action*. New York: McGraw-Hill.

Trist, E.L. & Bamforth, K.W. (1951). Some social and psychological consequences of the longwall method of coal-getting. *Human Relations*, **4**, 3–38.

Trist, E.L., Higgin, G.W., Murray, H. & Pollock, A.B. (1963). *Organisational Choice: Capabilities of Groups at the Coal Face under Changing Technologies*. London: Tavistock.

Wall, T.D. & Davids, K. (1992). Shop floor work organisation and advanced manufacturing technology. In C.L. Cooper & L.T. Robertson (eds), *International Review of Industrial and Organizational Psychology*, Vol. 7. Chichesker: Wiley.

Wall, T.D. & Jackson, P.R. (1995). New manufacturing initiatives and shopfloor job design. In A. Howard (ed.), *The Changing Nature of Work*. San Francisco: Jossey-Bass.

Wall, T.D., Jackson, P.R. & Davids, K. (1992). Operator work design and robotics system performance: a serendipitous field study. *Journal of Applied Psychology*, **77**, 353–362.

Wall, T.D., Jackson, P.R., Mullarkey, S. & Parker, S.K. (1995). The demand-control model of job strain: a more specific test. *Journal of Occupational & Organizational Psychology*, in press.

Wall, T.D., Kemp, N.J., Jackson, P.R. & Clegg, C.W. (1986). Outcomes of autonomous work groups: a long-term field experiment. *Academy of Management Journal*, **29**(2), 280–304.

Walton, R.E. & Susman, G.I. (1987). People policies for the new machines. *Harvard Business Review*, **March–April**, 98–106.

Walton, R.E. (1985). From control to commitment. *Harvard Business Review*, **March**, 77–84.

Warr, P.B. (1990). Decision latitude, job demands and employee well-being. *Work and Stress*, **4**(4), 285–294.

Wayne, S.J., Griffin, R.W. & Bateman, T.S. (1986). Improving the effectiveness of quality circles. *Personnel Administrator*, **March**, 79–88.

Wellins, R.S., Byham, W.C. & Wilson, J.M. (1991). *Empowered Teams: Creating Self-directed Work Groups that Improve Quality, Productivity and Participation*. San Francisco: Jossey-Bass.

Williams, K.J. & Lillibridge, J.R. (1992). Perceived self-competence and organizational behavior. In K. Kelley (ed.), *Issues, Theory & Research in Industrial/Organizational Psychology*. New York: Elsevier Science Publishers B.V., pp 155–184.

Wood, R.E. & Bandura, A. (1989). Social cognitive theory of organizational management. *Academy of Management Review*, **14**, 361–384.

Wood, R.E. Hull, F. & Azumi, K. (1983). Evaluating quality circles: the American application. *California Management Review*, **26**, 37–49.

Yorks, L. & Whitsett, D.A. (1985). Hawthorn, Topeka and the issue of science versus advocacy in organizational behavior. *Academy of Management Review*, **10**, 21–30.

Chapter 11

Dimensions, Criteria and Evaluation of Work Group Autonomy

Eberhard Ulich
and
Wolfgang G. Weber
Swiss Federal Institute of Technology, Zurich, Switzerland

Abstract

This contribution first of all describes structural features important in the designing of primary work systems, which are considered to be prerequisites of implementation of group work. Here the work task plays an outstanding role as the interface between the social and technical subsystems on the one hand and between the individual and the organization on the other. In order to reach the greatest degree of self-regulation possible and the development of a task orientation, the wholeness, or comprehensiveness, of tasks is of crucial significance. This fact is not discernible in all publications on group work, as definitions of work groups and group work as well as the criteria determining their autonomy frequently do not correspond. We compare the most widely held approach, that of Gulowsen, with our own task- or activity-oriented approach. This is amplified using two examples, which are reflected in a summary of previously available findings on work in partly autonomous groups. In deciding to implement such structures, technical, environmental and person-oriented contingencies as well as prevailing industrial relations must be taken into consideration, as their specific arrangement can promote or hinder various forms of individual and/or collective self-regulation.

DESIGNING SOCIO-TECHNICAL SYSTEMS AS A PREREQUISITE OF GROUP WORK

Socio-technical systems are open, dynamic systems (Bertalanffy, 1950), i.e. they receive inputs from the environment and deliver outputs to it. This applies to materials and energy; it is also true of information and rules.

Primary work systems are identifiable and definable subsystems within an organization, e.g. a production department, or an assembly department. Such systems may consist of a single group, or of a number of groups, sharing a recognizable common goal which combines the workers and their activities (Trist, 1981, p. 11). Primary work systems consist of a social subsystem and a technical subsystem. The social subsystem is made up of "the members of the organization, with their individual and group-specific physical and psychological needs—especially the demands which they place upon their work—and their knowledge and capabilities" (Alioth, 1980, p. 26). The technical sub-system consists in "the means of production, the installations and their layout, and, in general terms, the technological and spatial working conditions which place demands upon the social system" (loc. cit.). The social and technical subsystems are joined in two ways by the occupational roles of the employees: first, the occupational roles establish the functions which the employees must fulfil in the production process; second, they define the necessary cooperative relationships amongst the employees:

> Occupational roles express the relationship between a production process and the social organization of the group. In one direction they are related to tasks which are related to each other; in the other, to people who are also related to each other (Trist & Bamforth, 1951, p. 14).

The connection between the two sub-systems is reflected, for example, in different forms of division and interaction of functions between men and machines.

The unit of analysis is the whole primary work system, although particular attention is paid to the two sub-systems. The aim of work design is the joint optimization of these sub-systems, in the sense of the "best match" (Susman, 1976). The starting-point of the design process is the primary task, that is, the task for the performance of which the system or sub-system in question was created (Rice, 1958, p. 33). Admittedly, technological considerations relating to secondary tasks, e.g. control of inputs, can limit the scope for the design of the primary task. This means that increasing attention must be paid to secondary tasks when the introduction of advanced technology is being considered.

The concept of socio-technical systems design explicitly postulates the need for *joint* optimization of application of technology, organization and use of human resources. A late adjustment of the social to the technical sub-system, or *vice versa*, often leads to sub-optimal solutions.

A primary work system developed according to socio-technical concepts exhibits the following structural features:

1. *Relatively independent organizational units.* Relatively independent organizational units should receive assignments tasks which form integrated wholes. The independence of the units, together with the completeness of the tasks, puts them in a position to identify variances and disturbances at their source and regulate themselves. This can prevent the uncontrolled spread of variances and disturbances through other units in the organization, and the consequent time-consuming retrospective search for causes. Self-regulation of variances and disturbances also strengthens the independence of the organizational unit.
2. *Relatedness of tasks within the organizational unit.* The various sub-tasks within an organizational unit must be content-related, so that awareness of a common task can be evoked and maintained. Content-related sub-tasks also lead to work-related communication, which encourages mutual support. This in turn promotes collaboration in correcting variances and disturbances and broad and varied training across many parts of the whole task.
3. *Unity of product and organization.* Organizational structures must be designed so that work outputs can be assigned to organizational units in both qualitative and quantitative terms. "Input elements or disturbance factors which are produced by other units must be identifiable as such" (Alioth, 1986, p. 200). The unity of product and organization is a precondition for creating complete tasks and the rise of a shared task orientation. It permits identification with one's "own" product.

The formation of relatively independent organizational units is of predominant importance in the design of primary work systems. This is clear from the very early experiences in English coal-mining, and it has frequently been confirmed in recent decades.

THE PRIMACY OF THE TASK

According to Hacker (1986, p. 61), the work order (its interpretation or undertaking as a task) is "the central category of a psychological view of activity... because with the objective logic of its contents decisive determinations are made as to how the activity is regulated and organized". On the same subject, Volpert (1987, p. 14) says, "The character of an 'intersection' between organization and individual makes the task the psychologically most relevant part of the working conditions".

A connection may be made here with the concepts of socio-technical systems design, even if Hacker and Volpert did not do so explicitly. Blumberg (1988, p. 56) says: "... the task must be the point of articulation between the social and technical systems—linking the job in the technical system with its correlated role behaviour in the social system". This means that the task is not only the "point of intersection" between the organization and the individual, but at the same time the nucleus of the socio-technical system and the focus of work psychological design concepts.

Rice (1958) in his generalizing assumption also gives the task particular status, especially when considering the effects on motivation of participating in the performance of a complete task.

The Concept of Task Orientation

The term "task orientation" plays a significant role in the framework of the socio-technical systems approach. "Task orientation" denotes a state of interest and engagement evoked by certain characteristics of the task. Emery (1959, p. 53) gives two conditions which are necessary for the development of task orientation:

1. The individual should have control over the materials and processes of the task.
2. The structural characteristics of the task must be such as to induce forces on the individual towards aiding its completion or continuation[1].

However, according to Emery, the degree of control over the work processes depends not only on the features of the task or of the authority delegated, but primarily on the knowledge and competence that the individual brings to the task: "Thus, the knowledge that a skilled man brings to a job enables him to make choices between alternative modes of operation that are not obvious to an unskilled man" (Emery, 1959, p. 54). Jaques (1951, 1956) described the required degree of freedom of action as the "discretionary content" of a task.

It will already be clear how closely the concepts of scope for action, control and autonomy are connected. Jaques (1956, 34), for example, talks about "... all elements in which choice of how to do a job was left to the person doing it ... having to choose the best feeds and speeds for an impoverished job on a machine; having to decide whether the finish on a piece of work would satisfy some particular customer; ... having to plan and organise one's work in order to get it done within a prescribed time".

It is clear that "control" here means the freedom to choose between different possibilities, and/or the ability to influence processes. This accords perfectly with the concept of control as it has been defined in the German-language literature on work psychology since the 1970s. Here, too, a connection is made with characteristics of the work activity: "If the activity is split into parts, the individual does not have control of his or her own activity ..." (Frese, 1978, p. 165).

---

[1] In this context one might also consider examples from experimental social psychology, in which "... there is activity growing out of interest in the task itself, in the problems and challenges it offers. The task guides the person, steers his action, becomes the centre of concern" (Asch, 1957, p. 303).

In order to evoke the motivation which stimulates the individual to complete or continue the work, the task must be designed first and foremost so as to "... offer a challenge, combined with realistic demands" (Alioth, 1980, p. 31). It must not be too simple, since this would induce feelings of monotony and satiation. It must not be too complex, because too much complexity means too little feedback.

> ... if the task is too complicated for an individual he will display vicarious trial and error activity provided he is motivated to try to learn. If the task is so simple in structure as to appear structureless, learning will again only occur if rewarded or punished in a strictly scheduled fashion and will take the form of blind conditioning. Between these limits there is a recognized range of meaningfully structured material in which the individual learns by varying degrees of insight and, significantly, learns without extrinsic reward or punishment (Emery, 1959, p. 54).

Combining the conclusions of Emery & Emery (1974) with those of Cherns (1976, 1987) and Emery & Thorsrud (1976, 1982), we arrive at the following list of task characteristics which favour the development of task orientation: completeness; varied demands; opportunities for social interaction; autonomy; opportunities for learning; and development.

Although Hackman & Lawler (1971) and Hackman & Oldham (1976) arrive at their set of task characteristics in a theoretically different manner, nevertheless it agrees so well with the list just given that Trist (1981, p. 31) remarks: "This degree of agreement is exceptional in so new a field and has placed work redesign on a firmer foundation than is commonly realized".

Table 11.1 shows goals relating to the different task characteristics, together with ways of achieving them. It is clear from the early work of Rice (1958) and Emery (1959) that, among the characteristics listed in Table 11.1, completeness of a task is of paramount importance. Its operational relevance is explained below.

Whole Tasks

Rice (1958) and Emery (1959) make a number of comments on the motivational importance of the completeness or "wholeness" of tasks. In more recent psychological writings, Tomaszewski (1981) uses the term "whole task", while Hacker (1986, 1987) uses "whole activity", and Volpert (1987), "whole action".

Characteristics of task "wholeness" which should be taken into account in work design are summarized in Table 11.2. Activities which are not "whole"—or which are fragmented, in the sense in which Volpert (1974) uses the term—fail to offer "opportunities for independent goal-setting and decision-making, for the development of individual working styles or for sufficiently exact feedback" (Hacker, 1987, 44).

Table 11.1 Characteristics of task design which evoke task orientation

Design characteristic	Supposed effects	Realization through:
Completeness	Employees are aware of meaning and status of their work. Employees get feedback on their own progress from the activity itself	Tasks with planning, performing and checking activities and the possibility to check results of own work against requirements
Variety of demands	A variety of abilities, knowledge and skills can be applied. Unilateral strain can be avoided	Tasks with different sensory and physical demands
Opportunities for social interaction	Difficulties can be overcome together. Mutual support improves ability to cope with workloads	Tasks which suggest or require cooperation
Autonomy	Promotes feelings of self-worth and readiness to accept responsibility. Enables the experience that s/he is not without significance or influence	Tasks with opportunities for planning and decision-making
Opportunities for learning and development	Maintains general mental flexibility. Occupational qualifications are maintained and improved	Tasks which present problems, and require application and extension of existing qualifications or acquisition of new ones
Time elasticity and stress-free regulation possibilities	Avoids unsuitable density of work. Allows time for stress-free reflection and desired interactions	Inclusion of time buffers in scheduling
Meaningfulness	Gives employees the feeling of participating in the creation of socially useful products. Gives certainty of conformity between individual and social interests	Products of unquestionable social value. Products and production processes which can be shown to be ecologically harmless

From Ulich, 1994, with permission.

It is obvious that activities or tasks which are "whole" in the sense described here are of fairly broad scope. Often they may be tasks which cannot be designed as individual activities; they may need to be structured as group tasks. Researchers working on the basis of socio-technical concepts drew attention to this point at an early stage.

Table 11.2 Characteristics of whole tasks

1. Independent setting of goals, which can be embedded in superordinate goals.
2. Autonomous work preparation, i.e. planning functions.
3. Choice of means including interactions appropriate to goal attainment.
4. Performance functions accompanied by feedback of performance, enabling corrections to be made.
5. Checking with feedback of results and the possibility of checking results of one's own actions against the goals set.

Based on Hellpach 1992; Tomaszewski 1981; Hacker 1986; Volpert 1987; Ulich 1989a.

Group Tasks

Working in groups has particular psychological significance, for two related reasons:

1. In most modern working processes, "wholeness" of work can only be experienced if interdependent sub-tasks are combined to form complete and integrated group tasks.
2. The integration of interdependent sub-tasks into a common group task permits a higher degree of self-regulation and social support.

In connection with the first point, Wilson & Trist (1951) and Rice (1958) established very early that in cases where the individual sub-task does not permit this, satisfaction can result from cooperation in completing a "whole" group task. Regarding the second point, Wilson & Trist have suggested that the possible level of group autonomy is determined by the extent to which the group task constitutes an independent and "whole" entity. According to Emery (1959), common task orientation only develops in a work group if the group has a common task, for which it as a group can assume responsibility, i.e. the process of work within the group can be controlled by the group itself.

Awareness of a common task and common task orientation substantially determine the intensity and duration of group cohesion. Work groups whose cohesion is based mainly on socio-emotional relationships are therefore less stable than groups which are characterized by common task orientation (cf. Alioth, Martin & Ulich, 1976). These considerations are also reflected in the principles formulated by Emery & Thorsrud (1976, 1982) for the restructuring of activities. According to these principles, "interlocking" tasks or exchanges of activities within work groups are required primarily when individual activities have to be interdependent for technical or psychological reasons; individual activities make relatively high workloads; the work of the individual makes no clearly visible contribution to the usefulness of the end product.

When the members of a group are united by interlocking tasks or exchange of activities, these tasks or activities should be recognizable as a whole task which makes a contribution to the social usefulness of the product; offer some scope to set norms and obtain knowledge of results; and permit a measure of control over boundary tasks (Emery & Thorsrud, 1982, p. 34).

According to Emery & Thorsrud (1982, p. 35), these principles indicate that "... the restructuring of work activities goes beyond the realm of individual tasks and leads to the organization of work groups". The concept of partly autonomous work groups is particularly significant in this context.

Concerning the size of such groups, it is not the absolute size of groups, but the adequacy of their size, which is decisive in determining task orientation and optimal self-regulation. This has been stressed not only by Rice (1958) but most strongly by Greenberg (1979) in his discussion of "undermanning theory".

WORK GROUPS AND GROUP WORK

Since the beginning of the 1990s, the number of enterprises involved in the introduction of group work has been growing rapidly. This trend is especially apparent in the European car industry, and particularly in Germany. Well-known car producers, who until recently favoured a high level of division of production tasks and wide use of complex technology, have announced their intention of introducing a comprehensive system of group work. The main stimulus for this change in attitude is the result of an MIT study, (Womack, Jones & Roos, 1990), which showed amongst other things that European mass producers take twice as much time over the final assembly of a car as Japanese mass producers. Storage times were longer and quality problems more frequent amongst the European manufacturers. Furthermore, the proportion of the total working area occupied by repair facilities is three-and-a-half times as high in Europe as in Japan. Considerable differences are also noted in the time taken to develop new models and tools, and their time to market.

These differences were seen as a particular threat in the context of the opening of the European Market. The MIT study showed that the number of employees working in teams is more than a hundred times higher in Japanese car factories than in European factories. It was concluded from this that group work may be regarded as a decisive factor in the success of the Japanese car industry.

Admittedly, the study by Womack, Jones & Roos offers no evidence that group work has a decisive influence on success. Differences between the decades-old European concepts of group work and Japanese concepts are not considered. The remarks on Swedish car factories—which the authors admit they have not visited—seem more like subjective opinions and prejudices than established knowledge.

Unfortunately, it seems that in many cases group work is wrongly regarded as a simple determinant of success, promising rapid improvement of the competitive position. As yet there seems to be little understanding here of the fact that modern concepts of group work are aimed at a genuinely different way of organizing work. This is apparent in the discussions and efforts aimed at halving the span of control of the foremen in a German car factory, coinciding with the announcement of a comprehensive introduction of group work.

Group Work

The performance of tasks by groups and the interactions which take place in this context have been subjects of research in social psychology for several decades Schneider (1975) reported two decades ago that there existed almost 5000 publications in the area of small group research, of which about 3400 had appeared between 1967 and 1972. Measured against this, the state of knowledge about group work in industry is still far from satisfactory. One of the reasons for this is that the results of small group research in social psychology are not directly applicable to industrial reality because they are not sufficiently representative of it. The work consists mainly of experimental investigations in which researchers in laboratories carry out tasks of brief duration which are remote from everyday work activities.

> This research involved the study of groups in which there was no motive on the part of the members for the group's existence, and which had neither a past nor a future (Endres & Wehner, 1993, p. 22).

Investigations in which real industrial working conditions are created in the laboratory, and workers carry out tasks of the kind performed every day in industry, across a substantial period and for pay similar to that given in industry, are obviously the exception (e.g. Graf, 1954; Ulich, 1956; Graf, Rutenfranz & Ulich, 1956).

First, it is clear that these studies are not representative in terms of subjects, tasks and setting; indeed, this is often not attempted. Second, it seems that the social configurations studied are mostly not groups at all, as defined by Sherif & Sherif (1969). Rosenstiel derived from this definition the essential features according to which a social configuration may be defined as a group. A group would be defined as a number of people, in direct interaction over an extended period of time, having differentiated roles and common norms, and united by a "we-feeling" (cf. Rosenstiel, 1992, p. 261). According to Rosenstiel, the possibility of direct interaction over an extended period must be an essential feature of any definition, broad or narrow, since it is only under these conditions that there can be "experience and behaviour specifically coloured by the group". A further essential component of work-psychological formulations is the "pursuit of common goals", included by Sader (1991, p. 39) among frequently cited essential elements in definitions of groups.

Finally, "group working is only meaningful where participation in decision-making is possible" (Bungard & Antoni, 1993, p. 378). Lewin (1982, p. 283) has already stressed the particular psychological importance of participation in decision-making:

> The decision joins motivation to action, and seems at the same time to have a consolidating effect, partly because of the tendency of the individual to "stand by his decisions", and partly because of declared commitment to the group.

Accordingly, Demmer, Gohde & Kötter (1991, p. 20) postulate as a precondition for group work a "core task", which includes collective planning and decision-making processes, and which constitutes a "considerable part" of the total task (cf. Kötter, Gohde & Weber, 1989).

Autonomous setting of goals or sub-goals, making plans and arrangements, and the sharing of decisions determine the degree of "wholeness" of a task, and the level of regulation needed for its performance (cf. Oesterreich & Volpert, 1991). They also—in the case of group work—establish the degree of collective autonomy of the work group. Since, as a rule, this autonomy remains limited and does not include participation in decisions on investment, type of product, production location, etc., the term "partly autonomous work groups" will be used from now on.

Partly Autonomous Groups

The tasks for which partly autonomous work groups are given responsibility should be as "whole" as possible. In practice, varying levels of autonomy may be found, depending on how much decision-making authority the group receives.

The partly autonomous work group is a key concept for the implementation of socio-technical design principles (cf. Pasmore et al., 1982; Ulich, 1994). Partly autonomous group work serves both humane and economic goals: the direct regulation of fluctuations and disturbances (so-called "key variances") by qualified production groups on the spot at which they occur promotes the creation of whole tasks (see above) and in many cases increases production efficiency as well. In this section, we will examine more closely the organizational features that partly autonomous work groups require for desired positive effects to occur. Our aim is to illustrate the commonly accepted core of the concept as well as to show differences among the various representatives of the socio-technical approach.

Definitions and descriptions of components of partly autonomous group work which have been developed in the history of the socio-technical systems approach are compared in Table 11.3. It is not intended to give a complete synopsis of the history of this concept. Rather, some milestones of its development are compared in a summary. Partly, these elements of definition represent organizational prerequisites for realisation of group work; partly they build structural features and a core of criteria for the autonomy of work groups like Gulowsen's criteria. For the interpretation of Table 3 it is necessary to take into consideration that the rise of the concept of partly autonomous work groups encompasses four decades. At the beginning, characteristics of partly autonomous work groups appeared only implicitly in the form of descriptions that were given in case studies (e.g. Trist &

DIMENSIONS, CRITERIA AND EVALUATION OF WORK GROUP AUTONOMY

Table 11.3 Features of partly autonomous work groups proposed by various representations of the socio-technical systems approach

Proposed feature	Trist & Bamforth (1951)	Rice (1953)	Emery (1959)	Herbst (1976)	Emery & Emery (1974)	Susman (1976)	Cummings & Molloy (1977)	Pasmore et al. (1982); Pasmore (1988)	Pearce & Ravlin (1987)	Hackmann (1977); Hackmann (1986)	Wall & Clegg (1981); Kemp et al. (1983)	Alioth (1980); Alioth & Ulich (1981); Ulich (1994)
Spatial-organizational production unit	(X)	X	X		X	X	X	X	X	X	(X)	X
Common and integral primary tasks	(X)	(X)	X	(X)	X	X	X	(X)	X	X	X	X
Interdependency of subtasks	(X)	X	X	X	X	X	X	(X)	X	(X)	(X)	X
Common responsibility	(X)	(X)	(X)	X	X	X	(X)	X	X	X	X	X
Collective self-regulation: allocation of roles and functions	(X)	(X)	(X)	X	X	X	X	(X)		X	X	X
Collective self-regulation: coordination of manufacturing tasks								(X)				
Boundary maintenance by the group	X		(X)	X	X	X	X	X	X	X	X	(X)
Multifunctionality/polyvalence principle	(X)	(X)	(X)	X	X	(X)	(X)	(X)	(X)		(X)	X
Decision on internal leadership by the group												

Table 11.3 *Continued*

Proposed feature	Trist & Bamforth (1951)	Rice (1953)	Emery (1959)	Herbst (1976)	Emery & Emery (1974)	Susman (1976)	Cummings & Molloy (1977)	Pasmore et al. (1982); Pasmore (1988)	Pearce & Ravlin (1987)	Hackmann (1977); Hackmann (1986)	Wall & Clegg (1981); Kemp et al. (1983)	Alioth (1980); Alioth & Ulich (1981); Ulich (1994)
Decision on type of external representation	X		(X)			(X)	(X)	(X)				(X)
Common influence on group membership	(X)				X	(X)	(X)	(X)		(X)	(X)	(X)
Common influence on wage conditions	(X)	(X)				(X)		(X)				(X)
Group-level wage plan							(X)			X		X
Integration of meaningful secondary tasks	(X)		(X)		(X)	(X)	X		(X)			X
Job rotation	(X)	X	X	(X)		(X)	(X)	(X)			(X)	X

X = core feature/(X) = optional feature.

Bamforth, 1951; Rice, 1953, 1958). Later, its components were depicted more explicitly, precisely and in a more differentiated manner. With regard to the variations of the concept listed in the head of Table 3, it is not always clear which of the features mentioned by a single author are necessary and which of them are optional. For this reason we had to interpret some of their descriptions—therefore some interpretational uncertainty remains. Nevertheless, the presented variations in the history of the concept of autonomous group work build the foundation of the model which is described in this contribution.

As shown in Table 11.3, structural features of primary work systems are already systematized in Emery's concept (1959). But he does not specify the scope of self-regulation. The latter was done more exactly by Emery & Emery (1974) and especially by Susman (1976), who constructed a remarkable typology of "regulatory decisions". Alioth (1980), Alioth & Ulich (1981), and Ulich (1994) refer to Susman's concept but they stress the necessity of integrating meaningful secondary tasks in the primary work system of the group to promote personal development. Herbst (1976) accentuates the integration of relatively autonomous groups into cooperative structures of organizations, e.g. matrix organizations and networks. Moreover, he shows that autonomous work groups have the capacity to design single tasks which can be performed relatively independently by individual group members or by sub-sets of the group. Although partly stemming from another psychological tradition, the characterization of autonomous work groups given by Hackman (1977, 1986), Kemp et al. (1983) and Wall & Clegg (1981) has much in common with the socio-technical concept. They suggest using features of individual task design (cf. Table 11.1) for the analysis and design of shared group tasks. This is a very important proposal for the evaluation of sub-tasks in work groups but it is questionable if it is sufficient, because it presupposes that there are no structural inadequacies between individual tasks and collectively regulated group tasks, or between characteristics of individual and collective autonomy.

The comparative survey of the various authors' concepts in Table 11.3 shows, on the one hand, that there is satisfactory agreement with the following central features of relatively autonomous work groups: shared primary task, shared responsibility, interdependence ("interlocking") of sub-tasks, collective self-regulation (allocation of roles and functions; coordination of manufacturing tasks), multifunctionality principle/polyvalence of skills. On the other hand, certain features are of central interest according to some authors but not to others: boundary maintenance (i.e. regulation of the group's production input and output), internal decision on type of external representation, collective influence upon group membership, group-level wage plan, and the integration of meaningful secondary tasks. An influence of work groups on construction, product or production design is hardly mentioned by the authors listed.

Finally, the variations of the concept can be distinguished by the degree of individual autonomy that is considered as a necessary component of partly autonomous group work. The relation between individual and collective autonomy is theoretically and practically important because autonomous group work offers chances for differential and dynamic work design (Ulich, 1978, 1989b). This means that the internal assignment of tasks and roles can take into account individual competences, needs and moods. All authors more or less agree about the psychological importance of collective self-regulation with regard to the assignment of roles and tasks. However, not all of them discuss whether it is desirable that each member of the group who is interested, be allowed to perform challenging sub-tasks with a considerable degree of task integrity including requirements for individual self-regulation. Flexible assignment of integral subtasks, flexible job rotation and multifunctional, "polyvalent" qualification are methods to avoid internal hierarchy and an exaggerated internal "polarization" of skills (cf. Ulich, 1989b, 1984).

CRITERIA OF WORK GROUP AUTONOMY

Most of the work on criteria for determining the autonomy of work groups has been done by Gulowsen (1971, 1972) and Susman (1976).

The Gulowsen Approach

The criteria of autonomy were developed on a theoretical basis independent of, but following the collection of, the data for all the case studies. The criteria were not based on the empirical material in the cases, but were concerned with the "what, where, when, who and how of the groups' functions. Excluded were decisions regarding determination of norms, policy and doctrines, although such decisions would have great importance, e.g., in religious or political groups" (Gulowsen 1972, 375). Gulowsen's ways of putting these criteria into practice are given in Box 11.1. The list of criteria given in Box 11.1 was used to analyse the degree of autonomy of eight working groups in Norwegian firms. The results are shown in Table 11.4.

According to Gulowsen, the matrix reproduced in Table 11.4 shows that the criteria for autonomy follow the rules of a Guttman scale. This means that they form an ascending series, in which fulfilment of criteria for higher levels of autonomy always presuppose the fulfilment of those for lower levels.[2] Based on an analysis of the consequences of the respective decisions, Gulowsen draws the conclusion that the degree of autonomy is determined (a) by the time horizon of the autonomous decisions, and (b) the position in the system of the levels affected by the decisions.

Susman (1976) has allocated Gulowsen's types of autonomous decision to

---

[2] In analyses of 566 working groups with a total of 5700 members in 44 Siemens factories reported by Grob (1992), the hierarchical structure of the criteria for assessing autonomy as suggested by Gulowsen could not be confirmed in the given form, in spite of its plausibility. The question whether the criteria for autonomy form a hierarchical structure is in urgent need of an answer, because of its theoretical and practical importance.

> **Box 11.1 Criteria for the autonomy of work groups**
>
> 1. The group is able to influence the formulation of the goals valid for it:
>   (a) qualitatively, i.e. what the group is expected to produce, and;
>   (b) quantitatively, i.e. how much it is expected to produce and under what financial conditions. Criterion (b) is met only when both parts are fulfilled.
> 2. Provided that the boundary conditions are met, the group can decide the following:
>   (a) where to work;
>   (b) when to work; this criterion is met when the group can decide on the number of hours to be worked by the group as a whole, or when the group can decide whether a member may leave work during normal working hours, or when the group can decide whether and when overtime should be worked;
>   (c) in what further activities it wishes to engage. This criterion is met when the working group can interrupt its activity on its own responsibility, or when the members may engage in private or other work, provided they have fulfilled the set production goals.
> 3. The group makes the necessary decisions on selection of production method. This presupposes that:
>   (a) real alternatives exist, and that
>   (b) outsiders do not interfere in the choice of method (this criterion is irrelevant when (a) is not met).
> 4. The group decides on internal distribution of tasks. Presuppositions that this criterion can be met, are:
>   (a) there exist alternative patterns of task distribution, and;
>   (b) outsiders do not interfere in the decision process. This criterion is irrelevant if (a) is not met.
> 5. The group decides on its membership. This condition is met if the group can choose and engage new members, or if it can exclude undesired members.
> 6. The group takes decisions on two important aspects of leadership:
>   (a) whether it wishes to have a leader for procedures which take place within the group, and if so, who that leader shall be;
>   (b) whether it wishes to have a leader to regulate the boundary conditions, and if so, who that shall be.
> 7. Individual members of the group decide how to carry out their own tasks. This condition is not met if someone else makes the decision; it is irrelevant if the technology does not permit a decision.

three classes: (a) decisions on self-regulation (7, 6a, 5, 4), arising from the work process and serving to regulate the system; (b) decisions on self-determination (3, 2); these concern the outward independence of the working group, and do not necessarily arise from the work process; (c) decisions on self-management (6b, 1); these concern the position of the group in the power structure of the firm, and result from power politics or value judgements of management (numbers refer to Box 11.1).

Concerning the third class of autonomous decisions, it should be pointed out that the introduction of new technologies in many firms is accompanied by the

Table 11.4 Decision-making empowerment in eight partly autonomous work groups

Groups*	1a	1b	6b	2c	2b	3	4	5	6a	7
Logging group	−	+	+	+	+	+	+	+	+	+
Coal-mining group	−	+	+	+	+	+	+	+	+	+
Electrical panel-heater group	−	+	+	+	+	+	+	+	+	+
Alfa Lime Works oven group	−	−	−	+	+	+	+	+	+	+
Alfa Lime Works quarrier group	−	−	−	+	+	+	+	+	+	+
Rail-spring group	−	−	−	−	−	0	+	+	+	+
Ferro-alloy group	−	−	−	−	−	−	+	+	+	+
Galvanizing group	−	−	−	−	−	−	−	−	−	+

Criteria:
- 1a: The group has influence on its qualitative goals
- 1b: The group has influence on its quantitative goals
- 6b: The group decides on questions of external leadership
- 2c: The group decides what different tasks to take on
- 2b: The group decides when it will work
- 3: The group decides on questions of production methods
- 4: The group determines the internal distribution of tasks
- 5: The group decides on questions of recruitment
- 6a: The group decides on questions of internal leadership
- 7: The group members determine their individual production methods

From Gulowsen, 1972, with permission.

introduction of new working systems, the efficiency of which can only be ensured by appropriate opportunities for self-regulation (Bungard & Antoni, 1993; Bullinger, 1993; Ulich, 1993). In many cases, the rapid increase in customer-oriented production and the flexibility which this demands also make a functional necessity of work groups having extensive opportunities for self-regulation.

It is some time since Susman (1970) pointed out that, particularly under conditions of technical uncertainty—e.g. where there is increasingly complex automation—self-regulation within groups becomes a necessity. It may be reflected either in explicit organizational arrangements or in the tolerance of implicit ones.

Technical uncertainty concerns unforeseeable variances and disturbances, and means the (in)exactitude with which production or transformation processes can be controlled and checked by computer. Technical uncertainty therefore determines the extent of the informational and decision processes which confront workers in the process of task performance (cf. Cummings & Blumberg, 1987).

Criteria of Autonomy: An Activity-oriented Approach

Gulowsen's concepts about determining the autonomy status of work groups remain stimulating and of fundamental importance. But there are two further points to be made in connection with them:

1. As already pointed out, according to Gulowsen the "height" of the system level affected by decisions is one of the factors which determines degree of autonomy. However, in modern production organizations, an approach of this kind is no longer necessarily meaningful, since higher levels in the system by no means always have a greater influence on the structure of the organization, and thus on the possible autonomy of work groups. It is a fact that in many firms in recent years, the Information Technology (IT) Department, or the department responsible for production planning and control, has had a substantially greater influence than "higher system levels" on whether the structure moves in the direction of centralization or decentralization; which kinds of functional integration by means of IT linking are supported, and which obstructed; and which forms of man–machine division of functions are accepted, and which rejected. For this reason, it seems more meaningful to order the main activities or functions according to their influence on the production structure (cf. Figure 11.1). The matrix in Figure 11.1 is intended on the one hand to clarify the structuring power of the activities or functions, which decreases from top to bottom; on the other hand to depict the au-

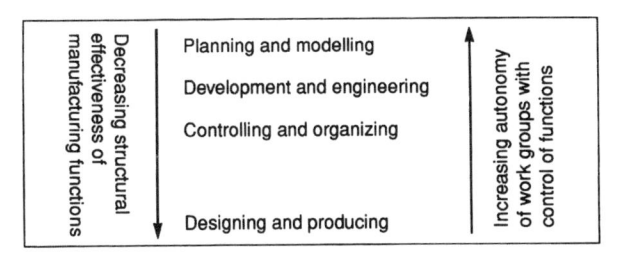

| Decreasing structural effectiveness of manufacturing functions ↓ | Planning and modelling
Development and engineering
Controlling and organizing
Designing and producing | ↑ Increasing autonomy of work groups with control of functions |

Figure 11.1 Functions with high structural effectiveness. From Ulich (1994), with permission

tonomy of work groups, which increases from bottom to top with increasing control of activities or functions.

2. The attempts to apply Gulowsen's operational features to the analysis and evaluation of the autonomy of work groups in modern production systems soon runs into difficulties (cf. Kirsch, 1993; Strohm et al., 1993; Weber & Ulich, 1993). These difficulties have to do with the fact that the method is not sufficiently task- or activity-oriented, so real work groups are difficult to classify according to degree of autonomy. Initially, the advantage of Gulowsen's concept appeared to lie in the fact that the method was independent of the activity, and thus permitted comparisons to be made across such different activities as assembly, electroplating, smelting, timber felling and coal-mining (cf. Table 11.4). However, the consequence of this is that means of self-regulation which are specific to activities or classes of activities can not be measured and their importance for personal development is either not recognized or is underestimated.

We therefore suggest the addition of an activity-oriented analysis grid to Gulowsen's method. It also seems useful to differentiate Gulowsen's scale according to whether decisions are made by the group or part of the group together, or by individual group members, and whether this is done without external interference or together with persons external to the group. Table 11.5 shows suggested activity-oriented categories.

It is clear from the list of activities in the analysis grid in Table 11.5 that task-oriented determination of the autonomy status of work groups must be preceded by investigation of the relevant sub-activities. This can be done by analysis of documents and/or observational interviews. Further differentiations may also be necessary, e.g. whether a particular task is always performed by the same group member alone, or together with people having other functions, or whether it is performed by several or all group members in turn.

In order to compare different activities or classes of activities, the activities may be ordered according to their sequential "wholeness", i.e. according to categories such as goal-setting, planning, preparation, organization, performance and checking; or according to their structural effectiveness (cf. Figure 11.1). Alternatively, the data can be entered in "Verfahren zur Ermittlung von Regulationserfordernissen in der Arbeit" (VERA) stages* (cf. Oesterreich & Volpert, 1991), so that a differently derived measure of autonomy is obtained by identifying collective regulation requirements. Finally, one might make a comparison using the Gulowsen items in a different formulation.

EVALUATION OF WORK GROUP AUTONOMY

An explorative study on the connection of socio-technical principles and characteristics of task design with analysis instruments stemming from the "action

---

* An instrument to identify regulation requirements in industrial work

Table 11.5 Example of activity-oriented categories for a profile of group work autonomy in manufacturing

The total group task includes:	+ − 0	The group alone	The group together with people having other functions	A particular group member alone	A particular group member together with people having other functions	The foreman or a person having other functions	Specify person having other functions
Layout of production area							
Arrangement of work places							
Planning of task sequence							
Setting of quality requirements for products							
Meeting deadlines							
Detailed dispositions							
Selection of production method							
Obtaining work means							
Selection of suitable work means							
Numerical control programming							
Setting up of machines							
Pre-adjustment of machines							

The decision is made by:

Table 11.5 Continued

		The decision is made by:				
The total group task includes:	+ − 0	The group alone	The group together with people having other functions	A particular group member alone	A particular group member together with people having other functions	The foreman or a person having other functions	Specify person having other functions
Servicing and maintenance							
Dealing with disturbances							
Carrying out small repairs							
Checking product quality							
Repair work							
Materials management							
Cleaning and transport							
Costs account							
Delivery of products to customer							
Internal task assignment							
Daily time-scheduling							
Regulation of presence and absence							

Decisions on overtime

Work tempo/Arrangement of breaks

Supply of personnel

Regulation of holidays

Decision on type of internal coordination

Choice of a group member for internal coordination

Decision on type of external representation

Selection of a group member for external representation

Regulation of boundaries with preceding and succeeding activities

Choice of new group members

Training of new group members

Training and further training of group members

Voting out undesired group members

Agreement on amount of production per time unit

Agreement of financial conditions

+ = Part of group task; − = Not part of group task; 0 = Non-existent.
From Ulich, 1994, with permission.

regulation theory" (cf. Hacker, 1986, 1994; Ulich, 1994; Volpert, 1987, 1992) will be elaborated. A brief description of two case studies in partly autonomous group work will be given. Theoretical consideration is given to the primacy of the task. Traditionally, work analysis instruments based on the theory of action regulation—such as VERA (Oesterreich & Volpert, 1986, 1991) and "Regulationshindernisse in der Arbeit"* (RHIA) (Greiner & Leitner, 1989; Leitner et al., 1987) focus on single work tasks. When they are used as an integral component of analysis and design strategy, this restriction can be overcome. In this way, these instruments are able to be utilized for the evaluation of "objective", task-related work group autonomy. Furthermore, in the next section some interim conclusions will be drawn about "subjective", person-related benefits as well as other selected results of partly autonomous group work.

Two Case Studies

From a sample of 60 case studies conducted in Swiss companies on the basis of document analysis, interviews with specialists and factory rounds, the authors chose two forms (cf. Weber & Ulich, 1993) in which two very different kinds of group work are practised (cf. Boxes 11.2 and 11.3). We evaluated the impact of certain task features using the following *categories of analysis* (based on observational interviews which, unfortunately, cannot be described in more detail here):

- *Individual autonomy* refers to the amount of planning and decision-making requirements the performed work tasks encompass. This is determined with the VERA instrument (Oesterreich & Volpert, 1986, 1991), whereby work tasks may be assigned to five levels of "regulation requirements" (each with two steps).
- *Task variety* occurs if an operator performs more than a single task, whether parallel or sequentially, as, for example, through job rotation.
- *Task-related opportunities for social interaction* occur if the work tasks performed by one worker necessitate coordination and synchronization with another. The maximal VERA-step of these parts of their tasks which require communication ("C") in the sense of common planning and decision-making are determined for each individual worker. It is called "VERA-C-step".

However, the amount of mental work load is an additional factor to consider: too high an amount can lead to discontent or psychophysiological disorders and threaten the acceptance of the group work overall. Task-related work load can be evaluated according to the empirically proven RHIA instrument (Leitner et al., 1987; Greiner & Leitner, 1989), which defines "regulation barriers". Whether determined by environment, technology or organization, these recurrent and

---

* An instrument to identify regulation hindrances in industrial work

> **Box 11.2 Case 1: Partly autonomous work group in a flexible manufacturing system for the sheet metal-working industry (FMS Group)**
>
> The FMS Group includes a foreman (skilled worker) as well as four operators (two of them skilled, two unskilled) who run a flexible manufacturing system (FMS). The FMS is used to produce sheet-metal parts for interior furnishings. The FMS consists of an automatic storage system for work pieces, a flexible transport system as well as two manufacturing lines. From the cell controller (workstation), Operator 1 calls up the sheet-metal parts (raw material) located on pallets from automatic storage (see Table 11.6) and directs them to a computerized numerical control (CNC) guillotine shear. The operator also programmes the very simple numerical control (NC) file to shear sheet-metal parts from the workstation, and ensures that sheared batches of parts travel over the automatic transport system (with pallet pool) near the FMS line machinery.

specific occurrences either render the given work task more difficult or interrupt it, in which case the worker is forced to engage in additional work, confront health or material risks, or overload his or her capabilities.

Table 11.6 shows that the amount of task-related mental load reaches considerable proportions for some members of the flexible manufacturing system (FMS) group. On average, approximately four regulation barriers occur for every operator at least several times a week. These necessitate an additional work effort of some 45 minutes in the working day. The four group operators alternate among the four work zones of the FMS weekly (systematic job rotation). While the foreman's tasks are not included in the job rotation, he does assist, given a personnel shortage on the FMS. This organizational form effects a marked "polarization" of *individual autonomy*. While the foreman's tasks (numerical control (NC) programming, production control, maintenance) require personally challenging planning and decision-making skills (VERA step 4), the operator's tasks, with one exception, simply require mental processing of the foreman's directions in advance (Step 2R) or completion of them (Step 2).

The notion of "polarization" also marks the *collective autonomy* of the FMS group to a great extent. Primarily the foreman enjoys frequent and personally challenging task-related opportunities for communication (VERA-C Step 4). The foreman, rather than the group itself, takes decisions regarding nearly all criteria for the collective autonomy of work groups. This form of "partly autonomous group work" has little to do with the socio-technical concept.

The amount of mental work load is markedly less than in the FMS group (cf. Table 11.6). On the average, a little less than three regulation barriers occur at least several times a week, costing the operator around 25 additional minutes' work a day. As to the work load, "polarization" of group members occurs. Two operators, who are not a part of work rotation, suffer considerable overload. In contrast to the FMS group in Case 1, the production island (PI) operators do not rotate systematically among the various work-places; the PI group is only a few weeks old and seems to require a certain degree of specialization, based on the

> **Box 11.3 Case 2: Partly autonomous work group in a flexible CNC production island for mould manufacturing (PI group)**
>
> The PI group consists of eight skilled metal workers without a foreman. The revision and repair of moulds make up their common primary task, i.e. the manufacture of complicated spare parts and, periodically, working new moulds. The group has the following at its disposal: a computerized numerical control (CNC) lathe, two direct numerical control (DNC) milling machines, two CNC surface grinding machines, a CNC machining centre for spark erosion, as well as twelve conventional machine tools. The group-technological structure of the machine tools permits workers to perform nearly all machining processes for each of the mould components. Highly qualified operators create most of the NC programmes directly on the CNC control station (partially with graphic display Support).

complexity of the work order. Because the group has many machine tools at its disposal, certain of them, where needed, are used by numerous PI group members. Rather than being strictly schematic, job rotation depends on the situation and is flexible in the sense of differential and dynamic work design (Ulich, 1989b, 1994).

Compared to the FMS group, operators of the PI group have considerably more *individual autonomy*. All of the operators perform challenging secondary tasks. For example they programme NC-files, or plan the steps of operations on conventional machine tools, set up the machines and occasionally even maintain them. Therefore, planning and decision-making requirements in keeping with "qualified labour" characterize the activities performed ("sub-goal planning", VERA level 3). This also applies, incidentally, to operator 7, who frequently alternates work places with operator 6. The *collective autonomy* is also more strongly pronounced: Every work task requires collective planning, understandably at different levels (steps 2 to 4R). The number of communication partners for every operator in the group is much greater than that in Case 1 (averaging 6.9 versus 1.3). There is no foreman to block information channels; instead, a network communication structure extends even beyond the limitations of the group itself. The PI group represents a partly autonomous group work to a considerably greater degree than the FMS group. Particularly with respect to several criteria affecting shop floor organization and control, the PI group takes autonomous group decisions. The level of individual autonomy guarantees challenging possibilities for learning and promoting personal development.

Interim Conclusions

Unfortunately failures are not generally published, even though there is often more to be learned from analysing failures than from reading reports of success. Nevertheless, the reports which are available indicate a number of possible benefits arising from the introduction of group work (cf. Table 11.7).

DIMENSIONS, CRITERIA AND EVALUATION OF WORK GROUP AUTONOMY

Table 11.6 Task features of two work groups

	Autonomy	Social interaction		Work load	Variety	
	VERA step	VERA-C step	No. of partners	No. of regulation barriers	No. of tasks	No. of workplaces
Case 1 (FMS group)						
Foreman	4	4	10	4	8	14
Operators (Work places):						
1 (Storing and transport system/shearing)	2	2R	2	7	5	12
2 (FMS line 1)	2R	2R	1	5	5	12
3 (FMS line 2)	3R	3R	2	3	5	12
4 (Punching/press brake)	2R	—	—	2	5	12
Average	2R/2	1/2R	1.25	4.25	5	12
Case 2 (PI group)						
Operators (Work places):						
1 (Lathes)	3	2	5	5	2	2
2 (Milling)	3	2	9	1	6	8
3 (Milling)	2	2	5	3	1	4
4,5 (Cylinder grinding)	3	3	6/9	3	2/5	2/5
6,7 (Surface grinding, etc.)	2/3	2	4/7	1	4	4
8 (Spark erosion, etc.)	4R	4R	10	5	3	5
Average	3R/3	2/3R	6.9	2.7	3.4	4.25

Table 11.7 Possible benefits of the introduction of partly autonomous work groups

Employee	Organization	Production
Intrinsic motivation through task orientation	Reduction in hierarchical levels	Improvement in product quality
Improvement of qualifications and skills	Changed supervisory roles	Decreased throughput times
Increase in flexibility	Changes in spans of control	Decrease in waiting times caused by work sequence
Qualitative change in work satisfaction	Functional integration	Decrease in periods of down time
Reduction of one-sided loads	Increased flexibility	Increased flexibility
Reduction of stress through mutual support	Redefinition of positions	Reduction of absenteeism
More active use of leisure time	New wage concepts	Reduction in turnover

From Ulich, 1994, with permission.

Admittedly, the positive effects described in Table 11.7 can only be expected if attention is paid to certain conditions, e.g. participation and timely training of participants, and if appropriate wage policies are developed at an early stage.

Macy et al. (1986) conducted a methodically careful meta-analysis of a total of 56 innovation projects which were carried out between 1970 and 1981 and which may be classified as methodologically convincing field studies. They concluded (a) that work in partly autonomous groups leads to an increase in productivity, and (b) that the introduction of group work raises productivity more than other innovations. However, they also found (c) negative relationships between group work and work satisfaction. Goodman, Devadas & Hughson (1990, p. 311), who reported on these findings, considered it surprising that work satisfaction did not show a positive relationship with group work. However, one should only be surprised at this if one considers work satisfaction simply from the quantitative point of view, as being more or less pronounced. It was this kind of experience which led to distinctions being made two decades ago between qualitatively different forms of work satisfaction (Bruggemann, 1974; Bruggemann, Groskurth & Ulich, 1975), and to a warning against expecting an increase in work satisfaction as a result of broadening of tasks and introducing group work (Ulich, 1976). According to the arguments presented in an earlier work, one should, for example, be more inclined to expect the appearance of progressive work (dis)satisfaction, which in response to simple enquiries can appear as a lack of satisfaction (Ulich, 1976).

In several cases of implementing self-regulating work groups we have found a change from a rather resigned job satisfaction, which is produced by a reduction of the level of aspiration, to a progressive job (dis)satisfaction, which is characterized by an increase in the level of aspiration and extended goals. The employees were trained to be able to manage their work system on their own. The aspiration level has risen during the process of change and competence has grown. Therefore, their attitudes to the work situation were based on a higher level and consequently became more critical.

Incidentally, Goodman, Devadas & Hughson expect a slow but accelerating spread of group work. They give three reasons for this: (a) a continuous cultural trend towards increasing participation; (b) varied and widespread experience with less complex forms of group work, e.g. quality circles, and the "evolutionary powers" resulting from them; (c) progressive technology, which—as in CIM concepts—makes increasing integration and flexibility possible, or even brings it about. Finally, the authors also expect a further spread of group work outside industrial production.

> "We expect more growth of these teams in nonmanufacturing environments. Also, we expect these teams to be found more frequently at the managerial level... We also expect greater use of self-managing teams in service or support settings. Airline crews, sales teams, and maintenance teams seem ripe for this self-management intervention." (Goodman, Devadas & Hughson, 1990, p. 324)

The authors justify their expectation that the spread of "self-managing teams" will be a slow process by the argument that it involves very complex organizational interventions, which must be consistent both with the values of an organization and with the technology. This should urge caution upon all those who believe that group work can be introduced within a short time.

Hackman (1990, p. 499), names three structural prerequisites for the success of work groups: (a) a "well designed" group task, which stimulates and maintains the motivation of the group members; particular attention should be paid to the "meaningfulness" of the activity, the measure of autonomy, and the feedback which results directly from task performance; (b) a "well composed" group. This should be as small as the task permits, have clear boundaries, and consist of members having appropriate professional and social qualifications—"neither as similar as peas in a pod nor so different that they will have trouble working together"; (c) a clear and explicit specification of the group's authority and its limits and, correspondingly, the group's accountability.

In order to make full use of the opportunities for self-regulation in work groups, the group's work must be actively supported by organizational structures. According to Hackman (1990, p. 500), the key elements of such support include:

1. A reward system which places the greatest emphasis not on the achievement of the individual, but on identification and reward of the achievement of the group.
2. An educational system which makes available all forms of training and technical advice which the members need to complete their knowledge and expertise.
3. An information system which provides the group with all the data and forecasts which it needs for the proactive management of its work.

4. The material resources—equipment, tools, space, financial and personal means—which the group needs to carry out its work.

Finally, allowance must be made for the fact that there are considerable individual differences between the employees in a firm, and that "there can be no single optimal working structure for all employees" (Zink, 1978, p. 46).

A CONTINGENCY MODEL

Cummings & Blumberg (1987) have formulated a contingency model based on socio-technical systems concepts. Their model might also explain why, under certain conditions, the Taylorist concept could succeed (see Taylor, 1911).

Cummings & Blumberg (1987) extend and elaborate the socio-technical concept by formulating technical, environmental and person-related contingencies. The two key technological features which can influence the success of work or task design are termed "technical interdependence" and "technical uncertainty". *Technical interdependence* means the extent to which the technology for creating a product or delivering a service requires cooperation between workers. The measure of technical interdependence determines whether the work should be designed as individual or group activity. When the degree of technical interdependence is low and there is little necessity for cooperation, the tasks should be structured as individual activities. However, if there is a high level of technical interdependence, the work should be structured as a group activity, in which the group members carry out tasks which are related or interconnected. *Technical uncertainty* means the amount of information processing and decision-making with which the employees are confronted in the course of performing the task. The degree of technical uncertainty determines whether control functions are part of the task, or whether they are fulfilled from outside through superiors, standards or time limits. When the level of uncertainty is low and little information processing is needed, external controls should be provided. However, if the level of technical uncertainty is high, controlling and decision-making functions should be transferred to the workers.

The feature of the *environment* which is important for work or task design is the degree of environmental stability or lability; this is known as "environmental dynamics." Every socio-technical system maintains exchange relationships with its environment. The dynamics of the environment partly determine how tasks must be structured, so that these exchange relationships can be adequately regulated. If the environment is relatively stable, exchange—e.g. of energy or information—can be take place in a standard manner. In this respect, work sequences can become routine. However, if the task environment is more dynamic, if changes are difficult to foresee, and the management of exchange relationships requires flexible adaptation to changing demands, then informational and decision processes must be included in the task in large measure.

With regard to personal characteristics which have a bearing on work design, Cummings & Blumberg refer to the work of Brousseau (1983) and Hackman

& Oldham (1980). They include "the desire for significant social relationships" and "the desire for personal accomplishment, learning and development". The extent of social needs is an important factor in deciding whether tasks should be structured as individual or group activities. The level of need for personal development determines the degree of division of tasks or "wholeness" of tasks.

Work psychologists who, like the authors of this chapter, feel committed to concepts of personality promoting work will be inclined at this point to raise questions about the technology itself and its design.

Table 11.8 shows the relationships between the technological, environmental, and personal features already described and a total of four "pure" forms of activity/task design. From the information in Table 11.8 we can derive the following statements:

1. The design of tasks as traditional, individual activities can be successful if technical interdependence, technical uncertainty, environmental dynamics, social and developmental needs are all low.
2. Traditional group work, with extensive division of labour, is particularly effective when technical interdependence is high but technical uncertainty is low; the environment is stable; and there is little desire for personal development, but marked social needs.
3. Individual job enrichment with varied demands, high autonomy and feedback promises success where there is low technical interdependence combined with high technical uncertainty, high environmental dynamics, a strong wish for personal development, and low social needs.
4. Self-regulating groups are especially successful where technical interdependence and technical uncertainty are high, the environment is not stable and there are strong needs for personal development and social interaction.

In their further analysis, Cummings & Blumberg refer to particular cases to show that advanced production technology substantially raises the level of tech-

Table 11.8 Work designs and Contingencies From Cummings & Blumberg (1987)

Work designs	Technical interdependence Low	Technical interdependence High	Technical uncertainty Low	Technical uncertainty High	Environmental dynamics Low	Environmental dynamics High	Growth needs Low	Growth needs High	Social needs Low	Social needs High
Traditional jobs	X		X		X		X		X	
Traditional work groups		X	X		X		X		X	
Enriched jobs	X			X		X		X	X	
Self-regulating workgroups		X		X		X		X		X

nical interdependence, technical uncertainty and environmental dynamics. The authors draw the logical conclusion that with regard to work design, the only answer is :

> ...self-regulating work groups, composed of multi-skilled employees who can jointly control technical and environmental variances. Such work designs are best suited to employees with high growth and social needs and may require upgrading employee skills and making changes in selection practices, training programmes, reward systems, and management styles (Cummings & Blumberg, 1987, p. 59).

WORK GROUP AUTONOMY AND INDUSTRIAL RELATIONS

When making international comparisons, it should be borne in mind that industrial relations, which are determined by cultural and/or legal norms, create conditions which may differ in the extent to which they favour self-regulation in production (cf. Figure 11.2).

Following Flanders (1965), the "Industrial Relations System" is considered as a system of rules, rights and obligations, and contractual relationships. Central to this is the relationship between employer and employee, with respect to their organizations. These rules, rights and obligations are established singly or in combination in institutions, and appear in different forms.

> For example, in the form of state laws and decrees, rules of unions or employers' organizations, collective agreements of social partners, rulings made by courts or boards of arbitration, decisions made by leadership of enterprises, and all generally accepted customs and traditions (Hotz-Hart, 1989).

Still following Flanders, we may distinguish two categories of rules. First, there are formal rules or, as Flanders puts it, "procedural rules" according to which conflicts of interest are resolved. They are aimed at the behaviour of whole companies and have an ordering function. They establish how material rules, or "substantive rules", which apply to the individual worker or position, are negotiated. Material rules have a regulatory function. Formal and material rules give rise to a network of rights and obligations, a network of contractual relationships. These rights are protected, defended, traded, bought and sold by the participants according to their interests" (Hotz-Hart, 1989, p. 28).

The statements about person-centred production systems in Table 11.8 may be taken as an approximate picture of the differences between the countries of the European Community.

Even if they cannot be interpreted exactly to scale, nevertheless the relationships make it clear that the development and implementation of human-centred or work-centred production systems—and with them, the introduction of partly autonomous groups—comes up against widely varying requirements at the level of statutory industrial relations.

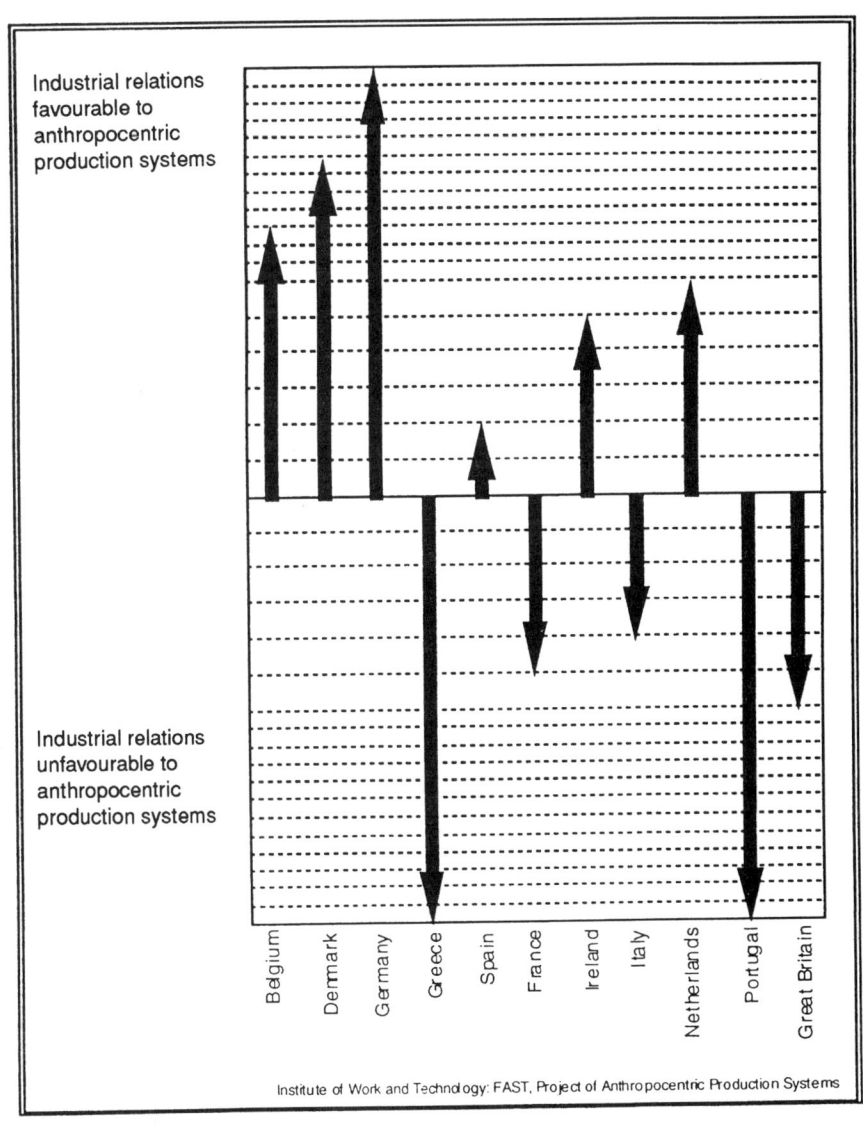

DIMENSIONS, CRITERIA AND EVALUATION OF WORK GROUP AUTONOMY 277

Figure 11.2 Influence of industrial relations on the development of person-centred production systems. From Lehner (1991), with permission

CONCLUSIONS

Successful implementation of group work in the sense defined here is possible only when it is a component of a comprehensive, socio-technically oriented concept of production. Here the design of the work task plays a key role in that it determines the division of functions between person and machine and also fosters or impedes the development of a task orientation. The wholeness of a task assigned to a group is ultimately decisive with regard to the possible degree of self-regulation of the individual and the collective. Self-regulation can be assessed empirically using task-oriented categories. Numerous investigations confirm the positive effects of work in partly autonomous groups both in terms of the personality development of the employees involved and of economy. In making decisions on the questions of the feasibility of group work and the form of group work to be realized, it is important, among other contingencies, to take the particular shape of industrial relations into account.

REFERENCES

Alioth, A. (1980). Entwicklung und Einführung alternativer Arbeitsformen. In E. Ulich (ed.), *Schriften zur Arbeitspsychologie*, Vol. 27. Bern: Huber.

Alioth, A. (1986). Technik—kein Sachzwang. In W. Duell & F. Frei (eds), *Arbeit gestalten—Mitarbeiter beteiligen*. Frankfurt: Campus, pp. 195–202.

Alioth, A. & Ulich, E. (1981). Gruppenarbeit und Mitbestimmung am Arbeitsplatz. In F. Stoll (ed.), *Anwendungen im Berufsleben: Arbeits-, Wirtschafts- und Verkehrspsychologie (Die Psychologie des 20. Jahrhunderts, Bd. 13)*. Zürich: Kindler, pp. 863–885.

Alioth, A., Martin, E. & Ulich, E. (1976). Semi-autonomous work groups in warehousing. *Proceedings of the 6th Congress of the International Ergonomics Association*. Washington D.C., pp. 187–191.

Asch, S.E. (1957). *Social Psychology*. New York: Prentice-Hall.

Bertalanffy, L.V. (1950). The theory of open systems in physics and biology. *Science*, **111**, 23–29.

Blumberg, M. (1988). Towards a new theory of job design. In W. Karwowski, H.R. Parsaei & M.R. Wilhelm (eds), *Ergonomics of Hybrid Automated Systems*, Vol. I. Amsterdam: Elsevier, pp. 53–59.

Brousseau, K.R. (1983). Toward a dynamic model of job-person relationships: findings, research questions and implications for work system design. *Academy of Management Review*, **8**, 33–45.

Bruggemann, A. (1974). Zur Unterscheidung verschiedener Formen von "Arbeitszufriedenheit". *Arbeit und Leistung*, **28**, 281–284.

Bruggemann, A., Grosskurth, P. & Ulich, E. (1975). Arbeitszufriedenheit. In E. Ulich (ed.), *Schriften zur Arbeitspsychologie*, Vol. 17. Bern: Huber.

Bullinger, H.-J. (1993). Human computer interaction and lean production: the shop floor example. Paper presented to the 5th International Conference on Human–Computer Interaction, Orlando, Florida, August 8–13.

Bungard, W. & Antoni, C. (1993). Gruppenorientierte Interventionstechniken. In H. Schuler (ed.), *Lehrbuch Organisationspsychologie*. Bern: Huber, pp. 377–404.

Cherns, A. (1976). The principles of organizational design. *Human Relations*, **29**, 783–792.

Cherns, A. (1987). Principles of sociotechnical design revisited. *Human Relations*, **40**, 153–162.

Cummings, T. & Blumberg, M. (1987). Advanced manufacturing technology and work design. In T. Wall, C. Clegg & N. Kemp (eds), *The Human Side of Advanced Manufacturing Technology*. Chichester: Wiley, pp. 37–60.

Cummings, T.G. & Molloy, E.S. (1977). *Improving Productivity and the Quality of Working Life*. New York: Praeger.

Demmer, B., Gohde, H.-E. & Kötter, W. (1991). Komplettbearbeitung in eigener Regie. *Technische Rundschau*, **83**(4), 18–26.
Emery, F.E. & Emery, M. (1974). *Participative Design*. Canberra: Centre for Continuing Education, Australian National University.
Emery, F.E. & Thorsrud, E. (1976). *Democracy at Work*. Leiden: Martinus Nijhoff.
Emery, F.E. & Thorsrud, E. (1982). Industrielle Demokratie. In E. Ulich (ed.), *Schriften zur Arbeitspsychologie*, Vol. 25. Bern: Huber.
Emery, F.E. (1959). Characteristics of Socio-technical Systems. London: Tavistock Institute of Human Relations, Document No. 527.
Endres, E. & Wehner, T. (1993). Kooperation — die Wiederentdeckung einer Schlüsselkategorie. In J. Howaldt & H. Minssen (eds), *Lean, Leaner, ...? Die Veränderung des Arbeitsmanagements zwischen Humanisierung und Rationalisierung*. Dortmund: Montania, pp. 201–222.
Flanders, A. (1965). *Industrial Relations: What is Wrong with the System?* cited by Hotz-Hart 1989.
Frese, M. (1978). Partialisierte Handlung und Kontrolle: zwei Themen der industriellen Psychopathologie. In M. Frese, S. Greif & N. Semmer (eds), *Industrielle Psychopathologie Schriften zur Arbeitspsychologie* (ed. E. Ulich), Vol. 23. Bern: Huber, pp. 159–183.
Goodman, P.S., Devadas, R. & Hughson, T.L. (1990). Groups and productivity: analyzing the effectiveness of self-managing teams. In J.P. Campbell & R.J. Campbell (eds), *Productivity in Organizations*. San Francisco: Jossey-Bass, pp. 295–327.
Graf, O. (1954). *Studien über Fliessarbeitsprobleme an einer praxisnahen Experimentieranlage*. Köln, Opladen: Westdeutscher Verlag.
Graf, O., Rutenfranz, J. & Ulich, E. (1956). Nervöse Belastung bei industrieller Arbeit unter Zeitdruck. *Forschungsberichte des Landes Nordrhein-Westfalen*, N. 1425. Stuttgart: Kohlhammer.
Greenberg, C.I. (1979). Toward an integration of ecological psychology and industrial psychology: undermanning theory, organization size, and job enrichment. *Environmental Psychology and Non-verbal Behaviour*, **3**, 228–242.
Greiner, B. & Leitner, K. (1989). Assessment of job stress: the RHIA-Instrument. In K. Landau & W. Rohmert (eds), *Recent Developments in Job Analysis*. London: Taylor & Francis, pp. 53–66.
Grob, R. (1992). Teilautonome Arbeitsgruppen. Bilanz der Erfahrungen in der Siemens AG. *Angewandte Arbeitswissenschaft*, **134**, 1–31.
Gulowsen, J. (1971). *Selvstyrte Arbeidsgrupper*. Oslo: Tanum.
Gulowsen, J. (1972). A measure of work group autonomy. In L.E. Davis & J.C. Taylor (eds), *Design of Jobs*. Harmondsworth: Penguin, pp. 374–390.
Hacker, W. (1986). Arbeitspsychologie. In E. Ulich (ed.), *Schriften zur Arbeitspsychologie*, Vol. 41. Bern: Huber.
Hacker, W. (1987). Software-Ergonomie: Gestalten rechnergestützter Arbeit? In W. Schönpflug & M. Wittstock (eds), *Software Ergonomie' 87: Nützen Informationssysteme dem Benutzer?* Stuttgart: Teuber, pp. 31–54.
Hacker, W. (1994). Action regulation theory and occupational psychology. Review of german empirical research since 1987. *The German Journal of Psychology*, **18**(2), 91–120.
Hackman, J.R. (1977). Work design. In J.R. Hackman & J.L. Suttle (eds), *Improving Life at Work*. Santa Monica: Goodyear, pp. 96–162.
Hackman, J.R. (1986). The psychology of self-management in organizations. In M.S. Pallak & R.O. Perloff (eds), *Psychology and Work: Productivity, Change and Employment*. Washington, DC: American Psychological Association, pp. 85–136.
Hackman, J.R. (ed.) (1990). *Groups That Work (and Those That Don't)*. San Francisco: Jossey-Bass.

Hackman, J.R. & Lawler, E.E. (1971). Employee reactions to job characteristics. *Journal of Applied Psychology*, **55**, 259–286.

Hackman, J.R. & Oldham, G.R. (1976). Motivation through the design of work: test of a theory. *Organizational Behaviour and Human Performance*, **60**, 250–279.

Hackman, J.R. & Oldham, G.R. (1980). *Work Redesign*. Reading, MA: Addison-Wesley.

Hellpach, W. (1922).'Sozialpsychologische Analyse des betriebstechnischen Tatbestandes "Gruppenfarikation". In R. Lang & W. Hellpach (eds), *Gruppenfabrikation*. Berlin: Springer, pp. 5–186.

Herbst, P.G. (1976). *Alternatives to Hierarchies*. Leiden: Martinus Nijhoff.

Hotz-Hart, B. (1989). *Modernisierung von Unternehmen und Industrien bei unterschiedlichen industriellen Beziehungen*. Bern: Haupt.

Jaques, E. (1951). *The Changing Culture of a Factory*. London: Tavistock.

Jaques, E. (1956). *The Measurement of Responsibility*. London: Tavistock.

Kemp, N.J., Wall, T.D., Clegg, C.W. & Cordery, J.L. (1983). Autonomous work groups in a greenfield site: a comparative study. *Journal of Occupational Psychology*, **56**, 271–288.

Kirsch, C. (1993). *Autonomie von Arbeitsgruppen und Qualitätszirkeln in japanischen Produktionsbetrieben*. Zürich: Institute of Work Psychology, Swiss Federal Institute of Technology.

Kötter, W., Gohde, H.-E. & Weber W.G. (1989). Technological and organizational options for skill-based task design in a group technology project. In P. Kopacec, M. Moritz & R. Genser (eds), *Skill-based Automated Production*. Preprints of the IFAC-/IFIP-/IMACS-Symposium, Austria, November 15–17. Vienna: Austrian Center for Productivity and Efficiency, pp. TS 12/1–TS 12/6.

Lehner, F. (1991). Anthropocentric production systems. The european response to advanced manufacturing and globalisation. *APS Research papers*, Vol. 4. Brussels: Commission of the European Communities, Programme FAST.

Leitner, K., Volpert, W., Greiner, B., Weber, W.G. & Hennes, K. (1987). *Analyse psychischer Belastung in der Arbeit. Das RHIA-Verfahren. Handbuch und Manual*. Köln: TÜV Rheinland.

Lewin, K. (1982). In C.F. Graumann (ed.), *Werkausgabe*, Vol. 4, *Feldtheorie*. Bern: Huber.

Macy, B.A., Hurts, C.C., Hurts, C.C., Izumi, H., Norton, L.W. & Smith, R.R. (1986). Meta-analysis of united states empirical organizational change and work innovation field experiments: methodology and preliminary results. Paper presented at the 46th Annual Meeting of the National Academy of Management. Chicago: August.

Oesterreich, R. & Volpert, W. (1986). Task Analysis for Work Design on the Basis of Action Regulation Theory, *Economic and Industrial Democracy*, **7**, 503–527.

Oesterreich, R. & Volpert, W. (1991). VERA Version 2. In R. Oesterreich & W. Volpert (eds), *Forschungen zum Handeln in Arbeit und Alltag*, Vol. 3. Berlin: Technische Universität, Institut für Humanwissenschaften in Arbeit und Ausbildung.

Pasmore, W.A. (1988). *Designing Effective Organizations: The Socio-technical Systems Perspective*. Chichester: Wiley.

Pasmore, W., Francis, C., Haldeman, J. & Shani, A. (1982). Sociotechnical systems: a North American reflection on empirical studies of the seventies. *Human Relations*, **35**, 1179–1207.

Pearce, J.A. & Ravlin, E.C. (1987). The design and activation of self-regulating work groups. *Human Relations*, **40**, 751–782.

Rice, A.K. (1953). Productivity and social organization in an indian weaving shed: an examination of the socio-technical system of an experimental automated loom shed. *Human Relations*, **6**, 297–329.

Rice, A.K. (1958). *Productivity and Social Organization: The Ahmedabad Experiment*. London: Tavistock.

Rosenstiel, L.V. (1992). *Grundlagen der Organisationspsychologie*, 3rd Edn. Stuttgart: Schäffer/Poeschel.
Sader, M. (1991). *Psychologie der Gruppe*, 4th Edn. Munich: Juventa.
Schneider, H.-D. (1975). *Kleingruppenforschung*. Stuttgart: Teubner.
Sherif, M. & Sherif, C. (1969). *Social Psychology*. New York: Harper & Row.
Strohm, O., Kirsch, C., Kuark, J.K., Leder, L., Louis, E., Pardo, O., Schilling, A. & Ulich, E. (1993). Computer aided manufacturing systems: work psychological aspects. *Proceedings of the European Conference on Computer Science, Communications and Society: A Technical and Cultural Challenge*. Bern, pp. 221–238.
Susman, G. (1970). The impact of automation on work group autonomy and task specialisation. *Human Relations*, 23, 567–577.
Susman, G.I. (1976). *Autonomy at Work: A Socio-technical Analysis of Participative Management*. New York: Praeger.
Taylor, F.W. (1911). *Principles of Scientific Management*. New York: Hanper & Brothers.
Tomaszewski, T. (1981). Struktur, Funktion und Steuerungsmechanismen menschlicher Tätigkeit. In T. Tomaszewski (ed.), *Zur Psychologie der Tätigkeit*. Berlin: Deutscher Verlag der Wissenschaften, pp. 11–33.
Trist, E.L. (1981). *The Evolution of Socio-technical Systems. Issues in the Quality of Working Life*. Occasional Papers No. 2. Toronto: Ontario Quality of Working Life Centre.
Trist, E.L. & Bamforth, K.W. (1951). Some social and psychological concequences of the longwall method of coal getting. *Human Relations*, 4, 3–38.
Ulich, E. (1956). Gruppenbildung am Fliessband. *Psychologische Rundschau*, 7, 260–269.
Ulich, E. (1976). Über mögliche Auswirkungen von Arbeitsstrukturierungen auf Zufriedenheit und Beanspruchung. *Fortschrittliche Betriebsführung*, 25, 343–345.
Ulich, E. (1978). Über das Prinzip der differentiellen Arbeitsgestaltung. *Industrielle Organisation*, 47, 566–568.
Ulich, E. (1989a). Arbeitspsychologische Konzepte der Aufgabengestaltung. In S. Maas & H. Oberquelle (eds), *Software-Ergonomie '89: Aufgabenorientierte Systemgestaltung und Funktionalität*. Stuttgart: Teubner, pp. 51–65.
Ulich, E. (1989b). Humanization of work—concepts and cases. In J. Fallon, H.P. Pfister & J. Brebner (eds), *Advances in Industrial and Organizational Psychology*. Amsterdam: Risevier North-Holland, pp. 133–143.
Ulich, E. (1993). CIM—eine integrative Gestaltungsaufgabe im Spannungsfeld von Mensch, Technik und Organisation. In G. Cyranek & E. Ulich (eds), *CIM—Herausforderung an Mensch, Technik, Organisation. Schriftenreihe Mensch—Technik—Organisation* (ed. E. Ulich), Vol. 1. Zürich: Verlag der Fachvereine; Stuttgart: Teubner, pp. 29–43.
Ulich, E. (1994). *Arbeitspsychologie*, 3rd Edn. Zürich: Verlag der Fachvereine/Stuttgart: Schäffer-Poeschel.
Volpert, W. (1974). *Handlungsstrukturanalyse als Beitrag zur Qualifikationsforschung*. Köln: Pahl-Rugenstein
Volpert, W. (1987). Psychische Regulation von Arbeitstätigkeiten. In U. Kleinbeck & J. Rutenfranz (eds), *Arbeitspsychologie. Enzyklopädie der Psychologie, Themenbereich D*, Series III, Vol. 1. Göttingen: Hogrefe, pp. 1–42.
Volpert, W. (1992). Work design for human development. In C. Floyd, H. Züllighoven, H. Budde, & R. Keil-Slawik (eds), *Software Development and Reality Construction*. Berlin: Springer, pp. 336–348.
Wall, T.D. & Clegg, C.W. (1981). A longtudinal field study of group work redesign. *Journal of Occupational Behavior*, 2, 31–49.
Weber, W.G. & Ulich, E. (1993). Psychological criteria for the evaluation of different

forms of group work in advanced manufacturing systems. In M.J. Smith & G. Salvendy (eds), *Human–Computer Interaction: Application and Case Studies*. Amsterdam: Elsevier, pp. 26–31.

Wilson, A.T.M. & Trist, E.L. (1951). *The Bolsover System of Continuous Mining.* London: Tavistock Institute of Human Relations, Document No. 290.

Womack, J.P., Jones, D.T. & Roos, D. (1990). *The Machine that Changed the World.* New York: Macmillan.

Zink, K. (1978). Zur Begründung einer zielgruppenspezifischen Organisationsentwicklung. *Zeitschrift für Arbeitswissensschaft*, **32**, 42–48.

Section IV

Group Outcomes

Chapter 12

Criteria for the Study of Work Group Functioning

Felix C. Brodbeck
Department of Psychology, University of Munich, Germany

Abstract

In this chapter current criterion concepts and measurement practices are explored by reviewing theories and empirical studies about work group functioning. The conceptual issues raised pertain to the distinction between process criteria (performance) and outcome criteria (effectiveness); to their dimensionality; and to factors that modify the performance–effectiveness relationship such as situational constraints, work group autonomy and temporal changes. The measurement issues raised concern the integration of global and fine-grained criteria, composite measures, procedures for criteria selection, multiple levels of analysis and the use of subjective data for the study of work group functioning. Throughout the chapter issues from the individual performance and the organizational effectiveness literatures are explored in relation to how they can be used to develop theories of effective work group functioning. Overall, the status of the work group performance and effectiveness concept is examined and critically evaluated. A criterion model of work group functioning is outlined.

INTRODUCTION

In 1986 McGrath explored the feasibility of building a research domain that concentrates on task performance of groups in organizations. He described putting more emphasis on theory building as one of ten critical needs for studying groups at work. If we are to build theories of performance, the same degree of effort should be applied to develop criterion measures as has been applied to the development of predictor tests (Borman, 1991). However, there is little conceptual clarity about performance criteria in industrial and organizational psychology (Campbell, 1990; Pritchard, 1992). Campbell & Campbell (1988) see this as not a definitional problem. They perceive a need for a better conceptual understanding of performance and suggest that the lack of criterion-related research has considerably hindered theoretical development. In recent publications, examining individual job performances (e.g. Bormann, 1991; Campbell, 1990) and organizational productivity (e.g. Campbell & Campbell, 1988; Pritchard, 1992), systematic accounts of criterion-related issues are given. Even though reviews about group performance in organizations have been recently published (e.g. Guzzo & Shea, 1992; Sundstrom, De Meuse & Futrell, 1990), no specific account of the criteria of work group functioning is currently available.

In this chapter a first step towards such an account is taken by analyzing how theoretical models of work group functioning delineate the criteria they use and what the communalities and differences are. Only theories that view work groups as performing units within organizational contexts are examined. The analysis also describes current theoretical and methodological developments that are relevant for studying work group functioning within organizations. Eight areas are discussed with respect to conceptual and methodological ramifications for theory development and measurement of work group performance (see Table 12.2). In the first two sections the difference between process criteria (performance) and outcome criteria (effectiveness) and their underlying dimensions are described. In the third and fourth sections, factors are identified that can affect the relationship between work group performance and effectiveness: situational constraints, work group autonomy and time. The propositions derived from the discussions of these topics flow into a criterion model for the study of work group functioning, which is summarized in the fifth section. The next four sections address specific problems of criterion measurement in work groups and methods currently used*: (a) global vs. specific criteria in composite measures; (b) value and policy capturing by multiple constituency models; (c) individual vs. group level constructs and multiple-level analysis, and (d) subjective criterion measures. In the final section, suggestions to meet standards for delineating and measuring criteria of work group functioning are summarized.

What is discussed in this chapter is not meant to give a complete account of all criterion-related issues. It reflects a subjective selection of current problems. By discussing them, the author wishes to further theoretical understanding and to improve measurement practice for the study of work group functioning within organizations.

---

*For a discussion of general issues and methods for criterion measurement the reader is asked to refer to the excellent reviews on organizational effectiveness (Smith, 1976; Campbell & Campbell, 1988; Pritchard, 1992), on individual performance (Bormann, 1991; Campbell, 1990), on psychometric aspects of criterion measurement (Bormann, 1991; Landy & Farr, 1983), and on the "criterion problem" (Austin & Villanova, 1992).

A CRITERION MODEL FOR THE STUDY OF WORK GROUP FUNCTIONING

Performance vs. Effectiveness

In all work group theories reviewed a distinction between intermediate (process) criteria and final (output) criteria of performance is identifiable (see Table 12.1). The distinction is explicitly made in some models (cf. Cummings, 1981; Gladstein, 1984; Hackman, 1987; Pearce & Ravlin, 1987; Weldon & Weingart, 1993) and supplemented by the theoretical assumption that final performance is a function of intermediate performance. Other models make the same distinction implicitly by restricting the performance concept to either intermediate criteria (Nieva, Fleischman & Rieck, 1978, as described in Goodman, Ravlin & Argote, 1986) or to final criteria only (cf. Goodman, 1986; Kollodny & Kiggundu, 1980; Shea & Guzzo, 1987a,b; Sundstrom, De Meuse & Futrell, 1990).

Sometimes the same variables refer to different criterion concepts, "performance", "effectiveness" or "productivity". For example, "delivery of products and services per specification" is referred to by Shea & Guzzo (1987a,b) as an indicator of "group productivity" and by Sundstrom, De Meuse & Futrell (1990) as an indicator of "group performance". In Hackman's (1987) model it would be considered to be an indicator of "group effectiveness". A conceptual distinction made by Campbell & Campbell (1988) gives a clear-cut criterion delineation that is consistent with definitions within the organizational productivity and the individual performance domains (see also Campbell et al., 1970). The authors define "performance" as an aggregate of those behaviors that are relevant for achieving the goals specified; "effectiveness" as the degree to which the performance outcomes approach the goals specified; and "productivity" as how efficiently a particular level of effectiveness is achieved.

The distinction between work group performance and effectiveness is an essential feature of the criterion model developed in this chapter (see Figure 12.1), for several reasons. It has been argued that independent assessment of performance and effectiveness enables the researcher to portray when high performance does not correspond with high effectiveness. If there is disparity, it invites investigation of the reasons why (Cummings, 1981; Campbell & Campbell, 1988). The distinction illustrates that the so-called "unmodified linear assumption"—more performance means more effectiveness (cf. Kahn, 1977)—held by many work group models, is not necessarily true (Goodman, Ravlin & Schminke, 1987). Under a "modified linear assumption", the criterion relevance of the variables used to study work group functioning is of particular concern. Deficiency and contamination are two important aspects of criterion relevance (Borman, 1991). Deficiency comes about when a set of criteria does not measure all important areas of performance. Contamination exists when criterion measurement taps variance irrelevant to performance.

Table 12.1 Performance vs. effectiveness dimensions in work group theories

Work group models	Dimensions of work group performance	Dimensions of work group effectiveness
Cummings, 1981	Effort, psychological arousal, task commitment. Knowledge and skill. Performance strategies, expectations and beliefs.	Workers' values (growth needs, social needs). Managers' values (theory X vs. theory Y). Organization values (quantity vs. quality, innovation vs. tradition).
Gladstein, 1984	Open communication, supportiveness, conflict. Weighting individual inputs, discussion of strategy, boundary management.	Performance (sales revenue, self reported performance). Satisfaction (with team, with meeting customer needs, with extrinsic rewards and work).
Goodman, 1986	Not specified.	Production (number of products).
Hackman, 1987	Level of effort expended for task completion. Knowledge and skill members bring to bear on the task. Performance strategies used by the group.	Productive output (according to the standards of those who review the product). Social criteria (ability of members to work together). Personal criteria (satisfaction of members' needs).
Kolodny & Kiggundu, 1980	Not specified.	Productivity (high output, efficiency, e.g. cost per cord of wood). Maintenance of skilled labor. Satisfaction (e.g. pride in performance, work group cohesiveness).
Nieva, Fleishman & Rieck, 1978 (from Goodman, Ravlin & Argote, 1986)	Individual task performance (e.g. monitoring a machine). Team performance functions (e.g. interaction, coordination).	Not specified.
Pearce & Ravlin, 1987	Commitment to group. Variety of member's responses, coordination of members.	Productivity. Safety, absenteeism, turnover, satisfaction. Innovation.
Shea & Guzzo, 1987a,b	Not specified.	Productivity (delivery of products and services per specification).
Sundstrom, DeMeuse & Futrell, 1990	Not specified.	Performance (delivery of products and services per specification). Viability (satisfaction, participation and willingness to continue working together).
Weldon & Weingart, 1993	Effort, concern for performance aspects unrelated to the goal. Planning, cooperation, morale building.	Performance (productive outcome).

```
                    ┌──────────────┐  ┌──────────────┐
                    │ Situational  │  │  Work group  │
                    │ constraints  │  │   autonomy   │
                    └──────┬───────┘  └──────┬───────┘
┌────────────────────┐     │                 │     ┌────────────────────┐
│ Performance        │     ▼                 ▼     │ Effectiveness      │
│ dimensions         │                             │ dimensions         │
│                    │←────────────────────────────→│                    │
│ -Motivation        │                             │ -Productive output │
│ -Knowledge and skills                            │ -Personal criteria │
│ -Internal and external                           │ -Social criteria   │
│  collective strategies                           │ -Innovations       │
└────────────────────┘                             └────────────────────┘
              ↖                                   ↗
                       ┌──────────────────────┐
                       │ Development and time │
                       │                      │
                       │ -Social dynamics     │
                       │ -Shifts in abilities, task,
                       │  technology and product
                       │ -Time-lag of measurement
                       └──────────────────────┘
```

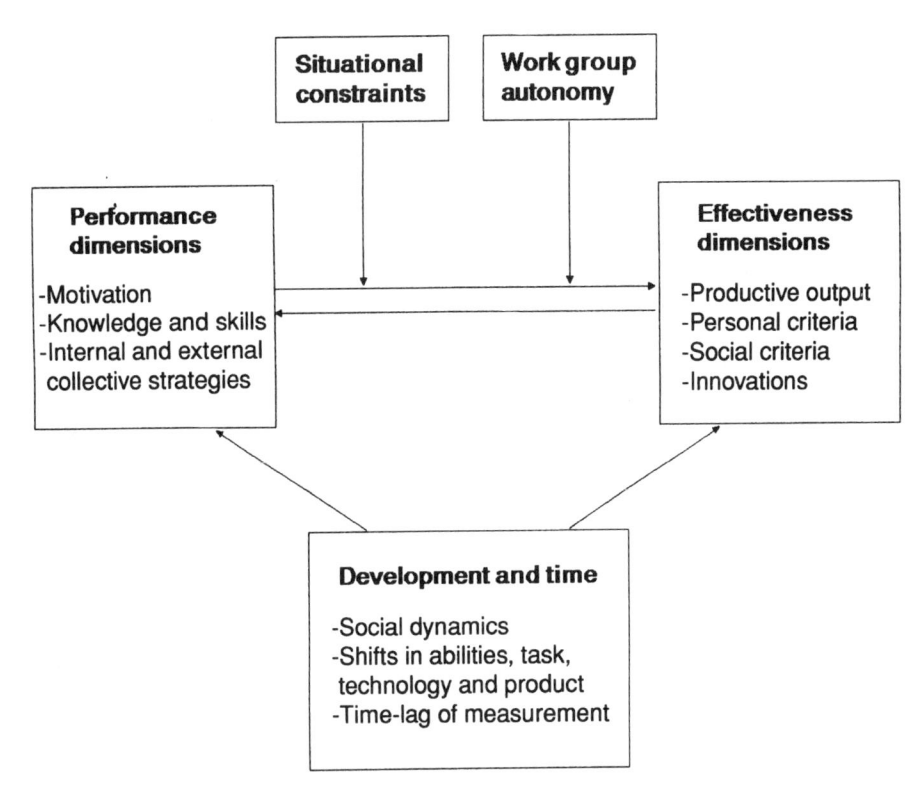

Figure 12.1 A criterion model for the study of work group functioning

Dimensions of Performance and Effectiveness

Performance Dimensions

The theories that specify intermediate criteria pertain to what Campbell & Campbell (1988) define as performance: an aggregate of those behaviors that are relevant for achieving the goals specified. Most commonly the distinctions made by Hackman (1987) are drawn between three dimensions: motivation to work (e.g. effort), knowledge and skill brought to bear on the task (e.g. how a machine is monitored) and performance strategies used by the group (e.g. coordination techniques).

Many theories reviewed use the heuristic input-process-output model (McGrath, 1964) of work group performance as a frame of reference. It relates a set of contextual determinants which affect work group effectiveness through the mediation of only *internal activities* of work groups. However, some authors argue, that for environmental integration *external activities* need to be performed by the work group. For instance, Gladstein (1984) uses boundary management as a performance dimension and Sundstrom, De Meuse & Futrell (1990) suggest the way work groups are "integrated into larger systems through coordination and synchronization with suppliers, managers, peers and customers" (p. 124) is a key aspect of group performance. Teams actively managing external demands are shown to be more effective (Pfeffer, 1986; Pfeffer & Salancik, 1978). In this respect, a fruitful line of research has been reopened by Gladstein-Ancona (1990) by looking at the collective performance strategies work groups and their leaders enforce to relate to their external environment. For teams with new unstructured tasks facing external task demands, she shows that a so-called "probing strategy" ("a lot of interaction with outsiders to diagnose their needs and experiment with solutions", p. 344), as compared to "informing" and "parading" strategies (only internal information is used to map environmental needs and requirements), is associated with higher levels of effectiveness in the long run, when rated by outsiders. However, in the short run, when rated by team members, making use of the probing strategy is associated with lower levels of personal criteria (e.g. members' satisfaction) and lower levels of social criteria (e.g. group cohesiveness). Gladstein-Ancona's (1990) research calls for the inclusion of external interaction strategies within work group performance research. The mutual influence between environmental constraints and team action should be of more concern to work group theorizing and research (see "Situational Constraints," below; see also Allen, this volume). Moreover, the differential effects of external probing on different effectiveness dimensions rated by different constituents call for the use of multiple effectiveness dimensions and multiple-constituency approaches (see "Value and Policy Capturing with Multiple Constituency Approaches", below). In summary, it is suggested that work group performance should be conceptualized with at least three dimensions in mind; motivation to work, individual knowledge and skill brought to bear on the group task, and collective performance strategies used by the group for internal and for external activities (see Figure 12.1).

Effectiveness Dimensions

All of the work group theories but one (Nieva, Fleishman & Rieck, 1978) incorporate what Campbell & Campbell (1988) define as effectiveness: the degree to which the performance outcomes approach the goals specified. Usually, distinctions are drawn between productive output (e.g. sales revenue, tons of coal), social criteria (e.g. willingness to work together, satisfaction with the team) and personal criteria (e.g. member satisfaction, personal development, individual safety and health). Disparities among the theories exist where it comes to the question of what dimensions should be part of an effectiveness concept. For instance, Goodman's (1986) model makes use of only one effectiveness dimension, namely productive output. Goodman suggests concentrating on one dimension only. He argues that this allows for the development of different models depending on what effectiveness criterion is used. In Hackman's

(1987) and in Cummings' (1981) models, the workers' values (e.g. growth needs, social needs, satisfaction), and in Hackman's (1987) and Sundstrom, De Meuse & Futrell's (1990) models, work group viability (e.g. member's willingness to continue working together) are perceived to be essential parts of the effectiveness criterion, in addition to task completion. However, Shea & Guzzo (1987a) argue for task accomplishments to be the only important components, "The *sine qua non* of organizational work groups is the successful completion of tasks, hence determining their effectiveness should turn on just that." (p. 330).

Sundstrom, De Meuse & Futrell (1990) explicitly go beyond such a task completion model, by stating that it "overlooks the possibility that a team can 'burn itself up' [Hackman & Oldham, 1980, p. 169] through unresolved conflict or divisive interaction" (p. 122). Task completion models use a "top down" perspective on group effectiveness. They view work groups predominantly as parts of an organization, consequently a group's ultimate goal is to serve the predefined organizational goals. This perspective is not only likely to neglect theoretically and practically relevant dimensions of work group functioning—the problem of criterion deficiency (Borman, 1991). It is also likely to neglect aspects of humanization of work. Since the perspective taken here is meant to serve theorizing about all relevant aspects of work group functioning, social and personal criteria are included in the effectiveness concept, in addition to criteria of task completion (see Figure 12.1).

Innovation is suggested as another effectiveness dimension by Cummings (1981) and Pearce & Ravlin (1987). Team innovation can be divided into two successive components, idea generation and implementation (West, 1990). They mirror the distinction between performance and effectiveness. The number and quality of innovative ideas (idea generation) as a result of group interaction, motivation, knowledge and skill fits into the concept of work group performance. The transformation of innovative ideas into some new product, method or service (implementation) is part of the effectiveness criterion. Whereas the idea generation aspect of innovation can be subsumed under the three performance dimensions already discussed, I do not see how this could be done for the implemention aspect of innovation. Thus, within the conceptual model, innovation implementation is used as a separate effectiveness dimension.

Situational Constraints

Effectiveness can be attributed to work group performance plus measurement error, only if a work group has complete control over *all* resources needed to accomplish the goals used for determining work group effectiveness. Effectiveness measures, when used as indicators of work group performance, are usually contaminated because work groups within organizations do not have complete control. Therefore, factors not under control of the work group that might moderate the relationship between performance and effectiveness need to be taken into account in a criterion model of work group functioning.

Peters & O'Connor (1980) have examined situational constraints and individual performance. They note that even though individuals may be willing (motivated) and able (knowledgeable and skillful) to successfully accomplish a task, they can be prevented from doing so by situational characteristics beyond their control. They identify three dimensions of situational constraints that affect the relationship between individual ability, performance and effectiveness as the unavailability, inadequate quantity or inadequate quality of resources needed.

There are two major categories of situational constraints that can affect work group effectiveness. First, group members may impose situational constraints on each other (e.g. production blocking, Diehl & Stroebe, 1987; social loafing, Latané, Williams & Harkins, 1979). Second, work groups as performing units can face situational constraints within the organizational context which are not under their control. The first type has been explored predominantly within social psychological research with *ad hoc* groups (cf. Hill, 1982) and within the domain of individual job performance (Schoorman & Schneider, 1988). Work flow interdependence (Weldon & Weingart, 1993) is a factor that can influence the constraints group members impose on each other. Examples of the second type of external situational constraints imposed on work groups as a whole are material resources (Hackman, 1987), task complexity, environmental uncertainty, market growth (Gladstein, 1984) and technology (Goodman, 1986).

Goodman (1986) reports that physical conditions (situational constraints) moderate the relationships between work group performance and effectiveness. In bad physical conditions, well coordinated mining crews (high group performance) produce more tons of coal (high outcome effectiveness) than other mining crews. No such differences appear in average or good physical conditions. In Gladstein's (1984) empirical test of her work group theory, based on about 100 sales teams, sales revenue (outcome effectiveness) was predicted predominantly by market growth, a contextual factor, and not by any of the group performance variables measured. From the perspective taken here, market growth serves as a situational constraint. It is not controllable by the sales teams and it strongly predicts work group effectiveness independently from work group performance. These empirical studies show that situational constraints can moderate the relationship between work group performance and effectiveness.

Another way to incorporate the mutual influence between environmental constraints and team action into a criterion model of work group functioning is to account for the degree work groups exert control over situational factors, e.g. by changing them or by adequately coping with them. The more control is exerted the less a situational factor can directly determine work group effectiveness and the less it can moderate the performance–effectiveness relationship. In other words, the higher the work group's control over situational factors, the more variance in work group effectiveness can potentially be attributed to their performance. Physical conditions, market growth or technology are situational constraints which are difficult for work groups to control. However, more or less adequate strategies for coping with them could be employed. Work flow interdependence or task complexity seem to be factors work groups are more likely to actively control. However, the degree to which they are able to do this, depends on how much autonomy they have, e.g. in structuring their group tasks or in developing their communication style.

Measuring the degree of work group autonomy can be helpful for theorizing. Work group autonomy, a dimension used within socio-technical-systems theory, is defined by Gulowsen (1979) as the degree to which a work group can influence the formulation of its goals, can decide where and when to work, what production methods are used, how the tasks are internally distributed, who should be part of the group, what kind of leadership for internal and external affairs is required, and how the particular work operations shall be performed. By use of a Guttman scale, Gulowsen (1979) aligns different types of work groups (e.g. coal-mining, or galvanizing groups) on an autonomy dimension. A more recent approach, that is based on Gulowsen's work and action theoretical approaches to job analysis (cf. Hacker, 1986; Frese & Zapf, 1994; Ulich, 1991) is reported by Weber (1994).

In summary, both uncontrollable situational constraints and work group autonomy can moderate the relationship between work group performance and effectiveness, as is shown in Figure 12.1. Thus, for investigating the relationship between work group performance and effectiveness it is argued that situational constraints not under control of the work group should be taken into account as well as situational factors over which work groups can exert more or less control, depending on the degree of work group autonomy.

Temporal Aspects of Work Group Functioning

In general, work group theories concentrate on static aspects of work group performance, effectiveness and their determinants. Some models explicitly acknowledge temporal aspects, but mainly to the extent that reciprocal relationships between work group effectiveness and its determinants are assumed (cf. Cummings, 1981; Hackman, 1987; Kolodny & Kiggundu, 1980; Shea & Guzzo, 1987a,b; Sundstrom, De Meuse & Futrell, 1990). The latter, for instance, emphasize reciprocal interdependence between determinants and effectiveness criteria that may result in either "self-reinforcing spirals of increasing effectiveness" (cf. Hackman, 1987) or of increasing process losses (cf. Steiner, 1972). Shea & Guzzo (1987a,b) describe a group's "potency" (the collective belief that it can perform well) as determined, among other factors, by the work group's level of effectiveness. For the remaining models reviewed one can assume that the authors have some implicit appreciation of group effectiveness influencing its own determinants over time. Reciprocal relationships between performance and effectiveness are empirically demonstrable. For instance, Mullen & Copper (1994) conducted a meta-analysis of studies of the relationship between group cohesiveness (viewed here as a performance dimension) and group effectiveness*. The authors give evidence that changes in cohesiveness brought about by group effectiveness are stronger ($r = 0.51$) than changes in group effectiveness that can be brought about by group cohesiveness ($r = 0.25$). Further temporal issues of work group functioning were only recently theoretically related to work group effectiveness: synchronization within groups, group developmental processes and time-lag effects. However, empirical evidence is rare (cf. Argote & McGrath, 1993).

Synchronization Within Groups

McGrath (1991) presented a theory (time, interaction and performance, TIP) that gives special attention to temporal issues of synchronization within groups (see also McGrath & O'Connor, this volume). Among other propositions TIP states that all collective action is confronted with problems of temporal ambiguity about the occurrence, recurrence and duration of events; conflicting temporal requirements and interests; and scarcity of temporal resources. Work group effectiveness is assumed to depend on how well deadlines are established and reinforced, how well group norms are established that reinforce smooth synchronization, and how well differential demands and capabilities among team members are matched by regulating the temporal flow of tasks. These temporal aspects can be considered to be aspects of work group functioning not discussed within the work group theories reviewed above.

Group Developmental Processes

Temporal aspects of work group functioning that reflect the social dynamics of work group development have been recently reported, e.g. social entrainment, a group performance strategy by which temporal patterning is acquired within groups (cf. McGrath & Kelley, 1992); the development of collective habitual behavior in groups (Gersick & Hackman, 1990); group learning (Argote & Epple, 1990); the development of transactional memory systems within groups (Wegner, 1987); the development of norms about the group's task (Bettenhausen & Murnighan, 1985; Gersick, 1988); and life cycle phenomena, like "midpoint transitions" within project groups (Gersick, 1988, 1989), that contradict the often cited group development sequence—forming, storming, norming, performing (Tuckman, 1965) and adjourning (Tuckman & Jensen, 1977).

---

*Mullen & Copper (1994) use the term "performance" for variables that belong to "group effectiveness" as defined here.

Variables of importance to work group functioning, but less intimately related to the social dynamics of groups, are also shown to co-vary with work group development, e.g. shifts in abilities and technology over time resulting in a reduction of uncertainty (Adams & Barnd, 1983), and shifts in task requirements, e.g. in project teams (Pinto & Prescott, 1988). More specifically, for research and product development teams (R&D projects), not only do task demands change dramatically (from conceptual tasks to planning to construction to implementation), but also the product itself can change some of its attributes over time. For instance, the further down the road the less likely is it that design changes can be implemented easily. This is particularly true in software development projects (cf. Pressman, 1987; Brodbeck & Frese, 1994). Pinto & Prescott (1988) demonstrated that strength of predictor–effectiveness relationships varies according to a project's life cycle stage and that only some factors predict performance during all stages (e.g. mission clarity). In software-development projects, a hypothesized positive relationship between amount of communication (a performance dimension) and work group effectiveness was demonstrable only when project life cycle was statistically controlled for (Brodbeck, 1993), in contrast to a similar study that did not control for the project life cycle as a co-variate. There, no relationship between amount of communication and project effectiveness was found (Allen, Lee & Tushman, 1980).

Time-lag Effects

According to Smith (1976), the time-span covered by criterion measurement is crucial. Depending on whether a short or a long time-span is chosen, different underlying processes might determine differences in effectiveness. For instance, Mullen & Copper (1994) demonstrated by use of meta-analytical methods that it is possible to empirically test assumptions about the effects of different time-lags between measurement. They report that group effectiveness predicts cohesiveness more strongly when the time-lag is relatively short. No effect was found when cohesiveness is used as a predictor of effectiveness. There is no theoretical guidance for determining the appropriate time-lag between measurement of performance, effectiveness and its determinants. Goodman & Pennings (1980) suggest relying on what the dominant coalition describes as the proper time-lag, and carefully delineating the interrelationships between predictors, performance and effectiveness variables. Pinto & Slevin (1988) describe the influence of external factors on project effectiveness as a function of time after the work group product or service has been delivered to the client. Thus, questions such as, "How long would it take for the group product to be visible to the relevant constituents?", and, "How long does it take for the group product to be changed considerably as a consequence of external factors?" should be asked for identifying adequate time-lags.

As indicated in Figure 12.1 social dynamics and shifts in group members' ablity, in technology, in group task demands and in the group product itself can have consequences for both work group performance and effectiveness. They should be taken into account as co-variates when relationships between work group performance and effectiveness are under investigation. Additionally, when longitudinal studies are undertaken, the selection of an appropriate time-lag becomes crucial for proper hypothesis testing. The arrows in Figure 12.1 are not meant to be exclusive. Group developmental processes can also serve as direct determinants of performance and effectiveness and as mediators of bidirectional relationships between the two (cf. Argote & McGrath, 1993).

Summary of the Criterion Model

The criterion model of work group functioning above describes common, contradictory and complementary components of ten different work group theories. It incorporates the distinction between work group performance and effectiveness, explicitly or implicitly made by all of the theories. In order to minimize the likelihood of criterion deficiency, the performance dimensions, commonly described as comprising motivation, knowledge and skill, and collective strategies for internal activities, are supplemented by collective strategies for external activities. For the same reason, task completion models of effectiveness that make use of only one effectiveness dimension (outcome productivity) are complemented by social and personal criteria and by innovation implementation as further effectiveness dimensions. Contrary to many of the work group theories reviewed, a "modified" relationship between performance and effectiveness is a central assumption of the model. Thus, the model incorporates factors that account for criterion contamination: situational constraints and work group autonomy. To further reduce criterion contamination and to account for dynamic properties of criteria, the model also incorporates temporal aspects of work group functioning that affect either performance or effectiveness, or both, concordantly: social dynamics and shifts in task, technology, ability and the group product itself.

The criterion model differs from so-called input-process-output models (McGrath, 1964; Steiner, 1972; cf. Hackman, 1987). The latter are more concerned with the determinants of work group functioning. They direct attention to factors (input) that directly determine work group performance (process), which in turn determines work group effectiveness (outcome). The underlying assumption, that determinants are of importance to work group functioning, is not refuted by the criterion model. However, by concentrating on the criteria of work group functioning, the criterion model directs attention to situational factors that determine work group effectiveness (outcome) either beyond or under partial control of a work group. The underlying assumption postulates the existence of situational factors that modify the relationship between work group performance (process) and effectiveness (outcome). In this respect, the criterion model complements input-process-output models.

MEASUREMENT ISSUES AND CURRENT METHODS

The conceptual propositions made in the criterion model are meant to foster work group theory development in meeting standards for criteria (cf. Borman, 1991), and thus, in identifying determinants and processes of effective work group functioning in a richer and more meaningful way. However, not much has been said about what methods should be employed for appropriate criterion measurement. Therefore, the remaining sections address current methods developed to solve some of the criterion measurement problems raised by studying work group functioning:

1. Composite measures for integrating global vs. specific criteria.
2. Multiple constituency models for value and policy capturing within work groups and organizations.
3. Multiple-levels analysis for testing individual level, group level and cross level constructs.
4. Advantages and concerns about the use of subjective criterion measures.

Integrating Global vs. Fine-grained Criteria within Composite Measures

In order to improve our understanding of predictor–criterion relationships, multiple criteria should be used, because combining criteria that stem from different performance areas in a composite measure masks relationships between individual predictors and criteria (Borman, 1991; Goodman, Ravlin & Schminke, 1987; McGrath, 1986). This notion is consistent with the scaling down of the search for an "ultimate" criterion within psychological assessment over the past decades (Austin & Villanova, 1992). Most of the work group theories reviewed make use of multiple-dimension effectiveness concepts. However, among these models there is considerable dissent concerning the use of global vs. fine-grained effectiveness criteria.

Hackman's (1987) normative model is intended to apply to a variety of work groups. Thus, he uses multiple global dimensions of effectiveness. Other work group theories use fine-grained effectiveness criteria applicable only to specific types of work groups, e.g. self-regulating work groups (Pearce & Ravlin, 1987), wood harvesting teams (Kolodny & Kiggundu, 1980) or sales teams (Gladstein, 1984). Goodman (1986) summarizes the rationale for the use of fine-grained criteria: "Properties of the criterion variables are different and different models are needed for different criteria ... quantity, quality, downtime, satisfaction, group stability over time, and so on" (p. 145). He also presents a model based on only one type of work group (mining crews) that explains one effectiveness criterion (tons of coal) and argues for a much more idiographic approach than is contemporarily used within work group research. However, McGrath (1986) criticizes this extreme position, in saying, "If he [Goodman, 1986] were right, then we should each set about developing a 'science of mine shaft 32', or 'mine shaft 46'" (p. 370), and "... we would be out of the science business altogether and in the history business" (p. 371). This is not meant to discredit the use of fine-grained criteria, but it does remind us that at some point fine-grained criteria need to be recast into global criteria so that comparisons and generalizations across different types of work groups are possible.

Integration of fine-grained models within global models seems to be necessary because the former are better suited for testing hypotheses about particular predictor–criterion relationships, and the latter apply to a wider domain of work groups and allow for the development of general work group theories. Furthermore, multiple dimensions of work group effectiveness should be used, otherwise not very much can be said about how the determinants investigated affect work group effectiveness in the whole. I see two possible strategies. One is to develop a general criterion model of work group functioning. It serves as a reference system for empirical research using either multiple fine-grained criteria or multiple global criteria. Another strategy is to integrate global and fine-grained effectiveness criteria within the same studies, making it possible to give an empirical rationale for the attachment of fine-grained criteria to global criteria. For doing this, composite measures seem to be an adequate method.

Composite Measures

Composite measures have been repeatedly suggested for criterion evaluation within the domain of organizational productivity as a device for integrating global and fine-grained effectiveness criteria (Campbell & Campbell, 1988; Pritchard, 1992). The rationale for merging different effectiveness dimensions within one composite measure or the transformation to a single measure (e.g. the dollar) is that the effectiveness of several performing units within an organization needs to be combined and adequately weighted in order to evaluate the overall productivity of an organization. Within work group research composite measures have been neglected widely because they were thought to mask theoretically relevant relationships between individual predictors and criteria. Recently, Sundstrom, De Meuse & Futrell (1990) advocated the use of Pritchard et al.'s (1988, 1989) measurement system for solving the problem of integration by merging specific indicators into an index of percentage of maximum effectiveness. Since this method also fulfills other requirements for group performance and effectiveness measurement (Pritchard, 1990) and satisfies psychometric principles (Hesketh, 1993) it is discussed in more detail below.

The *pro*ductivity *m*easurement and *e*nhancement *s*ystem (ProMES) is based on the motivational concept of Naylor, Pritchard & Ilgen (1980). It is basically an intervention technique for improving motivation by giving feedback and thereby improving performance in organizations (Pritchard, 1995a). Effectiveness criteria (so-called products) and specific variables (so-called indicators) are established in group discussions by group members and supervisors. Higher management has to approve the criteria and variables identified. The variables are then "psychologically scaled" (Hesketh, 1993) to a common effectiveness scale. Based on group consensus about the expected levels of effectiveness, which are given a zero value, maximum effectiveness levels (+100), and minimum effectiveness levels (−100) are established by use of contingency tables. A contingency is a graphic display of the relationship between the value of a variable and the contribution to overall effectiveness (utility). This relationship may be a non-linear function. Empirical results support the assertion that non-linear utility functions often exist and that they add important information to composite measures of work group effectiveness (Pritchard et al., 1988, 1989). The feature of accounting for non-linear utility functions is unique among productivity measurement systems (Pritchard, 1990). The contingency tables are fed back to management. After approval, the overall effectiveness index is calculated based on the indicators and their utility functions. Data at several points in time (before, within and after the feedback period) are evaluated. Feedback is given to the work group and managers in order to identify improvement strategies.

As an intervention technique, ProMES has been demonstrated to improve productivity of different types of work groups within different organizations with an average effect size of approximately $d = 2.3$ (Pritchard, 1995b). However, to employ ProMES for the purpose of criteria measurement some further issues need to be considered. First, ProMES is a fairly labour-intensive intervention technique. The calendar time it takes is reported to be about 18–20 weeks, including about 20 hours for the design team within the organization and another 50–60 hours preparation time (Pritchard, 1995b). However, when used as a criterion measurement system, rather than as a feedback system, it can be simplified considerably, being much less time-consuming (Jones & Ourth, 1995). Second, during baseline assessment, productivity improvement occurs with an average effect size of approximately $d = 0.75$ (Pritchard, 1995b) which is comparable to treatment effect sizes of organizational interventions: $d = -0.03-0.78$ (Guzzo, Jette & Katzell, 1985), $d = 0.18-0.70$ (Tett, Meyer & Roese, 1994, pp. 102–105). This might be a result of role clarification and motivation through participation. If used for criterion measurement only, the use of indicators on which prior data is available is suggested (Jones & Ourth, 1995). Additionally, equal levels of participation in the ProMES procedure should be maintained among the work groups investigated. This can be approached by creating a design team of representatives, who subsequently facilitate contingency development in the work groups they belong to (Watson et al., 1995). This procedure is also time-saving. Third, the use of ProMES can have effects on variables that are used as performance or effectiveness criteria. ProMES has positive effects on job satisfaction and morale; work groups become more aware of their interdependencies with its environment; existing conflicts surface in ProMES development (e.g. distrust between workers and management, between specific individuals, between different shifts doing the same work, disagreement about goals); and positive attitudes towards ProMES are reported (Pritchard, 1995b).

Since any performance and effectiveness dimension can be expressed on the basis of specific indicators and their contingency functions, ProMES could enable attachment of fine-grained criteria to global criteria within individual studies. ProMES also allows for combining effectiveness and efficiency measures. Thus, productivity—the ratio between input or costs and output or effectiveness (cf. Mahoney, 1988; Campbell & Campbell, 1988)—can also be measured. By use of efficiency measures, indicating how well a system can exploit the available resources, work group theory could relate more strongly to systems resource models of effectiveness. When costs and inputs can be incorporated by use of a ratio measure, situational constraints could be incorporated in a similar way. It also seems to be possible to develop a composite measure of work group autonomy by use of ProMES. The authors of the method state that it allows for cross-unit comparison of work groups performing different tasks and facing different situational factors (cf. Pritchard, 1990, 1995a).

Value and Policy Capturing with Multiple Constituency Approaches

Theories differ in their views of appropriate strategies for deriving performance and effectiveness dimensions and criteria. Criteria derivation is perceived to be a matter of theoretical considerations (e.g. Goodman, Ravlin & Schminke, 1987; Hackman, 1987) or practical convenience, policy capturing and local appropriateness (e.g. Kolodny & Kiggundu, 1980; Shea & Guzzo, 1987a,b). One model uses both strategies (Pearce & Ravlin, 1987). So-called multiple constituency approaches make use of the values of different interest groups involved with a work group. Criterion derivation can be based on the values from the dominant coalition within organizations—usually the management (e.g. Goodman, Ravlin & Schminke, 1987), or it can be based on several different constituencies, e.g. work group members and managers (e.g. Cummings, 1981).

The way through which work groups are rewarded and promoted depends on others' assessments of the group's output (cf. Hackman, 1987). The values of these other persons and the policy used within organizations for the assessment of work group effectiveness can serve as a source for criteria selection. For theoretical reasons, some authors assert that only the dominant coalition in an organization should be used for value and policy capturing (cf. Goodman, Ravlin & Schminke, 1987). They argue that members of the dominant coalition define what construct underlies successful completion of tasks. Thus, their view should be adopted by the researcher. However, conceptualizing effectiveness criteria on the basis of only one predominant constituent can lead to a fragmented view of work group functioning—the problem of deficient criteria (Borman, 1991). From a broader theoretical view, many constituencies can profit or suffer from the work groups' products and services, in a way not visible to the dominant coalition. In Hackman's (1987) model the latter line of argumentation is enforced: "The productive output of the work group should meet or exceed the performance standards of the people who receive and/or review the output" (p. 323). That includes clients, managers, co-workers from other work groups and departments, etc. Additionally, use can be made of personal and social criteria of effectiveness, as perceived by group members and constituents outside the work group. This is done by social justice and relativistic multiple constituency approaches.

Multiple Constituency Approaches

In a multiple constituency approach criterion dimensions are generated by use of different stakeholders that interact with, are affected by, or evaluate work groups (e.g. suppliers, customers, clients, managers, group members, economists). Within a multiple constituency approach effectiveness is perceived to be a set of several statements, each of which reflects the views and values of a constituent involved with a work group, because "an answer to the question 'How well is entity x performing?' is inevitably contingent on whom one is asking" (Conolly, Conlon & Deutsch, 1980, p. 212). Different multiple constituency approaches are described in the literature. The power approach suggests the use of values from the dominant coalition (usually the managers) within an organization for selection of effectiveness criteria. Shea & Guzzo's (1987a,b) work group theory makes use of such a power approach. Other work group theories make use of a power approach in combination with a social justice approach (Keeley, 1978) that reflects the values of the least advantaged constituents (e.g. group members, clients). Examples of work group theories that use this particular combination are the models of Hackman (1987), Pearce & Ravlin (1987) and Cummings (1981). A relativistic multiple constituency approach (e.g. Conolly, Conlon & Deutsch, 1980), where all identifiable constituents are used for criteria selection, is not used in any of the work group theories reviewed.

Poulton & West (1993, 1994), though not presenting explicitly a work group theory, apply a relativistic constituency approach for deriving effectiveness criteria for primary health care teams. The authors identify altogether 15 stakeholder groups as constituents in judging health care teams' effectiveness. They show that the major groupings of effectiveness dimensions they found can be related to three different conceptualizations of organizational effectiveness. The consumers' perspective, and the quality of care dimensions they found, relate to a goal model of organizational effectiveness. This model defines effectiveness as the degree to which desired goals, as specified by consumers, are achieved. It matches with goal-oriented concepts of work group effectiveness that use "production" or "quality of service" as final effectiveness criteria. The staff development and team viability dimensions Poulton & West found relate to an internal process model of organizational effectiveness. This model defines effectiveness in terms of how well problems are collectively solved and how well employee well-being is maintained. It matches with the use of social and personal effectiveness criteria within work group theories from Hackman (1987), Sundstrom, De Meuse & Futrell (1990), Pearce & Ravlin (1987), and Kolodny & Kiggundu (1980). The management and planning of care dimensions found by Poulton & West relates to a systems resource model, which is input-focused, by defining effectiveness in terms of how well a system can exploit the available resources. Only one of the work group theories reviewed makes explicit use of an efficiency measure ("cost per cord of wood"), indicating an underlying systems resource model (Kolodny & Kiggundu, 1980).

Some drawbacks of constituency approaches need to be mentioned. It is nearly impossible to identify all relevant constituents for derivation of effectiveness criteria and weight them properly. Therefore, one needs to make value judgments concerning the set of effectiveness dimensions used and their relative importance (Mark & Shotland, 1985). The perceptions of effectiveness depend on the constituent's personal values and frame of reference (Zammuto, 1984), which is difficult to explicate. Furthermore, divergence and conflict within the set of criteria proposed by different constituents are to be expected. Finally, Poulton & West (1993, 1994) show that depending on what constituent one is asking, different concepts of effectiveness are preferred. This is in line with Goodmann & Penning's (1980) notion that up to now, no singular conceptualization of organizational effectiveness can be preferred on the basis of empirical evidence. The same might be true for the concept of work group effectiveness. Despite these reservations, multiple constituency approaches are seen as an alternative to the common view of work group effectiveness as an objective concept (Poulton & West, 1994).

Two further applications of the policy capturing methods deserve mention. The first pertains to policy capturing as a criterion of effective work group functioning, and the second addresses the value of multiple constituency approaches for work group research in general. Zammuto (1984) states that it is not the question of *whose* preferences should be satisfied by a working unit at a given time but *how* divergent preferences can be satisfied over the long run (an evolutionary multiple constituency approach). How well a work group manages to satisfy different constituents in the long run can be viewed as a further dimension of work group effectiveness. Policy capturing activities, e.g. external probing as identified by Gladstein-Ancona (1990), can be viewed as collective performance strategies that help work groups to approach that goal. Based on many constituents' views, effectiveness criteria can be identified, some of which a singular class of constituents (e.g. the management or work group researchers) might not be aware of, or might not acknowledge as relevant to the organization's, the work group's, the members' or the clients' prosperity. Identifying work group performance dimensions that predict achievement of such effectiveness criteria might either promote further achievement of commonly known criteria, or foster achievement of other goals, not yet known to be of importance to work group functioning. Achievement of these goals may result in higher quality of work life, higher quality of products and services, and in acknowledgement of new functions to be served by work groups. Thus, multiple constituency approaches could help to identify new goals and performance dimensions, which in turn could open whole new lines of research as to what are the determinants of the newly defined criteria.

Level of Constructs and Multiple-levels Analysis

For all theories reviewed the work group as a performing unit is the focus of analysis, although some acknowledgement is given to the difference between individual and group level phenomena. A closer look at the performance criteria indicates that some models are concerned with how individual level phenomena might combine into group level phenomena, e.g. variety of members' responses (Pearce & Ravlin, 1987) or weighting of individual inputs (Gladstein, 1984). Two work group theories explicitly distinguish between individual and group level criteria: individual vs. collective performance (Nieva, Fleischman & Rieck, 1978) and individual vs. collaborative effectiveness dimensions (Cummings, 1981).

The perspective of group effectiveness as an aggregate of individual effectiveness is favored within experimental research on the difference between individual vs. group effectiveness (for reviews, see Hill, 1982; Lorge et al., 1958). It draws primarily on Steiner's (1972) process loss model of work group productivity. According to this model actual productivity is a function of potential productivity minus process losses. Potential productivity is usually defined as some statistical aggregate of individual effectiveness, which is nearly impossible to operationalize properly within natural settings. This makes it difficult to transfer the process loss paradigm to work groups within organizations.

However, separating individual from group level performance and investigating the relationship between the two constructs is possible in natural settings. Jones (1974), for example, compared individual-performance-to-group-effectiveness regression models of four different competitive sports: tennis, baseball, American football and basketball. Correlations between individual performance and group effectiveness ranged from a modest but substantial $r = 0.60$ in basketball teams to a high $r = 0.90$ in American football and baseball teams. Even though the sum of individual performance predicted group level effectiveness strongly in tennis, baseball and American football teams (only linear effects were found), for basketball teams there was no such association. In contrast, the effects tended strongly in the opposite direction, thus leaving variance to be explained by performance dimensions on the group level, e.g. collective performance strategies or social relations among the players, as Jones (1974) concludes.

Often work group models do not distinguish clearly between individual and group level constructs. For instance, models that make use of personal criteria of effectiveness (e.g. members' satisfaction, well-being), as defined by Hackman (1987), imply measurement at the individual level and aggregation to the work group level, using the group's mean value. Here, member satisfaction and well-being are perceived to be constructs generalizing across different levels (cross-level constructs). It is assumed that the group's mean values of individual well-being and satisfaction carry all criterion relevant information from the individual level onto the group level. However, this is not neccessarily true. From a systemic view, e.g. if only one or two group members' satisfaction and well-being scores are particularly low as a result of some determining group level factor, individual group members can be seen as the "symptom carriers" of the whole work group. Simple aggregation to a mean value would not carry this information onto the group level of analysis. For coping with such problems Sonnentag (this volume) suggests a mixed level strategy which takes individual as well as group level constructs of well-being, satisfaction and other personal criteria into account (see also Sonnentag et al., 1994).

Delineation of the concepts of work group performance and effectiveness requires work groups to be seen as composites of at least two levels, individual and group. However, further levels can be identified. Members of the same work group can be classified according to different job classes with different task demands and working conditions (e.g. user representatives vs. programmers in a software development project; medical doctors vs. nurses in a surgery team). Since constructs can generalize more or less across different levels of analysis, the desired level of the theoretical constructs needs to be specified prior to investigation.

Consideration of multiple levels of analysis is important for hypothesis testing, theory development, reliability and validity estimation (Rousseau, 1985; Glick, 1985). Methods for multiple levels analysis have been suggested recently (see for example: George, 1992; George & James, 1993; Gollob, 1991; Kenney & LaVoie, 1985; Ostroff, 1993; Yammarino & Markham, 1992; Yammarino & Naughton, 1988). They seem to be helpful for testing multiple level models. However, they do not free the researcher from clearly specifying on what level of analysis the theoretical constructs are meant to be and what the causal links between them are.

For measuring group level constructs with individual level data some methodological justification for aggregation needs to be given by measures of consensus among group members (James, 1982; James, Demaree & Wolf, 1984). However, there is some debate about the best method (cf. James, 1982; James, Demaree & Wolf, 1984; Kozlowski & Hattrup, 1992; James, Demaree & Wolf, 1993; Schmidt & Hunter, 1989). In my view the debate has not been resolved. Additionally, it was found that the often suggested within-group-consensus measure (r_{wg}; James, Demaree & Wolf, 1984) does not produce the significant differences, to be expected when r_{wg} measures of real work groups are compared with r_{wg} measures of statisticized groups, similar in size and randomly drawn from the same samples (West, Brodbeck & Patterson, in preparation). Therefore, it is suggested that the intraclass-correlation statistics, ICC (1) and ICC (2), from James (1982) should be used for reliability and consensus estimates as long as the methodological debate remains unresolved. However, high ICC (1) and ICC (2) values cannot be used as the sole basis for justification of aggregation. One needs to make sure that individual level measurement of group level phenomena is justified. This can be done, for instance, by using items that specifically and exclusively address group level phenomena (content validity), and by use of multiple methods, e.g. comparing statistical consensus of nominal groups with social consensus as a result of group discussion (Moeller et al., 1988).

Subjective Criterion Measures

Objective measures are better than subjective measures in that certain classes of judgmental bias cannot occur (e.g. leniency, halo, restriction of range). However, as Pritchard (1992) states, all effectiveness measurement within organizations is an "operational definition[s] of organizational policy, and policy is by nature subjective" (p. 459). Independent from the source of data—objective or subjective—the criterion selection and weighting procedures within the natural setting of work groups depend on subjective judgments. Therefore, there can be no totally objective measurement system for work group effectiveness.

Hackman (1987) deliberately prefers subjective measurement methods for estimating effectiveness of work groups for two reasons. First, only for a limited class of work groups do reliable and valid objective criteria exist. Restricting models to a narrow class of work groups would not serve the development of general work group effectiveness theories. Second, what happens to work groups depends more strongly on the constituents' and the members' subjective assessment of the work group than on any objective performance index, even though constituents and group members may rely in part on objective measures.

However, aside from psychometric issues (cf. Borman, 1991; Landy & Farr, 1983) some additional precautions must be taken when relying on subjective criterion estimates for the study of work group functioning. Subjective assessment should not allow for deliberate fake, inflation or deflation in relative contribution of the work groups involved (Pritchard, 1992). Subjective client assessment of group output is less reliable when clients are highly competitive or ethnocentric with the work groups to be assessed (Hackman, 1987). Another threat to the validity of work group performance and effectiveness measures is the evaluators' implicit theories of group performance, whether they are group members, other constituents or researchers external to the organization. Implicit theories of group performance and effectiveness lead individuals to make inferences about relationships between group performance and effectiveness indicators. Staw (1975) argues that attribution processes lead to an overestimation of the relationship between performance and effectiveness. However, DeNisi & Pritchard (1978) show that this assertion does not hold for long-standing work groups in organizations. Gladstein (1984) commented on her finding of no relationship between objective (sales revenues) and subjective measures of work group outcome (self-reported effectiveness and satisfaction): "The variables shown to influence self-reported effectiveness read like a textbook on team building" (p. 511). Her explanation of the results, however, differs from Staw's (1975) assertion. Even though the subjects did not know their actual outcome effectiveness, they may have attributed high effectiveness to their group when it displayed group performance behavior theoretically expected to be effective.

Guzzo et al. (1986) distinguish between response bias and memory bias when group performance behavior is subjectively measured. A negative response bias is shown when informants are exposed to negative feedback about group effectiveness. When exposed to positive feedback, behavior evaluations are not different from those made without feedback. Martell & Guzzo (1991) show that a more liberal decision criterion for the occurrence of behavior consonant with the implicit group theory (a set of assumptions about behavior–performance–effectiveness relationships) is used than for dissonant behavior (see also Martell, Guzzo & Willis, 1995). This indicates a memory bias. To cope with memory bias, Martell & Guzzo (1991) suggest making use of recognition rather than recall methods. Decision criteria for judging whether a certain behavior has occurred or not should be explicitly given and reality-monitoring training can help to improve subjective performance assessment (cf. Lord, 1985). Response bias can also be reduced, when observers external to the groups are involved and are unaware of the work group's outcome effectiveness.

For assessing social and personal effectiveness criteria and for the detection of relevant group performance measures, group members' estimates have some advantages. Group members should know best what is going on within their team, because they are the task experts and they are most strongly involved in the social dynamics of the group. Thus, for estimates pertaining to performance and social effectiveness dimensions group members have first-hand information. They tend to use this information accurately, and the more first-hand information they have, the less they tend to use implicit theories of work group behavior (DeNisi & Pritchard, 1978).

In summary, Hackman (1987) gives two good reasons for using subjective measures of assessment of work group performance: (a) avoidance of restricting research to narrow class of work groups where objective measures are readily available, and (b) taking account of the fact that what happens to work groups depends strongly on the constituents' and the members' subjective assessments. Additionally, the group members' expert knowledge is useful for identifying particular collective performance strategies, for measuring individual motivation, as well as social and personal criteria of effectiveness. One should also bear in mind that objective effectiveness criteria, readily to be found within organizations, are not necessarily reliable and valid estimates of work group performance. This can be due to local policy, value judgments and situational constraints. Furthermore, identifying the meaningfulness of objective measures often needs careful observation and interpretation (cf. Hesketh, 1993).

SUMMARY

The central propositions in the criterion model of work group functioning and the suggestions for measurement practice made are summarized below. The propositions and suggestions are related to criterion standards which should be met more rigorously in future research studies about work group functioning (an overview is given in Table 12.2).

In the introductory section it is argued that in order to further theoretical understanding the criterion of work group functioning needs to be conceptually delineated prior to investigation and development of operational measures. The implied ordering is meant to prevent "the common practice of using criterion measures simply because they are available or easily developed" (Borman, 1991, p. 275). Evaluation of the extent to which operational measures reflect the underlying conceptual criterion is necessary to reflect upon criterion relevance (e.g. deficiency and contamination).

The following four propositions are made within the criterion model of work group functioning:

- *Work group performance and effectiveness should be explicitly distinguished and separately measured.* With this proposition the model adopts the criterion delineation suggested by Campbell et al. (1970) and Campbell & Campbell (1988). It helps to raise criterion relevance by reducing criterion deficiency and criterion contamination. Deficiency is reduced by defining both process and outcome criteria as part of work group functioning. Furthermore, the proposition helps to portray when high performance does not correspond with high effectiveness. Criterion contamination can be accounted for by operating under the assumption that a "modified" relationship between work group performance and effectiveness exists. In doing so, factors can be explicitly considered that might be confounded with work group performance and effectiveness measures.
- *Performance contains three dimensions: (a) motivation, (b) knowledge and skill, (c) internal and external collective strategies. Effectiveness contains four dimensions: (a) task completion, (b) personal criteria, (c) social criteria, (d) innovation implementation.* These dimensions portray the relevant areas of the criterion to the best of our theoretical knowledge. Consideration of the dimensions described helps to reduce criterion deficiency.
- *Situational constraints not under control of the work group and work group autonomy are factors that can modify the relationship between work group performance and effectiveness.* Accounting for situational constraints (e.g. market growth, environmental uncertainty) and work group autonomy, allowing work groups to exert more control over situational factors (e.g. task structure, group composition) helps to reduce criterion contamination. The use of these factors helps to identify more precisely the amount of effectiveness variance predictable by variance in work group performance.

Table 12.2 Criterion-related concerns in the study of work group functioning

Chapter sections	Criterion standards involved	Suggestions made
Introduction	Criterion relevance (contamination, deficiency)	Develop conceptual criteria first, criterion measures second.
Conceptual model		
Process vs. outcome criteria	Criterion relevance (contamination, deficiency)	Measure performance and effectiveness separately. Check for factors that "modify" their relationship.
Criterion dimensionality	Criterion relevance (deficiency)	Consider performance dimensionality (motivation, knowledge and skill, internal and external collective strategies) and effectiveness dimensionality (task completion, social and personal criteria, innovation).
Situational factors	Criterion relevance (contamination)	Consider situational constraints and work group autonomy as moderators of performance–effectiveness relationships.
Temporal aspects	Dynamic criteria	Consider or control for social dynamics, shifts in task, technology, ability and the group product (if applicable).
Measurement practice		
Global vs. fine-grained criteria	Hypothesis specificity. Generalizability	Attach fine-grained to global criteria in single studies (e.g. with utility functions). Attach criteria to dimensions in criterion models of work group functioning.
Value and policy capturing	Practical usefulness and acceptance of criteria and values	Identify differential values about criteria (multiple constituency models). Consider "satisfying multiple constituencies" as an effectiveness criterion.
Level of constructs	Criterion relevance (contamination)	Identify single/cross-level constructs. Give conceptual and methodological justification for aggregation.
Subjective measures	Sample restriction Factual consequences	Check for general psychometric properties. Check for implicit theories of group performance.

- *Temporal aspects can influence performance or effectiveness, or both, concordantly.* This proposition reflects the dynamic nature of criteria (Ghiselli, 1956). It helps to portray when determinants affect criteria only within certain periods in time, due to social dynamics and to shifts in task, technology, ability or the group product itself. Furthermore, the proposition points to the need to control for temporal aspects in the analysis of performance–effectiveness relationships.

The following four suggestions for measurement practice in the study of work group functioning are made:

- *Attach fine-grained to global criteria by use of conceptual criterion models of work group functioning and by use of composite criterion measures within individual studies.* The use of fine-grained criteria is necessary for hypothesis specificity, that is criterion relevance to a particular predictor–criterion hypothesis (rather than to work group effectiveness in the whole), that would lead to a greater understanding of predictor–criterion relationships (Wallace, 1965). On the other hand, the use of global criteria is necessary for generalizability of research findings to different types of work groups. Integration of fine-grained and global criteria is important for building theories that generalize across different types of work groups.
- *Identify the constituents and their values in relation to the criteria employed.* The criterion can be perceived to be a set of several statements each of which reflects the values of a constituent involved—including the researcher. If it is true that no singular conceptualization of work group effectiveness can be preferred on the basis of empirical evidence, there is an idefinite number of theoretically relevant effectiveness criteria. Limiting this indefinite array, on grounds other than the researcher's theoretical orientation, can be achieved by determining the practical usefulness and acceptability to constituents of the criteria. Pearce & Ravlin (1987) describe criteria selection as a matter of theoretical interest as well as relevant to value and policy capturing. They suggest that the selection of work group performance criteria should follow the theoretical assumptions of the researcher, whereas the selection of effectiveness criteria should be predominantly a matter of practical usefulness and acceptability. However, when effectiveness measures are used for validation of performance criteria, they need to be selected according to theoretical assumptions as well.
- *Indicate clearly the level of analysis at which the criteria are meant to be located. Give conceptual and methodological justification for aggregating lower level data for measuring group level constructs.* Criterion contamination comes about when measures of group level criteria tap variance irrelevant to work group performance requirements. More particularly, effectiveness measures can be confounded in the sense that they reflect both work group performance and other factors on the individual level, the job class level or some wider organizational levels of analysis that determine work group effectiveness.
- *Make use of objective and subjective measures.* For both subjective and objective measures great care needs to be taken to establish their meaningfulness. The psychometric properties of subjective measures and their relevance to

implicit theories of group performance need to be established. However, subjective measures have some advantage over objective measures. They help to avoid sample restriction, due to the exclusion of work groups where objective measures are not readily available. They reflect the fact that what happens to work groups depends strongly on the constituents' and the members' subjective assessments. Also, they make use of the constituents'—especially the group members'—expert knowledge about the functioning of "their" work group.

References

Adams, J.R. & Barnd, S.E. (1983). Behavioral implications of the project life cycle. In D.I. Cleland & W.R. King (eds), *Project Management Handbook*. New York: Van Nostrand Reinhold, pp. 222–244.

Allen, T.J., Lee, D.M. & Tushman, M.L. (1980). R&D performance as a function of internal communication, project management, and the nature of work. *IEEE Transactions on Engineering Management*, **27**, 2–12.

Argote, L. & Epple, D. (1990). Learning curves in manufacturing. *Science*, **247**, 920–923.

Argote, L. & McGrath, J.E. (1993). Group processes in organizations: continuity and change. In C.L. Cooper & I.T. Robertson (eds), *International Review of Industrial and Organizational Psychology*, Vol. 8. Chichester: Wiley, pp. 333–389.

Austin, J.T. & Villanova, P. (1992). The criterion problem: 1917–1992. *Journal of Applied Psychology*, **77**, 836–874.

Bettenhausen, K. & Murnighan, J.K. (1985). The emergence of norms in competitive decision-making groups. *Administrative Science Quarterly*, **30**, 350–372.

Borman, W.C. (1991). Job behavior, performance and effectiveness. In M.D. Dunette & L.M. Hough (eds), *Handbook of Industrial and Organizational Psychology*, Vol. 2. Palo Alto: Consulting Psychologists Press, pp. 271–326.

Brodbeck, F.C. (1993). Kommunikation und Leistung in Projektarbeitsgruppen. Eine empirische Untersuchung an Software-Entwicklungsprojekten [Communication and performance. An empirical investigation of software-development projects]. Dissertation, University of Giessen. (Requests for an English abstract of the dissertation should be send to the author's address: Dept. of Psychology, University of Munich, Leopoldstr. 3, D-80802 Munich, Germany).

Brodbeck, F.C. & Frese M. (1994). *Produktivität und Qualität in Software-Projekten: Psychologische Analyse und Optimierung von Arbeitsprozessen in der Software-Entwicklung.* [Productivity and Quality in Software Projects: Analysing and Optimizing Work Processes for Software Development]. Munich: Oldenbourg-Verlag.

Campbell, J.P. (1990). Modelling the performance prediction problem in industrial and organizational psychology. In M.D. Dunette & L.M. Hough (eds), *Handbook of Industrial and Organizational Psychology*, Vol. 1. Palo Alto: Consulting Psychologists Press, pp. 687–732.

Campbell, J.P. & Campbell, R.J. (1988). Industrial–organizational psychology and productivity: the goodness of fit. In J.P. Campbell & R.J. Campbell (eds), *Productivity in Organizations*. San Francisco: Jossey-Bass, pp. 82–93.

Campbell, J.P., Dunnette, M.D., Lawler, E.E., III & Weick, K.E. (1970). *Managerial Behavior, Performance, and Effectiveness*. New York: McGraw-Hill.

Conolly, T., Conlon, E.J. & Deutsch, S.J. (1980). Organizational effectiveness: a multiple-constituency approach. *Academy of Management Review*, **5**, 211–217.

Cummings, T.G. (1981). Designing effective work groups. In P.C. Nystrom & W.H. Starbuck (eds), *Handbook of Organizational Design*, Vol. 2. New York: Oxford, pp. 250–271.

DeNisi, A.S. & Pritchard, R.D. (1978). Implicit theories of performance as artifacts in survey research: a replication and extension. *Organizational Behavior and Human Performance*, **21**, 358–366.

Diehl, M. & Stroebe, W. (1987). Productivity loss in brainstorming groups: towards the solution of a riddle. *Journal of Personality and Social Psychology*, **53**, 497–509.

Frese, M. & Zapf, D. (1994). Action as the core of work psychology: a German approach. In H.C. Triandis, M.D. Dunette & J.M. Hough (eds), *Handbook of Industrial and Organizational Psychology*, Vol. 4. Palo Alto: Consulting Psychologists Press, pp. 271–340.

George, J.M. (1992). Personality, affect and behavior in groups. *Journal of Applied Psychology*, **75**, 107–116.

George, J.M. & James, L.R. (1993). Personality, affect and behavior in groups revisited: comment on aggregation, levels of analysis, and a recent application of within and between analysis. *Journal of Applied Psychology*, **78**, 798–804.

Gersick, C.J.G. (1989). Time and transition in work teams: toward a new model of group development. *Academy of Management Journal*, **31**, 9–41.

Gersick, C.J.G. (1988). Marking time: predictable transitions in task groups. *Academy of Management Journal*, **32**, 274–309.

Gersick, C.J.G. & Hackman, J.R. (1990). Habitual routines in task-performing groups. *Organizational Behavior and Human Decision Processes*, **47**, 65–97.

Ghiselli, E.E. (1956). Dimensional problems of criteria. *Journal of Applied Psychology*, **40**, 1–4

Gladstein, D.L. (1984). Groups in context: a model of task group effectiveness. *Administrative Science Quarterly*, **29**, 499–517.

Gladstein-Ancona, D.L. (1990). Outward bound: strategies for team survival in an organization. *Academy of Management Journal*, **33**(2), 334–365.

Glick, W.H. (1985). Conceptualizing and measuring organizational and psychological climate: pitfalls in multilevel research. *Academy of Management Journal*, **10**, 601–616.

Gollob, H.F. (1991). Methods for estimating individual- and group-level correlations. *Journal of Personality and Social Psychology*, **60**, 376–381.

Goodman, P.S. (1986). Impact of task and technology on group performance. In P.S. Goodman & Associates (eds), *Designing Effective Work Groups*. San Francisco: Jossey Bass, pp. 120–167.

Goodman, P.S. & Pennings, J.M. (1980). Critical issues in assessing organizational effectiveness. In E.E. Lawler III, D.A. Nadler & C. Cammann (eds), *Organizational Assessment: Perspectives on the Measurement of Organizational Behavior and the Quality of Work Life*. New York: Wiley, pp. 185–215.

Goodman, P.S., Ravlin, E.C. & Argote, L. (1986). Current thinking about groups. In P.S. Goodman & Associates (eds), *Designing Effective Work Groups*. San Francisco: Jossey Bass, pp. 1–133.

Goodman, P.S., Ravlin, E. & Schminke, M. (1987). Understanding groups in organizations. *Research and Organizational Behavior*, **9**, 121–173.

Gulowsen, J. (1979). A measure of work-group autonomy. In L.E. Davis & J.C. Taylor (eds), *Design of Jobs*. Santa Monica: Goodyear, pp. 206–218.

Guzzo, R.A., Jette, R.D. & Katzell, R.A. (1985). The effects of psychologically based intervention programmes on worker productivity: a meta analysis. *Personnel Psychology*, **38**, 275–291.

Guzzo, R.A. & Shea, G.P. (1992). Group performance and intergroup relations in organizations. In M.D. Dunette & M. Hough (eds), *Handbook of Industrial and Or-

ganizational Psychology, Vol. 3. Palo Alto: Consulting Psychologists Press, pp. 269–313.
Guzzo, R.A., Wagner, D.B., Maguire, E., Herr, B. & Hawley, C. (1986). Implicit theories and the evaluation of group process and performance. *Organizational Behavior and Human Decision Processes*, **37**, 279–295.
Hacker, W. (1986). *Arbeitspsychologie [Work psychology]*. Bern: Hans Huber.
Hackman, J.R. (1987). The design of work teams. In J. Lorsch (ed.), *Handbook of Organizational Behavior*. Englewood Cliffs: Prentice Hall, pp. 315–342.
Hackman, J.R. & Oldham, G.R. (1980). *Work Redesign*. Reading: Addison-Wesley.
Hesketh, B. (1993). Measurement issues in industrial and organizational psychology. In C.L. Cooper & I.T. Robertson (eds), *International Review of Industrial and Organizational Psychology*, Vol. 8. Chichester: Wiley, pp. 133–172.
Hill, G.W. (1982). Group versus individual performance: are n + 1 heads better than one? *Psychological Bulletin*, **91**, 517–539.
James, L.R. (1982). Aggregation bias in estimates of perceptual aggreement. *Journal of Applied Psychology*, **67**, 219–229.
James, L.R., Demaree, R.G. & Wolf, G. (1984). Estimating within-group reliability with and without response bias. *Journal of Applied Psychology*, **69**, 85–98.
James, L.R., Demaree, R.G. & Wolf, G. (1993). r_{wg}: An assessment of within-group interrater agreement. *Journal of Applied Psychology*, **78**, 306–309.
Jones, M.B. (1974). Regressing group on individual effectiveness. *Organizational Behavior and Human Performance*, **11**, 426–451.
Jones, S.D. & Ourth, L. (1995). Linking training evaluation to productivity. In R.D. Pritchard (ed.), *Productivity Measurement and Improvement: Organizational Case Studies*. Westport: Praeges, pp. 299–311.
Kahn, R.L. (1977). Organizational effectiveness: an overview. In P.S. Goodman & J.M. Pennings (eds), *New Perspectives on Organizational Effectiveness*. San Francisco: Jossey Bass, pp. 235–248.
Keeley, M.A. (1978). A social justice approach to organizational evaluation. *Administrative Science Quarterly*, **22**, 272–292.
Kenney, D.A. & LaVoie, L. (1985). Separating individal and group effects. *Journal of Personality and Social Psychology*, **48**, 339–348.
Kolodny, H.F. & Kiggundu, M.N. (1980). Towards the development of a sociotechnical systems model in woodlands mechanical harvesting. *Human Relations*, **33**, 623–645.
Kozlowski, S.W.J. & Hattrup, K. (1992). A disagreement about within-group agreement: disentangling issues of consistency versus consensus. *Journal of Applied Psychology*, **77**, 161–167.
Landy, F.J. & Farr, J.L. (1983). *The Measurement of Work Performance: Methods, Theory, and Application*. New York: Academic Press.
Latané, B., Williams, K. & Harkins, S. (1979). "Many hands make light the work": the causes and consequences of social loafing. *Journal of Personality and Social Psychology*, **37**, 822–832.
Lord, R.G. (1985). Accuracy in behavioral measurement: an alternative definition based on raters' cognitive schema and signal detection theory. *Journal of Applied Psychology*, **70**, 66–71.
Lorge, I., Fox, D., Davitz, J. & Brenner, M. (1958). A survey of studies contrasting the quality of group performance and individual performance, 1920–1955. *Psychological Bulletin*, **55**, 337–372.
Mahoney, T.A. (1988). Productivity defined: the relativity of efficiency, effectiveness, and change. In J.P. Campbell & R.J. Campbell (eds), *Productivity in Organizations*. San Francisco: Jossey-Bass, pp. 13–39.
Mark, M.M. & Shotland, R.L. (1985). Stakeholder-based evaluation and value judgements. *Evaluation Review*, **9**, 605–626.
Martell, R.F. & Guzzo, R.A. (1991). The dynamics of implicit theories of group perfor-

mance: when and how do they operate? *Organizational Behavior and Human Decision Processes*, **50**, 51–74.

Martell, R.F., Guzzo, R.A. & Willis, C.E. (1995). A methodological and substantive note on the performance-cue effect in ratings of work group behavior. *Journal of Applied Psychology*, **80**, 191–195.

McGrath, J.E. (1964). *Social Psychology: A Brief Introduction*. New York: Holt, Rinehart and Winston.

McGrath, J.E. (1986). Studying groups at work: ten critical needs for theory and practice. In P.S. Goodman & Associates (eds), *Designing Effective Work Groups*. San Francisco: Jossey-Bass, pp. 362–392.

McGrath, J.E. (1991). Time, interaction and performance (TIP): a theory of groups. *Small Group Research*, **22**, 147–174.

McGrath, J.E. & Kelley, J.R. (1992). Temporal context and temporal patterning in social psychology. *Time and Society*, **1**, 399–420.

Moeller, A., Schneider, B., Schoorman, F.D. & Berney, E. (1988). Development of the work-facilitation diagnostic. In F.D. Schoorman & B. Schneider (eds), *Facilitating Work Effectiveness*. Massachusetts: Lexington Books, pp. 79–103.

Mullen, B. & Copper, C. (1994). The relation between group cohesiveness and performance: an integration. *Psychological Bulletin*, **15**, 210–227.

Naylor, J.C., Pritchard, R.D. & Ilgen, D.R. (1980). *A Theory of Behavior in Organizations*. New York: Academic Press.

Nieva, V.F., Fleishman, E.A. & Rieck, A. (1978). *Team Dimensions: Their Identity, Their Measurement, and Their Relationships*. Final Technical Report for Contract No. DAHC19-78-C-0001. Washington, D.C.: Advanced Research Resources Organizations.

Ostroff, C. (1993). Comparing correlations based on individual-level and aggregated data. *Journal of Applied Psychology*, **78**, 569–582.

Pearce, J.A. & Ravlin, E.C. (1987). The design and activation of self-regulating work groups. *Human Relations*, **40**, 751–782.

Peters, L.H. & O'Conner, E. (1980). Situational constraints and work-outcomes: the influences of a frequently overlooked construct. *Academy of Management Review*, **5**, 391–397.

Pfeffer, J. (1986). A resource dependence perspective on intercorporate relations. In M.S. Mizruchi & M. Schwartz (eds), *Structural Analysis of Business*. New York: Academic Press, pp. 117–132.

Pfeffer, J. & Salancik, G.R. (1978). *The External Control of Organizations: A Resource Dependence Perspective*. New York: Harper & Row.

Pinto, J.K. & Prescott, J.E. (1988). Variations in critical success factors over the stages in the project life cycle. *Journal of Management*, **14**, 5–18.

Pinto, J.K. & Slevin, D.P. (1988). Project sucess: definition and measurement techniques. *Project Management Journal*, **19**, 67–71.

Poulton, B. & West, M.A. (1993). Effective multidisciplinary teamwork in primary health care. *Journal of Advanced Nursing*, **18**, 918–925.

Poulton, B. & West, M.A. (1994). Primary health care team effectiveness: developing a constituency approach. *Health & Social Care*, **2**, 77–84.

Pressman, R.S. (1987). *Softward Engineering. A Practitioner's Approach*. New York: McGraw-Hill.

Pritchard, R.D. (1990). *Measuring and Improving Organizational Productivity*. New York: Praeger.

Pritchard, R.D. (1992). Organizational productivity. In M.D. Dunette & M. Hough (eds), *Handbook of Industrial and Organizational Psychology*, Vol. 3. Palo Alto: Consulting Psychologists Press, pp. 443–471.

Pritchard, R.D. (1995a). *Productivity Measurement and Improvement: Organizational Case Studies*. Westport: Praeger.

Pritchard, (1995b). Lessons learned about ProMES. In R.D. Pritchard (ed.), *Productivity*

Measurement and Improvement: Organizational Case Studies. Westport: Praeger, pp. 325–366.

Pritchard, R.D., Jones, S.D., Roth, P.L., Stuebing, K.K. & Ekeberg, S.E. (1988). Effects of group feedback, goal setting, and incentives on organizational productivity. *Journal of Applied Psychology*, **73**, 337–358.

Pritchard, R.D., Jones, S.D., Roth, P.L., Stuebing, K.K. & Ekeberg, S.E. (1989). The evaluation of an integrated approach to measuring organizational productivity. *Personnel Psychology*, **42**, 69–115.

Rousseau, D.M. (1985). Issues of level in organizational research: multi-level and cross-level perspectives. *Research in Organizational Behavior*, **7**, 1–37.

Schmidt, F.L. & Hunter, J.E. (1989). Interrater reliability coefficients cannot be computed when only one stimulus is rated. *Journal of Applied Psychology*, **74**, 368–370.

Shea, G.P. & Guzzo, R.A. (1987a). Groups as human resources. *Research in Personnel and Human Resources Management*, **5**, 323–356.

Shea, G.P. & Guzzo, R.A. (1987b). Group effectiveness: what really matters? *Sloan Management Review*, **Spring**, 25–31.

Schoorman, F.D. & Schneider, B. (1988). *Facilitating Work Effectiveness*. Massachusetts: Lexington Books.

Smith, P.C. (1976). Behaviors, results and organizational effectiveness: the problem of criteria. In M.D. Dunette (ed.), *Handbook of Industrial and Organizational Psychology*. Chicago: Rand McNally, pp. 745–775.

Sonnentag, S., Brodbeck, F.C., Heinbokel, T. & Stolte, W. (1994). Stressor–burnout relationship in softwar development teams. *Journal of Occupational and Organizational Psychology*, **67**, 327–341.

Staw, B.M. (1975). Attribution of the "causes" of performance: a general alternative interpretation of cross-sectional research on organizations. *Organizational Behavior and Human Performance*, **13**, 414–432.

Steiner, I.D. (1972). *Group Process and Productivity*. New York: Academic Press.

Sundstrom, E., De Meuse, K.P. & Futrell, D. (1990). Work teams: applications and effectiveness. *American Psychologist*, **45**, 120–133.

Tett, R.P., Meyer, J.P. & Roese, N.J. (1994). Applications of meta-analysis: 1987–1992. In C.L. Cooper & I.T. Robertson (eds), *International Review of Industrial and Organizational Psychology*, Vol. 9. Chichester: Wiley, pp. 71–112.

Tuckman, B. (1965). Development sequence in small groups. *Psychological Bulletin*, **63**, 384–399.

Tuckman, B. & Jensen, M. (1977). Stages of small-group development. *Group and Organizational Studies*, **2**, 419–427.

Ulich, E. (1991). *Arbeitspsychologie [Work psychology]*. Stuttgart: Poeschel.

Wallace, S.R. (1965). Criteria for what? *American Psychologist*, **20**, 411–417.

Watson, M.D., Hedley, A., Clark, K., Paquin, A., Noga, G. & Pritchard, R.D. (1995). Using ProMES to evaluate university teaching effectiveness. In R.D. Pritchard (eds), *Productivity Measurement and Improvement: Organizational Case Studies*. Westport: Praeger, pp. 190–208.

Weber, W.G. (1994). Autonomie und restriktive Gruppenarbeit in der Produktion [Autonomous and restrictive group work on the shop floor]. *Zeitschrift für Arbeitswissenschaft*, **48**(3), 147–156.

Wegner, D.M. (1987). Transactive memory: a contemporary analysis of the group mind. In B. Mullen & G.R. Goethals (eds), *Theories of Group Behavior*. New York: Springer, pp. 185–208.

Weldon, E. & Weingart, L.R. (1993). Group goals and group performance. *British Journal of Social Psychology*, **32**, 307–334.

West, M.A. (1990). The social psychology of innovation in groups. In M.A. West & J.L. Farr (eds), *Innovation and Creativity at Work: Psychological and Organizational Strategies*. Chichester: Wiley.

West, M.A., Brodbeck, F.C. & Patterson, M. (in prep.). *Agreeing to disagree: The inadequacy of standard measures of within-group consensus*. Manuscript. Institute of Work Psychology, The University of Sheffield, Sheffield, S10 2TN, UK.

Yammarino, F.J. & Markham, S.E. (1992). On the application of the within and between analysis: are absence and affect really group based phenomena? *Journal of Applied Psychology*, **77**, 168–176.

Yammarino, F.J. & Naughton, T.J. (1988). Time spent communicating: a multiple levels of analysis approach. *Human Relations*, **41**, 655–676.

Zammuto, R.F. (1984). A comparison of multiple constituency models of organizational effectiveness. *Academy of Management Review*, **9**, 606–616.

Chapter 13

Innovation and Creativity in Work Groups

Anders Agrell
and
Roland Gustafson
University of Örebro, Sweden

Abstract

Analysis is conducted on three levels, the individual, the group and the organizational context, in order to explain innovation and creativity in work groups. Facilitating and inhibiting characteristics and processes are identified on each level. Innovation is facilitated if group members exhibit creativity, self-efficacy and cognitive abilities in support of creative production and inhibited if they adher to defensive attitudes called single-loop learning. Group structure variables such as size, diversity and longevity are not sufficient to explain innovativeness. Group climate factors such as visions and shared objectives, participative safety, task orientation/climate for excellence and norms in support of innovation have more explicatory value. Processes that inhibit innovation can be identified on different levels of awareness in groups, at a subconscious level such as basic assumption functioning, at preconscious level as a result of mixed messages, and on a conscious level as a result of innovation colliding with group interests. Interventions to overcome opposition to innovation are described. Organizational context factors that facilitate innovation are job discretion, leadership in support of innovation, appropriate work group boundaries and rewards. Consequences of bureaucracy in terms of hierarchy, formalization and centralization are inhibiting. The review is summed up by a synthetic model describing different outcomes such as successful innovation, abandoned innovation or failing appropriate innovation as dependent on multifaceted variables operating within the organizational context, the group and the individual in a dynamic interplay. Concluding remarks emphasize the importance of trusting dialogue between colleagues, group leadership and participation in problem-solving by group members to achieve innovation.

INTRODUCTION

In order to study innovation and creativity in the work group there are three levels of analysis to consider, namely, the individual, the group and the organizational context. For example, the individual in the work group may develop an idea and may want to implement an innovation. He or she may become encouraged by the group climate and so starts to influence other members of the work group to try new things. The enthusiasm of this specific individual employee may further be encouraged by conditions around the group, i.e. the discretion level, the reward system, the leadership and the whole organizational culture.

As well as forces facilitating innovation in the work-place, there are also forces inhibiting new ideas and new applications. These inhibiting forces can also be conceptualized on an individual level, such as fear; on a group level, such as a norm for hard work; and on an organizational level, such as bureaucracy (see Table 13.1).

Thus, this chapter will explore the facilitating and the inhibiting factors within the individual, the group itself and the organizational context of the work group. Further, the purpose is to analyse tentatively possible relations between these levels. We are aware that some of the factors in Table 13.1 are dimensions and so have positive and negative poles. The division of concepts into facilitating and inhibiting columns might also be, to some extent, arbitrary. However, we believe that such a model provides a useful organizing framework. It is not intended to be a complete description, but is used as a first step towards developing a more comprehensive understanding of innovation and creativity in work groups.

Table 13.1 The general design of the chapter and the model of analysis

Level	Facilitating	Inhibiting
Individual	Creativity Traits related to creativity Creative ability Self-efficacy	Cognitive limitations Defence mechanisms
Group	*Structure*: size, tenure, diversity *Climate*: the four-factor model *Group belief*: potency	Defensive routines Basic-assumption functioning
Organizational context	Leadership Boundary Rewards Job discretion	Bureaucracy Centralization Formalization

In this review, creativity is considered to be mainly a cognitive process within the individual, as conceptualized by Wallas (1926). The surrounding social context plays a motivational role, as elaborated by Amabile (1983), and others' views add cognitive richness to the individual. Innovation is postulated to be a social process and the definition of innovation we have reflects this:

> ... the intentional introduction and application within a role, group or organization of ideas, processes, products or procedures, new to the relevant unit of adoption, designed to significantly benefit the individual, the group, the organization or wider society (West & Farr, 1990, p. 9).

The definition emphasizes that innovation is restricted to intentional attempts to arrive at anticipated benefits in contrast to routine change. Further, the definition encompasses innovations in technology as well as in administration and work organization. The definition also requires an application component, which will almost always imply a social element of the innovation process.

INDIVIDUAL LEVEL

Individual Characteristics Facilitating Work Group Innovation

In order to discover individual factors, a first approach would be to look for creativity as a trait among work group members. Creativity has been considered a personality trait in itself (Guilford, 1959) but Nicholls (1972) has argued that this approach has not proved successful. The concept of trait has long been challenged. However, the development of research and instruments to measure creativity continue. A definition that has attracted wide acceptance states:

> Creativity means a person's capacity to produce new or original ideas, insights, restructurings, inventions, or artistic objects, which are accepted by experts as being of scientific, aesthetic, social, or technological value (Vernon, 1989, p. 94).

A second approach would be to study traits associated with creative achievement: desire for autonomy (McCarrey & Edwards, 1973), social independence (Coopey, 1987), high tolerance for ambiguity (Child, 1973), a propensity for risk-taking (Michael, 1979) and a moderate anxiety level (Wallach & Kogan, 1965). This research provides a consistent picture of the creative individual. However, it is based on correlational studies and King (1990) has cautioned us against concluding that creative achievement is a simple function of a certain trait. For instance, is a moderate level of anxiety necessary for creativity or is it an effect of the difficulties inherent in creative productions?

A third approach to consider could be to study self-efficacy, defined as self-perceptions about one's ability to produce and regulate events in one's life (Bandura, 1986). Our hypothesis is that the recognition of a problem, a performance gap or a need for change in the workplace is approached with enthusiasm and positive expectations by individuals with strong perceptions of self-efficacy.

Farr & Ford (1990) suggest that perceptions of self-efficacy regarding innovation and change at work are affected by past relevant job experiences and formal training. For instance, in a study by Wiersma & Bantel (1992; see Box 13.2 below) the more innovative management teams included members with more academic scientific training. Positive experiences of former innovations should lead to stronger efficacy beliefs when facing a new obstacle. Bandura (1986) also argues that individualized instructions and evaluations, that focus on an individual's relative learning and progress, enhance self-efficacy.

The final approach would be to consider cognitive abilities that might influence creative production, such as the ability to make random associations between ideas; to see divergent uses for a single idea; to access one's subconscious in the service of the ego; and to visualize potential solutions (Barron & Harrington, 1981).

The concept of creativity and traits associated with creative production, self-efficacy and creative abilities all explain how individuals' characteristics might facilitate work group innovation. We now turn to individual characteristics which may inhibit innovation.

Individual Characteristics Inhibiting Innovation

Individuals often resist innovation regardless of the arguments in favour of an innovation, such as improved efficiency, profitability and even greater well-being. This resistance might be associated with personality traits, e.g. a strong need for control, rule dependence and authoritarianism (Winter, 1973). The tendency to resist could also result from previous negative experience of innovation. Thus, the resistance of the individual is an attitude containing components of information, emotion and behavioural tendencies.

A Cognitive-learning Approach

Argyris (1968) has argued that hierarchical organizations often create a defensive attitude towards learning and change among staff. Argyris & Schön (1974, 1978) have studied the individual's defensive cognitive schemes and behavioural patterns and refer to two very different learning types: single- and double-loop learning. Single-loop learning (Argyris, 1990) refers to situations where individuals think and act out of given conditions, follow their habits and do not reflect much about what they are doing. Introduction of change in this case follows certain "rules" and is not innovative. Double-loop learning, on the other hand, refers to situations where individuals reflect more deeply on the conditions, values and norms that guide their thinking and acting in relation to their tasks, and leads to innovations. For an example of single-loop learning let us take a situation in a hospital ward in which a patient asks to wear his own clothing. The nurses do not particularly like this but decide to agree after having explored the arguments for and against, in terms of hygiene and laundry routines, as a one time exception. Had they taken this as an opportunity for double-loop learning they might have further explored patients' needs for keeping their integrity, and thus developed beneficial innovations in patients care.

Argyris & Schön (1974, 1978) also postulate a difference between what people say they stand for ("espoused theory") and how they actually act ("theories-in-use"). Individuals might express opinions about what is right and wrong and about how they would act in different situations. However, in these situations, they do not behave according to what they have said. They do not act out of the espoused theory, but according to their theory-in-use. For example, staff working with developmentally retarded people might have been trained to approach their patients with an emphasis on education rather than care. However, the training offered to them might not achieve the more thorough change of values and cognitive representations of their work that is needed (see Box 13.1 below). They know how to describe the new espoused theory, but in day-to-day practice they follow their old habits, their theory-in-use. When people exhibit such a discrepancy they illustrate single-loop learning, when double-loop learning was intended.

Van de Ven (1986) takes a different cognitive approach to innovation when he points out our limited capacity to deal with complexity. People have narrow spans of attention and will activate and concentrate on a specific cognitive scheme at work. Most individuals can perform routine tasks while at the same time paying attention to other things. In complex decision situations, individuals

---

Box 13.1 Innovation in work methods and goals among staff working with developmentally retarded people

In Sweden there has been in recent years a change of methods used to rehabilitate those who are developmentally retarded. Large institutions have closed down and patients have been moved to smaller, more home-like, units closer to society. These patients now live together four or five in a flat, with a group of staff attending to them. Along with this reorganization there is a retraining of staff. In the big institutions the staff "cared for" their "patients". Now they are supposed to "assist" their "guests". Scientific evaluations have been made of the progress of change of attitude among staff and the result is that, when interviewed, they know how to describe their new attitude (espoused theory), but observations show very little change in behaviour. Staff mainly continue caring, thus following their theory-in-use. To agree to the new objectives while in practice adhering to the old ones can be seen as a subconscious defensive routine. One reason for this might be the artificial character of the retraining scheme. Some staff never really understood this new way of helping their "guests".

create stereotypes as a defence mechanism to deal with complexity. In this way complexity is transformed into something simple. This, in many circumstances, appropriate way of functioning might sometimes inhibit individuals from innovating at work.

A third cognitive approach would be to acknowledge that people have widely varying adaptation levels (Helson, 1948). When exposed over time to a set of stimuli that deteriorate very gradually, people do not perceive the gradual changes, but unconsciously adapt to the worsening situation. An example is a situation where social workers in a neighbourhood do not observe their diminishing capability in communicating with the citizens. They fail to recognize in time that an important innovation would be for staff to learn a new language. This mechanism explains why people do not become dissatisfied with existing conditions and so are not motivated to innovate.

A Psychodynamic Approach

Psychoanalytic and psychodynamic theory mainly focus on and explore the irrational layers of the human mind. From this perspective, defensive reactions to innovations might be more or less obvious to us. First, defence mechanisms according to psychoanalytic theory operate on a subconscious level in the mind. Their function is to protect the self-concept of the individual and to stop information from reaching a level of conscious reflection that might damage individuals' perceptions of themselves and their environment. For example, we might fail to recognize an opportunity to innovate since this would mean, for example, a change of our role at work. Seeing ourselves in a different role at work might create a mental image that we subconsciously suppress to avoid anxiety. Team members may also project all their dissatisfaction with their own work performance onto colleagues and so fail to realize an opportunity to deal more efficiently with the task at hand through introducing appropriate innovations.

Second, also on a preconscious level, we might try to deny or oppose information that would provoke anxiety. For example it should be obvious to us that the present way of doing our job is not appropriate. However, we might be uncertain whether or not we have the necessary competence to handle it in another way. This uncertainty is something that we cannot bear to admit to ourselves, so we actively avoid the thought of adopting a new work method. Thus we fail to realize the possibility of an innovation or we oppose innovation implementation.

Third, on a conscious level, the individual might use rational arguments to hinder an innovation. An intended innovation might threaten the individual's interests in the work group, so he or she counteracts the idea. Another possibility is that the individual detects weaknesses in the innovation, and so appropriately criticizes the content. The conscious opposition of individuals can hinder work group innovation, but also may contribute to group performance since innovations are not necessarily beneficial.

GROUP LEVEL

Characteristics Facilitating Innovation

Historically, innovation at work was studied only at the individual or organizational levels, but in recent years the importance of work group characteristics has been emphasized. This part of our review will cover issues from structure to climate in work groups.

Group Structure Variables

Group Size

Wallmark (1973) studied the importance of size in research groups and found a positive correlation between group size and group productivity. This was interpreted as resulting from the greater number of possible contacts and consequent intellectual synergy. Stankiewicz (1979) examined group size in Swedish academic research groups and related this variable to scientific performance as a measure of creativity. In his study, 172 groups were randomly selected from the fields of natural science and technology. The groups in the sample ranged from 2 to 8 in size. The typical group contained 4–5 scientists. Stankiewicz (1979) confirmed a positive correlation between group size and productivity in groups high on cohesiveness and with very experienced leaders, but in groups with low cohesiveness he found an optimum size of seven members. So there seems to be an interaction effect between size and cohesiveness, since cohesiveness mediates between size and productivity.

The relation between "group age" (longevity) and performance is also mediated by cohesiveness, according to Stankiewicz (1979). Highly cohesive groups can quickly achieve high performance rates, while groups low in cohesion have to exist for a long time to reach the same performance level. Geshka (1983), in a theoretical article, proposed that specially trained innovation planning teams in organizations should contain 6–8 members from different functional areas and also include opinion leaders who can help in the implementation phase. The combination of a small work group and the presence of an opinion leader, who pays attention to dissenting minorities, should especially favour innovation (Geshka, 1983). The structural factors of size and longevity alone do not explain creative capacity in groups. They might create the basis for certain group processes leading to a high degree of cohesiveness, which in turn might favour innovation. These results might seem to direct attention away from structural factors and towards work group climate factors as explaining variables. However, other structural factors do have an influence on group innovation. These are described below.

Professional Diversity

As Andrews (1979) has pointed out, diversity is a multifaceted concept; a group is neither simply high or low on diversity. Andrews (1979) found 70 types of diversity in research and development (R&D) teams that could be divided into nine categories. Some of these categories relate to the group structure, e.g. interdisciplinary orientation; engagement in multiple scientific specialities; incorporation of multiple projects; arrangement of work so that scientists are engaged in multiple R&D activities. Other aspects are contextual, e.g. diversity in funding resources. The major finding from this study was that a combination of six diversity measures accounted for about 10% of the total variance in scientific recognition and number of publications (Andrews, 1979). This suggests that the variety of orientations and competence that people bring to a work group offers a small but significant contribution to work group performance and creative work.

Diversity in Tenure

Zenger & Lawrence (1989) argue that individuals who join an organization at the same time develop similar understandings of its events and of its technology. This "tenure homogeneity" has been positively related to frequency of communication, social integration within the group and innovation (O'Reilly & Flatt, 1989). Ancona & Caldwell (1992) found that tenure diversity had its effect more on internal group dynamics in the sense that it improved task work such as clarifying goals and setting priorities. This clarity was also related to high ratings of team performance. The conclusion from this study (Ancona & Caldwell, 1992) is that tenure diversity brings more creativity to problem-solving and product development but that there is less capability for implementing innovation.

Demographic Diversity

Demography encompasses variables such as age, company tenure, educational background and position. There is evidence that demographic diversity in groups increases conflict, reduces cohesion and complicates internal communication (see Jackson, this volume; Dougherty, 1987; Kiesler, 1978). Work groups made up of individuals of different age, experience and professional training may find it difficult to develop a shared purpose and an effective group process (Dougherty, 1987). Since diversity in this sense might counteract cohesiveness, it might inhibit innovation.

Functional Diversity

Diversity also relates to professional backgrounds and positions (Jackson et al., 1991). Souder (1987) has found that functionally diverse groups have difficulties in reaching agreements on implementing innovations. Zenger & Lawrence (1989) have suggested that functional diversity might influence work group performance through the increasing rate of external communication. Ancona & Caldwell (1992) found that when a work group recruited a new member from a certain functional area in an organization, communication went up dramatically in that area. This in turn might favour innovation through bringing in more and different ideas and models. Ancona & Caldwell (1992) studied 45 new product teams in five high technology companies. They found that the greater the functional diversity, the more team members communicated outside the work group's boundaries and the higher ratings they got on innovation.

Box 13.2 below provides a description of a recent study that illustrates that diversity is a multifaceted concept and that homogeneity might be important in some respects (e.g. age and educational level) and heterogeneity in other (e.g. functional).

Group Longevity

With time it is likely that a group becomes more cohesive and this could favour innovation (Nyström, 1979). On the other hand, Lovelace (1986) suggests that scientists need to work alone and that their social needs distract them from their work. He suggests that research scientists, when forced to function in groups, after some time will be less creative. Nyström (1979) argues for the advantages in

---

Box 13.2 What team is most capable of strategic change? A study of executive team demographics

In a management team at top level in an organization, innovation concerns strategic change. Should it diversify its line of products and expand into new areas? Should it take the opposite approach and narrow its focus on a smaller line of products? What quality objectives should be introduced? Is it possible to predict which of the organizations top teams will make strategic change decisions and which will not? A study by Wiersma & Bantel (1992) addresses this issue. They hypothesized that certain key demographic factors might be good predictors of when strategic change and innovation would occur. The investigators studied top management teams within 87 different Fortune 500 companies. In order to study innovation they took out a measure of diversification of products at two time points, 1980 and 1983. By comparing these figures they determined how much change took place with respect to diversification. The analysis showed which companies made decisions to change a great deal, e.g. by adding or dropping several product lines, and which did not. The degree of diversification was then related to several demographic data from the team members: age, organizational tenure, team tenure, education level, within-team heterogeneity of education, academic training in the sciences. These variables were extracted from large corporate databases. These variables did predict the amount of change in the teams' organizations. More change and innovation occurred in organizations whose top team members were younger, better educated, worked less time in their teams and in the organizations, were more diverse in educational specialization and had more academic scientific training compared to those who were opposite along these dimensions (Wiersma & Bantel, 1992).

relations to innovations of relatively short-lived groups, especially in the early stages of the innovation process. Katz (1982) found that work group longevity was negatively related to performance in R&D teams.

It seems that a single structural factor such as longevity does not explain innovative capacity in work groups. There are probably no strong relations at all between longevity or any other structural factors and innovative capacity in work groups. Structural factors can create the conditions for innovativeness, as in the case of functional diversity. However, innovation in work groups may well be more of a consequence of group climate, which in turn relies on an array of enabling conditions within and around the work group.

The Concept of Group Climate

Schneider & Reichers (1983) assert that it is meaningless to apply the concept of climate without a particular referent (e.g. climate for change, climate for quality, climate for innovation). Rousseau (1988) has argued similarly and advocates the study of "facet-specific climates". As Anderson & West (1994) emphasize, this approach to the concept of climate seems more promising as opposed to earlier ambitions to find a "catch-all" concept.

Many measures of climate take the whole organization as the unit of analysis (Patterson, West & Payne, 1992). There seems to be more justification for the assumption that demonstrable and discriminable climates exist within work groups, that is, smaller units of an organization. It is within a work group that staff

---

Box 13.3 The development of a team climate measure predicting innovation

The psychometric properties of the Team Climate Inventory (TCI) were first studied in a longitudinal study of 27 management teams of British hospitals (Anderson & West, 1994). Exploratory factor analysis supported a four-factor model of group climate (a total of explained variance of 61.7%). This robust factor structure was later replicated on a bigger sample with confirmatory factor analysis using linear structural relationships (LISREL) techniques. The internal homogeneity and reliability of the four sub-scales were acceptable. The concurrent validities were tested by correlating the self-reports on the TCI with coded behaviour on team meetings in nine of the 27 management teams. The results showed positive correlation between the two measures. Scores on the TCI were also related to the quantity and quality of innovation implemented by the teams. According to regression analysis, 42% of the variance in innovation could be explained by differences in TCI scores (Anderson & West, 1994). The team climate measured by the TCI seems to predict a substantial part of the innovation capacity. These results have, to some extent, been replicated by Agrell & Gustafson (1994) on a Swedish sample of 17 teams operating on different levels in organizations. The TCI was translated into Swedish and the four-factor model was confirmed through exploratory factor analysis. The reliability was good and the correlations between TCI scores and independent ratings of the innovativeness of the teams were acceptable (Agrell & Gustafson, 1994).

interact and communicate with one another, whereas medium and large organizations are almost certainly characterized by widely differing sub-cultures, departments and hierarchical levels. West (1990) has developed a model of group climate predicting innovation in organizations (the empirical test is described in Box 13.3). The model comprises four climate factors.

Vision and Shared Objectives

A vision is an idea of a valued outcome, a higher order goal, which is a motivating force for a work group (West, 1990). The concept of vision contains a component of value added to the objective. For example, staff at a department of occupational medicine might feel committed to finding occupational health hazards in the workplace and controlling or eliminating them.

There are certainly important qualities or dimensions within this concept of vision and shared objectives. The clearer the vision, the more effective it is likely to be as a facilitator of innovation, since new ideas can be assessed against it (West, 1990). The more the vision is negotiated and shared within a group, the more the group members are committed to implement an innovation. It is also important that visions are attainable, since otherwise steps towards its achievement cannot be envisaged.

Participative Safety

Participation and safety are characterized by West (1990) as a single psychological concept. The contingencies are such that involvement in all the team's work is motivated and reinforced when occurring in an environment that is perceived as interpersonally non-threatening. This climate factor has a quantitative dimension: the more group members share information and involve each other in decision-making, the higher the likelihood of appropriate innovation. Quality of participation concerns the relevance and importance of ideas exchanged in the group. A feeling of safety in the group climate probably enables the exploration of radical ideas (West, 1990).

Task Orientation and a Climate for Excellence

Task orientation in a work group would be evidenced by a shared concern with excellence of quality of task performance in relation to shared visions or outcomes (West, 1990). Further, it would be addressed by appraisal of and constructive challenges to the group's performance; a concern for standards of performance; tolerance of diversity; exploration of opposing opinions; and a monitoring of each other's performance. Tjosvold (1982) also has demonstrated positive effects of allowing constructive controversy in decision-making. This implies encouraging diversity of opinions and at the same time ensuring high quality of innovation by careful examination of ideas proposed.

Group Norms in Support for Innovation

This dimension comprises the expectation, approval and practical support for innovation in groups. Are new ideas routinely rejected or ignored, or do they find both articulated and enacted support in the group? The support might be verbal within and outside meetings. It can also be in the form of cooperation in the development and application of new ideas. It can appear in the form of members providing time and resources to others in trying to implement an innovation (West, 1990). If a climate is supportive in this sense it also implies a tolerance of errors made by an innovator, who knows that he or she will not be penalized when risk-taking does not pay off. Peters & Waterman (1982) found that members of organizations often were encouraged to innovate, but only "safe experimentation" was supported.

The Group Belief in Potency

A concept related to the concept of climate is that of group belief. A group belief is shared among the members of the group and is a collective belief in, for example, the effectiveness of the group (Guzzo et al., 1993). Potency shares a certain similarity with the individual motivational construct of self-efficacy (Bandura, 1986). Since this concept probably is of importance to understanding innovation (see above, and Farr & Ford, 1990), it might be argued that a work group with a strong belief in its potency would be more innovative.

Group Characteristics Inhibiting Innovation

Communication Style

To achieve innovation there must be ideas and these appear from among individuals in the work-place. When these ideas are further developed, refined, tested and in the end implemented, the result rests on interaction among individuals. Senge (1990) underlines the importance of how people talk to each other and the difference between "having a discussion" and "having a dialogue". In a discussion we argue for our case and try to change that of others, but in a dialogue we actively listen and we are open to changing our opinions. It is primarily through dialogue that we are likely to change our basic assumptions. Otherwise we get stuck in our own arguments, as in the case of a work group that has become the victim of groupthink (Janis, 1972). Argyris & Schön (1974) make a similar distinction between arguing and inquiring. Gupta, Ray & Wilemon (1985) found, when studying R&D groups, that communication barriers and insensitivity towards other members' capacities and viewpoints were major obstacles to efficiency.

A Psychodynamic Approach

Bion (1961) differentiates between two levels of functioning in groups: the rational "working" group and the "basic-assumption" group. On the latter level, the goals and tasks are secondary to the emotional needs of members. A particular group might vary between the state of "working group" and the state of "basic assumption". A "neurotic" group stays or functions in the latter state more often than a "sound" group.

> Participation in basic-assumption activity requires no training, experience or mental development. It is instantaneous, inevitable and instinctive: I have not felt the need to postulate the existence of a herd instinct to account for such phenomena as I have witnessed in a group (Bion, 1961, p. 153).

The basic-assumption functioning appears spontaneously, is elicited by a perceived threat, is subconscious and primitive. Taking part in a group means to be subconsciously aware of emotional needs expressed by group members and adjust to these needs so that they become the needs of the group.

Defensive routines as defined by Argyris (1990) could be seen as an extension of the original examples of basic-assumption functioning described by Bion (1961). The work group may be exposed to a demand for change and innovation. For example, the group is required by senior management to implement a new work method. Work gruop members are trained in applying the new method and they agree to its application only verbally and not in action. The strategy agreeing to an innovation verbally but not putting it into action can be seen as a defensive routine (Argyris, 1990). The case in Box 13.1 above is an illustration of this. In that example, staff confronted with demands of innovation learned the lesson in theory but regressed to their old habits and ways of working in practice. The maintenance of the old habit was secured through collective action patterns of defensive routines. The emotional needs of the group to survive when faced with demands they could not cope with made them minimize the primacy of the task.

First, defensive routines in groups can be categorized in terms of the degree of awareness among the members (Kylén, 1993). If they exist at the level of the subconscious of the group, they can be referred to as defence mechanisms and are similar to such mechanisms among individuals. Groups can project, deny, repress and rationalize in order to avoid threats. In this case the defensive reaction is collective.

Second, on a preconscious level, groups might oppose innovation. One cause of this opposition might be found in the concept of "mixed messages" as developed by Argyris (1990). This concept describes how "bad news" in organizations often is presented in a way everybody can accept. Individuals say: "I do not mean to interrupt you" or "I do not want to upset you". The respondent is then forbidden to express a natural feeling of frustration and upset. Argyris (1990) calls some mixed messages "organizational lies", such as, "Thank you for the feed-back", when we do not like or agree with it, or, "I'm offering you a developmental opportunity", when a supervisor means, "I don't like your performance and am moving you elsewhere to do less harm". There are strong norms in the workplace not to disclose the underlying genuine message, so the recipient is left with an uncomfortable feeling and with the cognition of a meta-message saying that direct constructive controversy is impossible. A frequent use of mixed messages in a work group is likely to inhibit a group climate favouring innovation.

Third, resistance to innovation might be completely conscious in a work group. A particular group may not agree to an innovation as agreeable because it is not in accordance with its interests. This may be very rational from the group's point of view. It might also be to the benefit of the organization if the innovation is inappropriate. Groups might consciously use political tactics to resist innovation. For example, Frost & Egri (1991) describe the political process in technological, social and scientific innovation. People who innovate might collide with power interests from other members of a group and face tactics used to resist innovation, such as "rule-citing", where members start going by the book and referring to rules, regulations and policy documents.

Interventions to Overcome Opposition to Innovation

Kylén (1993) has conducted process studies in work groups at three youth correction institutes to remove defensive routines in order to facilitate innovation. He observed interactions in staff group meetings and identified different types of

---

Box 13.4 An example of the development of a defensive routine (Kylén, 1993)

The setting is a staff group in a youth correction institution.
1. A problem creates unease—"Bob refuses to get out of bed in the morning".
2. How does the staff group cope with this?—"We must decide on an action plan and stick to it".
3. Agreement:—"When the other clients have gone to their duties we get Bob out of bed!"
4. One team-member does not comply and avoids the situation.
5. Silence—the colleagues fail to correct the team member. The incident becomes undiscussable in formal meetings. It is, however, discussed man-to-man. If taken up in a meeting the subject is covered up (defensive routine of avoidance).
6. Different types of defences appear in the group—projection, "This client is impossible".
7. More deviations from professional responsible behaviour of the same kind occur.
8. Similar situations are affected by the same deficiency of functioning in the group.
9. Chaos in the ward, resulting in patients absconding and absenteeism among staff.

defensive routines. His conclusions were reflected back to the group and tailored exercises were used to "work through" observed resistance. The result indicated that success was dependent on the "development level" of the group (Tuckman & Jensen, 1977). In two of the three staff groups Kylén (1993) found that his "mirroring" of the group process had no effect on their climates. At the third institution, however, the work group became aware of its defensive routines and managed to abandon some of them. Kylén (1993) concludes that the first two groups were in forming and adjourning phases respectively (Tuckman & Jensen, 1977). The third and successful group, however, was in a storming phase and this made them open to the possibility of help from outside. The research was also supported by management in this group. In Box 13.4 above we describe an example of the development of a defensive routine from Kylén's results (1993).

ORGANIZATIONAL CONTEXT

Characteristics Facilitating Innovation in the Work Group

In the research literature on group performance there has been a bias towards looking only for within-group factors, which predict performance only within the group. There now seems to be a growing awareness of the importance of variables in the organizational context (Guzzo & Shea, 1992). Group dynamic variables might be of less importance than the conditions offered by the organizational context for work group effectiveness and innovation. This is the issue which is addressed in the last part of this chapter.

Job Discretion

A positive antecedent to creative or innovative performance is discretion of freedom of choice (Amabile, 1983). An autonomous work situation seems to be important as a background condition for idea exploration and creativity. High job discretion was a necessary condition for role innovation among individuals in a study by West (1987).

Leadership

Maier (1970a) has conducted a series of well designed experiments with laboratory groups exploring the influence of different kinds of leadership on problem-solving and creativity. College students and supervisors from industry have been randomized to experimental and control conditions. Large samples of groups have been exposed to the same tasks. The quality of solutions was determined through standardized procedures and so the result of different strategies of leadership could be determined. Problem-solving processes in groups and the group leaders' support of these processes seem to have major relevance for understanding the influence of leadership on innovation in work groups.

Maier (1970b) has studied several leadership principles that increase the ability for a group to solve problems; they have all received empirical support in experimental studies A first principle is that the leader should introduce "problem-mindedness". Maier (1970b) claims that the starting point of a problem is richest in solution possibilities. Once one starts in a particular direction one moves away from certain alternatives (Hoffman & Maier, 1970). Each route confronts the group with obstacles along the way. Because the group is involved in removing these obstacles, the partial success prevents the group from turning back to the starting point. Once a task is begun, psychological forces are set up to push the task to completion and people tend to progress too rapidly toward a solution—"solution-mindedness" (Maier, 1970b). A second principle states that the idea-getting phase should be separated from the idea-evaluation phase, since the latter inhibits the former (Maier, 1970b). To demand proof of new ideas at the time of their inception is to discourage the creative process (Maier, 1970b). The discussion leader can delay a group's criticism of an idea by asking for alternative contributions and he or she can encourage the search for something different and new. Thirdly, the leader can and should use his position in the group to protect minority individuals so that their opinions will reach evaluation (Maier & Solem, 1970a). A fourth leadership principle studied by Hoffman, Harburg & Maier (1970) suggests that leaders should encourage disagreement by turning this into factual considerations and thus avoid interpersonal conflict and injured pride among members. A fifth principle says that leaders' positive expectations of group members lead to more innovative ideas in group discussions (Maier & Hoffman, 1970). A sixth principle concerns the following: a group may interpret a situation as one of making a choice between alternatives, a "choice-situation", and as a consequence much discussion is blocked until one of the alternatives is selected (Maier & Solem, 1970b). A skilful leader can turn this into a "problem-situation" and thereby help the group to find further alternatives. A seventh principle is about the "problem-situation", a situation in which the group is confronted with an obstacle in reaching a goal (Maier, 1970b). A natural reaction in a problem-situation is to act on the first possible solution and leaders can encourage search for other alternatives. Also, studies have shown that if a leader demands a "second solution" from the group after they have reached a first one, this second one is often superior in quality (Maier & Hoffman, 1970). An eighth principle states that leaders should keep their own solutions to themselves for as long as possible, since propositions from leaders are improperly evaluated and tend either to be accepted or rejected rather than evaluated (Hoffman & Maier, 1970). A ninth principle implies that leaders must be able to diagnose and separate when they are dealing with facts and feelings in the group. The skills for removing obstacles in the form of feelings and in the form of facts are quite different (Maier, 1970b). The problem-solving skills studied by Maier (1970a) are concentrated more on the intellectual than on the emotional aspects of group discussions.

Maier (1970c) concludes that the leader should function as "the group's central nervous system": receive information, facilitate communication, relay messages, and integrate the incoming responses so that a single unified response occurs. The leader must be receptive to information but not impose his solutions. He or she must concentrate on the group process, listen in order to understand rather than to appraise or refute, assume responsibility for accurate communication, be sensitive to unexpressed feelings, protect minority views, keep the discussion moving and develop skills in summarizing (Maier, 1970c).

The leadership literature identifies two superordinate dimensions of leadership: task structure and consideration (Fleishman & Harris, 1962; Fiedler, 1967; Yukl, 1981). Are these two dimensions in leadership sufficient in a context where there are strong demands for change and innovation in the workplace? Ekvall, Arvonen & Nyström (1987) studied leader behaviour in four divisions of a Swedish chemical industry. Factor analysis of questionnaire responses from supervisors and white-collar workers loaded on three factors. Tow of them corresponded with task structuring and showing consideration. The items loading positively on the third factor were related to creating visions, accepting new ideas and making quick decisions when necessary. And some items loaded negatively on that factor, e.g. conscientiousness in performance; wanting everything to work out according to plan. Ekvall (1988) concludes that the emergence of this new factor, termed support for creativity, might be a result of the quicker pace of change in working life today.

Anderson & King (1993) conclude in a review on leadership and innovation in organizations that a participative/collaborative leadership style is likely to foster innovation. They also suggest that a key element of successful leadership for innovation is the leader's clear vision or sense of mission for the organization (Anderson & King, 1993). Knorr et al. (1979) found that group climate, innovativeness and general performance in R&D teams were predicted by the leader's planning and coordinating activities; ability to integrate the team; emphasis on career promotion; and the leader's overall professional status.

Kolb (1992) studied 16 research teams and 16 non-research teams testing the hypothesis that the important functions of leadership in a research team are in the area of public relations and coordination. Managers knowledgeable of, but not involved in, team activities rated the teams' performance. The results supported the hypothesis; there were significant correlations between leadership behaviour such as representation, superior relations, good standing and the exhibition of trust on one hand, and autonomy and research team performance on the other hand. There were no significant relationships between these behaviours as rated by team members using the Ohio State University's Leader Description Questionnaire and performance in the 16 non-research teams (Kolb, 1992). The study by Kolb (1992) suggests one general conclusion, that a leader of an innovative work group must manage external relations, enabling the work group to concentrate on their objectives.

Work Group Boundaries

Sundstrom, de Meuse & Futrell (1990) have discussed the relationship between work groups and their surrounding organizations, which can be conceptualized in terms of team boundaries. They suggest that group boundaries mediate between organizational context and team development and are tied to effectiveness. Boundaries help to define what constitutes effectiveness for the work group. One key aspect of the group–organization boundary is integration through coordination and synchronization with suppliers, colleagues, managers and customers. For a work group to fulfill its objectives, it might be dependent on the pace and timing of other work units. A second key aspect of group–organization boundaries is differentiation, which includes the degree of specialisation, independence and autonomy of a work group in relation to others (Sundstrom, De Meuse & Futrell, 1990). When a work group is highly differentiated, this means that some of its activities are protected from outside interference. It could also mean that it is differentiated through exclusive membership, extended working time, or team life-span, or exclusive access to physical facilities. Sundstrom, De Meuse & Futrell (1990) conclude that there are different types of work groups with diverse boundaries. Project and developmental groups whose products are innovations are likely to be high in differentiation and low in integration.

Rewards

A potentially important contextual factor for work group innovation is reward for innovation. Outcomes like money, fringe benefits, public recognition and preferred work assignments should not be overlooked. Abbey & Dickson (1983), in a study of 40 successful R&D teams in different companies, found that reward systems had a strong positive relationship with performance.

Stolte-Heiskanen (1979) studied the relation between financial resources and the effectiveness of research units. She found no relation in objective terms between funding and measures of effectiveness. However, there was a strong relation between satisfaction with the material conditions and performance. This result might support our hypothesis that work group climate is of major importance to creativity and innovation.

Bureaucracy

Thompson (1965) described the relative inability of bureaucratic organizations to produce innovations. In bureaucratic organizations opposition is oppressed, conflicts are not accepted, and pluralism in opinions is lost. Competition, not co-operation, is rewarded; ideas have to be approved by someone higher up in the hierarchy with a veto possibility. In bureaucracies there tends to be a conservative atmosphere, where new ideas stand out as threatening. The organization is thus divided into departments and groups who all look after their own interests (Thompson, 1965).

Zaltman, Duncan & Holbek (1973) propose that high centralization in bureaucratic organizations inhibits the initiation of innovations because of restrictions in communication. In a decentralized structure there are more viewpoints brought into consideration and this is likely to produce a greater variety of ideas. King (1990) concludes in a review that stratification is negatively related to innovation since many levels lead to much preoccupation with status.

Zaltman, Duncan & Holbek (1973) emphasize that rigid rules and procedures and a high degree of formalization in organizations inhibit decision-makers from seeking new sources of information. King (1990) argues for the advantages of complexity in organizations, supporting the idea that a work group in a modern decentralized organization needs to be located in a culture supportive of innovation.

Conclusions

Job discretion and rewards seem to be basic conditions to motivate a work group. Leadership might influence the interaction in the group most and thereby influence group climate. A leader should be participative and exert moderate control. He or she should also encourage and support new ideas in the group and be able to formulate objectives and visions. This leadership style coincides to a large extent with the dimensions in the four-factor model of group climate, which can predict innovation. Furthermore, the leader should guard the boundaries of the group, and enable the group to work effectively without organizational distractions. But the group also needs to be in contact with relevant outside partners in order that collaboration possibilities can be exploited. The leader could also take care of relations between the group and the bureaucratic context, minimizing their involvement in unhelpful bureaucratic procedures.

A SYNTHESIS AND CONCLUDING MODEL

The theoretical concepts and empirical results analysed so far are now related to each other in a tentative model (for the following discussion, refer to Figure 13.1).

On an organizational level the characteristics of the context surrounding the work group can be either beneficial or non-beneficial to work group innovation. The most beneficial context is decentralized, offering job discretion and rewards for innovation. The non-beneficial context is inflexible, hierarchical and bureaucratic. The characteristics of most organizations are somewhere in between these two poles.

On a group level, climate can be beneficial to innovation, as characterized by

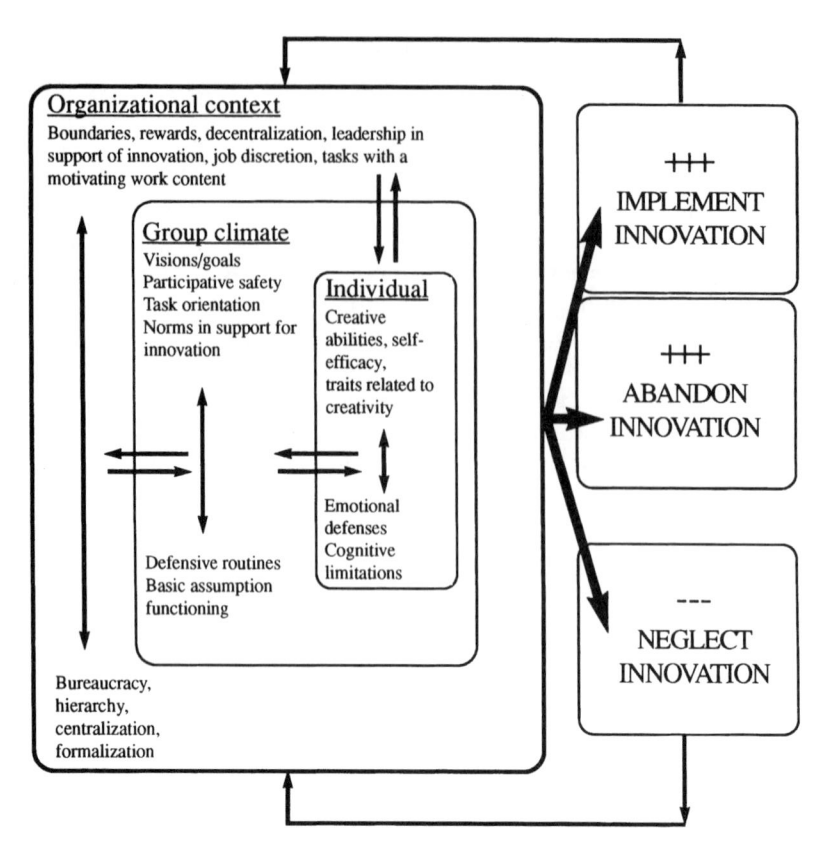

Figure 13.1 A model describing the relations between variables within and around the work group determining the degree of successful innovation

the four-factor model, or non-beneficial when burdened by negative interactions, such as defensive routines and basic assumption functioning. When these latter conditions dominate, the articulation of visions and goals, participative safety, task orientation and norms in support for innovation are weak. The climate in most work groups is likely to be in between those conditions.

On an individual level, work group members might be characterized by creativity, self-efficacy and creative abilities or, when these characteristics are not apparent, show signs of emotional defences and cognitive limitations in relation to possible innovations.

Resulting from interdependent activity on all three levels, the model further depicts three possible outcomes in terms of innovation. At the top is illustrated the successful outcome of implementation of an objectively appropriate innovation. In the middle alternative, an objectively inappropriate innovation is abandoned. Both these cases are successful outcomes in terms of innovation. In the third type of outcome, the work group is perhaps confronted with a performance gap but fails to meet that demand for change, which is a negative outcome. These different outcomes have an impact upon the organizational context, the work group and the individuals. When the outcome is successful, all three levels find support for appropriate innovation. When there is a failure to innovate there is likely to be a strengthening of the negative characteristics in the organizational context, in the group and within the individual.

The model further depicts an exchange of influence between the contextual factors and work group climate, the individual and the group and directly between the context and the individual. Research and theory are not currently available which would enable analyses of all these six possible relations. The following analysis concentrates on the influence of the work group on the individual and secondly on effects on the work group of the organizational context.

The Influence on the Individual of the Work Group

Individual members of a work group in an organization are exposed to two kinds of stimulation, according to Hackman (1992). Ambient stimuli are directed to all group members and consist of the workplace environment, the task materials and other members of the group. Ambient stimuli pervade the group setting and provide the individual with cues as to what contributions will be reinforced by social satisfaction (Hackman, 1992). Discretionary stimuli consist of stimulation directed to particular group members, sometimes as responses to specific actions.

This behaviourist analysis can be used to formulate hypotheses about the effect on individuals from the group climate specified by the four-factor model (West, 1990). Ambient and discretionary stimulation together can be seen to form work group climate. Hackman (1992) argues that stimulation supplied by the group affects the individuals' informational, affective and behavioural states.

Let us elaborate this with a few hypothetical examples. Participative safety (West, 1990) consists of an ambient stimulation of reinforcement of behaviours, of information-sharing and behaviours of acceptance of contributions and ideas from individuals in the group. When a group is characterized by a high degree of participative safety this will positively influence the informational states of individuals by providing them with more and better information. This enables them to produce more and better ideas, which could lead to innovation. In the longer perspective it might also strengthen their creative ability.

The climate dimension "visions and goals" (West, 1990) includes ambient stimuli concerning group goals and perhaps also discretionary stimuli of individual goals. When this aspect of climate is pronounced it impacts upon the affective state of the individual by causing arousal (Hackman, 1992) and thereby motivation and commitment to the task. If this ambient stimulation is too high it causes anxiety, and could be balanced by ambient stimulation of participative safety. Task orientation/climate for excellence (West, 1990) operates partly through discretionary stimuli in the form of feedback of praise or blame to individuals. If positive affective states are created frequently for individual team members, it might enhance their self-efficacy and so influence their capacity to innovate (Farr & Ford, 1990). The factor of norms in support of innovation (West, 1990) is primarily an ambient stimulus that influences the individual's behavioural state (Hackman, 1992). When climate is favourable in this respect, the stimulation might lead the individuals to respond positively to ideas for innovation and also offer their enacted support.

Ambient stimulation might also operate within defensive routines (Argyris, 1990). When a group is characterized by a high degree of defensive routines, the ambient stimuli reinforce the members' responses that are not beneficial to task performance. They are instead reinforced for being passive and avoiding efficient goal-directed behaviour. A group might be locked in this passive state, since defensive routines and ambient stimulation are difficult for the group to identify and reflect upon. Hackman (1992) has conceptualized this as social inertia. In the longer term, this might shape the individuals not to observe the performance gaps that can be significant stimuli for innovation processes.

The Effect of Organizational Context on Group Climate

The predominant organizational context factor influencing work group performance is task design (Hackman & Morris, 1975; McGrath, 1991; Guzzo & Shea, 1992; Tschan & von Cranach, this volume) since it offers the basic prerequisite for collaboration. If task design implies a high degree of job discretion, it should affect work group climate favourably, according to the four-factor model. The goals and visions of the work group would be discussed more and negotiated both within the group and with superiors. If there is job discretion for the group as a whole and task interdependence within the group, this should support the development of both a higher degree of participative safety and task orientation/climate for excellence (West, 1990).

The second important factor is hypothesized to be the quality of leadership for the group in terms of a high degree of consideration, structure and support for innovation. This type of leadership should have a pervasive effect on all four climate factors. An important task for the leader is to clarify goals and visions. If he or she has high status they will also influence norms in support of innovation positively (West, 1990).

A third concept of relevance is group boundaries. These are highly appropriate if they are flexible, and so can both guard the group and enable exchange with the surrounding organization (Sundstrom, De Meuse & Futrell, 1990). The more the group is well guarded, the better are the possibilities that they can concentrate on the objectives of the group and develop collaboration. And if the exchange outside the group is appropriate, this would provide the group with more information, diversity in views and a higher degree of task orientation/climate for excellence (West, 1990).

Finally, it is hypothesized that to the extent that the work group is rewarded for being innovative, this will correlate positively with all four factors of work group climate (West, 1990).

Innovation Influences the Team Climate

The innovation cycle has been outlined by West (1990) as containing four phases. The first phase is the *recognition* by an individual or a group of, for example, a performance gap. The second phase is represented by an *initiation*, i.e. a discussion in the work group. The third phase is the *implementation* of an innovation, and the fourth phase is *stabilization*, i.e. the innovation is found to be appropriate. In each of these phases there is a possible abandonment of the innovation for good or bad reasons (West, 1990). It is highly probable that work group climate is influenced positively by successful innovation.

Support for this is found in a meta-analysis of more than 200 studies of the relation between cohesiveness and group performance, conducted by Mullen & Copper (1994). Cohesiveness was conceptualized as consisting of interpersonal attraction among group members, commitment to task and group pride. Mediating variables were the degree of interaction in the group, the group size and whether the group was a real work group. A small but significant effect of cohesiveness on group performance was found. However, a stronger effect was demonstrated in the reverse direction. Changes in cohesiveness "that can be brought about by performance are likely to be even stronger than the changes in performance that can be brought about by cohesiveness" (Mullen & Copper, 1994, p. 224).

FINAL CONCLUSIONS

Multifaceted variables have been identified within the organizational context, the group climate and the individual. Innovation results from interdependence between the three levels of analysis and the variables within each one in a dynamic interplay.

Innovation, according to our definition, can be conceptualized in terms of a process. In the beginning of this process the production of ideas from individuals take place. When in a dialogue at work you face another work-mate who, verbally and non-verbally, reacts with much interest and sympathy, joy and eagerness to what you have to say; this constitutes a fundamental feed-back influence on your thinking and emotions. It will enable you to get many more and quicker associations; you will dare more; it will relieve you from anxieties and your thinking will cross over borders.

When the work-mate actively listens to you speculating on possible ventures for the business you are both in, the work-mate's imagination is activated. He or she is being taken on a "journey" and will experience possibilities that fill him or her with enthusiasm, which is fed back to the "story-teller". The dialogue is a carrier of the creative process.

In a work group there are a number of possibilities for genuine dialogues. These are, however, endangered by the fears of the individuals to expose themselves and be rejected by the other group members or expelled from the organization. A skilful discussion leader can "contain" and thereby relieve the members from these fears. He or she can further ask each person and the group the right questions, summarize the present discussion, support the right kind of disagreement and on the whole have a powerful influence over the group climate.

Innovation, however, is not restricted to creative thinking. It implies the effective realization of ideas in organizational settings. In order for an individual to be able to elaborate, adjust and apply the ideas evoked in different dialogues, it is necassary that he or she has actively taken a part in the whole process. When an idea encounters the realities from different forces operating in an organization, it might need to be adjusted and also to be argued for and defended. Innovations will often be unfairly abandoned or defeated if people who are trying to introduce them have not taken part in the whole process.

REFERENCES

Abbey, A. & Dickson, J.W. (1983). R&D work climate and innovation in semiconductors. *Academy of Management Journal*, **26**, 362–368.

Agrell, A. & Gustafson, R. (1994). The Team Climate Inventory: a psychometric test on a Swedish sample. *Journal of Occupational and Organizational Psychology*, **67**, 143–151.

Amabile, T.M. (1983). *The Social Psychology of Creativity*. New York: Springer Verlag.

Ancona, D.G. & Caldwell, D.F. (1992). Demography and design: predictors of new product team performance. *Organization Science*, **3**, 321–341.

Anderson, N. & King, N. (1993). Innovation in organizations. In C.L. Cooper & I.T. Robertson (eds), *International Review of Industrial and Organizational Psychology*. Chichester: Wiley, pp. 1–34.

Anderson, N.A. & West, M.A. (1994). *The Team Climate Inventory, Manual*. Windsor: ASE Press.

Andrews, F.M. (1979). Motivation, diversity and the performance of research units. In F.M. Andrews (ed.), *Scientific Productivity*. Cambridge: Cambridge University Press, pp. 252–287.

Argyris, C. (1968). Conditions for competence and therapy. *Journal of Behavioural Science*, **4**, 147–179.

Argyris, C. (1990). *Overcoming Organizational Defenses, Facilitating Organizational Learning*. Boston, MA: Allyn and Bacon.

Argyris, C. & Schön, D. (1974). *Theory in Practice—Increasing Professional Effectiveness*. San Francisco, CA: Jossey-Bass.

Argyris, C. & Schön, D. (1978). *Organizational Learning: A Theory of Action Perspective*. Reading, MA: Addison-Wesley.

Bandura, A. (1986). *Social Foundations of Thought and Actions*. Englewood Cliffs, NJ: Prentice-Hall.

Barron, F. & Harrington, D.M. (1981). Creativity, intelligence and personality. *Annual Review of Psychology*, **32**, 439–476.

Bion, W.R. (1961). *Experiences in groups*. London: Tavistock.

Child, D. (1973). *Psychology and the Teacher*. New York: Holt-Rinehart.

Coopey, J.G. (1987). Creativity in complex organizations. Paper presented at the Annual Occupational Psychology Conference of the British Psychological Society, University of Hull, January.

Dougherty, D. (1987). New Products in Old Organizations: The Myth of the Better Mousetrap in Search of the Beaten Path. PhD dissertation, Sloan School of Management, MIT.

Ekvall, G., (1988). Förnyelse och friktion, Om organisation, kreativitet och innovation [Renewal and Friction: On Organization, Creativity and Innovation]. Stockholm: Natur och Kultur.

Ekvall, G., Arvonen, J. & Nyström, H. (1987). Organisation och innovation. En studie av fyra divisioner vid EKA Kemi AB (Organization and Innovation. A Study of Four Divisions of EKA Kemi AB). Lund: Studentlitteratur.

Farr, J.L. & Ford, C.M. (1990). Individual innovation. In M.A. West & J.L. Farr (eds), Innovation and Creativity at Work. New York: Wiley, pp. 63–80.

Fiedler, F.E. (1967). A Theory of Leadership Effectiveness. New York: McGraw-Hill.

Fleishman, E.A. & Harris, E.F. (1962). Patterns of leadership behavior related to employee grievances and turnover. Personnel Psychology, 15, 43–56.

Frost, P.J. & Egri, C.P. (1991). The political process of innovation. Research in Organizational Behavior, 13, 229–295.

Geschka, H. (1983). Creativity techniques in product planning and development: a view from West Germany. R&D Management, 13, 169–183.

Guilford, J.P. (1959). Traits of Creativity. In H.H. Anderson (ed.), Creativity and its Cultivation. New York: Harper, pp. 142–161.

Gupta, A.K., Ray, S.P. & Wilemon, D. (1985). The R&D marketing interface in high-technology firms. Journal of Product Innovation Management, 2, 12–24.

Guzzo, R.A. & Shea, G.P. (1992). Group performance and intergroup relations in organizations. In M.D. Dunnette & L.M. Hough (eds), Handbook of Industrial and Organizational Psychology, Vol. 3. Palo Alto, CA: Consulting Psychologists' Press, pp. 269–313.

Guzzo, R.A., Yost, P.R., Campbell, R.J. & Shea, G.P. (1993). Potency in groups: articulating a construct. British Journal of Social Psychology, 32, 87–106.

Hackman, R. (1992). Group influences on individuals in organizations. In M.D. Dunette & L.M. Hough (eds), Handbook of Industrial and Organizational Psychology, Vol. 3. Palo Alto, CA: Consulting Psychologists' Press, pp. 199–267.

Hackman, J.R. & Morris, C.G. (1975). Group tasks, group interaction process and group performance effectiveness: a review and proposed integration. In L. Berkowitz (ed.), Group Processes. New York: Academic Press.

Helson, H. (1948). Adaptation-level as a basis for a quantitative theory of frames of reference. Psychological Review, 55, 294–313.

Hoffman, L.R., Harburg, E. & Maier, N.R.F. (1970). Differences and disagreements as factors in creative group problem solving. In N.R.F. Maier, (ed.), Problem Solving and Creativity in Individuals and Groups. Monterey, CA: Brooks/Cole, pp. 377–389.

Hoffman, L.R. & Maier, N.R.F. (1970). Valence in the adoption of solutions by problem solving groups. II. Quality and acceptance as goals of leaders and members. In N.R.F. Maier (ed.), Problem solving and Creativity in Individuals and Groups. Monterey, CA: Brooks/Cole, pp. 230–241.

Jackson, S.E., Brett, J.F., Sessa, V.I., Cooper, D.M., Julin, J.A. & Peyronnin, K. (1991). Same differences make a difference: individual dissimilarities and group heterogeneity as correlates of recruitment, promotions and turnover. Journal of Applied Psychology, 76, 675–689.

Janis, I.L. (1972). Victims of Groupthink: A Psychological Study of Foreign Policy Decisions. Boston: Houghton Miffin.

Katz, R. (1982). The effects of group longevity on project communication and performance. Administrative Science Quarterly, 27, 81–104.

Kiesler, S.B. (1978). *Interpersonal processes in Groups and Organizations*. Arlington Heights, IL: AHM Publishing.

King, N. (1990). Innovation at work: the research literature. In M.A. West & J.L. Farr (eds), *Innovation and Creativity at Work*. Chichester: Wiley, pp. 15–60.

Knorr, K.D., Mittermeier, R., Aichholzer, G. & Waller, G. (1979). Leadership and group performance: a positive relationship in academic research units. In F.M. Andrews (ed.), *Scientific Productivity: The Effectiveness of Research Groups in Six Countries*. Cambridge: Cambridge University Press, pp. 95–120.

Kolb, J.A. (1992). Leadership of creative teams. *Journal of Creative Behavior*, 26(1), 1–9.

Kylén, S. (1993). Arbetsgrupper med utvecklings- och förändringsuppdrag—från defensiva till offensiva rutiner (Work groups with tasks of development and change—from defensive to offensive routines). Licentiatavhandling, Psykologiska Institutionen, Göteborgs Universitet.

Lovelace, R.F. (1986). Stimulating creativity through managerial interventions. *R&D Management*, 16, 161–174.

Maier, N.R.F. (1970a). *Problem Solving and Creativity in Individuals and Groups*. Monterey, CA: Brooks/Cole.

Maier, N.R.F. (1970b). Leadership principles for problem solving conferences. In N.R.F. Maier (ed.), *Problem Solving and Creativity in Individuals and Groups*. Monterey, CA: Brooks/Cole, pp. 266–276.

Maier, N.R.F. (1970c). Assets and liabilities in group problem solving. The need for an integrative function. In N.R.F. Maier (ed.), *Problem Sovling and Creativity in Individuals and Groups*. Monterey, CA: Brooks/Cole, pp. 431–444.

Maier, N.R.F. & Hoffman, L.R. (1970). Quality of first and second solutions in group problem solving. In N.R.F. Maier (ed.), *Problem Solving and Creativity in Individuals and Groups*. Monterey, CA: Brooks/Cole, pp. 368–376.

Maier, N.R.F. & Solem, A.R. (1970a). The contribution of a discussion leader to the quality of group thinking: the effective use of minority opinions. In N.R.F. Maier (ed.), *Problem Solving and Creativity in Individuals and Groups*. Monterey, CA: Brooks/Cole, pp. 219–229.

Maier, N.R.F. & Solem, A.R. (1970b). Improving solutions by turning choice situations into problems. In N.R.F. Maier (ed.), *Problem Solving and Creativity in Individuals and Groups*. Monterey, CA: Brooks/Cole, pp. 390–395.

McCarrey, M.W. & Edwards, S.A. (1973). Organizational climate conditions for effective research scientist role performance. *Organizational Behaviour and Human Performance*, 9, 439–459.

McGrath, J.E. (1991). Time, interaction and performance (TIP): a theory of groups. *Small Group Research*, 22, 147–174.

Michael, R. (1979). How to find and keep creative people. *Research Management*, **September**, 43–45.

Mullen, B. & Copper, C. (1994). The relation between group cohesiveness and performance: an integretion. *Psychological Bulletin*, 115(2), 210–227.

Nicholls, J.G. (1972). Creativity in the person who will never produce anything original and useful: the concept of creativity as a normally distributed trait. *American Psychologist*, 27, 717–727.

Nyström, H. (1979). *Creativity and Innovation*. New York: Wiley.

O'Reilly, C.A. & Flatt, S. (1989). Executive team demography, organizational innovation and firm performance. Working paper, University of California, Berkeley.

Patterson, M., West, M.A. & Payne, R.L. (1992). Collective climates: a test of their sociopsychological significance. Paper presented at Academy of Management Conference, Los Angeles.

Peters, T.J. & Waterman, R.H. (1982). *In Search of Excellence: Lessons from America's Best Run Companies*. New York: Harper and Row.

Rousseau, D.M. (1988). The construction of climate in organization research. In C.L.

Cooper & I.T. Robertson (eds), *International Review of Industrial and Organizational Psychology*, Vol. 3. Chichester: Wiley, pp. 58–88.
Schneider, B. & Reichers, A.E. (1983). On the etiology of climates. *Personnel Psychology*, **36**, 19–39.
Senge, P.M. (1990). *The Fifth Discipline*. New York: Double Day/Currency.
Souder, W.E. (1987). *Managing New Product Innovations*. Lexington MA: Lexington Books.
Stankiewicsz, R. (1979). The effectiveness of research groups in six countries. In F.M. Andrews (ed.), *Scientific Productivity*. Cambridge: Cambridge University Press, pp. 191–221.
Stolte-Heiskanen, V. (1979). Externally determined resources and the effectiveness of research units. In F.M. Andrews (ed.), *Scientific Productivity*. Cambridge: Cambridge University Press, pp. 121–154.
Sundström E., De Meuse, K.P. & Futrell, D. (1990). Work teams: applications and effectiveness. *American Psychologist*, **45**(2), 120–133.
Thompson, V.A. (1965). Bureaucracy and innovation. *Administrative Science Quarterly*, **10**(1), 1–20.
Tjosvold, D. (1982). Effects of approach to controversy on superiors' incorporation of subordinates' information in decision making. *Journal of Applied Psychology*, **67**, 189–193.
Tuckman, B.W. & Jensen, M.A. (1977). Stages of small group development revisited. *Group and Organizations Studies*, **2**, 419–427.
Van de Ven, A.H. (1986). Central problems in the management of innovation. *Management Science*, **5**, 590–607.
Vernon, P.E. (1989). The nature–nurture problem in creativity. In J.A. Glover, R.R. Roming & C.R. Reynolds (eds), *Handbook of Creativity: Perspectives on Individual Differences*. New York: Plenum Press, pp. 92–125.
Wallmark, J.T. (1973). The increase in efficiency with the size of research teams. *Transaction on Engineering Management*, **3**, 80–86.
Wallach, M.A. & Kogan, N. (1965). A new look at the creativity–intelligence distinction. *Journal of Personality*, **33**, 348–369.
Wallas, G. (1926). *The Art of Thought*. London: Cape.
West, M.A. (1987). Role innovation in the world of work. *British Journal of Social Psychology*, **26**, 305–315.
West, M.A. (1990). The social psychology of innovations in groups. In M.A. West & J.L. Farr (eds), *Innovation and Creativity at Work. Psychological and Organizational Strategies*. Chichester: Wiley, pp. 309–334.
West, M.A. & Farr, J.L. (1990). Innovation at work. In M.A. West and J.L. Farr (eds), *Innovation and Creativity at Work. Psychological and Organizational Strategies*. Chichester. Wiley, pp. 3–14.
Wiersma, M.F. & Bantel, K.A. (1992). Top management team demography and corporate strategic change. *Academy of Management Journal*, **35**, 91–121.
Winter, D.G. (1973). *The Power Motive*. New York: Free Press.
Yukl, G.A. (1981). *Leadership in Organizations*. Englewood Cliffs, NJ: Prentice Hall.
Zaltman, G., Duncan, R. & Holbek, J. (1973). *Innovations in Organizations*. New York: Wiley.
Zenger, T.R. & Lawrence, B.S. (1989). Organizational demography: the differential effects of age and tenure distributions on technical communication. *Academy of Management Journal*, **32**, 353–376.

Chapter 14

Work Group Factors and Individual Well-being

Sabine Sonnentag
University of Amsterdam, The Netherlands

Abstract

In this chapter work group factors are discussed in their relationship to individual well-being, namely job satisfaction and other work-related well-being measures. Methodological and conceptual problems associated with this research are addressed. The chapter shows how far group work is related to individual well-being. Literature concerning the relationship between group composition factors, group task characteristics, group process factors, group development interventions, and well-being is reviewed. Existing studies suggest that autonomous group work and aspects of the group process are indeed associated with individual well-being. However, parts of this research suffer from methodological problems. Therefore, open questions for future research are discussed.

INTRODUCTION

This chapter deals with work group factors and individual well-being. Existing literature on the effects of work groups factors has mainly concentrated on performance-related issues (e.g. Gladstein, 1984; Goodman, 1986; Guzzo & Shea, 1992; Hackman & Morris, 1975; Worchel, Wood & Simpson, 1992; Brodbeck, this volume). Compared to this large area of research, the relationship between work group factors and well-being has received far less attention. Work-related well-being has been mainly studied with respect to the work situation of individuals, focusing on stressful working conditions and lack of control at work (e.g. Frese, 1989; Karasek & Theorell, 1990).

Handbook of Work Group Psychology. Edited by M.A. West.
© 1996 John Wiley & Sons Ltd.

There might be at least two reasons for the "dissociation" between work group factors and well-being in the empirical literature: First, research on work group factors and research on well-being belong to two different research traditions. Researchers established in both group research and research on stress and individual job design are rare. Second, research on work group factors and research on well-being are conducted at different levels of analysis: research on work group factors is mainly done at the group level, i.e. an aggregate of several individuals, while research on well-being is almost always performed at the individual level. Considering both work group factors and individual well-being in one line of research may cause conceptual and methodological problems.

However, there is research in both areas that can contribute to our knowledge about the relationships between work group characteristics and individual well-being. Findings from this research will be presented in this chapter. In the first section, the concept of well-being will be described. Then conceptual and methological issues associated with the study of work group factors and individual well-being will be discussed. The following section addresses the question of whether group work in itself has any effect on individual well-being at all. Then selected work group characteristics will be described in their relationship to individual well-being. This section starts with a framework of work group characterteristics and then well-being effects of group composition, group tasks, group process and group development will be considered. The chapter closes with an integrative discussion of research findings.

CONCEPT OF WELL-BEING

Well-being refers to a person's subjective positive experience of life and is closely related to happiness, satisfaction, morale and positive affect (Diener, 1984). Within the psychological literature, well-being is a broad term covering variations in mood and affect as well as major mental health issues, such as anxiety and depression (Edwards, 1992). For the purpose of this chapter, well-being will be mostly used in the latter sense. Recent research suggests that both low negative affectivity and favourable objective conditions influence a person's subjective well-being through his or her interpretation of these objective conditions (Brief et al., 1993). Warr (1987) conceptualized affective well-being as one of five components of mental health. Within the well-being component, Warr differentiates between context-free and job-related well-being. Under job-related well-being he subsumes concepts such as job satisfaction, organizational commitment, job-related tension, job-related depression, job-related burnout, and morale. Empirical relationships between context-free and job-related well-being have also been found (Judge & Hulin, 1993; Kelloway & Barling, 1991).

A great portion of research on job-related well-being—especially that dealing with work group factors—has concentrated on job satisfaction. However, as Bruggemann, Groskurth & Ulich (1975) have pointed out by describing "resigned satisfaction", job satisfaction might not be the best indicator of a person's well-being and mental health. Therefore, studies including job satisfaction measures have to be discussed cautiously. Another shortcoming related to studies on job-related well-being should be mentioned. Diener (1984) stressed that research on well-being should include positive measures, "not just the absence of negative factors" (p. 543). However, most studies—using other measures than job satisfaction—derived their conclusion about well-being and mental health from the absence of negative symptoms, such as burnout or psychosomatic complaints. Therefore, strictly speaking, we know more about the harms caused by negative work group factors than about the well-being benefits caused by favourable factors.

CONCEPTUAL AND METHODOLOGICAL ISSUES

Research on the relationship between work group factors and well-being has to deal with various conceptual and measurement levels. Work group factors are usually seen as concepts at the group level. For example, a group's size or cohesiveness are shared among all members of the group. Hackman (1992) calls such factors that are potentially available to all group members "ambient stimuli". The most adequate measurement level for these factors is the group level. However, it is also possible to measure them at the individual level. Additionally, there are work group factors that are not the same for all group members. Hackman (1992) refers to them as "discretionary stimuli". Thus, they should be conceptualized at the individual level. Typical examples are social support or the experience of interpersonal conflicts. Measurement of these work group factors only make sense at the individual level (cf. Repetti, 1987, for a related argument).

Because individuals are part of the work group, there is a great overlap between the individuals' and the group's work situation. For example, it can be assumed that in a highly cohesive and highly supportive group, social support in the individuals' work situations will be higher than in a group with low cohesion and low supportiveness. However, high cohesion and high supportiveness does not imply that for *every* group member high social support will be provided. One can imagine highly cohesive groups where several individuals suffer from low social support. Therefore, it is necessary to differentiate between these two conceptual levels of work group factors.

Well-being is an experience of the individual (Campbell, 1976). It is the individual who is satisfied with his or her job, who experiences tension or burnout, or who suffers from psychosomatic complaints. Therefore, well-being should be measured at the individual level. However, there are also concepts of well-being at the group level. For example, McGrath (1991) describes the group well-being function as one important function of the group, besides the production function and the member support function. However, his group well-being function refers to the development and maintenance of the group as a system. Although possibly empirically related, this group well-being function is conceptually different from individual well-being as it is used within this chapter.

Table 14.1 summarizes possible study designs examining the relationship between work group factors and individual well-being. The second column shows the conceptual level of work group factors. In the third and forth columns the measurement level of work group factors and well-being are displayed. Column five indicates the level of analysis when relating work group factors to individual well-being.

Within Type A and Type B studies, work group factors conceptualized at the group level (e.g. size, climate) are measured at the group level. Two levels of analysis are possible: a group-level analysis where individual well-being scores are aggregated at the group level (Type A); and an individual-level analysis where the same group-level scores of group factors are assigned to every group member (Type B). An example of the Type A approach is a study by Campion, Medsker & Higgs (1993). In this study, data from 78 work groups of a large financial services company were analysed. Measures of group characteristics were provided by five randomly selected group members and the groups' managers and then aggregated across groups. Satisfaction measures were provided by all employees and also aggregated across groups. Analysis was performed at the group level. The Type B approach was used by Sonnentag et al. (1994). Here, members of 29 software development teams assessed the quality of team interaction (e.g. openness to criticism, competition) and provided data concerning their well-being. Individual perceptions of quality of team interaction were aggregated

Table 14.1 Taxonomy of study designs relating work group factors to individual well-being

Type of study	Conceptual level of work group factor	Measurement level of work group factor	Measurement level of well-being	Level of analysis
Type A Pure group level approach	Group	Aggregated work group factor score	Aggregated well-being score	Group
Type B Mixed approach	Group	Aggregated work group factor score	Individual well-being score	Individual
Type C Mixed approach	Group	Individual measure of group work factor	Individual well-being score	Individual
Type D Pure individual level approach	Individual	Individual measure of group work factor	Individual well-being Score	Individual

across teams. Analysis was done at the individual level by assigning the aggregated team interaction score to every individual member of the corresponding team.

Most empirical studies examining the relationship between work group factors and well-being are Type C studies. Group level factors conceptualized at the group level are measured at the individual level. An example for this research is a study by Leiter (1992), in which individual perceptions of cohesion within the team were correlated with individual burnout measures. In this type of study, analysis is only possible at the individual level. However, now this is associated with a major conceptual problem: within these studies only individual perceptions of work group factors are used without testing if these perceptions reflect group phenomena. One central condition for the assumption of a group phenomenon is that there is a certain degree of agreement about this phenomenon within the group (James, 1982). Because Type C studies rely only on individual measures the question of agreement can not be answered.

Type D studies include research conceptualizing and measuring both well-being and work group factors at the individual level. For example, this is done when social support experienced by individual group members is related to these persons' well-being scores. The level of analysis is the individual, too. This procedure is also the usual and appropriate level of analysis when examining the relationship between other working conditions and mental health. Although both level of analysis and level of concept and measurement correspond, this type of analysis has its pitfalls (Kasl, 1978): if working conditions and well-being are assessed by self-report measures—as is frequently the case—they share common method variance (Campbell & Fiske, 1959) leading to an overestimation of the true correlation. Cross-sectional research designs do not allow conclusive causal interpretations and do not offer any adequate control for selection and self-selection effects.

EFFECTS OF GROUP WORK ON WELL-BEING

The fact that working in a group vs. working individually has an impact on a person's behaviour and feelings is a well-known finding within research on real work groups (e.g. Roethlisberger & Dickson, 1939; Trist & Bamforth, 1951). For example, Trist & Bamforth (1951) reported the dispanding of small stable working groups associated with a new coal-getting method that resulted in irritation, psychosomatic and other neurotic disorders in the now isolated workers. Hackman (1992) distinguishes between informational, affective and behavioral impacts of groups on individuals. Concerning the affective impact that has some overlap with the well-being concept within this chapter, Hackman states that membership in a group can contribute directly to an individual's satisfaction if the stimuli provided by the group fit the person's needs.

Being a member of a work group offers opportunities for social contact and other rewards that are controlled by the group, for example rewards influencing one's self-esteem (Hackman, 1992). Additionally, work groups can be seen as providers of social support (Richman, 1989), which is assumed to be an important resource in coping with stressors (House, 1981). From an action theory approach (Frese & Zapf, 1994; Hacker, 1986), one can argue that the opportunity for cooperation—which can be best realized within group work—is an important feature of completeness of action. Completeness of action is regarded to be essential for high performance and individual well-being.

There is empirical evidence that group work is associated with better individual well-being and motivation. For example, Moch (1980) studied 522 employees of an assembly and packaging plant and found that those who were involved in networks of work relationships showed higher internal motivation than did isolated employees. This result remained stable when controlling for other job characteristics. Greller, Parsons & Mitchell (1992) reported a relationship between the experience of group work and well-being in police employees. Employees in a large metropolean police department had to indicate the degree to which they perceived their work as teamwork. This teamwork measure was correlated $r = -0.28$ with a psychosomatic complaints scale.

In a validation study of a job analysis instrument, Rudolph, Schönfelder & Hacker (1987) found correlations of $r = 0.27$ between type of cooperation (group work vs. isolated work) and satisfaction measures. Clerical workers in cooperative settings were more satisfied with their work and their relationship to colleagues than were employees in settings that did not require cooperation. Similarily, an experimental study by Rau (1994) suggests stress-compensation effects of teamwork.

Framework of Work Group Characteristics

Within an input–process–output framework describing work groups (cf. Hackman, 1987; Guzzo & Shea, 1992), individual well-being can be seen as one specific form of a group's output. Hackman (1987) explicitly regards satisfaction of individual group members' needs as one indicator of group effectiveness. In the past decades, various models have been developed to explain work group effectiveness (Gladstein, 1984; Hackman, 1987; Hackman & Morris, 1975; Kolodny & Kiggundu, 1980; Shea & Guzzo, 1987; Sundstrom, DeMeuse & Futrell, 1990; Tannenbaum, Beard & Salas, 1992; cf. Goodman, Ravlin & Argote, 1986; Guzzo & Shea, 1992, for reviews). These models differ in their assumptions about the most relevant group factors responsible for group effectiveness and in their assumptions about relationships among these factors. For example, Hackman & Morris (1975) regarded group task characteristics as one important input factor that is related to outcome factors through group interaction processes as mediators. Contrarily, Gladstein (1984) conceptualized the group task as a moderator of the process–effectiveness relationship.

Despite these differences among the models, there are some common factors that are incorporated in almost every model of group effectiveness. Such central components in most models are: group composition; group task; group interaction process; group development. In the following sections these work group characteristics will be discussed in their relationship to individual well-being.

Group Composition

Composition of the group refers to issues such as size, homogeneity vs. heterogeneity in members' skills and personal attributes, and other personal characteristics of team members. Concerning performance criteria, it is recommended not to overpopulate the group and to find a balance between homogeneity and heterogeneity of group members (Hackman & Oldham, 1980). However, empirical research shows that heterogeneous groups outperform homogeneous groups on tasks that require innovation and creativity (Jackson, 1992; King & Anderson, 1990; Payne, 1990).

With regard to individual well-being, Campion, Medsker & Higgs (1993) found relative group size to be positively correlated with employee satisfaction at the group level. Within this study, relative group size referred to the perception that the number of people in one's team was not too small for the work to be done. Further studies suggest that group size does not have a direct effect on well-being but affects cooperation within the group and other intragroup process variables, with small groups experiencing better interaction (Gladstein, 1984; Stahelski & Tsukuda, 1990). However, in a group level analysis, George (1990) did not find significant correlations between group size and positive or negative affective tone within a group.

Does homogeneity among group members have any effect on individual well-being? Here, a mediator effect of group cohesion seems to be an adequate explanation because homogeneity within the group is associated with high cohesion (Terborg, Castore & DeNinno, 1976) and cohesion shows a postive relationship to members' satisfaction (Lott & Lott, 1965). However, a recent study by Watson, Kumar & Michaelsen (1993) showed that compared to culturally diverse groups, homogeneous groups experienced a better interaction process only in the beginning of cooperation. As group work continued, the interaction scores of the two types of groups converged. Research shows that high heterogeneity within work groups was related to high turnover rates (Jackson et al., 1991; McCain, O'Reilly & Pfeffer, 1983). Because turnover and satisfaction are interrelated (Cotton & Tuttle, 1986) one can assume that satisfaction co-varies also with heterogeneity within the work group. However, no such relationship was found by Campion, Medsker & Higgs (1993).

Additionally, group members' attitudes towards team work could be regarded as a predictor of group members' well-being. One could argue that group work is associated with better individual well-being if group members are in favour of group work. Empirical findings are inconsistent. Campion, Medsker & Higgs (1993) found that the preference for team work within a group correlated positively with a satisfaction measure at the group level. In a study of physicians in Dutch hospitals, preference for team work was not related to satisfaction with the work environment, including descriptions of cooperation (Stevens, Diederiks & Philipsen, 1992).

Summarizing this research on the relationship between group composition and individual well-being, no clear pattern emerges. Existing findings suggest that *if* there is indeed a relationship between group composition and well-being it is mediated by the group process or group cohesion.

Group Tasks

Characteristics of the task a person performs is related to his or her well-being. Studies on individual work situations showed that persons in jobs with a low amount of stressors and high autonomy experienced better well-being than did persons in stressful jobs and in work situations with low autonomy. This was found both in cross-sectional and longitudinal studies (Frese, 1985; Karasek et al., 1981; Leitner, 1993). Models by Hackman (1987), Gladstein (1984), and Sundstrom, De Meuse & Futrell (1990) suggest that characteristics of the group task are also related to group members' well-being.

There are two areas of research that examined the relationship between group task characteristics and individual mental health: research on autonomous work groups, mainly focusing on participation; and research examining several characteristics of the group task and relating it to individual outcome measures.

Research on Autonomous Work Groups

The concept of autonomous work groups has its origins in work by Lewin (1951) and in socio-technical theory (Trist & Bamforth, 1951). Central aspects of autonomous group work are the group's responsibility for a relatively whole task; the group's involvement in coordination and decision-making; a relatively great variety of tasks that offer learning possibilities for all group members; and the availability of feedback (Cummings, 1978; Pearce & Ravlin, 1987). Concepts similar to that of autonomous work groups are self-regulating work groups, semi-autonomous work groups, and self-managing teams. These terms are mostly used interchangeably (Goodman, Devadas & Hughson, 1988; Guzzo & Shea, 1992; cf. Sundstrom, De Meuse & Futrell, 1990 for a discussion of differences among these concepts).

Research on the effects of autonomous work groups has mainly concentrated on performance criteria, absenteeism and turnover. Reviews of these studies are provided by Pearce & Ravlin (1987), Goodman, Devadas & Hughson (1988), and Beekun (1989). However, there are also studies examining the effect of autonomous work groups on job satisfaction and other indicators of well-being. Trist,

Susman & Brown (1977) described an action research project that aimed at the introduction of autonomous work groups in a US coal mine. Within this project, union members reported that workers "no longer felt tired when they got home from work" (p. 224), indicating an improvement of individual well-being. However, no exact data were given and it can not be ruled out that this finding was reported for political reasons.

Wall & Clegg (1981) evaluated the implementation of semi-autonomous work groups in a British confectionery company. It was found that workers' mental health improved within a 6-month period after work redesign. A further improvement of mental health scores occurred within the following 18 months. Wall & Clegg (1981) reported also an increase in general job satisfaction. However, a significant change in this variable was not apparrent at 6 months, but only 18 months after the implementation of the group work concept. A second study using a quasi-experimental design was performed by Wall et al. (1986). Data were collected 6, 18 and 30 months after implementation of autonomous group work. In this study, it was found that members of autonomous work groups showed both higher intrinsic and extrinsic job satisfaction than did subjects in traditionally designed work. However, initial high extrinsic job satisfaction within autonomous work groups declined over time. No improvements in mental health associated with autonomous group work were found.

Berggren (1991) examined job satisfaction and other indicators of well-being in five Swedish automobile plants. One plant was characterized by traditional work organization with short cycles, the other four plants practised group work. Workers involved in traditional work organization expressed lower job satisfaction and more discomfort before going to work than did those who were involved in group work. There was a tendency for more psychosomatic complaints associated with traditional work organization. Additionally, workers with long task-cycles experienced fewer psychosomatic complaints than did workers with short cycles.

A longitudinal study of autonomous work groups is reported by Cordery, Mueller & Smith (1991). Analysis showed that workers in semi-autonomous groups had higher intrinsic and extrinsic job satisfaction. In contrast to the findings of Wall et al. (1986), no changes in job satisfaction over time (6 months compared to 20 months after introduction) were found. Pearson (1992) compared autonomous group work with traditional work design using a Solomon four-group design with two pre-test and four post-test measurements. Concerning job satisfaction, there were no differences in pre-test scores between autonomous and non-autonomous groups. After implementation of autonomous group work, job satisfaction in autonomous groups increased, while it decreased in non-autonomous groups. This was reflected in significantly higher post-test satisfaction scores within autonomous groups compared to non-autonomous groups.

The question arises whether changes in well-being are due to the fact that *group* work was introduced or to the specific task characteristics associated with autonomous group work. The studies by Wall & Clegg (1981), Wall et al. (1986) and Cordery, Mueller & Smith (1991) show that the implementation of autonomous work groups was accompanied by changes in task characteristics—especially high group autonomy.

Summarizing the results of these studies, it can be concluded that the implementation of autonomous work groups has a positive effect on group members' job satisfaction. Members of autonomous work groups showed higher job satisfaction than did members in control groups with traditional work design. However, the temporal patterns of changes in job satisfaction within autonomous work groups are inconsistent. This might be due to other simultaneously occurring economic and organizational factors that are not directly related to the implementation of autonomous group work and that differ across various studies. This assumption is supported by a study by Antoni (1994) in which members of autonomous work groups reported generally positive attitudes towards this kind of work design but, at the same time, expressed negative feelings about work overload due to the economic situation of the company.

Concerning indicators of well-being other than job satisfaction, the empirical basis is too small to reach a definitive conclusion. However, existing findings suggest that autonomous work groups do have such well-being effects. But these effects seem to be less prominent than benefits within the performance area.

Studies Relating Group Task Characteristics to Individual Well-Being

In the study by Campion, Medsker & Higgs (1993), job design variables were related to employee satisfaction scores. It turned out that participation, task variety and task significance were positively related to employee satisfaction, while there were no significant relationships between self-management and task identity on the one hand and employee satisfaction on the other.

Besides these more traditional job design variables, task interdependence is one important element of a group's task. Task interdependence refers to the amount of interaction and mutual dependence that is required for task accomplishment (Shea & Guzzo, 1987). Empirical studies show that although high interdependence is associated with satisfaction with the work *team* (Fandt, 1991) there is no (linear) relationship between task interdependence and individual satisfaction (Campion, Medsker & Higgs, 1993). This could be due to an inverted U-shaped relationship between task interdependence and affective outcomes, as reported by Wong & Campion (1991).

GROUP PROCESS

Group process refers to interaction patterns within the group and can be seen as a mediator between input factors and group outcome (Gladstein, 1984; Hackman

& Morris, 1975). Main features of the group process are communication, cooperation, conflict and supportiveness. Within this section, group cohesiveness and group climate will also be discussed as group process variables because they reflect the interaction within the group (cf. Guzzo & Shea, 1992). However, other approaches (e.g. Hackman & Morris, 1975) regard cohesiveness as both an input and an output variable.

As outlined in an earlier section, there are group process variables at both the conceptual level of the group and the individual. In this section, research will first be described that relates group process factors conceptualized at the group level to individual well-being. Then, studies on the relationship between group process as characteristics of the individual work situation, namely social support, interpersonal conflicts and well-being, will be presented.

Group Process as a Feature of the Whole Work Group

In most studies examining group process variables as work group characteristics, relationships between these variables and individual well-being, especially job satisfaction, were found. The most frequently studied group process variables were global measures of group interaction, climate, cohesion, communication and cooperation.

Mossholder & Bedeian (1983) studied 112 nursing employees in 18 groups and found that favourable peer group interaction was positively correlated with high satisfaction and low tension. Similarily, Zalesny, Farace & Kurchner-Hawkins (1985) found a correlation of 0.46 between a global social environment measure and job satisfaction in a sample of 420 state government employees. In two samples of teachers, Hart (1994) reported correlations of $r = 0.50$ and $r = 0.38$ respectively between poor staff relations and psychological distress. However, in another study with teachers (Lachman & Diamant, 1987) social relations were found to be related to burnout in men but not in women.

Peiró, González-Romá & Ramos (1992) examined the relationship between work-team climate, tension and satisfaction. They found that members of teams with a positive climate, for example concerning mutual support and goal-oriented information flow, experienced less tension and a higher job satisfaction than did members of teams with an unfavourable climate. However, positive climate was only associated with low tension and high job satisfaction in those teams in which various climate dimensions were balanced. In a study by Repetti (1987), a global measure of general climate at work was negatively related to depression and anxiety and positively to self-esteem. Also Jackofsky & Slocum (1988) found positive climate among co-workers to be correlated with job satisfaction.

The relationship between group cohesiveness and performance is a frequently studied question within work group research (cf. Evans & Dion, 1991; Mullen & Copper, 1994, for recent meta-analyses). Besides this large amount of research on cohesiveness and performance there are also studies examing the relationship between cohesiveness and group members' well-being. For example, Greller,

Parsons & Mitchell (1992) studied police employees and found that low work group cohesiveness was positively correlated with psychosomatic complaints. Both Leiter (1992) and Kruger, Botman & Goodenow (1991) reported negative relationships between cohesion within the team and indicators of burnout in samples of health and social service workers. Additionally, in multiple regression analyses, team cohesion turned out to be a significant predictor for high personal accomplishment and low depersonalization (Kruger, Botman & Goodenow, 1991). Similar correlations between cohesion and burnout were found in studies by Gaines & Jermier (1983) and Pretty, McCarthy & Catano (1992). Multiple regression analysis revealed that in female managers of a telecommunications corporation, low peer cohesion was the only significant predictor of depersonalization (Pretty, McCarthy & Catano, 1992). In a sample of 181 male cardiac patients, Pfaff (1989) found negative correlations between work group cohesion and depression and feelings of worthlessness, while work group cohesion and self-confidence were positively related.

Manning & Fullerton (1988) examined various units in the US Army. They found the highest cohesion scores within so-called A-Teams. At the same time, members of these teams showed higher general well-being, reported better physical health and a higher Army satisfaction than did members of other kinds of units. However, members of A-Teams did not show higher social desirability scores than did others. This indicates that the coincident report of high cohesion and high mental health in A-Teams can not be explained by higher social desirability within A-Teams. Positive relationships between cohesion and satisfaction scores were also reported by Skaret & Bruning (1986) and Zaccaro & Dobbins (1989). Keller (1986) analysed the relationship between group cohesiveness and job satisfaction at the group level and found a correlation of $r = 0.35$ between cohesiveness and satisfaction in a sample of 32 R&D project groups.

So far, these studies clearly show that group cohesiveness is related to individual well-being. However, a study by Martin (1984) in two hospitals produced equivocal findings. Low group cohesiveness predicted acute and chronic mental health problems in one but not the other hospital. Maslach & Jackson (1984) reported findings of a study showing that in nurses, work-group cohesiveness was negatively correlated with depersonalization but not with the other burnout factors.

Another group process factor that was studied in its relationship to individual well-being is communication and cooperation. However, these studies also lead to inconsistent results. Yammarino & Naughton (1988) studied 54 employees embedded in 13 work groups of a law enforcement agency of an university. It was found that work groups that spent more time communicating were more satisfied with their work than were other groups. In a study by Rosse et al. (1991), high quality of communication was negatively related to burnout in a sample of 256 hospital workers. In a sample of 93 nurse managers, Frone & Major (1988) found that communication quality with co-workers and subordinates, i.e. members of their own working group, was not correlated with job satisfaction at the zero-order level but moderated the relationship between job involvement and job satisfaction. Finally, in the study by Campion, Medsker & Higgs (1993), who measured group characteristics at the group level, communication/cooperation was not correlated with satisfaction.

The examination of further group process variables yielded substantial relationships to well-being scores. In the study by Rosse et al. (1991) interpersonal trust was negatively correlated to burnout. Sonnentag et al. (1994) found low openness to criticism within the team to be a significant predictor of burnout. Additionally, the study by Campion, Medsker & Higgs (1993) showed that potency within teams was related to employee satisfaction.

As well as the described zero-order correlations between group process factors and individual well-being, in some studies moderator effects of group process factors were found. Frone & Major (1988) performed a moderated regression analysis with communication quality and job involvement as predictors of job satisfaction. They found significant interaction terms of communication quality and job involvement for the following communication sources: immediate supervisor, subordinate and co-workers. When job involvement was high, communication quality was positively related to job satisfaction; when job involvement was low, communication quality showed a weak relationship to job satisfaction. A study by Sonnentag et al. (1994) revealed that *low* competition among team members enhanced the relationship between stressors in the work situation and burnout. This indicates that a positive interaction within the work group can put additional demands upon team members that make it difficult to cope with a stressful situation. These results show that group process variables that are generally assumed to be favourable are not always positively related to mental health or job satisfaction. It turned out that under conditions of low job involvement or high stressors a "good" group process can have its own pitfalls.

Although the findings concerning zero-order relationships between group process factors and individual well-being show a relatively consistent pattern, this research has some shortcomings concerning methodological soundness. In most studies, both group process variables and mental health measures were assessed at an individual level. With such a procedure it can not be ruled out that correlations between work process factors and mental health are due to individual response bias, for example persons with good mental health or high job satisfaction perceive the group process more positively than do colleagues with poor mental health and low satisfaction.

However, there are some studies in which group level measures of group process variables were used. Mossholder & Bedeian (1983) used both individual and group level measures of peer group interaction. Compared to the individual level results, for group measures of peer group interaction, lower but still significant correlations with both satisfaction and tension were found. Repetti (1987) correlated both individual scores and consensual measures of climate with individual well-being. Consensual scores of climate showed correlations of $r = -0.26$ and $r = -0.20$ with depression and anxiety. Sonnentag et al. (1994) measured group process variables at the team level and reported significant negative correlations between democracy and openess to criticism on the one hand and burnout on the other. Campion, Medsker & Higgs (1993) only referred to group level measures. However, with the exception of potency, they reported only small and non-significant correlations between group process and satisfaction.

To sum up, the results of these studies show that there is still a relationship between group process variables and team members' well-being if group level data are used. Members of work groups with a more favourable group process show better individual well-being than those of groups with a more negative kind of group process. This indicates that not all findings reported in this section can be explained by individual response bias. However, the magnitude of the group level correlation coefficients suggests that this relationship is indeed weaker than one could conclude from studies relying only on individual level data.

Group Process Variables as Features of the Individual Work Situation

Characteristics of the group process can be also regarded as features of the individual work situation. Such factors include social support and interpersonal conflicts at the work place. These variables differ from those described in the previous section because they are not necessarily shared among all members of the group.

Social support refers to resources that are provided by other persons (Cohen & Syme, 1985) including support from supervisors, co-workers and also persons off the job. The concept of social support encompasses support at an emotional, evaluative, informational and instrumental level (House, 1981). Reviews of the large body of research on social support suggest that there is some evidence for a direct effect of social support on individual well-being and mental health (Cohen & Wills, 1985; Kahn & Byosiere, 1992). Additionally, studies have examined the question whether social support buffers the negative effects of stressors on individual well-being. Research findings are inconsistent (Cohen & Wills, 1985; Kahn & Byosiere, 1992). Besides studies that found buffer effects of social support on the relationship between work stress and well-being (e.g. LaRocco, House & French, 1980), there are studies reporting enhancer effects (e.g. Kaufman & Beehr, 1986). This indicates that social support can even increase the negative effects of a stressful work situation. Although the findings concerning social support are not unequivocal, it can be concluded that the social support a person experiences within the work situation has a positive effect on his or her well-being.

Other group-related characteristics of the individual work situation that might be related to individual well-being are the amount of contacts one has to deal with and interpersonal conflicts. A study by Leiter (1988a) showed that the number of work contacts can have an ambiguous effect on individual well-being. Within a mental health team, having a high amount of work contacts was positively related to feelings of personal accomplishment, and at the same time showed a rather strong positive relationship to emotional exhaustion.

In contrast, findings from studies on interpersonal conflicts showed a consistent pattern. For example, Leiter (1988b) and Richardsen, Burke & Leiter (1992) found positive relationships between conflict and burnout scores. Based on a study of secretaries and their supervisors, Spector, Dywer & Jex (1988) reported positive correlations between the frequency of conflict secretaries were involved in and levels of anxiety, frustration, satisfaction and health symptoms.

TEAM DEVELOPMENT

Team development refers to changes within groups over time. Broad conceptualizations of team development (e.g. Sundstrom, De Meuse & Futrell, 1990) subsume also questions of group structure and interaction processes—because both develop over time. However, within this section, team development is used in a narrower sense, concentrating on effects of team development interventions on individual well-being. More general issues of team development are reviewed by McGrath & O'Connor (this volume).

Team development procedures can be considered as one type of organizational development intervention, aimed at changing social factors within a work group in order to improve the group's competence in dealing with problems and making decisions (Porras & Robertson, 1992). Additionally, the improvement of group members' individual well-being is one (side-)effect that is expected from team development interventions (e.g. Dyer, 1987; Numerof, 1987). Team development comprises various approaches. Porras & Robertson (1992) refer to team-building, goal-setting, process consultation and various kinds of meetings, among others.

Evaluations of group development procedures that assessed the effects on individual well-being mostly focused on job satisfaction. Literature reviews show no clear pattern concerning the effects of group development on job satisfaction and related measures. De Meuse & Liebowitz (1981) reviewed 36 team-building studies published from 1962 to 1980. Concerning attitudinal and perceptual changes including job satisfaction as outcome measures, mainly positive effects of team-building interventions were found. However, the authors regard their findings as inconclusive, due to a lack of methodological rigour in the studies reviewed. Sundstrom, De Meuse & Futrell (1990) reviewed 13 team development studies published between 1980 and 1988. Five of these studies used satisfaction measures as dependent variables. In two studies, no changes in satisfaction were found; two reported increased satisfaction; one found decreased job satisfaction associated with team development (cf. Tannenbaum, Beard & Salas, 1992 for a similar review). A literature review by Porras & Robertson (1992) on team-building and related interventions, including 29 studies—reviewing some of the same as Sundstrom, De Meuse & Futrell (1990)—found an even more ambiguous result. Out of those studies that used job satisfaction as criteria for the success of team development, 65.6% resulted in no change in individual outcome, while

17.8% found an improvement in these measures, and 16.6% reported negative change.

However, a meta-analysis by Neuman, Edwards & Raju (1989) came to more positive findings. The authors reported an uncorrected effect size of 0.351 on the relationship between team-building interventions and overall satisfaction based on 916 subjects in 8 studies. The lower bound of the 90% confidence interval was 0.191. For the relationship between survey feedback interventions and overall satisfaction, an uncorrected effect size of 0.173 resulted. For this kind of intervention, 0 was included in the 90% confidence interval.

Taking these findings together, it can be concluded that there is only weak support for the assumption that group development procedures have a positive effect on individual well-being.

INTEGRATIVE DISCUSSION OF RESEARCH FINDINGS

Summarizing the research on work group characteristics and their relationship to individual well-being, it is clear that it is mainly task characteristics associated with autonomous group work and features of group processes which seem to be related to job satisfaction and other well-being measures. Team development methods produce only weak and inconsistent effects on well-being. If at all, group composition seems to be related to well-being through the group process.

However, before we can conclude that work group task and process factors have a substantial effect on individual well-being, some questions have to be answered: the question of causality; the question of relative importance of various work group factors; and the question of the importance of work group factors compared to other work characteristics.

Concerning the question of causality, empirical findings do not give a clear answer. With respect to autonomous work groups, research designs of at least some studies allow a causal interpretation of the results, indicating that autonomous group work has indeed a causal positive effect on job satisfaction. Studies examining group process variables mainly applied cross-sectional designs. Therefore, at least three rival explanations additional to the possible causal effect of group process on individual well-being have to be taken into account (cf. Kasl, 1978, for a related argument within stress research).

The first explanation refers to individual and group response bias, influencing both the perception of group processes and individual well-being. However, some studies tried to rule out individual response bias by using group-level data (e.g. Mossholder & Bedeian, 1983; Repetti, 1987) and still arrived at significant correlations between group process variables and individual well-being. Second, one can imagine a causal path from individual well-being to work group factors. It is possible that group members with higher job satisfaction and better well-being contribute to a better interaction within the group and that this leads to high group level scores of process measures. This argument is consistent with the approach by George (1990), who found individual affect to be related to the affective tone of the work group. Third, one could argue that the relationship between group processes and individual well-being can be explained by third variables that have an effect both on the group process and a person's well-being. For example, one can assume that, under stressful working conditions that are known to be negatively related to individual well-being, group process also becomes worse. There is some empirical evidence for this hypothesis (e.g. Beehr, 1981). However, as will be shown in the discussion of the third question concerning the relative importance of work group factors compared to other working conditions, group process variables are related to well-being measures also when other work characteristics are taken into account. Taking these arguments together, it becomes clear that not all rival explanations can be ruled out. Therefore, the question whether work group factors have a causal effect on individual well-being can not be answered finally.

The second question refers to the relative importance of various work group factors. Until now, it is unanswered whether group task characteristics have a stronger relationship to individual well-being than do group process variables, or *vice versa*. We also do not know whether these various work group factors are related independently to individual well-being or if one relationship is mediated or moderated by another work group factor. Most studies included only group task characteristics *or* group process variables. An exception is the study by Campion, Medsker & Higgs (1993), in which a wide range of work group characteristics were assessed. Within this study individual level correlations ranging from $r = 0.10$ to $r = 0.50$ between job design measures (i.e. task characteristics) and process variables were found. However, in further analyses every work group characteristic was related separately to satisfaction measures. Therefore, this study, also, allows no conclusion about the relative importance of various work group characteristics.

The third question concerns the contribution of work group factors to individual well-being compared to other work characteristics. Strictly speaking, research on work group factors in its relationship to individual well-being is only relevant if it can be shown that these factors explain variance in individual outcome measures that can not be explained by other features of the work situation. Again, the empirical basis for coming to a conclusive answer is rather small. Existing studies that controlled for other work characteristics, such as work load, control at work, job complexity and skill use found significant relationships between group process variables and individual well-being (Lachman & Diamant, 1987; Richardson, Burke & Leiter, 1992; Sonnentag et al., 1994). Additionally, Repetti (1987) reported an interaction effect of a consensual climate measure and supervisor support on depression. Negative climate increased the negative relationship between supervisor support and depression. Taken together, these results indicate that group process factors can explain additional variance in individual well-being measures that is not explained by other work characteristics.

Thus, it becomes clear that work group characteristics show relationships to individual well-being that can not be simply reduced to the effects of other working conditions. However, as the discussion of the first question showed, the causality within this relationship is still unknown. Additionally, the relative importance of the various work group factors needs clarification. Therefore, further research is necessary.

There is a strong need for longitudinal studies examining the causal effects of work group characteristics on individual well-being. In order to come to a deeper and more complete understanding of the effects of group factors on the individual it is also necessary to consider the relationships among these group factors and their relative importance in predicting well-being, as well as their effects in combination with other work characteristics. For arriving at conclusive results concerning work group characteristics, group level measures should be used whenever dealing with constructs conceptualized at the group level.

Although not all questions concerning the well-being effects of work group factors can be answered by existing research, it becomes obvious that work group characteristics play a significant role for a person's well-being. The experiences an individual has within his or her working group are important for both satisfaction with the job and the experience of well-being outside work. Favourable work group factors can not be completely substituted by other work characteristics. Therefore, they must be taken into account when (re-)designing jobs in order to improve the quality of working life.

ACKNOWLEDGEMENTS

I wish to thank Felix C. Brodbeck, Michael Frese, Sabine Remdisch and Michael West for helpful comments on a first draft of this chapter.

REFERENCES

Antoni, C. (1994). Auswirkungen von teilautonomen Arbeitsgruppen auf Kriterien humaner Arbeit und ökonomischer Effizienz. In K. Pawlik (ed.), *Bericht über den 39. Kongreß der Deutschen Gesellschaft für Psychologie, Hamburg, 25–29 September 1994*, Vol. 1. Hamburg: Psychologisches Institut I der Universität Hamburg, p. 32.

Beehr, T.A. (1981). Work-role stress and attitudes toward co-workers. *Group & Organization Studies*, **6**, 201–210.

Beekun, R.I. (1989). Assessing the effectiveness of sociotechnical interventions: antidote or fad? *Human Relations*, **42**, 877–897.

Berggren, C. (1991). *Von Ford zu Volvo: Automobilherstellung in Schweden*. Berlin: Springer.

Brief, A.P., Butcher, A.H., George, J.M. & Link, K.E. (1993). Integrating bottom-up and top-down theories of subjective well-being: the case of health. *Journal of Personality and Social Psychology*, **64**, 646–653.

Bruggemann, A., Groskurth, P. & Ulich, E. (1975). *Arbeitszufriedenheit*. Bern: Huber.

Campbell, A. (1976). Subjective measures of well-being. *American Psychologist*, **31**, 117–124.

Campbell, D.T. & Fiske, D.W. (1959). Convergent and discriminant validation by the multitrait–multimethod matrix. *Psychological Bulletin*, **56**, 81–105.

Campion, M.A., Medsker, G.J. & Higgs, A.C. (1993). Relations between work group characteristics and effectiveness: implications for designing effective work groups. *Personnel Psychology*, **46**, 823–850.

Cohen, S. & Syme, S.L. (1985). *Social Support and Health*. New York: Academic Press.

Cohen, S. & Wills, T.A. (1985). Stress, social support, and the buffering hypothesis. *Psychological Bulletin*, **98**, 310–357.

Cordery, J.L., Mueller, W.S. & Smith, L.M. (1991). Attitudinal and behavioral effects of autonomous group working: a longitudinal field study. *Academy of Management Journal*, **34**, 464–476.

Cotton, J.L. & Tuttle, J.M. (1986). Employee turnover: a meta-analysis with implications for research. *Academy of Management Review*, **11**, 55–70.

Cummings, T.G. (1978). Self-managing work groups: a socio-technical synthesis. *Academy of Management Review*, **3**, 625–634.

De Meuse, K.P. & Liebowitz, S.J. (1981). An empirical analysis of team-building research. *Group & Organization Studies*, **6**, 357–378.

Diener, E. (1984). Subjective well-being. *Psychological Bulletin*, **95**, 542–575.

Dyer, W.G. (1987). *Team building. Issues and alternatives*. Reading, MA: Addison-Wesley.

Edwards, J.R. (1992). A cybernetic theory of stress, coping, and well-being in organizations. *Academy of Management Review*, **17**, 238–274.

Evans, C.R. & Dion, K.L. (1991). Group cohesion and performance: a meta-analysis. *Small Group Research*, **22**, 175–186.

Fandt, P.M. (1991). The relationship of accountability and interdependent behavior to enhancing team consequences. *Group & Organization Studies*, **16**, 300–312.

Frese, M. (1985). Stress at work and psychosomatic complaints: a causal interpretation. *Journal of Applied Psychology*, **70**, 314–328.

Frese, M. (1989). Theoretical models of control and health. In S.L. Sauter, J.J. Hurrell Jr & C.L. Cooper (eds), *Job Control and Worker Health*. Chichester: Wiley, pp. 107–127.

Frese, M. & Zapf, D. (1994). Action as the core of work psychology: a German approach. In H.C. Triandis, M.D. Dunnette & J.M. Hough (eds), *Handbook of Industrial and Organizational Psychology*, Vol. 4. Palo Alto, CA: Consulting Psychologists Press, pp. 271–340.

Frone, M.R. & Major, B. (1988). Communication quality and job satisfaction among managerial nurses: the moderating influence of job involvement. *Group & Organization Studies*, **13**, 322–347.

Gaines, J. & Jermier, J.M. (1983). Emotional exhaustion in a high stress organization. *Academy of Management Journal*, **26**, 567–586.

George, J.M. (1990). Personality, affect, and behavior in groups. *Journal of Applied Psychology*, **75**, 107–116.

Gladstein, D. (1984). Groups in context: a model of task group effectiveness. *Administrative Science Quarterly*, **29**, 210–216.

Goodman, P.S. (ed.) (1986). *Designing Effective Work Groups*. San Francisco, CA: Jossey-Bass.

Goodman, P.S., Devadas, R. & Hughson, T.L.G. (1988). Groups and productivity: analyzing the effectiveness of self-managing teams. In J.P. Campbell & R.J. Campbell (eds), *Productivity in Organizations: New Perspectives from Industrial and Organizational Psychology*. San Francisco, CA: Jossey-Bass, pp. 295–327.

Goodman, P.S., Ravlin, E.C. & Argote, L. (1986). Current thinking about groups: setting the stage for new ideas. In P.S. Goodman (ed.), *Designing Effective Work Groups*. San Francisco, CA: Jossey-Bass, pp. 1–33.

Greller, M.M., Parsons, C.K. & Mitchell, D.R.D. (1992). Additive effects and beyond: occupational stressors and social buffers in a police organization. In J.C. Quick, L.R. Murphy & J.J. Hurrell Jr (eds), *Stress & Well-being at Work. Assessments and Interventions for Occupational Mental Health*. Washington, DC: American Psychological Association, pp. 33–47.

Guzzo, R.A. & Shea, G.P. (1992). Group performance and intergroup relations in organizations. In M.D. Dunnette & L.M. Hough (eds), *Handbook of Industrial and Organizational Psychology*, Vol. 3. Palo Alto, CA: Consulting Psychologists Press, pp. 269–313.

Hacker, W. (1986). *Arbeitspsychologie*. Bern: Huber.

Hackman, J.R. (1987). The design of work teams. In J.W. Lorsch (ed.), *Handbook of Organizational Behavior*. Englewood Cliffs, NJ: Prentice-Hall, pp. 315–342.

Hackman, J.R. (1992). Group influences on individuals in organizations. In M.D. Dunnette & L.M. Hough (eds), *Handbook of Industrial and Organizational Psychology*, Vol. 3. Palo Alto, CA: Consulting Psychologists Press, pp. 199–267.

Hackman, J.R. & Morris, C.G. (1975). Group tasks, group interaction process, and group performance effectiveness: a review and proposed integration. In L. Berkowitz (ed.), *Advances in Experimental Social Psychology*, Vol. 8. New York: Academic Press.

Hackman, J.R. & Oldham, G.R. (1980). *Work Redesign*. Reading, MA: Addison-Wesley.

Hart, P.M. (1994). Teacher quality of work life: integrating work experiences, psychological distress and morale. *Journal of Occupational and Organizational Psychology*, **67**, 109–132.

House, J.S. (1981). *Work Stress and Social Support*. Reading, MA: Addison-Wesley.

Jackofsky, E.F. & Slocum, J.W. Jr (1988). A longitudinal study of climates. *Journal of Occupational Behavior*, **9**, 319–334.

Jackson, S. (1992). Team composition in organizational settings: issues in managing an increasingly diverse work force. In S. Worchel, W. Wood & J.A. Simpson (eds), *Group Process and Productivity*. Newbury Park: Sage, pp. 138–173.

Jackson, S.E., Brett, J.F., Sessa, V.I., Cooper, D.M., Julin, J.A. & Peyronnin, K. (1991). Some differences make a difference: individual dissimilarity and group heterogeneity as correlates of recruitment, promotions, and turnover. *Journal of Applied Psychology*, **76**, 675–689.

James, L.R. (1982). Aggregation bias in estimates of perceptual agreement. *Journal of Applied Psychology*, **67**, 219–229.

Judge, T.A. & Hulin, C.L. (1993). Job satisfaction as a reflection of disposition: a multiple source causal analysis. *Organizational Behavior and Human Decision Processes*, **56**, 388–421.

Kahn, R.L. & Byosiere, P. (1992). Stress in organizations. In M.D. Dunnette & L.M. Hough (eds), *Handbook of Industrial and Organizational Psychology*, Vol. 3. Palo Alto, CA: Consulting Psychologists Press, pp. 571–650.

Karasek, R.A., Baker, D., Marxer, F., Ahlbom, A. & Theorell, T. (1981). Job decision latitude, job demands, and cardiovascular disease: a prospective study of Swedish men. *American Journal of Public Health*, **71**, 694–705.

Karasek, R. & Theorell, T. (1990). *Healthy Work. Stress, Productivity, and the Reconstruction of Working Life*. New York: Basic Books.

Kasl, S.V. (1978). Epidemiological contributions to the study of work stress. In C.L. Cooper & R. Payne (eds), *Stress at Work*. New York: Wiley, pp. 3–48.

Kaufman, G.M. & Beehr, T.A. (1986). Interactions between job stressors and social support: some counter-intuitive results. *Journal of Applied Psychology*, **71**, 522–526.

Keller, R.T. (1986). Predictors of the performance of project groups in R&D organizations. *Academy of Management Journal*, **29**, 715–726.

Kelloway, E.K. & Barling, J. (1991). Job characteristics, role stress and mental health. *Journal of Occupational Psychology*, **64**, 291–304.

King, N. & Anderson, N. (1990). Innovation in working groups. In M.A. West & J.L. Farr (eds), *Innovation and Creativity at Work. Psychological and Organizational Strategies*. Chichester: Wiley, pp. 81–100.

Kolodny, H. & Kiggundu, M.N. (1980). Towards the development of a sociotechnical systems model in woodland mechanical harvesting. *Human Relations*, **33**, 623–645.

Kruger, L.J., Botman, H.I. & Goodenow, C. (1991). An investigation of social support and burnout among residential counselors. *Child & Youth Care Forum*, **20**, 335–352.

Lachman, R. & Diamant, E. (1987). Withdrawal and restraining factors in teachers' turnover intentions. *Journal of Occupational Behaviour*, **8**, 219–232.

LaRocco, J.M., House, J.S. & French, J.R.J. Jr (1980). Social support, occupational stress, and health. *Journal of Health and Social Behavior*, **21**, 202–218.

Leiter, M.P. (1988a). Burnout as a function of communication patters: a study of a multidisciplinary mental health team. *Group & Organization Studies*, **13**, 111–128.

Leiter, M.P. (1988b). Commitment as a function of stress reactions among nurses: a model of psychological evaluations of work settings. *Canadian Journal of Community Mental Health*, **7**, 117–133.

Leiter, M.P. (1992). Burnout as a crisis in professional role structures: measurement and conceptual issues. *Anxiety, Stress, and Coping*, **5**, 79–93.

Leitner, K. (1993). Auswirkungen von Arbeitsbedingungen auf die psychosoziale Gesundheit. *Zeitschrift für Arbeitswissenschaft*, **47**, 98–107.

Lewin, K. (1951). *Field Theory in Social Science*. New York: Harper & Row.

Lott, A.J. & Lott, B.E. (1965). Group cohesiveness and interpersonal attraction: a review of relationships with antecedent and consequent variables. *Psychological Bulletin*, **64**, 259–302.

Manning, F.J. & Fullerton, T.D. (1988). Health and well-being in highly cohesive units of the U.S. Army. *Journal of Applied Social Psychology*, **18**, 503–519.

Martin, T.N. (1984). Role stress and inability to leave as predictors of mental health. *Human Relations*, **37**, 969–983.

Maslach, C. & Jackson, S.E. (1984). Burnout in organizational settings. In S. Oscamp (ed.), *Applied Social Psychology Annual*, Vol. 5. Beverly Hills: Sage, pp. 133–153.

McCain, B.R., O'Reilly, C.C. III & Pfeffer, J. (1983). The effects of departmental demography on turnover. *Academy of Management Journal*, **26**, 626–641.

McGrath, J.E. (1991). Time, interaction, and performance (TIP): a theory of groups. *Small Group Research*, **22**, 147–174.

Moch, M.K. (1980). Job involvement, internal motivation, and employees' integration into networks of work relationships. *Organizational Behavior and Human Performance*, **25**, 15–31.

Mossholder, K.W. & Bedeian, A.G. (1983). Group interactional processes: individual and group level effects. *Group & Organization Studies*, **8**, 187–202.

Mullen, B. & Copper, C. (1994). The relation between group cohesiveness and performance: an integration. *Psychological Bulletin*, **115**, 210–227.

Neuman, G.A., Edwards, J.E. & Rahu, N.S. (1989). Organizational development interventions: a meta-analysis of their effects on satisfaction and other attitudes. *Personnel Psychology*, **42**, 461–489.

Numerof, R.E. (1987). Team-building interventions: an organization stress moderator. In J.C. Quick, R.S. Bhagat, J.E. Dalton & J.D. Quick (eds), *Work stress. Health care Systems in the Workplace*. New York: Praeger, pp. 171–194.

Payne, R. (1990). The effectiveness of research teams: a review. In M.A. West & J.L. Farr (eds), *Innovation and Creativity at Work. Psychological and Organizational Strategies*. Chichester: Wiley, pp. 101–122.

Pearce, J.A. II & Ravlin, E.C. (1987). The design and activation of self-regulation work groups. *Human Relations*, **40**, 751–782.

Pearson, C.A.L. (1992). Autonomous workgroups: an evaluation at an industrial site. *Human Relations*, **45**, 905–936.

Peiró, J.M., González-Romá, V. & Ramos, J. (1992). The influence of work team climate on role stress, tension, satisfaction and leadership perceptions. *European Review of Applied Psychology*, **42**, 49–58.

Pfaff, H. (1989). *Streßbewältigung und soziale Unterstützung. Zur sozialen Regulierung individuellen Wohlbefindens*. Weinheim: Deutscher Studien Verlag.

Porras, J.I. & Robertson, P.J. (1992). Organizational development: theory, practice, and research. In M.D. Dunnette & L.M. Hough (eds), *Handbook of Industrial and Organizational Psychology*, Vol. 3. Palo Alto, CA: Consulting Psychologists Press, pp. 719–822.

Pretty, G.M.H., McCarthy, M.E. & Catano, V.M. (1992). Psychological environments and burnout: gender considerations within the corporation. *Journal of Organizational Behavior*, **13**, 701–711.

Rau, R. (1994). Team- versus Einzelarbeit: Handlungssicherheit in Abhängigkeit von der Arbeitsform. *Zeitschrift für Arbeits- und Organisationspsychologie*, **38**, 62–70.

Repetti, R.L. (1987). Individual and common components of the social environment at work and psychological well-being. *Journal of Personality and Social Psychology*, **52**, 710–720.

Richardson, A.M., Burke, R.J. & Leiter, M.P. (1992). Occupational demands, psychological burnout and anxiety among hospital personnel in Norway. *Anxiety, Stress, and Coping*, **5**, 55–68.

Richman, J.M. (1989). Groupwork in a hospice setting. *Social Work with Groups*, **12**, 171–184.

Roethlisberger, F.J. & Dickson, W.J. (1939). *Management and the Worker*. Cambridge, MA: Harvard University Press.

Rosse, J.G., Boss, R.W., Johnson, A.E. & Grown, B.F. (1991). Conceptualizating the role of self-esteem in the burnout process. *Group & Organization Studies*, **16**, 428–451.

Rudolph, E., Schönfelder, E. & Hacker, W. (1987). *Tätigkeitsbewertungssystem Geistige Arbeit. TBS-GA*. Berlin: Psychodiagnostisches Zentrum der Humboldt-Universität.

Shea, G.P. & Guzzo, R.A. (1987). Groups as human resources. In K.M. Rowland & G.R. Ferris (eds), *Research in Personnel and Human Resources Management*, Vol. 5. Greenwich, CT: JAI Press, pp. 323–356.

Skaret, D.J. & Bruning, N.S. (1986). Attitudes about the work group: an added moderator of the relationship between leader behavior and job satisfaction. *Group & Organization Studies*, **11**, 254–279.

Sonnentag, S., Brodbeck, F.C., Heinbokel, T. & Stolte, W. (1994). Stressor–burnout relationship in software development teams. *Journal of Occupational and Organizational Psychology*, **67**, 327–341.

Spector, P.E., Dwyer, D.J. & Jex, S.M. (1988). Relation of job stressors to affective, health, and performance outcomes: a comparison of multiple data sources. *Journal of Applied Psychology*, **73**, 11–19.

Stahelski, A.J. & Tsukuda, R.A. (1990). Predictors of cooperation in health care teams. *Small Group Research*, **21**, 220–233.

Stevens, F., Diederiks, J. & Philipsen, H. (1992). Physician satisfaction, professional characteristics and behavior formalization in hospitals. *Social Science and Medicine*, **35**, 295–303.

Sundstrom, E., De Meuse, K.P. & Futrell, D. (1990). Work teams: applications and effectiveness. *American Psychologist*, **45**, 120–133.

Tannenbaum, S.I., Beard, R.L. & Salas, E. (1992). Team building and its influence on team effectiveness: an examination of conceptual and empirical developments. In K. Kelley (ed.), *Issues, Theory, and Research in Industrial/Organizational Psychology*. Amsterdam: Elsevier, pp. 117–153.

Terborg, R.R., Castore, C. & DeNinno, J.A. (1976). A longitudinal field investigation of the impact of group composition on group performance and cohesion. *Journal of Personality and Social Psychology*, **34**, 782–790.

Trist, E.L. & Bamforth, K.W. (1951). Some social and psychological consequences of the longwall method of coal-getting. *Human Relations*, **4**, 3–38.

Trist, E.L., Susman, G.I. & Brown, G.R. (1977). An experiment in autonomous working in an american underground coal mine. *Human Relations*, **30**, 201–236.

Wall, T.D. & Clegg, C.W. (1981). A longitudinal field study of group work redesign. *Journal of Occupational Behavior*, **2**, 31–49.

Wall, T.D., Kemp, N.J., Jackson, P.R. & Clegg, C.W. (1986). Outcomes of autonomous workgroups: a long-term field experiment. *Academy of Management Journal*, **29**, 280–304.

Warr, P. (1987). *Work, Unemployment, and Mental Health*. Oxford: Clarendon Press.

Watson, W.E., Kumar, K. & Michaelsen, L.K. (1993). Cultural diversity's impact on interaction process and performance: comparing homogeneous and diverse task groups. *Academy of Management Journal*, **36**, 590–602.

Wong, C.S. & Campion, M.A. (1991). Development and test of a task level model of motivational job design. *Journal of Applied Psychology*, **76**, 825–837.

Worchel, S., Wood, W. & Simpson, J.A. (eds) (1992). *Group Process and Productivity*. Newbury Park, CA: Sage.

Yammarino, F.J. & Naughton, T.J. (1988). Time spent communicating: a multiple levels of analysis approach. *Human Relations*, **41**, 655–676.

Zaccaro, S.J. & Dobbins, G.H. (1989). Contrasting group and organizational commitment: evidence of differences among multilevel attachments. *Journal of Organizational Behavior*, **10**, 267–273.

Zalesney, M.D., Farace, R.V. & Kurchner-Hawkins, R. (1985). Determinants of employee work perceptions and attitudes: perceived work environment and organizational level. *Environment and Behavior*, **17**, 567–592.

Section V

Groups in Organizations

Chapter 15

Affective Reactions to the Group and the Organization

Natalie J. Allen
*Centre for Administrative and Information Studies,
The University of Western Ontario, Canada*

Abstract

Many employees have two important, and inextricably linked, identities: they are members of both a work group (or team) and a larger organization. Such employees will learn to operate within, make psychological sense of, and develop affective reactions toward, both these domains. Evidence within the work attitude research suggests two premises that guide this chapter. The first is that employees can and do draw a meaningful affective distinction between their work groups and their organizations. The second premise is that affective reactions to both domains have important consequences. Employees who have positive attitudes toward their organizations are more likely to behave in a manner consistent with organizational goals than are those with negative attitudes. Similarly, those with positive attitudes toward the group will work toward group goals more than those with negative attitudes. Just as important are the psychological implications of work attitudes; quite simply, it "feels better" to have positive, rather than negative, attitudes toward one's group and organization. Taken together this suggests an important challenge: to create workplaces in which employees feel positively towards *both* their work group and the organization as a whole. This may well require us to focus on the interplay between group and organizational variables—something that has received very little attention from researchers or practitioners. More specifically, it is argued that strong affective reactions to both domains can only be assured when attention is paid to the congruence between group-level and organization-level variables. Three issues of "group-organization congruence" are explored here: (1) employees' understanding of how their own, and other groups, fit together within the organization, (2) congruence between work group practices and organizational practices, and (3) the extent to which the group leader is also an organizational leader.

INTRODUCTION

> When I joined my organization, I was assigned to a team and told that the organization valued teamwork—that developing an *esprit de corps* amongst team members was an important goal. Yet there was nothing done, either within the group or by the company, that suggested that this was really the case. If anything, the place seemed designed to confuse us and divide our loyalties. In the end, I had little real affection for my team. If I was loyal to anything, it was to the organization—and that was just because they signed the pay cheques.
>
> Employee A
>
> When I began my job, I was led to believe that I should think about the organization in a "big picture" sort of way—and become attached to it as well as to my department and co-workers. I never really developed that feeling because no one in my department had any regard for head office or anything that it stood for. We were constantly made to feel, one way or another, that we were the "good guys" and head office people were the "bad guys" and that our department's survival depended on keeping that in mind. It didn't seem right that we felt this way, but we did and nothing ever changed.
>
> Employee B

Researchers and practitioners interested in work groups must recognize an important fact of working life. Employees who are members of a defined work group, or team, are also members of a larger organization. They "belong" to both. Thus, they must grapple with the structures, policies, practices and values of both to determine what form that belonging will take. In short, organizational members who also belong to work groups must make psychological sense of their dual membership and try to behave in accordance with it.

The affective reactions, or attitudes, that employees develop toward the group and the organization represent an important aspect of this sense-making. Admittedly, few areas within the psychological study of work have been fraught with as much conceptual and operational blurring as the study of work attitudes. One thing, however, seems fairly clear: work attitudes and behaviour are related. Employees who have positive attitudes toward their organizations are more likely to behave in a manner consistent with organizational goals than are those with negative attitudes. Similarly, those who have positive attitudes toward their groups are more likely to behave in a manner consistent with group goals than are those with negative attitudes. In addition, work attitudes can have psychological implications; quite simply; it "feels better" to have positive, rather than negative, attitudes toward one's group and organization.

Clearly, then, an important challenge for organizations is to create situations in which the attitudinal effects of group membership and organizational membership are optimized—in other words, to create workplaces in which the employee feels positively toward both the work group and the organization as a whole. In meeting this challenge, one encounters two problems. First, there is very little suggestion in the practitioner-oriented literature that systematic thought has been put into the interplay between these two domains; indeed, a cynic could argue that some organizations seem specifically designed to thwart group attachment and some groups seem designed to thwart organizational attachment. Second, though there are exceptions (e.g. Becker, 1992; Becker & Billings, 1993; Reichers, 1985, 1986), very few work attitude researchers have examined the interplay between attitudes toward these two domains. Indeed, the frequently issued admonition that groups are not examined in organizational context (Goodman, Ravlin & Schminke, 1987; Guzzo & Shea, 1992) applies well to the work attitude literature. Much of the research examining the affective meaning of group membership has taken place in isolation from the organization in which the group is nested. It is also the case, though perhaps to a lesser extent, that research examining attitudes toward the organization has ignored group variables.

Despite the dearth of attention given to the dual membership issue, however, it seems quite likely that employee attitudes toward the work group and the organization are both influenced by the interplay between group and organizational variables. Indeed, the central theme of this chapter is that in order to understand how best to develop strong positive employee attitudes to both the work group and the organization, we need to consider the work group in organizational context. Failure to do so may jeopardize the development of strong positive attitudes to one, and possibly both, of these domains.

The chapter begins with some comments about terminology and the two basic premises on which the chapter is based. Following this, it is organized around three general issues, each of which deals with the notion of fit or congruence between the work group and the organization.

Terminology

Throughout the chapter, "work group", "group" and "team" are used interchangeably to refer to a set of employees who belong to a defined unit within the organization and who work together in an interdependent fashion. "Organization" is used to refer to the larger institution which employs these group members and within which the group is embedded.

Finally, although research psychologists have conceptualized, labelled and measured affective reactions to the workplace in various ways, the focus here is not on fine-grained distinctions. This is not because they are unimportant, but rather, since the propositions forwarded here are of a very general nature, it makes sense to paint with a somewhat broader brush. Consistent with research in the areas of organizational commitment (Meyer & Allen, 1991) and, more recently, attachment to the group (Korsgaard, Schweiger & Sapienza, 1995), the focus here is at the individual level of analysis and not, as with research on group cohesiveness (Mullen & Copper, 1994), at the group level of analysis. Thus, throughout the chapter, the terms "affective reactions", "affective attachment" and "attitudes" are used interchangeably to refer to the affect that *individual* employees associate with the specific domain of interest.

Premise 1: Organizations and Work Groups are Psychologically Distinct Domains

The first premise on which the chapter is based is that employees can draw a meaningful distinction, affectively, between their work groups and their organizations. Clearly, if this were not true, discussions about how to deal with this dual identity and how best to strengthen affective reactions to both domains would be unnecessary.

One form of evidence relevant to this issue comes from studies in which affective reactions toward both domains have been examined using the same sample. Two of the three studies referred to here used quite comparable measures to assess affective reactions to the two domains. Becker (1992) administered three affective measures using both the organization and the work group as the focal domain; correlations between the three pairs of comparable measures ranged from 0.36 to 0.45 ($p < 0.001$, for each). Zaccaro & Dobbins (1989) also reported a positive correlation between two parallel measures of affective commitment, one with an organizational focus and the other with a work group focus ($r = 0.45$, $p < 0.001$). Finally, Yoon, Baker & Ko (1994) used measures of affective attachment to the work group and the organization that, though conceptually similar, were made up of quite different items. Their measure of the interpersonal attachment employees felt toward members of their work group correlated significantly with a measure of affective attachment to the organization ($r = 0.41$, $p < 0.001$).

Given the diversity of affective measures and samples, the narrow range of correlations produced by these studies is quite striking (0.36–0.45). Certainly, affective reaction to the work group and the organization are related and, apparently, quite consistently so. The link between them, however, is a modest one, suggesting that employees are indeed able to make an affective distinction between the two domains.

Related to this is evidence that affective reactions to the two domains are predicted by somewhat different variables. This has been examined explicitly in only one study. Zaccaro & Dobbins (1989) reported that organization-related variables contributed significantly to the prediction of affective commitment to the organization, but not to the group. Group-related variables, on the other hand, contributed to affective commitment to the group but, with one exception, did not predict commitment to the organization.

Finally, both anecdotal and empirical evidence suggests that employees can experience psychologically important conflicts between these (and other) work-related domains. Though there is disagreement in the empirical literature as to the magnitude and/or frequency of these conflicts (Hunt & Morgan, 1994;

Reichers, 1986), the fact that such conflicts exist at all supports the notion that the work group and organization have distinguishable meaning for employees.

Premise 2: Attitudes Toward both the Group and the Organization Have Important Consequences

The second premise is that the workplace and individual employees will be better served if employees feel positively toward both the group *and* the organization to which they belong. The body of evidence on which this premise is based has some limitations. First, there are very few studies in which potential consequences of attitudes toward both domains have been examined. Thus, most of the evidence relating to this premise comes from examinations of affect toward the organization or the group, but not both considered jointly. Second, studies examining the correlates of individually held attitudes toward the organization far outnumber those that focus on individually held attitudes toward the group. (In the group literature, the focus is much more closely directed at group-level indices of affect, such as cohesiveness.) Finally, although the behavioural correlates of work attitudes are described as "consequences", it must be recognized that few studies use research designs that fully justify such causal language.

These limitations aside, what evidence is there in support of the basic premise that attitudes toward the domains in question are important? First, as is self-evident, feeling positively toward the organization for which one works and the group with which one works is valuable in its own right—psychologically, it "feels better" to spend time where one's sentiments are positive, rather than negative. The psychological value of positive work attitudes is acknowledged, at least implicitly, in the vast collection of studies in which measures of satisfaction with, or emotional attachment to, the organization and/or the group are used as dependent variables. Further, recent research illustrating the stress-buffering role that can be played by affective commitment to organization (Begley & Czajka, 1993) suggests the possibility that positive attachments may have some psychological health benefits for the individual. Finally, there is evidence suggesting that affective attachment to the organization has positive consequences for non-work aspects of the employee's life (Romzek, 1989).

A second type of evidence comes from studies linking affective reactions to turnover behaviour. Studies with an organizational focus clearly dominate this research. Although requests to transfer out of the work group might be the obvious analogue to voluntary turnover from the organization, researchers have not examined the links between affective attachment to the group and such requests. Within the organizational literature, however, there is considerable evidence supporting the prediction that those with strong affective commitment to the organization have weaker intentions to leave the organization and, indeed, are less likely to leave, than those with weak affective commitment (Allen & Meyer, in press; Cohen, 1993; Mathieu & Zajac, 1990).

A third area in which the value of attitudes toward the group or organization has been examined involves performance toward domain-specific goals. The assumption is made that affect directed toward the organization (or the group) should "translate" into enhanced levels of individual performance. Although this often goes unsaid, the theoretical mechanism through which this is presumed to occur is motivational in nature. Feeling positively toward the organization (or group) predisposes the individual to *want* to work harder in the service of organizational (or group) goals (Angle & Lawson, 1994). Whether these goals are articulated clearly enough for the individual to recognize them as such (Shim & Steers, 1994), whether the individual has the skills and ability to achieve the goals, and whether technological and structural constraints limit their achievement (Goodman, Ravlin & Schminke, 1987) are not involved, theoretically, in the "affect breeds performance" notion. Unfortunately, these limiting factors are rarely considered when researchers examine attitude–performance links (Johns, 1991). Despite this, there is considerable evidence suggesting that affective commitment to the organization is related to job performance, organizational citizenship behaviour and attendance (see Allen & Meyer, in press; Meyer & Allen, 1991, for summaries). Similarly, affective attachment to the group is associated with greater cooperation with other group members and greater efforts directed toward the achievement of group goals (Becker & Billings, 1993; Deutsch, 1949; Janis, 1982). Although separate streams of research (i.e. "organization" and "group" research) illustrate that desirable consequences are associated with positive attitudes toward each domain, these links are rarely examined within the same study. An exception is research by Becker & Billings (1993), who compared employees with strong affective commitment to both the organization and the work group with three other groups: those committed to neither, those committed primarily to the work group, and those committed primarily to the organization. Across several dependent measures (e.g. turnover intention, prosocial behaviour), employees committed to both domains either "outperformed" or were as good as employees committed primarily to only one domain. On all dependent variables, those with a dual commitment outperformed those committed to neither domain.

Based on this evidence, and that pieced together from the two separate streams of research referred to above, we proceed with the premise that a reasonable goal, for both the workplace and the employee, would be to develop positive attitudes toward both domains.

Developing Positive Affect toward Both Domains: Issues of Group–Organization Congruence

How can strong positive attitudes toward *both* domains be developed and sustained? This is a challenging question and one, unfortunately, for which there are few empirical answers.

One reason for this is that most work attitudes studies have focused on the hypothesized antecedents of attitudes toward either the organization or the group, but not both. An important limitation of these studies is that they cannot be used to determine whether a particular variable will create trade-offs between the employee's attitude toward one domain and his/her attitude toward the other. It is possible that a particular variable contributes to strong positive feelings for the group, for example, but does so at the expense of positive feelings for the organization as a whole. Another limitation of the empirical work attitude research is its failure to acknowledge explicitly that groups are embedded in organizational contexts and that employees experience, and must make sense of, group and organizational factors in concert. The consequence of this is that few studies examine variables that assess how the employee's experiences in one domain colour, or are interpreted in light of, experiences in the other. Though such variables could take several forms, and address different aspects of working life, the common thread between them is the notion of congruence.

As indicated earlier, the central theme of this chapter is that it is very difficult to develop and sustain strong positive attitudes toward the group and the organization without considering issues of "group–organization congruence". In the remainder of the chapter, three congruence-related themes are explored. These are: (a) the employee's understanding of how their own, and other groups, fit together within the organization; (b) congruence between work group practices and organizational practices; and (c) the extent to which the group leader is also an organizational leader.

THE IMPORTANCE OF UNDERSTANDING "GROUP–ORGANIZATION FIT"

Work group members frequently complain about the role that their group plays, or is seen to play, in the organization. Some of these complaints involve the belief that "others" in the organization don't understand their group's position in, and value to, the organization ("Don't they understand what a mess this organization would be without us?"). Some complaints involve group members' own confusion about the role their group occupies in the organization ("How do we fit in the scheme of things?"). Still other complaints betray ignorance about the position occupied by other groups ("Why on earth does this organization even need Department X?").

Complaints such as these remind us that, while work groups facilitate the performance of complex tasks, they also put up walls, figuratively speaking, between people within the same organization (Ashforth & Mael, 1989). Such complaints also suggest that knowledge about why these walls (groups) exist, and how they fit together, may be an important variable in the study of dual work attitudes. Used in this context, an understanding of what we will call "group–organization fit" refers to the extent to which employees understand two related issues: how their groups' goals fit with, or serve, the goals of the organization and how the various groups within the organization fit together.

Interestingly, no empirical research has examined the link between the employee's understanding of group–organization fit and his/her attitudes toward either the work group or organizational domain. It seems quite reasonable to suggest, however, that strong positive affect toward one, or both, domains will be blunted in the absence of an understanding of how the two fit together. The logic for this general proposition is outlined below.

Understanding Group–Organization Fit: Implications for Attitudes Toward the Organization

A good understanding of the fit between the goals of the group and those of the organization may be particularly important in the development of positive attitudes toward the organization. There are several reasons for this suggestion.

First, such understanding can help buffer bad news, something the organization often must communicate to work groups. Consider, for example, an organizational initiative that appears to disadvantage, or even just inconvenience, one's own work group (e.g. budget cut, change of reporting arrangements, procedural change). Group members with an appreciation of the larger picture will be better able to understand the initiative and "forgive" the organization for its impact on the work group. Group members with little such appreciation, however, can be expected to be particularly resentful of such changes and, therefore, of the organization.

Second, a good understanding of group–organization fit can reduce the likelihood that the employee will inadvertently make errors and put him/herself in politically, or interpersonally, awkward situations within the organization. Employees who have such experiences are quite likely to point the finger of blame at the organization, attributing their errors (perhaps correctly) to poor organizational communication. Clearly, such attributions will not enhance positive attitudes toward this domain.

Finally, we must acknowledge the more general fact that people simply find it easier to criticize, and develop negative attitudes toward, entities that are distal (in this case, "the organization") rather than proximal ("the group"). Indeed, given how easily very localized social identities seem to develop (Tajfel, 1981), it may be that members of groups with little understanding of the larger picture will develop antipathy for, rather than emotional attachment to, the organization. This will be especially true, of course, if events (such as making organizational *faux pas*) make salient to employees that they know little about the links between the distal and proximal domains.

Understanding Group–Organization Fit: Implications for Attitudes Toward the Group

The impact of a poor understanding of group–organization fit on employee attitudes toward the group is somewhat less predictable. One possibility is that having little sense of the bigger picture will cause the employee to develop negative attitudes toward the work group. There are at least three processes through which this could occur. First, it could occur via mere association: in the absence of strong reasons to do otherwise, the employee may simply generalize his or her sense of isolation from the organization and its goals to the entire work situation, including the work group. A second process is more attributional in nature. Faced with a choice of attributing one's vague understanding of group–organization fit to the organization, the group, or oneself, the employee may choose to blame the group ("I am supposed to be part of this team; if they really cared about me, they would explain this..."). Finally, it is possible that employees will take their own uncertainty about the group-in-context as evidence that the group goals are, in fact, relatively unimportant compared to those of the larger organization. This not-very-flattering attribution is unlikely to enhance the employee's affective attachment to the group.

The other possibility, of course, is that a poor understanding of group–organization fit will increase one's attitudes toward the group. Assuming that all else is well within the work group, those who have little understanding of the big picture may see the work group as the "only home" they know. As such they may turn inwards and develop particularly strong attachments to the group. This may be particularly true of work group members who feel that their group is relatively powerless within the organization (Kanter, 1977).

Developing an Understanding of Group–Organization Fit

The above analysis suggests that the development of strong positive attitudes toward both domains may require that work group members have a reasonable understanding of links between the various constituent groups—including their own—within the larger organization and an understanding of how their proximal (group) goals fit with more distal (organizational) goals. The focus turns now to a consideration of how organizations and groups can effectively develop and maintain this understanding.

Communicating Group–Organization Fit Information

One way in which information about the organization and its constituent parts (groups) is conveyed to organizational newcomers is through the use of orientation sessions. Though the details vary, newcomers in a typical orientation session spend a day or half-day with members of the human resource (HR) department who provide them with information about the organizational structure, its HR policies, its physical lay-out and the like (McShane & Baal, 1984). Introductions to key people may be made and the employee will likely be given a welcome-to-the organization message as well as various written documents (e.g. policy manuals, the organizational chart). The employee is then sent to the work group and gets on with his or her job.

Although there seems little doubt that the materials provided in such sessions are helpful in providing new employees with simple, practical information that they need before beginning work (Louis, Posner & Powell, 1983), it has not been demonstrated that they contribute much to their understanding of how groups within the organization fit together or how group goals serve organizational goals. Timing may be the primary culprit here. Indeed, just as youth is said to be wasted on the young, much of this information may well be wasted on newcomers. There are two reasons for this. First, during the bewildering first few days with the organization, the newcomer is less likely to pay very close attention to information of this sort; instead, attention will be focused on the practical issues (e.g. learning names, discovering where to park). Second, without some experience of the group in its organizational context, it may simply be impossible to make much real sense of such information (Louis, 1980; Ostroff & Kozlowski, 1992).

One solution would be to dispense with information of this sort during early orientation and leave it to newcomers to learn, on their own, from other "clues" in the environment. Though recent research suggests that newcomers are quite proactive in acquiring information (Morrison, 1993a, 1993b), this strategy may leave a bit too much to chance—particularly with respect to information about the organization (Ostroff & Kozlowski, 1992). Instead the organization should consider the following. First, it should give serious thought to how orienting information is timed and how it is reinforced as the newcomer's experience with the organization and the group grows. Regardless of whether or not explicit group–organization fit information is provided during early orientation sessions, it *must* be given after the newcomer has had some experience with the group. By then, newcomers will be able to pay closer attention and, more importantly, will have some frame of reference in which to interpret the information. Second, the organization should ensure that the information provided rings true to group members. Otherwise, group members may encourage the newcomer to disregard what is being conveyed, a situation that either can harm affective reactions to the organization directly, or can do so indirectly by providing the newcomer with confusing information about group–organization fit. To ensure that both the organizational and group perspectives are represented, any planned sessions should involve members of the relevant work group as well as "organizational" personnel (e.g. HR staff members). Finally, given the key role that supervisors and co-workers play in the socialization of newcomers, attention should be paid to a recent suggestion made by Ostroff & Kozlowski (1992) that organizations focus less on developing formal orientation/socialization programmes for newcomers and more on training "organizational insiders" to provide newcomers with appropriate,and appropriately timed, information.

Another mechanism through which information about group–organization fit can be conveyed involves the various written (and, increasingly, electronic) devices that organizations use to communicate with their employees: newsletters, corporate newspapers, electronic bulletin boards and the like. Virtually every time organizational "news" about a group is communicated through one of these devices—whether it be about an accomplishment, a change of personnel, or a new project—the organization also has an opportunity to convey something about how the group fits into the larger context. Such messages need not be lengthy or complex, nor do they need to be repeated with every communication about a particular group. They should, however, be seen as an important tool for providing employees with "big picture" information and for drawing explicit links between group and organizational goals (e.g. "The ABC team provides essential consultative services to the XYZ Department and other departments involved in new product development").

Experiencing Group–Organization Fit

It is one thing, however, to hear or read about how group and organizational goals converge; it is quite another to learn this in a more direct fashion through contact and experience with various members within the organization. Particularly apt here is the distinction made in the socialization literature between acquisition of information and gaining of knowledge (Ostroff & Kozlowski, 1992). Both group and organizational policies must allow for, and encourage, activities that help sustain and enhance the employee's knowledge of the role (and goals) of groups in organizational context. One way to do this is by increasing the contact that work group members have with those in other groups (Nelson, 1989). Here we are not referring simply to making it possible for people to "get to know" each other—for example, by locating them proximally or by hosting frequent social events. Rather, both the organization and the group must be designed to encourage *meaningful* goal-oriented contact and information sharing across groups. Without such contact, the individual has a rather secondhand view of the larger context and may feel only peripherally related to the organization (Ibarra & Andrews, 1993).

There are a number of strategies that contribute to this goal. One organizational-level strategy, that provides employees with much contextual information about their own and other groups within the organization, is job rotation or secondments. At one university with which I am familiar, for example, administrative staff are occasionally seconded to other departments in order to learn about their operations. Anecdotal evidence suggests that this enriches the staff members' sense of their roles in both their "home" departments and the university as a whole. Though it is often thought of as a training technique, and reserved for newcomers, Campion, Cheraskin & Stevens (1994) recently examined the correlates of job rotation in an organization that used the technique for all levels of employees. They showed that employees' rate of job rotation was associated with a number of work-related outcomes, including a sense of integration into the organization. It is important to note, however, that rotated employees in this particular study did not necessarily "come from" an intact work group, neither did they typically return to their "old" jobs. Specific research is needed, therefore, to determine how well job rotation (and the group–organization fit information it can provide) can be incorporated into team-based organizations.

Mentoring is another organization-level strategy that has the potential to increase the employee's understanding of group–organization fit. In a recent study comparing mentored and non-mentored employees, for example, Ostroff & Kozlowski (1993) found that the most significant differences between the two groups was that mentored newcomers learned more about organizational issues and practices. Like job rotation, however, the implications of mentoring for organizations with teams have not been examined. It may be that work group members will not be particularly well served by mentors who, themselves, have not worked as part of a group and/or have had little direct experience with the group to which the protégé belongs.

CONGRUENCE BETWEEN THE POLICIES AND PRACTICES OF THE ORGANIZATION AND THE GROUP

Two general, and parallel, questions are addressed here. First, does the organization provide a group-friendly context for its members? Second, does the work group provide an organization-friendly context for its members? In both cases, attention is focused on whether the policies and practices of one domain meaningfully acknowledge the existence and importance of the other. Failure to do so, it is argued, will weaken the employee's affective attachment to the organization, to the group, or to both domains.

Do Organizational Human Resource Management Practices Acknowledge the Value of Groups?

In addressing the first question, three human resource management issues are examined: staffing, training and rewarding performance. At issue in each case is whether organizational practices complement, or collide with, the idea of group-based work.

Staffing Issues

Recruiting and Selecting Newcomers

Increasing attention is being given to the notion of "fit" between the culture of the organization and the values of those who aspire to join it (e.g. Chatman, 1991). In paying attention to this type of fit, it is argued, the organization will help newcomers adjust more readily to the organization, become more attached to it, and become productive employees more quickly. Although this same logic can be applied easily to the group, this is rarely done. Very often, decisions are made about who will join a particular work group or team without consultation with the membership of the team. Neither is much attention paid, during recruiting and selection, to the question of whether or not candidates have the characteristics necessary to work effectively as part of a team (Stevens & Campion, 1994a). Instead, the group newcomer is selected because he or she appears to have the particular combination of technical skills and experience deemed necessary for particular aspects of the job.

Both these organizational practices—excluding the work group from the selection process and ignoring group-relevant skills—are at odds with the reality of the group. Thus, they suggest that the organization is not very serious about the importance of work groups, regardless of what it may claim about "valuing teamwork". Over time, this is quite likely to have adverse effects on employees' attitudes toward the organization. Further, both practices reduce the likelihood that candidates most suited to the group in question will be selected. Employees who do not fit well into the group are unlikely to become attached to it or the organization. Neither is the arrival of a "poorly fitting" newcomer likely to enhance the attitudes toward either domain held by those who are already in the group.

How can organizational practices regarding selection become more congruent with group-based work? First, recruitment and selection strategies should be developed jointly by HR personnel and members of the group in question since, clearly, both parties have something meaningful to contribute. Armed with information from the group about the 'kind of person" the group needs, HR personnel ought to be able to do more effective recruiting. In addition, they can pre-screen applicants in a way that satisfies both the group's requirements and those of the organization. They can also provide support and advice to the group about how best to conduct selection interviews, how to make a selection decision, and the like. Popular press reports suggest that interviews conducted by group members are becoming more common (e.g. *The Financial Post*, 1994; Jenish, 1994). Though it seems likely that this practice will enhance attitudes toward both domains, it has not yet received much research attention.

Second, organizations should work toward incorporating the assessment of characteristics that facilitate group work into their selection strategies. Stevens & Campion (1994b) recently developed an instrument to assess the individual knowledge, skills and abilities that facilitate working in groups. Though work on this instrument is in its early stages, available validity evidence appears promising. Other approaches to selecting team players make use of personality assessment (Kinlaw, 1991), structured interviews and assessment centre techniques. This is a relatively new direction in selection research; not surprisingly, then, consensus does not yet exist as to the most effective way to assess team-relevant characteristics. It is encouraging to note, however, that organizations wishing to incorporate individual differences in "team playing" into their selection strategy have some viable options to explore.

Temporary Staffing of Groups

A related staffing issue that has also received relatively little attention in the research literature involves how the organization (or the group, for that matter) deals with the problem of temporarily replacing group members who are absent from work. In many cases, of course, group members are not replaced; the group simply does its work without the absent member(s). Where staffing of this nature is done, however, it can be done either with or without reference to group-relevant factors. Extrapolating from recent research showing that "familiarity" is related to group effectiveness (Goodman & Garber, 1988; Goodman & Leyden, 1991; Goodman & Shah, 1991), the former would seem preferable. Familiarity is conceptualized as the employee's knowledge about the unique configuration of features associated with a workplace (in this case, the group, its tasks and its environment). Given the importance of familiarity for effective group operation, staffing done without familiarity in mind may lead, via work disruptions, to increased stress and, perhaps, diminished attitudes toward the group. The more important point here, however, is that an organization that chooses to do staff replacement without consideration of how familiar the replacement worker is with the group and its constraints is communicating that the group, as an identifiable entity, is not very important. This is unlikely to have positive consequences for attitudes toward that organization.

Training Issues

Training is one human resource management activity around which there appears to be considerable sensitization about the need for congruence between the organization and the group. This is especially true if the organization in question is one that believes itself to have, or is working toward the creation of, a "team culture". Rarely does one see a description of an organization that thinks it has a team culture that does not include an exhortation about the importance of more and better employee training.

Do organizations that rely on groups actually emphasize training? Relative to organizations that care little about groups, it seems that they do, though the amount of training may be less than some organizations would like. A recent report from the Conference Board of Canada, for example, indicated that although most companies in the survey provide some training, "only 12% of companies consistently translate need into action" (Booth, 1994). Viewed from the perspective of organization–group congruence, however, the amount of training an organization does is perhaps not the most important issue. Instead, it is argued that organizations that want to be seen as actually valuing the groups that they claim to value should pay particular attention to two factors: appropriateness of the training and the contextual supports for the new behaviours that the training encourages.

Appropriateness

Lost, sometimes, in the "teams mean more training" mantra is a clear description of *which* skills need improving. Organizations need to remind themselves why it is that group-based organizations are believed to need more training (and determine whether this logic applies to them). A major part of the logic is that, at least in Western culture, individuals are not particularly good at working collaboratively (Nahavandi & Aranda, 1994). Thus, we need help developing the interpersonal skills that facilitate true team activity. Unless the organization has assiduously selected for these skills (as discussed above), it must make the interpersonal skills needed for group work the cornerstone of its training programme. Failure to do so means that the employees will quickly recognize an important incongruity: while group structure may characterize their organization, actually valuing group activity does not.

A second reason that team-based organizations are advised to emphasize training has to do with the notion of multi-skilling. There are many groups in which it is both possible and appropriate for all group members to learn to do most of the tasks a given group member might be called upon to do. In such cases, training aimed at multi-skilling makes sense. In other groups, however, it is *not* necessary (neither does it makes sense) for all members to have the same large set of skills. Instead of providing training aimed at multi-skilling in such groups (something doomed to failure in a group/task not suited to it), it may be much better to arm members with (a) the kind of pride in the group and its goals that will prevent them from saying "sorry, it's not my job", and (b) the resources (time, information, "permission") to locate and mobilize the person whose job it is.

Unfortunately, there has been a tendency for some organizations to overgeneralize the real need for multi-skilling. In attempting to provide "all skills for all people", the organization communicates that it does not really understand the group in question, but, instead, is just mindlessly buying into the prevailing enthusiasm for groups and the training strategies that have been associated with them. It is unlikely that any attitudinal impact of this sort of incongruence between organizational practices and group needs will be a positive one.

Contextual Supports

Here the main issue is whether or not the training provided is supported, and thus reinforced, by other features within the organizational and group contexts (e.g. reward system; technology). Clearly, mixed messages must be avoided. For example, an organization may encourage, through training, the development of interpersonal skills that mean team members will risk trusting each other, will sacrifice individual accomplishments for the good of the team, and so on. But what message is being sent if individual performance evaluation excludes any group-based outcomes? What message is being sent by the organization that provides group members with complex skills training, yet does not provide the group with the appropriate technology or resources to make use of the skills? Or provides training in participative decision-making but no group-based authority to make real decisions? Or couples intense team development training with a policy of frequent intra-organizational personnel transfers?

Appraising and Rewarding Performance

The performance of many complex jobs requires extensive interaction between, and coordination among, group members. Consequently, the outcomes associated with these efforts can rarely be attributed to any single individual but are, in fact, group outcomes. Indeed, if it is a "real group", it is for exactly these reasons that the group was formed in the first place. Organizational practices regarding performance appraisal and rewards, however, are often quite incongruent with this group reality. This manifests itself in two quite different ways.

Acknowledging Group Outcomes

First, appraisal and reward systems often deal with work performance only at the level of the individual. That is, individual accomplishments are appraised and rewarded, rather than group accomplishments. This puts the individual employee in a difficult and frustrating position. On the one hand, he or she is encouraged by the group, and by the constraints of the tasks, to work collaboratively with work group members. On the other, his or her "rewards" are reaped on the basis of an appraisal of individual accomplishments—measures which may not well reflect individual contributions to the group.

This incongruence between what the organization dictates, through its reward structure, and how group members really behave on the job is a major problem which has been discussed repeatedly in the literature. The focus of most discussions has been on the effects on group functioning and performance. It seems reasonable to suggest, however, that affective attachment to the group and, especially, to the organization will also suffer in the face of this incongruence. The "solution", of course, lies with incorporating group-level outcomes into the appraisal and reward system. This is by no means a solution without challenges (e.g. social loafing, how to reward "stars"). Viewed with the goal of sustaining positive attitudes toward *both* the organization and the group, however, the benefits of evaluating group-level outcomes (e.g. Booth, 1994; Hanlon, Meyer & Taylor, 1994; Pritchard et al., 1988) would seem to outweigh the difficulties.

Acknowledging "Team Players"

In suggesting that performance evaluation should incorporate group-level outcomes, however, few would argue that individual-level evaluation should be eliminated. Clearly, individuals need feedback about how they are doing, what behaviours are particularly valued, how they can improve, and so on. The second appraisal-related manifestation of incongruence between the organization and the group involves an important aspect of individual performance: behaving as a "team player". Internally, most groups recognize how valuable team players are. Thus, work group members who disrupt, rather than work with, the group are likely to be sanctioned informally by other group members. In a recent survey of over 100 Canadian organizations, for example, more than one-third of respondents indicated that individual contribution to team performance was assessed "on an informal or *ad hoc* basis" (Booth, 1994).

At the organizational level, however, few organizations explicitly incorporate this aspect of individual behaviour into their formal performance evaluation systems. (Within the same survey, for example, only 10% of respondents reported that individual contributions to the team were integrated formally into the performance evaluation systems.) This has two implications. First, the "team-playing" individual is given no formal recognition for his or her efforts to work as a member of a team. In cultures that, traditionally, have not emphasized teamwork, such efforts do not come naturally and, thus, may be especially deserving of recognition. Second, groups and their leaders are given no legitimate means by which the honing of the knowledge, skills, and abilities (KSAs) necessary for team-playing can be put on the employee development agenda. How can a group leader justify asking a particular group member to work on these KSAs, or justify allocating resources to KSA development, if the organization itself appears not to care about them?

The suggestion that individual performance evaluation should include an examination of the employee's team playing is entirely consistent with, and complements, two earlier suggestions about selection and training. What is being called for here is congruence—both across domains (organization and group) and within the organizational (HR) domain. These notions are not new. Indeed, though the focus has been on group functioning, rather than employee affect, the issues of congruence highlighted by these suggestions have been given considerable attention within the literature. We turn now to an area that, in contrast, has been given very little research attention.

Do Group Practices Acknowledge the Value of the Organization?

This relatively neglected question involves the extent to which group behaviours acknowledge the importance of the larger organization. Certainly, most group practices are less formalized than the organizational practices described above and many are shaped by the constraints of the tasks and by superordinate organizational policy. It would be naive to suggest, however, that the group has no control over the development of practices that can either complement, or be at odds with, organizational policies and practices.

Habitual Group Behaviour

Recent work on habitual behaviour within groups (Gersick & Hackman, 1990) illustrates how easily group habits develop, particularly under some conditions, and how tenaciously group members cling to these habits—even in the face of evidence that suggests that they are unjustified or dysfunctional. Such habits come to represent "truth".

There are several group habits that appear to disregard the importance of the larger organizational context or other groups within it and, as such, could be considered "unfriendly" to the idea of the organization. One that is commonly indulged in is that of "head-office bashing"—no matter what senior managers suggest, the first reaction of many groups is negative. Though senior management may be the favoured target of habitual derision, it is not the only one. Groups can, and do, extend this behaviour to any area of the organization (e.g. "the plant", "the people in finance", "administrators"). Another example of a group habit that could be considered incongruent with larger aims of the organization is that of spending department (group) funds at the budgetary year-end, regardless of real need, in order to avoid returning the funds to the central budget unit. Finally, groups can develop habitual ways of expressing their dissatisfaction. Those that express dissatisfaction through what Hirschman (1970) calls "voice" direct appropriately timed suggestions for change to the appropriate people within the organization. They are behaving, one could argue, in the interests of both the group and the organization. Other groups take a more passive, but equally habitual approach, developing almost ritualized "scripts" for complaining, but attempting no change-directed action.

External Activity

The extent to which the group acknowledges the importance of the larger organization is also reflected in the ways in which it chooses to interact with the environment beyond the group. Research by Ancona and her colleagues (Ancona, 1990; Ancona & Caldwell, 1992) describes the various external activities in which groups engage. Though this research has focused primarily on group performance, it seems reasonable to suggest that external activities, or boundary-spanning, will also influence individual attitudes.

One way in which external activity may have an impact upon attitudes toward the group and organization is by increasing the individual's knowledge about group–organization fit, as discussed above. The second is perhaps more straightforward. The more one interacts with people beyond the group, the more likely he or she is to develop positive interpersonal relationships within the wider organization. These, in turn, should promote a generalized feeling of belonging or affective attachment to the organization.

Considered with these processes (knowledge about fit; social contact) in mind, the *amount* of external activity in which the individuals and their groups engage is of particular importance. Unless contact is extremely superficial or extremely negative in tone, one would expect that amount of external activity will be correlated with affective attachment to the organization: the more, the better. Available evidence is generally supportive of this. Though Ancona & Caldwell (1992) did not directly compare the attitudes toward the organization held by individuals in "isolationist" groups with those whose groups had more external contacts, their description of isolationist groups suggest that these are not groups that are much concerned with their position in, or relation with, the larger organization. Specifically, we are told that isolationist groups have "impermeable boundaries that allow them a cocoon-like existence" (p. 663) and seem to be "oblivious to the negative feedback from other parts of the organization" (p. 662). It seems unlikely that such activity will produce strong individual affective attachment to the organization.

Interestingly, even more important than the *amount* of external activity are the *types* of activities in which a group engages. For example, all the highly successful groups that Ancona & Caldwell (1992) studied engaged in "ambassadorial activities" (e.g. lobbying for resources; garnering support for the group). In contrast, groups that engaged in prolonged "scouting activities" (e.g. scanning the external environment for ideas and information) were relatively unsuccessful. Interestingly, scouting activities were also negatively related to group-level cohesion, while ambassadorial activities were positively related to group cohesion.

It is important to note here that this research has not focused on individually held attitudes, toward either the group or organization. Thus, the comments made here are extremely speculative. Viewed from the perspective of congruence, however, the extension of the boundary-spanning notion to the study of dual attitudes would seem a fruitful one. There may well be patterns of external activity, adopted by groups, that provide a more organization-friendly context for group members than do others. Through these patterns the group may communicate, and make normative, particular views of the organization. For example, the technical scouting pattern identified by Ancona & Caldwell (1992) may be associated with a view of the larger organization as simply an information source to be mined, rather than a valuable goal-oriented entity in itself. Patterns of external activity, then, can be thought of as both antecedents and consequences of group members' attitudes toward the larger organization. Newcomers will take their attitudinal cues from them and old-timers will habitually enact them, perhaps having long since forgotten the reason they developed.

Clearly, whether or not external activity (both type and amount) has implications for the attitudes that group members have toward the two domains in which we are interested is a question that awaits further empirical study. Most useful would be research that explicitly examines the organization-friendliness of the activities that make up each pattern of activity.

GROUP LEADERSHIP IN ORGANIZATIONAL CONTEXT

Although not every group or team has someone who can be considered its leader, many do. The group leader can play a pivotal role in shaping positive employee attitudes toward both the group and the organization. In order to do this, however, the leader must be particularly mindful of the group's relation to the larger organizational context, must acknowledge that both domains are important and, of course, must have strong positive attitudes toward both. Further, the group leader must be someone who can successfully cross the various boundaries within the organization.

Interestingly, although much has been written about how best to lead groups, a quick review of texts or chapters on group psychology will demonstrate that the larger contextual nature of the leadership role is virtually ignored. Just as little emphasis is placed on the embedded nature of the group within the organization, little is placed on the embedded nature of the group leadership role within the organization. Despite this, it seems quite likely that the group leader's influence extends not only to employee attitudes and behaviour that are of relevance to the group, but also to the larger organization. In order to mobilize this influence successfully, he or she must be—and be seen to be—both a group leader *and* an organizational leader.

What can group leaders do to enhance, and help sustain, the attitudes of group members to *both* domains? Drawing on the logic of earlier sections of the chapter, it is argued here that they must engage in "congruence-enhancing" behaviours. Specifically, we are referring here to behaviours that increase employees understanding of group–organization fit and facilitate congruence between the policies and practices of the group and those of the organization.

Ambassadorial Behaviours

Of primary importance among congruence-enhancing behaviours are the messages the group leader sends about what the group is, what it does, why it is important, and how it fits with the rest of the organization. Groups leaders who want to enhance positive attitudes toward both domains must be able and eager to send such messages to *any* member of the organization (inside or outside the group). Such messages not only serve to enhance understanding of group–organization fit (both internally and externally), they also communicate that the leader is an advocate for the group and one who recognizes the importance of its organizational context. Thus, a distinction is drawn here between this approach and that taken by leaders who champion their groups' causes at all costs, regardless of the impact on the organization.

Also important are the messages the group leader delivers on behalf of the organization. He or she must be able to provide timely and accurate information about organizational-level issues, decisions and events and do so in a way that is meaningful to group members. Better still, group leaders should encourage group members to learn about the broader organization for themselves. Leaders that keep walls around their groups (the "isolationist groups"; the "overbounded groups") may increase positive attitudes toward the group—though perhaps only in the short term. It seems quite likely, however, that they do so at the expense of an understanding of group–organization fit and attitudes toward the organization.

Taken together, these behaviours resemble the "ambassadorial" behaviours described by Kraut and his colleagues; these include "communicating the needs of one's work group to others, helping subordinates interact with other groups, and acting as the work group's representative" (Kraut et al., 1989; p. 289). Kraut et al. examined the importance of various behaviours across several levels of management. Though there were many differences, one similarity was clear: ambassadorial behaviours were rated as important, and equally so across all levels of management.

Working Toward Congruence Between Group and Organizational Practices

The group leader is particularly well positioned to help achieve congruence between group and organizational practices of the sort outlined earlier. To do this, however, requires that the leader has considerable diagnostic and political skills and good knowledge of both internal (group) and external (organizational) processes. Most importantly, he or she must be willing to fight for congruence, whether that means working toward changes at the level of the group or the organization.

Interventions Within the Group

Earlier, it was suggested that the extent to which the group acknowledges the importance of the larger organization is reflected in two types of behaviours: its habitual routines (*vis à vis* other parts of the organization) and the more conscious choices it makes about interactions with the external environment. Both are potential sources of group–organization incongruence that may be influenced by interventions initiated by the group leader.

As Gersick & Hackman (1990) have noted, groups tend to maintain habitual routines unless explicitly impelled to do otherwise. Consider those habitual routines that characterize the group and other parts of the organization as being in a "we–they" relationship (e.g. head-office bashing; chronic, but passive complaining about other units). Given that such routines often have a socio-emotional basis, they may be particularly difficult to alter (Gersick & Hackman, 1990). Having identified the need to change a habitual routine within the group, therefore, the leader must be especially vigilant for, and/or willing to create, an appropriate impetus for change. These include reaching a milestone, experiencing failure, redesigning the group task, or experiencing personnel changes (including, for example, a new group leader). Even within that window of opportunity, however, the leader may have to time any intervention very carefully. The importance of timing is illustrated by the finding that how group leaders acted in initial meetings set lasting precedents for group interaction (Ginnett, 1987). It seems likely they will also set precedents for how group members interact with, talk about, and think about others in the external environment.

Research on external activity is in its relatively early stages and, as yet, has not directly examined the links between particular patterns of external activity and individual work attitudes. At the simplest level, and consistent with our arguments about enhancing employee understanding of group–organization fit, however, it seems likely that some external activity is better than none. Thus, group leaders who hoard, for themselves, all opportunities for boundary-spanning are doing few favours for the other members of their groups. Indeed, one could make the argument that a group leader is also an organizational leader to the extent that he or she encourages all members of the group to engage in meaningful boundary-spanning behaviour.

Beyond this, little information can be offered to group leaders about the specific implications, for work attitudes, of various patterns of external activity. In the absence of a larger research base, however, group leaders should be aware that patterns may make a difference and should attempt to monitor apparent links between patterns of activity and attitudes toward the group and organization. If the group leader truly is also an organizational leader, he or she will be mindful of the need to find a balance between underbounded and overbounded groups. Finally, it may be useful to think about the patterns of external activities that evolve in groups as particularly complex habitual routines (involving, not incidentally, the habitual routines of others outside the group). As such, they will be particularly resistant to change. Here the group leader might profitably intervene by encouraging the group to develop meta-routines (Gersick & Hackman, 1990) whereby they regularly review sets of behaviours to see if they are still functional. Gersick & Hackman argue that such interventions are unlikely to be successful in groups unless members have "logged a good measure of experience working together" (p. 94).

Interventions Beyond the Group

Organizations that structure work along group lines claim that they value groups and group-based activity, but often behave in a manner that is at odds with this claim. In order to effect congruence-related change that is external to the group (e.g. altering reward structures, providing support for training), group leaders must have two important sets of characteristics. First, the need for political skills, and boundary-spanning acumen, is particularly acute for such changes. In her analysis of organizational life, Kanter (1977) described the damage suffered by work group members whose leaders were relatively powerless outside the group. In addition to the concerns she expressed, we would add the following: without such power the group leader will be unable to convince others that their group, as a psychological reality, is important. Second, it is in this area that the comments made by Hackman & Walton (1990) about the critical need for group leaders with courage may be particularly important. In addition to political skill, group leaders need to be willing to take risks to ensure that the efforts they ask group members to put into their tasks are reinforced by a structure that recognizes and values those efforts. Some group leaders will have this courage and some, regrettably, will not.

Handling Conflict Between Domains

Obviously, it will not be possible to eliminate all conflict that arises as a result of the interplay between group and organizational concerns (Reichers, 1985). Neither is it reasonable, or desirable, to expect that group preferences and those of the larger organization will always coincide. Given this, an important task for group leaders is to assist group members in putting such conflict into perspective—by making it clear that conflict is an inevitable fact of organizational life, providing the group with extensive background information about a given conflict, and developing group-level and individual-level strategies for coping with the day-to-day stress of domain conflict.

Such activities are also important because they reduce the likelihood that tensions will escalate into serious, and often dysfunctional, antagonism and/or will create serious internal turmoil for individual employees. This latter concern is a particularly important one. At the beginning of the chapter, it was suggested that the development of strong affective attachment to both the group and organizational domains could benefit both the workplace and the individual. Unfortunately, we know very little about how serious conflict between domains is experienced by those employees who have strong attachment to both. It seems reasonable to suggest, however, that such situations may be the "exception to the rule". Indeed, unlike employees who have little attachment to either domain, or those with strong "partisan" attachments to only one domain, employees with strong attachments to *both* domains may find very painful those situations in which the organization and the group make competing demands. Group leaders cannot ignore this potential downside of strong dual attachment and must be prepared to deal with its implications for the individual. Indeed, perhaps above all else, the group leader who is also an organizational leader will work toward helping people make meaningful, and psychologically comfortable, sense of their dual membership.

CONCLUSIONS

The development of attitudes toward the group and the organization have been extensively researched and, indeed, many workplace interventions have been based on results of this largely single-domain research. Members of "real groups", however, do not belong to a single-domain workplace. This must be explicitly acknowledged if we wish to enhance employee attitudes toward, and enjoyment of, *both* the work group and the organization. Borrowing notions of congruence from the effectiveness/performance literature, it is suggested that we must begin by asking two sorts of questions: (a) Does the employee live in an organizational world that truly supports his or her group membership? and (b) Does the employee live in a group world that is meaningfully connected to the wider universe of the organization? If the answer to either of these questions is

"No", it seems unlikely that employees will develop strong positive attitudes to both, or possibly either, of their workplace worlds.

REFERENCES

Allen, N.J. & Meyer, J.P. (in press). Affective, continuance, and normative commitment to the organization: a examination of construct validity. *Journal of Vocational Behavior*.

Ancona, D.G. (1990). Outward bound: strategies for team survival in an organization. *Academy of Management Journal*, **33**, 334–365.

Ancona, D.G. & Caldwell, D.F. (1992). Bridging the boundary: external activity and performance in organizational teams. *Administrative Science Quarterly*, **37**, 634–665.

Angle, H.L. & Lawson, M.B. (1994). Organizational commitment and employees' performance ratings: both type of commitment and type of performance count. *Psychological Reports*, **75**, 1539–1551.

Ashforth, B.E. & Mael, F. (1989). Social identity theory and the organization. *Academy of Management Review*, **14**, 20–39.

Becker, T.E. (1992). Foci and bases of commitment: are they distinctions worth making? *Academy of Management Journal*, **35**, 232–244.

Becker, T.E. & Billings, R.S. (1993). Profiles of commitment: an empirical test. *Journal of Organizational Behavior*, **14**, 177–190.

Begley, T.M. & Czajka, J.M. (1993). Panel analysis of the moderating effects of commitment on job satisfaction, intent to quit, and health following organizational change. *Journal of Applied Psychology*, **78**, 552–556.

Booth, P. (1994). *Challenge and Change: Embracing the Team Concept*. Report 123–94. Ottawa: The Conference Board of Canada.

Campion, M.A., Cheraskin, L. & Stevens, M.J. (1994). Career-related antecedents and outcomes of job rotation. *Academy of Management Journal*, **37**, 1518–1542.

Chatman, J.A. (1991). Matching people and organizations: selection and socialization in public accounting firms. *Administrative Science Quarterly*, **36**, 459–484.

Cohen, A. (1993). Organizational commitment and turnover: a meta-analysis. *Academy of Management Journal*, **36**, 1140–1157.

Deutsch, M. (1949). An experimental study of the effects of cooperation and competition upon group process. *Human Relations*, **2**, 199–231.

Financial Post. (1994). Loyalty is the reward for good hiring. December 17.

Gersick, C.J. & Hackman, J.R. (1990). Habitual routines in task-performing groups. *Organizational Behavior and Human Decision Processes*, **47**, 65–97.

Ginnett, R.C. (1987). First Encounters of the Close Kind: The First Meetings of Airline Flight Crews. Unpublished doctoral dissertation, Yale University, New Haven, CT.

Goodman, P.S. & Garber, S. (1988). Absenteeism and accidents in a dangerous environment: empirical analysis of underground coal mines. *Journal of Applied Psychology*, **73**, 81–86.

Goodman, P.S. & Leyden, D.P. (1991). Familiarity and group productivity. *Journal of Applied Psychology*, **76**, 578–586.

Goodman, P.S., Ravlin, E. & Schminke, M. (1987). Understanding groups in organizations. *Research in Organizational Behavior*, **9**, 121–173.

Goodman, P.S. & Shah, S. (1991). Familiarity and work group outcomes. In S. Worchel, W. Wood & J.A. Simpson (eds) *Group Process and Productivity*. Newbury Park: Sage, pp. 276–298.

Guzzo, R.A. & Shea, G.P. (1992). Group performance and intergroup relations in organizations. In M.D. Dunnette & L.M. Hough (eds), *Handbook of Industrial and Organizational Psychology*. Palo Alto: Consulting Psychologists' Press, pp. 269–313.

Hackman, J.R. & Walton, R.E. (1990). Leading groups in organizations. In P.S. Goodman (ed.), *Designing Effective Work Groups*. San Francisco: Jossey-Bass, pp. 72–119.

Hanlon, S.C., Meyer, D.G. & Taylor, R.R. (1994). Consequences of gainsharing: a field experiment revisited. *Group and Organization Management*, **19**, 87–111.

Hirschman, A.O. (1970). *Exit, Voice and Loyalty: Responses to Decline in Firms, Organizations, and States*. Cambridge, MA: Harvard University Press.

Hunt, S.D. & Morgan, R.M. (1994). Organizational commitment: one of many commitments or key mediating construct? *Academy of Management Journal*, **37**, 1568–1587.

Ibarra, H. & Andrews, S.B. (1993). Power, social influence, and sense-making: effects of network centrality and proximity on employee perceptions. *Administrative Science Quarterly*, **38**, 277–303.

Janis, I.L. (1982). *Groupthink: Psychological Studies of Foreign Policy Decisions and Fiascos*. Boston: Houghton-Mifflin.

Jenish, D. (1994). Corporate culture club. *MacLean's*, December 12.

Johns, G. (1991). Substantive and methodological constraints on behavior and attitudes in organizational research. *Organizational Behavior and Human Decision Processes*, **49**, 80–104.

Kanter, R.M. (1977). *Men and Women of the Corporation*. New York: Basic Books.

Kinlaw, D.C. (1991). *Developing Surperior Work Teams: Building Quality and the Competitive Edge*. San Diego, CA: Lexington Books.

Korsgaard, M.A., Schweiger, D.M. & Sapienza, H.J. (1995). Building commitment, attachment, and trust in strategic decision-making teams: the role of procedural justice. *Academy of Management Journal*, **38**, 60–84.

Kraut, A.I., Pedigo, P.R., McKenna, D.D. & Dunnette, M.D. (1989). The role of the manager: what's really important in different management jobs. *The Academy of Management Executive*, **3**, 286–293.

Louis, M.R., Posner, B.Z. & Powell, G.N. (1983). The availability and helpfulness of socialization practices. *Personnel Psychology*, **36**, 857–866.

Louis, M.R. (1980). Surprise and sense-making: what newcomers experience in entering unfamiliar organizational settings. *Administrative Studies Quarterly*, **25**, 226–251.

Mathieu, J.E. & Zajac, D. (1990). A review and meta-analysis of the antecedents, correlates, and consequences of organizational commitment. *Psychological Bulletin*, **108**, 171–194.

McShane, S.L. & Baal, T. (1984). *Employee Socialization Practices on Canada's West Coast: A Management Report*. Burnaby, British Columbia: Simon Fraser University.

Meyer, J.P. & Allen, N.J. (1991). A three-component conceptualization of organizational commitment. *Human Resource Management Review*, **1**, 61–89.

Morrison, E.W. (1993a). Longitudinal study of the effects of information seeking on newcomer socialization. *Journal of Applied Psychology*, **78**, 173–183.

Morrison, E.W. (1993b). Newcomer information seeking: exploring types, modes, sources, and outcomes. *The Academy of Management Journal*, **36**, 557–589.

Mullen, B. & Copper, C. (1994). The relation between group cohesiveness and performance: an integration. *Psychological Bulletin*, **115**, 210–227.

Nahavandi, A. & Aranda, E. (1994). Restructuring teams for the re-engineered organization. *Academy of Management Executive*, **84**, 58–68.

Nelson, R.E. (1989). The strength of strong ties: social networks and intergroup conflict in organizations. *Academy of Management Journal*, **32**, 377–401.

Ostroff, C. & Kozlowski, S.W.J. (1992). Organizational socialization as a learning process: the role of information acquisition. *Personnel Psychology*, **45**, 849–874.

Ostroff, C. & Kozlowski, S.W.J. (1993). The role of mentoring in the information gathering processes of newcomers during early organizational socialization. *Journal of Vocational Behavior*, **42**, 170–183.

Pritchard, R.D., Jones, S.D., Roth, P.L., Stuebing, K.K. & Ekeberg, S.E. (1988). Effects of group feedback, goal setting, and incentives on organizational productivity. *Journal of Applied Psychology*, **73**, 337–358.

Reichers, A.E. (1985). A review and reconceptualization of organizational commitment. *Academy of Management Review*, **10**, 465–476.

Reichers, A.E. (1986). Conflict and organizational commitments. *Journal of Applied Psychology*, **71**, 508–514.

Romzek, B.S. (1989). Personal consequences of employee commitment. *Academy of Management Journal*, **32**, 649–661.

Shim, W. & Steers, R.M. (1994). Mediating Influences on the Employee Commitment–Job Performance Relationship. Unpublished manuscript.

Stevens, M.J. & Campion, M.A. (1994a). The knowledge, skill, and ability requirements for teamwork: implications for human resource management. *Journal of Management*, **20**, 503–530.

Stevens, M.J. & Campion, M.A. (1994b). Staffing teams: development and validation of the Teamwork KSA test. Paper presented at the annual meeting of the Society of Industrial and Organizational Psychology. Nashville, TN.

Tajfel, H. (1981). *Human Groups and Social Categories: Studies in the Social Psychology of Intergroup Relations*. London: Academic Press.

Yoon, J., Baker, M.R. & Ko, J. (1994). Interpersonal attachment and organizational commitment: subgroup hypothesis revisited. *Human Relations*, **47**, 329–351.

Zaccaro, S.J. & Dobbins, G.H. (1989). Contrasting group and organizational commitment: evidence for differences among multilevel attachments. *Journal of Organizational Behavior*, **10**, 267–273.

Chapter 16

Intergroup Relations in Organizations

Jean F. Hartley
Birkbeck College, University of London, UK

Abstract

The aim of this chapter is to review theoretical and empirical developments in intergroup relations, drawing on both social and organizational psychology. The gaps but also the links between social and work/organizational psychology will be critically examined. Intergroup relations is a large field of enquiry, covering collaboration, competition, negotiation, conflict, exclusion, mobility and discrimination between groups. Given this broad field, I will restrict my attention to issues concerning intergroup conflict. Strikes are examined as a form of intergroup conflict. They are a useful phenomenon to analyse because they are vivid and dramatic and so allow examination of processes occurring between groups that may be more hidden or implicit in less antagonistic conflict. The chapter argues that in some circumstances intergroup relations may contribute to and develop group relations rather than *vice versa*. Much social and organizational psychology has assumed that group relations colour intergroup processes. The chapter also argues for the importance of multiple rather than single identities as a factor in intergroup relations, and suggests that identification rather than social identity (as in social psychology theory) may be significant in organizational conflict.

INTRODUCTION

Intergroup relations have always been an important feature of organizational life, and there are indications that they will become more prominent as organizations undergo profound changes in their internal functioning and external interactions. Commentators argue that organizations are attempting to become less bureaucratic (less hierarchical and rule-bound) as they aim to become post-Fordist in their production and organization (e.g. Clegg, 1990; Hales, 1993; Osborne & Gaebler, 1992). If bureaucracy is a means of defining and controlling relations between groups (functions, departments, levels), then attempts to move to more "adhocratic" or organic organizations may mean that groups become more temporary and project-based. The growing use of groups, teams and task forces within many organizations means an increase in intergroup activity, as group members either represent their own group to other groups or must interact as a group with others in order to achieve goals. The potential, not only for cooperation between such groups but also the risk of conflict, is magnified because relations are less defined through hierarchy. Thus, issues of intergroup relations become more pressing to understand for policy reasons. In addition, many organizations are increasingly trying to achieve their aims through partnerships, joint ventures and alliances. For example, public, private and voluntary organizations are working together to provide a variety of community services, and car manufacturing companies combine in joint venture activities to design, produce and market new vehicle models. Such interorganizational relations mean that intergroup relations are likely to be more prominent than in the past as members of different organizations meet to work jointly. The opportunities for intergroup collaboration, but also conflict, are increased in these new ways of internal and external organizing.

Yet the development and use of theories of intergroup relations is very uneven. On the one hand, the theme of intergroup relations is vibrant in social psychology, with the prominence of social identity theory. However, while social identity theory has been applied a range of social issues, applications to the world of work and organizations are rare.

On the other hand, organizational psychologists devote more research attention to intragroup relations (e.g. processes of teambuilding, semi-autonomous work groups, groupthink decision-making) than to intergroup processes (e.g. collaboration, competition, negotiation, conflict) (e.g. Guzzo & Shea, 1992). There has, perhaps, been a tendency to apply existing knowledge to intergroup conflict (e.g. conflict resolution techniques and third-party intervention) rather than push forward the frontiers of theory. However, work and organizational psychology has a long history of interest in intergroup relations since research at the Western Electric company (e.g. Roethlisberger & Dickson, 1939; Lewin, 1948; Bion, 1961; Miller & Rice, 1967), and some commentators would argue that intergroup processes are more important than individual processes in organizations (e.g. Alderfer, 1986; Smith, 1983).

Management theory has long recognized the importance of intergroup relations, though it is largely phrased and conceptualized in structural terms. The structuring of the organization creates groups with varying degrees of interdependence (Thompson, 1967), with the organization defined, in part, by how the division of labour and the integration of tasks occurs (e.g. Lawrence & Lorsch, 1967; Burns & Stalker, 1968; Galbraith, 1973; Mintzberg, 1979). Organizational subcultures develop around the shared interactions of particular groups, whether these are formal or informal (e.g. Trice & Beyer, 1993; Frost et al., 1985; Schneider, 1990).

THE GROUP IN INTERGROUP RELATIONS

The definition of the group is important for how intergroup processes are conceptualized and investigated. McGrath (1984) distinguishes between natural, concocted groups and quasi-groups. The first are groups which exist independently of the researchers who are investigating them. Many or even most organizational groups fall into this category: teams, quality circles, departments and so forth. Concocted groups are either constructed for the purpose of the research (e.g. laboratory groups or allocation to experimental and control groups in an organization's off-the-job training sessions). Quasi-groups exist prior to the research but are constrained or directed by the researcher in their activity and setting (e.g. the reconstruction of negotiation studies in the laboratory using real negotiators, e.g. Balke, Hammond & Meyer (1973)). The distinctions between natural, concocted and quasi-groups are valuable in assessing the extent to which social psychological research, which has made great strides in understanding intergroup relations in an experimental setting, has relevance to the organizational context. In this chapter, we are concerned with the behaviours, attitudes, cognitions and feelings of the natural group in its intergroup relations, with evidence about concocted and quasi-groups used to the extent that the research throws light on natural groups. Organizational psychology has largely concerned itself with natural groups, while social psychology has largely concerned itself with concocted groups.

The classical psychological focus was on the small group and on its relations with other small groups. Such research had its origins in the laboratory and the therapy room (e.g. Bion, 1961; Shaw, 1976; Austin & Worchel, 1979). Here a group may be defined in terms of their interactions with each other (e.g. Homans, 1950), and intergroup relations when contact or actions affecting another (similarly constructed) group occur. Much of our understanding of intergroup conflict, notably from social psychology, derives from such small, closed groups (e.g. Tajfel, 1970; Turner & Giles, 1981).

However, groups in organizations are frequently larger and more complex than this. Some can be defined through the organizational structure, either through the organizational task (e.g. members of the marketing department, employees located at head office) or through their place in the organizational hierarchy (Alderfer, 1986; Smith, 1983). Alderfer (1986) calls these organization groups. Here, the groups are not conceptualized as closed groups but rather membership may change over time. Such organizational groups may be very large and they may not be based on all members knowing each other or on interacting with each other, as they may be geographically very spread (e.g. a national sales force) or their tasks may not bring them into contact with each other. Although such groups are defined by the organizational structure, they are given meaning and group identity both by members and non-members. Indeed, it can be argued that the group characteristics and group identity may differ between intragroup and intergroup relations. For example, those at the corporate centre of an organization may be defined as a coherent group with particular attitudes and values by those in direct service or product provision, while those at the corporate centre itself may perceive large differences and distinctions between their various components (Hartley, Cordingley & Benington, 1995).

This view of a group is more that of an open system. Organization structure and interactions with other groups are integral to the conceptualization. The definition of the group relies to some extent on interdependence of fate rather than similarity between group members (cf. Lewin, 1948). The group may develop identity and a sense of being a group in part through the actions and attitudes of non-members. This suggests that the group can be as much defined by intergroup processes as by intragroup processes. Thus the study of intergroup relations may not begin with the existence of groups, but rather with the proposition that interaction can lead to intra- and inter-group definition. This has important implications for how far the theorizing and empirical evidence which derives from intergroup processes in the laboratory may be useful for understanding intergroup relations in organizations.

Some groups may share the characteristic of interdependence of fate without being part of the organizational structure. For example, commuters may constitute a group relative to the railway organization, or social welfare clients may become a group as a result of their experiences with the social security organization, or citizens relative to the municipal authority. The extent to which they are a group rather than a crowd or collectivity may partly depend on social and psychological processes occurring both within but also importantly between groups.

Larger groups can also be based on identity groups (Alderfer, 1986), also called social categories (Taylor & Moghadam, 1994) where they are constituted through self-categorization or through other people's categorization:

> An identity group may be thought of as a group whose members share some common biological characteristic (such as gender), have participated in equivalent historical experiences (such as migration), currently are subjected to similar social forces (such as unemployment) and as a result have consonant world views. The coming together of world views by people who are in the same group occurs because of their having like experiences and developing shared meanings of these experiences through exchanges with other group members (p. 204).

Interestingly, while social psychologists have not, in the main, shown much interest in organizational groups, they have been prolific in their research on such identity groups, with many studies of intergroup relations between, for example, Jews and Arabs, Hindus and Muslims (e.g. Hewstone, Wagner & Machleit, 1989; Mogghadam, Taylor & Lalonde, 1987) or alternatively international conflict (e.g.

Fisher, 1990, 1994) Their work appears to have largely been focused *either* on the small, closed group *or* on the large social category, but to have neglected the middle ground in which much organizational group and intergroup relations is located.

Organizational psychology has addressed intergroup relations in large social categories. For example, Alderfer (1986) notes that, in practice, organizational and identity groups tend to overlap (e.g. those at the top of many organizational hierarchies are white males, while those at the middle and bottom tend to be women and/or black people). For both types of group he provides a definition (Alderfer, 1977) which pays attention to how intergroup relations shape the existence of the group:

> A human group is a collection of individuals (1) who have significantly interdependent relations with each other, (2) who perceive themselves as a group, reliably distinguishing members from non-members, (3) whose group identity is recognized by non-members, (4) who, as group members acting alone or in concert, have significantly interdependent relations with other groups, and (5) whose roles in the group are therefore a function of expectations from themselves, from other group members and from non-members (p. 230).

This definition includes both relatively objective characteristics (e.g. interdependency) and subjective elements. The group is partly defined from the inside by members but also, importantly, from the outside by non-members. Thus, intergroup relations is integral to the definition of the group.

Taylor & Moghaddam (1994) argue that intergroup relations are similar regardless of size, function or other features of the group (and therefore all theories of intergroup relations ought to be applicable to all groups). However, Rabbie & Horwitz (1988) believe, following Lewin's (1948) distinction between a compact unit and a loose mass, that there is a need to distinguish between groups and social categories in understanding intergroup relations. They argue that a social group is a "dynamic whole" which involves dynamic interrelations between persons in the group, while a social category consists of those who either self-categorize or are categorized by others as sharing some characteristics (this second is similar to Alderfer's identity groups). Rabbie & Horwitz (1988) note that a social category may become a social group in moving from a passive state to an active state where some, though not necessarily all, of its members may engage in dynamic interaction, accentuating, in the process, group properties. I argue that this change from a relatively passive state of social category to the active dynamic of social group is most likely to occur in the context of intergroup relations. Indeed, Rabbie & Horwitz' hypothetical example, of the social category of Brand X toothpaste users who experience a common fate of toxic side-effects having been discovered, illustrates this issue of intergroup relations:

> If the group moves from the passive state of having been acted upon into taking group action to improve its lot, some of its members, though not necessarily all, may

engage in face-to-face interaction, accentuating in the process such group properties as common norms... group identification... etc., culminating in a compact or organized group (p. 119).

There still remains some ambiguity among both social and occupational psychologists as to what they mean by group and intergroup relations, because the same term covers groups along a dimension from the small, face-to-face group to the large organizational or social category. This ambiguity contributes to the confusion about the validity of theories about the onset and progression of conflict.

THE SOCIAL CONSTRUCTION OF INTERGROUP RELATIONS

Much social psychology assumes that groups exist or are created and then intragroup processes lead to intergroup relations. The following is not untypical:

> The encoding and retrieval of these (cognitive) representations is (sic) assumed to underlie judgements about groups and group members, which *in turn* guide intergroup behavior (Messick & Mackie, 1989, p. 46—my emphasis).

Indeed, much of the work on social categorization which underpins some intergroup theory takes as its starting point individual and group cognitions, which are theorized to have a variety of effects at the intergroup level (e.g. Messick & Mackie, 1989; Turner, 1985; Hogg & Abrams, 1988; Brewer & Kramer, 1985). On this basis, Turner (1982) proposed that a group exists where "two or more individuals... perceive themselves to be members of the same social category" (p. 15). However, this definition ignores the public and sometimes intergroup nature of group classification. Brown (1988a) defines the group as existing when "two or more people define themselves as members of (the group) and when its existence is recognized by at least one other" (p. 3). This definition still appears to give primacy to the group's self-categorization and therefore the assumption that the group pre-exists intergroup relations.

However, it may be that groups develop not just in terms of self-categorization or even primarily in this way, as implied above. There are many occasions in organizations where a group is defined as much by non-members as by members. For example, women in organizations may not share an identity as women or perceive themselves as a group within the organization (e.g. Davidson & Burke, 1994; Donnellon & Kolb, 1994) and there are many examples of individuals trying to leave or deny their ascribed social categories (e.g. Taylor & Moghadam, 1994). Yet women may be treated by non-members of that social category (men) as constituting a group. This suggests that self-categorization is not a necessary condition for a group to exist or for intergroup relations to occur. This is an important development because so much of the definitional work by both social and organizational psychologists has arisen from studying the internal characteristics of groups, and then extending analysis to intergroup relations.

This view is reinforced by Taylor & Moggadham (1994), who define intergroup relations as:

> "any aspect of human interaction that involves individuals perceiving themselves as members of a social category, or being perceived by others as belonging to a social category" (p. 6).

This is an essentially psychological definition of intergroup relations, suggesting that a person does not have to be a member of a group (but only perceived to be so) for intergroup relations to occur. Thus, intergroup relations may precede group relations in some circumstances.

In addition, there are schools of social science which emphasize the importance of interaction in the social construction of group and intergroup relations. Mead (1934) and others (e.g. van Maanen, 1979) have shown how personal identity is shaped through interactions with other human beings, and it is quite plausible that social interactions, attributions, language and behaviours of others all may have a part to play in the development of intergroup relations and the group. For example, Moscovici's theory of social representations (Farr & Moscovici, 1984; Moscovici, 1988) is based on the development of shared understandings which emerge through language and conversation. Although his focus is primarily concerned with the development of groups, the approach can be applied to intergroup relations also, with intergroup understanding arising through social representations. Discourse analysis (Potter & Wetherell, 1987) also emphasizes the role of language in the development of social meanings, which may, by logical extension, include intergroup meanings. It has been argued that social identity theory in particular has paid insufficient attention to the temporal aspects of the development of group identity, and that a greater emphasis on the role of communication in intergroup relations would be valuable (e.g. Condor, 1990; Emler & Hopkins, 1990). Some organizational psychologists have tried to apply symbolic interactionism (McCall & Simmons, 1982) to understanding organizational phenomena (e.g. Hosking & Morley, 1991), though it is not clear how the processes of negotiation of identity are to be applied to intergroup relations. Nevertheless, this is a promising line of development. Of course, the work of Foucault (e.g. 1971) has been crucial in showing how subjectivity is shaped by social forces as well as vice versa. However, it is not always clear how a Foucauldian analysis can be applied outside the broad sweep of both history and society, and be used more concretely within specific organizational settings. Nevertheless, his work is providing a spur to a more socially constructed view of groups and intergroup relations. Taylor & Mogghadam (1994) develop a five-stage model of intergroup relations which presupposes the structural conditions in society of clearly stratified intergroup relations.

From the preceding discussion it should be clear that intergroup relations and processes cannot be fully categorized in isolation from the dynamic interrelations between groups. Indeed, the assertion that group dynamics and group identity may follow from, rather than precede, intergroup relations argues for a dynamic view.

THE ORGANIZATIONAL CONTEXT OF INTERGROUP RELATIONS

Much social psychology, as already noted, has avoided examining intergroup relations in an organizational context. Indeed, one aim has been to "isolate the minimal conditions that are sufficient to generate discriminatory ingroup–outgroup attitudes" (Rabbie & Horwitz, 1969, p. 270). This has been developed, in particular, in the minimal group paradigm (e.g. Tajfel, 1970), which has generated massive research activity on intergroup relations (e.g. Brewer, 1991; Brown, 1988a,b; Hogg & Abrams, 1988). However, the external validity of such research remains problematic for organizational psychologists, who wish to examine processes in their organizational context, in the recognition that the context itself may shape relations between groups, and may impart meanings for the actors which are absent from laboratory settings. Schiffman & Wicklund (1992) have argued for the need to develop a "maximal group paradigm", although their suggested variables are largely individualistic and still laboratory-based. However, this is a step in the right direction of developing theory in an appropriate social context.

Brett & Rognes (1986) argue that intergroup relations in organizations must be set in the structural context of the organization and its environment. They suggest that intergroup relations hold a great deal of potential for conflict because of the interdependence between groups to complete organizational tasks which cannot be done by one group alone, but where each group has differentiated skills, abilities and knowledge. Indeed, the work of management theorists (e.g. Lawrence & Lorsch, 1967; Burns & Stalker, 1968; Mintzberg, 1979; Hales, 1993) have noted that an increased level of differentiation can lead to increased problems of integration across teams, groups or departments. Brett & Rognes argue, in particular, that an analysis of power relations is essential to understanding intergroup relations because of the interdependency between groups. In addition, groups in organizations are generally competing for scarce resources in the organization, whether these are financial, staffing, status or other resources: so the potential for conflict is high. Furthermore, managers are often rewarded more for the performance of their teams or departments rather than the quality and effectiveness of lateral relations. In considering why the potential for conflict is endemic but not always expressed, Brett & Rognes argue that power assymetries deter some groups from engaging in conflict behaviours. They argue that power relations tend to be stable, at least in the short term, both because the groups are structurally located in the organization, so that power relations are slow to shift or change, and because perceptions of power relations tend to be stable over time. However, power relations may change as a function of changes in the environment in which the groups operate, which may increase the likelihood of overt conflict.

This concurs in its contextual emphasis with the theoretical work of Miller & Rice (1967) and others adopting an open systems approach to understanding group and intergroup behaviour. Intergroup relations cannot be understood simply as a function of the relations between the two (or more) groups but must be seen in their organizational and systemic context.

Alderfer's (1986) theoretical development of embedded intergroup relations theory also stresses the organizational context within which intergroup relations are enacted by group members. In particular, he notes some key features of intergroup relations, which affect how intergroup relations are likely to be conducted. These include:

1. *Group boundaries* (both physical and psychological). Some groups have relatively easier group entry and exit (permeability) than others.
2. *Power differences*, which in part affect permeability but also the strategies of intergroup relations. This aspect of intergroup relations is largely ignored by social psychologists (but see Sherif, 1966).
3. *Affective patterns*, notably the tendency to split feelings so that positive feelings are associated with own group and negative feelings are projected onto other groups.
4. *Cognitive formations*, including distortions. Alderfer points to the role of language and social categories in influencing perceptions and ideologies about groups and intergroup relations, drawing on the work of social psychologists such as Billig (1976) and Sherif & Sherif (1969).
5. *Leadership behaviour* is an important feature shaping intergroup relations.

These theoretical perspectives on intergroup relations are important because they suggest that intergroup relations do not take place in a vacuum but must be understood in terms of their political, economic, social and organizational context. This is a perspective largely missing from social and even organizational psychology.

INTERGROUP CONFLICT

Conflict within and between organizations can take many forms from interpersonal, through small group to intergroup, including the interorganizational. Some writers have stressed how conflict is endemic in organizations:

> Cooperation is too fragile and fleeting, purposiveness is too elusive, conflict is too frequently and too intensely directed at the very foundation of relationships for a model of benign, episodic conflict to be a valid representation of normal reality (Pondy, 1992, p. 259).

Pondy goes on to argue that organization is precisely a mechanism for internalizing and channelling conflict. Not all conflict is contained by structures, however, and Thomas & Schmidt (1976) found that managers reported spending 20% of their time dealing with conflict, though they did not indicate how much of this was intergroup conflict.

Much writing in organizational psychology has tended to favour explanations of conflict at the interpersonal level. For example, Thomas's (1992a) review of organizational conflict concentrates on the development and progression of conflict without distinguishing between interpersonal and intergroup conflict. His typology of managerial styles for conflict-handling does not refer to theories of intergroup conflict. This is despite a conclusion which notes that:

> Loyalties (cohesiveness)... within strong organizational cultures are often the dominant source of cooperative conflict intentions and behaviours (p. 702).

Mastenbroek (1993) and van der Vliert (1984) do not distinguish between conflict between individuals and groups in their analyses.

Conflict is a multi-faceted, ambiguous and value-laden term (Hartley, 1983) and a number of writers have discussed its meanings. Pondy (1967) notes that the term is used in at least two ways. First, it can refer to the antecedent conditions of conflict (scarce resources or incompatible goals) which may be called a conflict of interests, or latent conflict. Second, it can refer to overt conflict (i.e. expressed in behaviour). Pondy (1967, 1992) argues that for conflict to become overt, antecedent conditions must not just exist, they must be perceived by the parties. The material conditions for conflict are not inevitably translated into overt conflict but are mediated by perceptions. Kornhauser, Dubin & Ross (1954) were also aware of this:

> The reality of opposed interests *as seen by the parties* is, of course, the decisive fact. And the *perceived* relationship obviously depends not only on the "economic facts of life" but also on the social interpretations current among the people involved (p. 14).

In other words, there is an irreducible psychological component in conflict. The question remains as to how psychological theories may best explain the development and progression of conflict.

Thomas (1992a) defines the conflict process as:

> The process that begins when one party perceives that the other has negatively affected, or is about to negatively affect, something that he or she cares about (p. 653).

While this definition does not distinguish between interpersonal and intergroup conflict, it is nevertheless helpful in assessing what might be considered conflict. Putnam & Poole (1987) note that conflict requires interdependence between the parties, the perception of opposition or incompatibility of goals, and some form of interaction between the parties (see also Thomas, 1992b; Kolb & Bartunek, 1994).

In organizational settings, conflict based on intergroup relations can take many forms. Interestingly, not all of it may be expressed in intergroup terms. Donnellon & Kolb (1994) argue that as new social groups (identity groups) enter the workforce, conflicts rooted in class, gender, race and ethnicity have become more prominent, but that existing discourses of organizational conflict management mask the nature of such conflicts, making them appear interpersonal or role-based rather than intergroup-based. Organizational discourses which are based on individual achievement, appraisal and success, and organizational practices which are individualistic, such as many grievance procedures, means that much intergroup conflict may be minimized or avoided.

However, the focus of this section is on conflict which is perceived to be occurring between groups, either within or between organizations. This is therefore about collective rather than individual conflict (though some episodes of intergroup conflict may occur between representatives of the groups in conflict, and collective conflict can get transposed into interpersonal relations). This includes conflict between functional groups (e.g. marketing and production, development and production, business unit and corporate centre) and between groups of employees and managers (e.g. strikes, overtime bans, work-to-rules, lockouts).

I will examine intergroup conflict expressed through strikes (in particular, though not exclusively). Strikes are a useful phenomenon to analyse because they are vivid and dramatic and allow great visibility of intergroup dynamics in conflict (Hartley, 1983; Hartley, Kelly & Nicholson, 1983; Kelly & Kelly, 1992; Bluen, 1993). They allow us to consider some of the processes occurring between groups that may be more hidden or implicit in less antagonistic conflict.

THEORIES OF INTERGROUP CONFLICT

As I am concerned with intergroup processes, I will ignore those theories of conflict and participation in conflict which are based primarily on individual rather than group and intergroup processes (e.g. frustration-aggression theory, Dollard et al., 1939; dissatisfaction, Bluen, 1994; value-expectancy theory, e.g. Klandermans, in press). However, there are several theories and models for considering conflict from an intergroup perspective, especially in the context of industrial action.

Freud's Model of Intergroup Relations

Taylor & Moghaddam (1994) note the intellectual debt of intergroup researchers to Freud (1921) in that, although he had no proper model of group or intergroup processes (preferring instead to take individual unconscious processes to the group level), his work and that of his followers has been significant in its detailing of processes whereby groups tend to displace hostility onto outgroups as a result of in-group cohesion. This has been developed (although not necessarily with the same premises) by other writers who note the importance of unconscious processes, especially projection, in intergroup relations (e.g. Alderfer, 1986; Smith, 1983, 1989; Rice, 1969; see also Stein, this volume). Projective tendencies combined with internal cohesion have been a component of several social psychological and organizational theories, such as those of Sherif (1966). Indeed, in a test of this theory which created particular competitive conditions between groups, such hostility was generated that one field experiment had to be abandoned. Some writers, however, have shown that intergroup projection and hostility, while evident in Sherif's research, and in some organizational settings (e.g. Blake & Mouton, 1962; Blake, Shephard & Mouton, 1964; Shephard, 1965) is not inevitable. Nelson (1989) suggests, from a network and conflict analysis of groups in 20 organizations, that strong ties within groups can be conducive to organizational harmony where the intragroup ties are compensated for by strong ties (frequent contacts) linking groups. Furthermore, there is some debate as to whether the effects of intergroup conflict on in-group cohesion and intergroup hostility is best explained primarily in terms of unconscious processes, as the Freudian tradition would suggest, or primarily through amount of contact between groups (e.g. Hewstone & Brown, 1986; Allen & Stephenson, 1983; Kelly & Kelly, 1991) or through status and structural inequalitites (Kelly & Kelly, 1991). In addition, Freud's work is problematic in that it implies that it is intragroup dynamics which leads to intergroup hostility and conflict, whereas we have already noted from a more social constructionist perspective that, in some circumstances, intergroup relations may precede the group. Nevertheless, his work and that of researchers drawing on the Freudian (or Jungian) tradition of unconscious processes, has been valuable in highlighting the emotional concomitants of intergroup processes. This is in contrast to the perhaps overly cognitive emphasis of certain social psychologists (e.g. Turner, 1985; Hogg & Abrams, 1988; Messick & Mackie, 1989).

Realistic Conflict Theory

Sherif and associates developed a major theory of intergroup conflict in their field experiments with American pre-teenage boys attending summer camps (Sherif, 1966; Sherif & Sherif, 1969). Several experiments were carried out, each lasting 3 weeks. The boys attended camps and were isolated from outside contacts. There were three stages of group interaction: group formation, intergroup conflict (provoked through competition between teams) and the reduction of conflict (through the groups engaging in cooperative behaviours to achieve goals which could only be achieved by the groups working together). This work was a landmark, not only for its methodology (detailed and systematic study of perceptions, attitudes and behaviour in a natural field setting), but also because the cause of conflict was located in relationships between groups rather than in pre-existing motivations and frustrations of individuals. The theory is based on conflict occurring where groups are in competition with each other for scarce resources (a zero sum context), with intergroup antagonism and intragroup solidarity arising from this condition. Where groups were engaged in tasks which needed interdependent behaviour for the goal to be achieved, then cooperation would ensue. Sherif and colleagues were able to manipulate the level of conflict between groups on the basis of whether they were engaged in mutually incompatible or superordinate goals. The argument is that real, material conflicts of interest will (or can) lead to intergroup conflict. The best description of this work is in Sherif (1966), though useful accounts and analyses are available elsewhere (Jackson, 1993; Hartley, 1983; Skinner, 1978; Kelly & Kelly, 1992; Taylor & Moghaddam, 1994; Brown, 1988b). The impact of material competition on intergroup hostility and contact has been noted in research on conflict between employees and management or between groups of employees (e.g. Friedkin & Simpson, 1985; Brown et al., 1986; Blake & Mouton, 1962; Hartley, Kelly & Nicholson, 1983; Hartley et al., 1991; Stagner & Eflal, 1982). The impact of intergroup conflict on intragroup cohesiveness has been supported in some but not all cases of intergroup conflict. Intergroup conflict can lead to a degree of group disintegration (Hartley et al., 1991; Stein, 1976).

Social Identity Theory

This theory (which has also spawned self-categorisation theory, see Turner, 1985) is built on propositions about social categorisation, whereby individuals use categories to structure the social environment and define their own place in it (e.g. Tajfel et al., 1971; Brown, 1988a; Turner, 1975; Tajfel, 1982; Abrams & Hogg, 1990; Hogg & Abrams, 1988). Social identity, it is argued, is based on the knowledge that the person has that he or she belongs to certain social groups, combined with the values that person (and others) attach to that group membership. Individuals wish to belong to groups that compare favourably with, and are distinct from, other groups and that lead to positive evaluations of themselves, i.e. it is argued that social categorisation and comparison leads to increased self-esteem. This approach recognises that individuals may act not out of personal identity but a sense of themselves as representatives of a social group or category (Hogg & Abrams, 1988; Brown, 1988a; Taylor & Moghaddam, 1994). A key finding from social identity research was that group members behaved in a discriminatory manner (favourable to own-group, unfavourable to out-group) even where the group had only just been formed, where the group membership basis was "trivial" and where members did not interact with anyone from either their own or the other group (Tajfel et al., 1971). Individuals apparently behaved on the basis on some feature of group membership, even in conditions stripped of cues about group membership. Discrimination did not develop out of interaction, but because of cognitions about the person's own and the other group.

Social identity theory was developed to explain a range of intergroup behaviours, so it is only partly concerned with intergroup conflict (see Taylor & Moghaddam, 1994). However, it has been applied to the development of differential social identity between groups in a factory (Brown, 1978; Brown &

Williams, 1984) and processes inhibiting the development of equal opportunities (Liff & Aitkenhead, 1992). Social identity theory has also been employed in a model of the determinants of strike action (Kelly & Kelly, 1992), where it is suggested that some strikes will be shaped by the degree of group identification (in either an inhibitory facilitating manner).

Kelly & Kelly (1992) in their assessment of the contribution of social identity theory to understanding intergroup conflict between employees and managers, suggest it may be useful in two ways. First, social identity theory may explain the likelihood of employees taking part in conflict. Second, it may contribute to understanding how social identities are changed or transformed through participation in conflict.

Alderfer's Embedded Intergroup Relations Theory

Alderfer's (1986) work is also built on group identity (though its origins and meanings are different), but is set within organizational psychology. He argues that all people (including researchers) have their emotions, cognitions and behaviours shaped by their multiple group memberships, some of which are organizationally located (e.g. department, level, profession or occupation) and some of which have their origins outside the organization (e.g. race, gender, class). Taken with a clinical perspective (Alderfer, in press) this means that intergroup relations are a function of intrapersonal, intragroup and intergroup forces, and that multiple social identities may be in operation at one time. The theory argues that the group is the primary level of analysis (even where the focus is individual behaviour), and that groups are embedded within social systems, which affect their ways of functioning. Concepts from the theory apply to researchers as well as respondents so the approach is reflexive. Alderfer's approach has already been referred to earlier in the discussion about properties of groups in organizational settings. Group relations are embedded in that individuals carry images of their own and other groups as they serve in representational roles so that intergroup relations are a function of the individual's involvement in other group systems. In addition, parallel processing is likely to occur, which means that after interaction between groups, members may find that their roles and subgroups are changed by the experience and reflect the roles and subgroups of the group with which they have been relating. The empirical support for this model has mainly come from Alderfer and his colleagues (e.g. Smith, 1989) and so has not been widely tested. The approach does not make specific predictions about the course or quality of intergroup relations, but does suggest that in any situation, an understanding of the complex processes of interaction, including conflict, will be enhanced through experiential learning and careful uncovering of the layers of embeddedness of intergroup relations (Alderfer, 1992a,b). The meanings which individuals attach to their and other people's group memberships and social identities is relevant. Alderfer's theory has been used to explain intergroup conflict based on social identities (Alderfer, 1993; Alderfer, 1986; Smith, 1989).

AN ASSESSMENT OF INTERGROUP THEORIES OF CONFLICT

Both realistic conflict theory (RCT) and social identity theory (SIT) have appeal because they claim to explain some of the key intra- and intergroup dynamics involved in conflict between groups. One is based on competition for scarce resources, while the other is built on social identity of groups. One immediate problem with both these theories is that, on the basis of competition or group identity, one would predict much higher levels of intergroup conflict in organizations than currently exist. If it was simply social identity which led to discriminatory behaviours and possible conflict, then the plethora of group identities in the workplace would mean that researchers would be hard-pressed to explain any degree of organizational peace. While SIT is primarily concerned with discriminatory cognitions rather than conflict behaviours as such, this consideration is still relevant where SIT is drawn on to explain conflict. Thus neither theory alone is sufficient to explain the onset or inhibition of overt conflict.

Inhibitors of intergroup conflict, Brett & Rognes (1986) suggest, include structural characteristics of the organization (where hierarchy may be used to prevent conflict), as well as power inequalities. Alderfer (1986) also notes the impact of hierarchy and power on intergroup relations. Thus, intergroup conflict is more likely to occur where there are significant shifts in power relations or major shifts in competition for resources. To be fair, Sherif did recognize this, though many later accounts of his work overlook his view of power as being critical to understanding intergroup conflict:

"... it is important to specify differences from the model of our experiments ... (a) salient difference is that some groups in industry possess notably more power than others" (Sherif, 1966, p. 100)

Any analysis of intergroup conflict must therefore take account not only of group and intergroup dynamics, but must set this in a structural context. Giddens (1979) structuration theory may be one valuable way to examine the impact both of structure and action on behaviour, for example between groups (for a fuller explanation of this approach, see Kirkbride, 1992). Edwards & Scullion (1982), in examining a variety of forms of industrial conflict, have noted that the type and timing of overt conflict can be linked to the power bases of workers and managers, with worker conflict being more likely at that stage of bargaining when their own hand was strongest (see also Edwards, 1995). Batstone et al. (1977, 1978) also found that the threat of strikes was closely related to the bargaining round.

SIT predicts that disadvantaged groups are likely to take action to change a situation of disadvantage where intergroup relations are unstable (cf. Brett & Rognes, 1986) and where the ruling group's authority is seen to be illegitimate (Tajfel, 1978; Ashforth & Mael, 1989), though the research evidence on these conditions is contradictory, depending on whether laboratory or field (organizational) methods are employed (see Taylor & Mogghadam, 1994).

In addition, other factors may contribute to a lower level of intergroup conflict than predicted by RCT or by SIT alone. In the experiments which lead to both theories, the groups were closed (it was difficult if not impossible for subjects to leave the experiments), were temporary (from half an hour to three weeks) and were composed of children. It is likely, therefore, that behaviour is less constrained in organizational settings, where group members may be able to choose to leave the group as an alternative to engaging in conflict, or they may, as adults with a history and an ongoing relationship with other groups, have alternative strategies for dealing with conflict (negotiation, problem-solving, calling in third parties, developing coalitions, gaining support from superiors) or for avoiding conflict entirely (total avoidance, minimizing contact between groups, communicating formally, invoking procedures).

Furthermore, leadership (whether formal or informal) may shape perceptions of opportunities and constraints. For example, in Batstone, Boraston & Frenkel's (1978) study of the social organization of strikes in a vehicle factory, it was found that shop stewards were important not only in developing collective industrial action but also in avoiding it. Strikes were often avoided by convenors and more experienced shop stewards, who used other means, such as informal talks with management, to resolve issues. They were also more aware of the dangers of sectional disputes to strong trade union organization and so were prominent in arguing against strikes. Other researchers have also seen leadership as a key element in the development and focus of intergroup conflict (e.g. Edwards & Scullion, 1982; Hartley, Kelly & Nicholson, 1983; Hartley, 1989; Lane & Roberts, 1971; Alderfer, 1986).

These weaknesses of RCT and SIT may, therefore, suggest that they are less useful in understanding the onset of intergroup conflict than in the processes of conflict. SIT does not model conflict behaviours as such but it does suggest that group identification is sufficient to trigger discriminatory behaviours between groups. RCT shows how ingroup favouritism and the sharpening of ingroup norms of behaviours, attitudes and values, can lead to the projection of hostility and aggression onto the outgroup, and the use of stereotyping, biased perception and discriminatory evaluation of own and outgroup's performance (even where measures show that performance is equivalent). In this sense, we can all, on occasions, act like the children of Sherif's Robber's Cave experiments! There are many examples of intergroup conflict where biased perceptions and discriminatory evaluations of "the other side" are present (e.g. Hartley, Kelly & Nicholson, 1983; Waddington, 1986, 1987; Stagner & Eflal, 1982; Hiller, 1928; Karsh, 1958).

RCT and SIT may help to explain the de-escalation of intergroup conflict. Group identity, especially where it is heightened during the conflict itself, is related to in-group favouritism and outgroup bias, which are not conducive to the resolution or accommodation of conflict. Any conflict calming has to manage the processes which often occur of in-group favouritism and outgroup discrimination, even where this is not the original source of tension. Rational arguments for de-escalation of conflict or cooperative actions may be lost in biased perceptions and distorted cognitions. Indeed, the Sherif experiments showed clearly that having a superordinate goal did not lead immediately to the decline of conflict, but rather only a *series* of interdependent tasks led to the reduction of conflict. This has also been shown in organizational settings (e.g. Blake & Mouton, 1962; Lynn & Donaldson, 1976), where reductions in conflict only occur over time. Some applications of RCT are at variance with the theory in that they have put a premium on changing *perceptions* of group members about superordinate goals, while the theory itself emphasizes the existence of such goals. In addition, the Lynn & Donaldson research showed that material changes (e.g. improvements in payment systems and working conditions) had to be instigated by management for conflict to decline (i.e. which met at least in part the employees' grievances) as well as psychological measures to reduce conflict between the parties (e.g. sharing information, management keeping its word, increased contact between employees and managers).

THE IMPORTANCE OF SOCIAL IDENTITY IN INTERGROUP CONFLICT

Several theories of intergroup relations draw crucially on social or group identity as a mechanism influencing conflict. The industrial relations literature supports with empirical evidence the proposition that social identity is critical to the rhetoric and practices of worker groups in conflict with their managements. However, our consideration of social identity raises as many further questions as it answers (see also Taylor & Mogghadam, 1994; Schiffman & Wicklund, 1992). One question concerns how social identity is defined, while another concerns how it may change and be transformed over time.

While experimental research has shown that individuals can discriminate on the basis of minimal or "trivial" aspects of group categorization (supplied by the experimenters), this has not directly shown that it is a consequence of social identity, which remains largely an inferred concept. There is also the nagging question of why a trivial group membership, given only minutes before the experiment, should be part of a social identity contributing to self-esteem. Is social identity really so plastic? (see also Taylor & Mogghadam, 1994; also Schiffman & Wicklund, 1992; Farsides, 1993; Schiffman, 1993). In addition, once outside the laboratory, the empirical support for social identity as the basis of intergroup conflict is weak (although there are precious few studies). A study by Brown et al. (1986), in a paper-making factory and using departmental groups, is significant, in part, for its attempt to measure group identity, using a 10-item self-report measure. They found that while intergroup polarization was correlated with reported intergroup conflict, the contribution of group identification to polarization was weak, so clearly social identity in this context may not be as important as perhaps has been claimed by some of the experimental social psychological literature.

Research using the minimal group paradigm originally developed by Tajfel et al. (1971) and then extended by others (e.g. Sachdev & Bourhis, 1987) has tended to use either individuals allocated to concocted groups on the basis of trivial categories or identity groups, where group membership is stable and quickly evident (e.g. race, ethnicity, gender, class, linguistic group). In both cases, the group is relatively unambiguous and, for the duration of the experimental period, is usually the only salient group membership. In these settings too, there is generally only one other group present, a situation which is conducive to discrimination and even conflict. Yet, in organizational settings employees will have several group memberships, and hence a variety of social identities open to them. In addition, some of the groups may be ambiguous (for example, membership of a department or a trade union is rarely immediately obvious from the person's physical and linguistic characteristics). There will also be several other "outgroups" in the organization. So, key questions arise as to *how* and *why* individuals and groups draw on, change and use their multiple social identities.

Several pieces of research illustrate the importance of multiple and changing identities at the onset and during the progress of intergroup conflict. For example, in an intense conflict which occurred between UK steel workers and management a national strike was called and prosecuted by all the public sector steelworkers without (Hartley, Kelly & Nicholson, 1983). The "group" which went on strike across the country consisted of over 150 000 steelworkers. Group identity developed in the lead-up and early days of the strike and contrasted with a period of previously peaceful industrial relations. Strong group identity as strikers has been found in many accounts of strikes, especially long and large ones (e.g. Lane & Roberts, 1971; Adeney & Lloyd 1986; Hiller, 1928; Waddington, 1986; Hartley, Kelly & Nicholson, 1983; Fantasia, 1988; Winterton & Winterton, 1989). Group identity may be very important for workers during the "demobilisation" phase (Hiller, 1928) of a labour dispute, especially perhaps in the context where they are perceived as having not gained as much as had been hoped for from the conflict. At the end of the 1984–5 miners' strike in the UK, miners heightened group solidarity and identity by, in many locations, returning to working behind the trade union banner and band.

However, while identity as a national body of steelworkers was evident, the research by Hartley, Kelly & Nicholson (1983, see also Hartley, 1989) showed that other group memberships were or became salient during the strike and became the basis of explicit or implicit behaviours of intergroup conflict and discrimination. These included identities deriving from union, strike activities, closeness to the strike leadership, and values. In this context, what is the "group" which has "social identity" is open to some debate. What is more interesting than the mere fact of multiple groups and memberships is how these develop and change over time in the process of intergroup conflict. Group identities were crucial to the processes of decision-making, leadership and organization of the strike, and arose *during* the period of industrial action (see also Fantasia, 1988; Lane & Roberts, 1971). Boundaries of group membership and hence influence shifted and changed as the strike continued. Actions led to and reinforced identities (see also Ashforth & Mael, 1989).

This could not have been predicted on the basis of group memberships at the beginning of the strike, though it became interpretable in terms of the core values of the leadership of the strike, with these values having the effect of maintaining cohesion and morale in a hostile (external) environment (Hartley, Kelly & Nicholson, 1983). In addition, group identities were in part linked explicitly to the influence of the leadership, and the fact that leadership shifted slightly according to the tasks to be undertaken by the group (see also, Smith, 1983).

Another example serves to illustrate the shifting group identities and changing boundaries on membership. It also raises questions about the target of intergroup conflict. Vogelman (1989, 1995) studied a transport strike among several thousand black workers in South Africa during the Apartheid period. His research indicates that the strikers were initially cohesive and optimistic and that there were three "outgroups": the management, the police (who were often violent in their actions against strikers) and the non-strikers (other black workers who, for reasons of poverty or fear, were not on strike). As in some other strikes, but for reasons which have not been adequately theorized in intergroup terms, the non-strikers became the focus of aggression by those on strike. Is this because non-strikers are a threat to social identity, or because social comparison factors are operating, because they are more accessible, or because they are the least powerful outgroup? These are important questions for intergroup relations theorists to consider. Vogelman's research also illustrates the changing boundaries of group membership and group identity as the strike became more violent. This example again illustrates that social categories of group membership and group identity emerged through actions and interactions and may not be defined in the stable and unambiguous way suggested by many social psychological approaches to intergroup relations.

The issue of shifting identities, and subgroups in intergroup conflict, raises questions about how far such conflict should be characterized in terms of intragroup cohesion and intergroup hostility. While this may be a general pattern, especially with small, closed groups, and indeed is the case at a broad level within strikes (Hartley, Kelly & Nicholson, 1983), this can conceal considerable differentiation within the group itself. Different views and values about strategy and tactics, the management of the conflict, expectations and aspirations may contribute to more subtle group identities, and "inner circles" than is indicated from some intergroup theory. Furthermore, while social psychological theory has suggested decreased contact between groups and this is likely to be true for the group as a whole, some members of the in-group will be in direct working contact with the outgroup, either through dispensations to work (Hartley et al., 1983) or else through roles as negotiators or mediators (Friedman, 1992; Morley, 1992; Walton & McKersie, 1967). We need to learn more about how bargaining and negotiation contribute to group identities during intergroup conflict.

Social Identity or Group Identification?

Social identity theory and realistic conflict theory have been useful in highlighting the role of group categorizations and cognitions in intergroup processes, but perhaps the concept of *social identity* is too strong and stable. Social identity, developed as the group equivalent to personal identity, implies enduring cognition and affect. This is problematic even in the minimal group paradigm, for why should a fleeting allocation to a group cause social identity and contribute to self-esteem? Perhaps what we are witnessing is less a permanent social identity but rather the process of group identification. This may be characterized as more unstable, less enduring, and, importantly, arising in part out of the interactions, perceptions and practices of group and intergroup relations. Of course, individuals may have permanent and stable social identities based on personal or occupational characteristics, but the idea that all social identity is permanent and stable is not supported by the literature. A concept of group identification rather than social identity allows for a more socially constructed view of self as a member of a group. Group identification may be more similar to group commitment (cf. Ashforth and Mael, 1989) than to identity with its presumed links to self-esteem. There appears to be no reason (and indeed not a great deal of evidence) to link social identity to self-esteem, and group identification avoids this assumption.

CONCLUSIONS

This chapter has reviewed the theory and empirical research on intergroup relations, examining intergroup conflict in particular because of its importance and salience in intergroup relations. It has drawn on both social and psychological research and has attempted to marry the best parts of each, despite their uneven development. The first conclusion is that the identity and perceived existence of the group may arise out of intergroup relations rather than necessarily pre-existing. This reverses the implicit cause and effect models of much social psychology where groups are formed, which then engage in intergroup relations (especially discrimination and conflict). Group and intergroup relations cannot be separated, as they may both arise in a dialectical fashion together. This means that our theories of both group and intergroup relations need to be set in their organizational context and that groups should not, perhaps, be studied as isolated phenomena. The organizational context of group and intergroup relations is very important; in particular, organizational structures, power and leadership influence the extent to which conflict is perceived and expressed.

While research on strikes, as a particularly visible form of intergroup conflict, has shown that there are multiple and changing group affiliations and loyalties, there remains a considerable amount of research to undertake in this more socially constructed view of intergroup relations. We need to learn more about the boundaries of group membership in the context of intergroup relations. Some insight may be gained through examining those individuals who are boundary spanners during negotiations or during conflict (see, for example, Friedman, 1992). In addition, research is needed to develop more process rather than content theories of intergroup conflict, including the role of leadership.

The consideration of intergroup relations indicates that the behaviour and dynamics of groups cannot be separated from intergroup relations. There is a dialectical relationship between the processes occurring between and within groups, which may best be accessed through social constructionist theories. As organizations attempt to become more flexible and team-oriented, an understanding of intergroup relations becomes more crucial than ever.

Intergroup relations theories are potentially applicable to understanding a range of phenomena including organizational cultures and subcultures, labour–management conflict, collaboration and competition between teams, organizational and dual commitment, equal opportunities and discrimination, the use of power and conflict, and bargaining and negotiation. This chapter has concentrated on intergroup conflict, though in recognition that in organizations conflict and cooperation are often intertwined.

REFERENCES

Abrams, D. & Hogg, M.A. (1990). *Social Identity Theory: Constructive and Critical Advances.* Hemel Hempstead: Harvester Wheatsheaf.
Adeney, M. & Lloyd, J. (1986). *The Miners' Strike: Loss without Limit.* London: Routledge.
Alderfer, C. (1977). Group and intergroup relations. In J.R. Hackman & J.L. Suttle (eds), *Improving Life at Work.* Santa Monica: Goodyear, pp. 227–296.
Alderfer, C. (1986). An intergroup perspective on group dynamics. In J. Lorsch (ed.), *Handbook of Organizational Behavior.* Englewood Cliffs, NJ: Prentice-Hall.
Alderfer, C.P. (1992a). The race relations competence workshop: theory and results. *Human Relations,* **45**, 1259–1291.
Alderfer, C.P. (1992b). Changing race relations embedded in organizations: report on a long-term project with the XYZ Corporation. In S. Jackson (ed.), *Working with Diversity.* New York: Guilford Press.
Alderfer, C.P. (1993). A group psychological perspective on multiculturalism: what will it take for the high priests and priestesses to change their minds? Keynote address to the A.K. Rice Scientific Meeting, May, State University of New Jersey.
Alderfer, C. & Smith, K. (1982). Studying intergroup relations embedded in organizations. *Administrative Science Quarterly,* **27**, 35–65.
Allen, P.T. & Stephenson, G.M. (1983). Intergroup understanding and size of organization. *British Journal of Industrial Relations,* **21**, 312–329.
Ashforth, B. & Mael, F. (1989). Social identity theory and the organization. *Academy of Management Review,* **14**, 20–39.
Austin, W. & Worchel, S. (eds) (1979). *The Social Psychology of Intergroup Relations.* Monterey, CA: Brooks Cole.
Balke, W.M., Hammond, K.R. & Meyer, G.D. (1973). An alternative approach to labor–management relations. *Administrative Science Quarterly,* **18**, 311–327.
Batstone, E., Boraston, I. & Frenkel, S. (1977). *Shop Stewards in Action: The Social Organization of Workplace Conflict and Accommodation.* Oxford: Blackwell.
Batstone, E., Boraston, I. & Frenkel, S. (1978). *The Social Organization of Strikes.* Oxford: Blackwell.
Billig, M. (1976). *Social Psychology and Intergroup Relations.* London: Academic Press.
Bion, W.R. (1961). *Experiences in Groups.* London: Tavistock.
Blake, R.R. & Mouton, J.S. (1962). The intergroup dynamics of win–loss conflict and problem-solving collaboration in union–management relations. In M. Sherif (ed.), *Intergroup Relations and Leadership.* New York: Wiley, pp. 94–141.

Blake, R.P., Shepard, H.A. & Mouton, J.S. (1964). *Managing Intergroup Conflict in Industry*. Houston: Gulf.

Bluen, S.D. (1994). The psychology of strikes. In C.L. Cooper & I. Robertson (eds), *International Review of Industrial and Organizational Psychology*, Vol. 9. Chichester: Wiley, pp. 113–146.

Brett, J.M. & Rognes, J.K. (1986). Intergroup relations in organizations. In P.S. Goodman (ed.), *Designing Effective Work Groups*. San Francisco: Jossey-Bass.

Brewer, M.B. (1991). The social self: on being the same and different at the same time. *Personality and Social Psychology Bulletin*, **17**, 475–482.

Brewer, M.B. & Kramer, R.M. (1985). The psychology of intergroup attitudes and behaviour. *Annual Review of Psychology*, **36**, 219–243.

Brown, R. & Williams, J. (1984). Group identification: The same thing to all people. *Human Relations*, **37**, 547–564.

Brown, R. (1978). Divided we fall: an analysis of relations between sections of a factory workforce. In H. Tajfel (ed.), *Differentiation between Social Groups: Studies in the Psychology of Intergroup Relations*. London: Academic Press.

Brown, R. (1988a). *Group Processes: Dynamics Within and Between Groups*. Oxford: Blackwell.

Brown, R. (1988b). Intergroup relations. In M. Hewstone, W. Stroebe, J.-P. Codol & G.M. Stephenson (eds), *Introduction to Social Psychology*. Oxford: Blackwell.

Brown, R., Condor, S., Mathews, A., Wade, G. & Williams, J. (1986). Explaining intergroup differentiation in an industrial organization. *Journal of Occupational Psychology*, **59**, 273–286.

Burns, T. & Stalker, G.M. (1968). *The Management of Innovation*, 2nd edn. London: Tavistock.

Clegg, S. (1990). *Modern Organizations*. London: Sage.

Condor, S. (1990). Social stereotypes and social identity. In D. Abrams & M. Hogg (eds), *Social Identity Theory: Constructive and Critical Advances*. Hemel Hempstead: Harvester Wheatsheaf.

Davidson, M. & Burke, R.J. (1994). *Women in Management: Current Research Issues*. London: Paul Chapman.

Dollard, J., Doob, L., Miller, N., Mowrer, O. & Sears, R. (1939). *Frustration and Aggression*. New Haven: Yale University Press.

Donaldson, L. & Lynn, R. (1976) The conflict resolution process: The two factor theory and an industrial case, *Personnel Review*, **5**, 21–28.

Donnellon, A. & Kolb, D. (1994). Constructive for whom? The fate of diversity disputes in organizations. *Journal of Social Issues*, **50**, 139–155.

Edwards, P.K. (1995). Strikes and industrial conflict. In P.K. Edwards (ed.), *Industrial Relations: Theory and Practice in Britain*. Oxford: Blackwell.

Edwards, P.K. & Scullion, H. (1982). *The Social Organization of Industrial Conflict*. Oxford: Blackwell.

Emler, N. & Hopkins, N. (1990). Reputation, social identity and the self. In D. Abrams & M.A. Hogg (eds), *Social Identity Theory: Constructive and Critical Advances*. Hemel Hempstead: Harvester, pp. 113–130.

Fantasia, R. (1988). *Cultures of Solidarity: Consciousness, Action and Contemporary American Workers*. Berkeley: University of California Press.

Farr, R.M. & Moscovici, S. (1984). *Social Representations*. Cambridge: Cambridge University Press.

Farsides, T. (1993). Social identity theory—a foundation to build on, not undermine. *Theory and Psychology*, **3**, 207–215.

Fisher, R.J. (1990). *The social psychology of intergroup and international conflict resolution*. New York: Springer Verlag.

Fisher, R.J. (1994). Generic principles for resolving intergroup conflict. *Journal of Social Issues*, **50**, 47–66.

Foucault, M. (1971). *Madness and Civilisation.* London: Tavistock.
Freud, S. (1921). *Group psychology and the analysis of the ego.* London: Hogarth Press.
Friedkin, N.E. & Simpson, M.J. (1985). Effects of competition on members' identification with their subunits. *Administrative Science Quarterly*, **30**, 377–394.
Friedman, R. (1992). The culture of mediation: private understandings in the context of public conflict. In D.M. Kolb & J.M. Bartunek (eds), *Hidden Conflict in Organizations.* Newbury Park, CA: Sage.
Frost, P.J., Moore, L.F., Louis, M.R., Lundberg, C.C. & Martin, J. (1985). *Organizational Culture.* Beverley Hills, CA: Sage.
Galbraith, J. (1973). *Designing Complex Organizations.* Reading, MA: Addison-Wesley.
Giddens, A. (1979). *Central Problems in Social Theory.* London: Macmillan.
Guzzo, R. & Shea, G.P. (1992). Group performance and intergroup relations in organizations. In M. Dunnette & L. Hough (eds), *Handbook of Industrial and Organizational Psychology.* Palo Alto: Consulting Psychologists Press.
Hales, C. (1993). *Managing Through Organization.* London: Routledge.
Hartley, J.F. (1983). Industrial relations psychology. In M. Gruneberg & T. Wall (eds), *Social Psychology and Organizational Behaviour.* Chichester: Wiley, pp. 149–181.
Hartley, J.F. (1989). Leadership and decision-making in a strike organization. In B. Klandermans (ed.), *International Social Movement Research*, **2**, 241–265.
Hartley, J., Jacobson, D., Klandermans, B. & van Vuuren, T. (1991). *Job Insecurity: Coping with Jobs at Risk.* London: Sage.
Hartley, J.F., Kelly, J. & Nicholson, N. (1983). *Steel Strike.* London: Batsford Academic.
Hartley, J.F., Cordingley, P. & Benington, J. (1995). *Managing Organizational and Cultural Change.* Luton: Local Government Management Board.
Hewstone, M. & Brown, R. (1986). *Contact and Conflict in Intergroup Encounters.* Oxford: Blackwell.
Hewstone, M., Wagner, U. & Machleit, U. (1989). Self, ingroup and outgroup achievement attributions of German and Turkish pupils. *Journal of Social Psychology*, **129**, 459–470.
Hiller, E. (1928). *The Strike.* New York: Arno Press.
Hogg, M.A. & Abrams, D. (1988). *Social Identifications.* London: Routledge.
Homans, G. (1950). *The Human Group.* New York: Harcourt, Brace Jovanovich.
Hosking, D. & Morley, I. (1991). *A Social Psychology of Organizing: People, Processes and Contexts.* Hemel Hempstead: Harvester Wheatsheaf.
Jackson, J.W. (1993). Realistic group conflict theory: a review and evaluation of the theoretical and empirical literature. *Psychological Record*, **43**, 395–414.
Karsh, B. (1958). *Diary of a strike.* Urbana, II: University of Illinois Press.
Kelly, J. & Kelly, C. (1991). "Them and us": the social psychology of "the new industrial relations". *British Journal of Industrial Relations*, **29**, 25–48.
Kelly, J. & Kelly, C. (1992). Industrial action. In J.F. Hartley & G.M. Stephenson (eds), *Employment Relations: The Psychology of Influence and Control at Work.* Oxford: Blackwell, pp. 246–268.
Kirkbride, P. (1992). Power. In J.F. Hartley & G.M. Stephenson (eds), *Employment Relations: The Psychology of Influence and Control at Work.* Oxford: Blackwell, pp. 246–268.
Klandermans, B. (in press). The social psychology of union participation. In P. Pasture (ed.), *Trade Unions: The Lost Perspective?* Avebury Press.
Kolb, D.M. & Bartunek, J.M. (1992). *Hidden Conflict in Organizations.* Newbury Park, CA: Sage.
Kornhauser, A., Dubin, R. & Ross, A. (eds) (1954). *Industrial Conflict.* New York: McGraw-Hill.
Lane, T. & Roberts, K. (1971). *Strike at Pilkingtons.* London: Fontana.
Lawrence, P.R. & Lorsch, J. (1967). *Organization and Environment.* Cambridge, MA: Harvard University Press.
Lewin, K. (1948). *Resolving Social Conflicts.* New York: Harper and Row.

Liff, S. & Aitkenhead, M. (1992). Equal opportunities: an attempt to restructure employment relations. In J.F. Hartley & G.M. Stephenson (eds), *Employment Relations: The Psychology of Influence and Control at Work*. Oxford: Blackwell, pp. 246–268.

Mastenbroek, W. (1993). *Conflict Management and Organization Development*. Chichester: Wiley.

McCall, G.J. & Simmons, J.L. (1982). *Identities and Interactions*. New York: Free Press.

McGrath, J.E. (1984). *Groups: Interaction and Performance*. Englewood Cliffs, NJ: Prentice-Hall.

Mead, G.H. (1934). *Mind, Self and Society*. Chicago: University of Chicago Press.

Messick, D.M. & Mackie, D.M. (1989). Intergroup relations. *Annual Review of Psychology*, **40**, 45–81.

Miller, E.J. & Rice, A.K. (1967). *Systems of Organization*. London: Tavistock.

Mintzberg, H. (1979). *The Structure of Organizations*. Englewood Cliffs, NJ: Prentice-Hall.

Moghaddam, F.M., Taylor, D.M. & Lalonde, R.N. (1987). Individualistic and collective intergration strategies among Iranians in Canada. *International Journal of Psychology*, **22**, 301–313.

Morley, I. (1992). Intraorganizational bargaining. In J.F. Hartley & G.M. Stephenson (eds), *Employment Relations: The Psychology of Influence and Control at Work*. Oxford: Blackwell, pp. 246–268.

Moscovici S. (1988) Notes towards a description of social representations. *European Journal of Social Psychology*, **18**, 211–250.

Nelson, R.E. (1989). The strength of strong ties: socia networks and intergroup conflict in organizations. *Academy of Management Journal*, **32**, 377–401.

Osborne, D. & Gaebler, T. (1992). *Reinventing Government: How the Entrepreneurial Spirit Is Transforming the Public Sector*. Reading, MA: Addison-Wesley.

Pondy, L. (1967). Organizational conflict: concepts and models. *Administrative Science Quarterly*, **12**, 296–320.

Pondy, L. (1992). Reflections on organizational conflict. *Journal of Organizational Behavior*, **13**, 257–261.

Potter, J. & Wetherell, M. (1987). *Discourse and Social Psychology: Beyond Attitudes and Behaviour*. London: Sage.

Putnam, L.L. & Poole, M.S. (1987). Conflict and negotiation. In F.M. Jablin, L.L. Putnam, K.H. Roberts & L.W. Porter (eds), *Handbook of Organizational Communication*. Beverley Hills, CA: Sage, pp. 549–599.

Rabbie, J.M. & Horwitz, M. (1988). Categories versus groups as explanatory concepts in intergroup relations. *European Journal of Social Psychology*, **18**, 117–123.

Rice, A.K. (1969). Individual, group and intergroup processes. *Human Relations*, **22**, 565–584.

Roethlisberger, F.J. & Dickson, J.J. (1939). *Management and the Worker*. Cambridge, MA: Harvard University Press.

Sachdev, I. & Bourhis, R.Y. (1987). Status differentials and intergroup behaviour. *European Journal of Social Psychology*, **17**, 277–293.

Schiffman, R. (1993). Social identity notions and theories: a reply to Farsides. *Theory and Psychology*, **3**, 217–222.

Schiffman, R. & Wicklund, R.A. (1992). The minimal group paradigm and its minimal group psychology: on equating social identity with arbitrary group membership. *Theory and Psychology*, **2**(1), 29–50.

Schneider, B. (1990). *Organizational Culture and Climate*. San Francisco: Jossey-Bass.

Shaw, M.E. (1976). *Group Dynamics: The Psychology of Small Group Behaviour*, 2nd Edn. New York: McGraw-Hill.

Sherif, M. (1936). *The Psychology of Social Norms*. New York: Harper and Row.

Sherif, M. & Sherif, C. (1969). *Social Psychology*. New York: Harper and Row.

Sherif, M. (1966). *Group Conflict and Cooperation*. London: Routledge.

Skinner, M. (1979). The social psychology of intergroup conflict. In G.M. Stephenson & C. Brotherton (eds), *Industrial Relations: A Social Psychological Approach*. Chichester: Wiley.

Smith, K. (1983). An intergroup perspective on individual behavior. In J.R. Hackman, E. Lawler & L. Porter (eds), *Perspectives on Behavior in Organizations*. New York: McGraw-Hill.

Smith, K. (1989). The movement of conflict in organizations: the joint dynamics of splitting and triangulation. *Administrative Science Quarterly*, **34**, 1–20.

Stagner, R. & Eflal, B. (1982). Internal union dynamics during a strike: a quasi-experimental study. *Journal of Applied Psychology*, **67**, 37–44.

Stein, A.A. (1976). Conflict and cohesion: a review of the literature. *Journal of Conflict Resolution*, **20**, 143–172.

Tajfel, H. (1970). Experiments in intergroup discrimination. *Scientific American*, **223**(5), 96–102.

Tajfel, H. (1978). *Differentiation Between Social Groups: Studies in the Psychology of Intergroup Relations*. London: Academic Press.

Tajfel, H. (1982). *Social Identity and Intergroup Relations*. Cambridge: Cambridge University Press.

Tajfel, H., Flament, C., Billig, M. & Bundy, R. (1971). Social categorisation and intergroup behaviour. *European Journal of Social Psychology*, **1**, 149–177.

Taylor, D.M. & Moghaddam, F.M. (1994). *Theories of Intergroup Relations*, 2nd Edn. Westport, CT: Praeger.

Thomas, K. & Schmidt, W. (1976). A survey of managerial interests with respect to conflict. *Academy of Management Journal*, **19**, 315–318.

Thomas, K. (1992a). Conflict and negotiation processes in organizations. In M. Dunnette & L. Hough (eds), *Handbook of Industrial and Organizational Psychology*. Palo Alto: Consulting Psychologists Press.

Thomas, K. (1992b). Conflict and conflict management: reflections and update. *Journal of Organizational Behavior*, **13**, 265–274.

Thompson, J.D. (1967). *Organizations in Action*. New York: McGraw-Hill.

Trice, H.M. & Beyer, J.M. (1993). *The Cultures of Work Organizations*. Englewood Cliffs, NJ: Prentice-Hall.

Turner, J.C. (1975). Social comparison and social identity: some prospects for intergroup behaviour. *European Journal of Social Psychology*, **5**, 5–34.

Turner, J.C. (1982). Towards a cognitive redefinition of the social group. In H. Tajfel (ed.), *Social Identity and Intergroup Relations*. Cambridge: Cambridge University Press.

Turner, J.C. (1985). Social categorisation and the self-concept: a social cognitive theory of group behaviour. In E.J. Lawler (ed.), *Advances in Group Processes*, Vol. 2. Greenwich, CN: JAI Press, pp. 77–122.

Turner, J.C. & Giles, H. (1981). *Intergroup Behaviour*. Oxford: Blackwell.

van der Vliert, E. (1984). Conflict and conflict management. In P.J. Drenth, H. Thierry, P.J. Willems & C.J. de Wolff (eds), *Handbook of Work and Organizational Psychology*. Chichester: Wiley.

van Maanen, J. (1979). The self, the situation and the rules of interpersonal relations. In W. Bennis, J. van Maanen, E. Schein & F. Steele (eds), *Essays in Interpersonal Dynamics*. Homewood, IL: Dorsey Press, pp. 43–101.

Vogelman, L. (1995). The pathways to murder. Unpublished PhD thesis, Department of Organization Psychology, University of London.

Vogelman, L. (1989). Strike violence: some factors to consider. *South African Labour Bulletin*, **14**(3), 47–56.

Waddington, D. (1987). *Trouble Brewing: A Social Psychological Analysis of the Ansell's Brewery Dispute*. Aldershot: Gower.

Waddington, D. (1986). The Ansells' brewery dispute: a social-cognitive approach to the study of strikes. *Journal of Occupational Psychology*, **59**, 231–246.

Walton, R.E. & McKersie, R.B. (1965). *A Behavioral Theory of Labor Negotiations: An Analyis of a Social Interaction System*. New York: McGraw-Hill.

Winterton, J. & Winterton, R. (1989). *Coal, Crisis and Conflict: The 1984–5 Miners' Strike in Yorkshire*. Manchester: Manchester University Press.

Chapter 17

Work Group Socialization

Neil Anderson
and
Helena D.C. Thomas
Goldsmiths College, University of London, UK

Abstract

In this chapter we review existing research into work group socialization. Contrasting the socialization of newcomers into the wider organization with their assimilation into their proximal work group, we argue that the work group often forms the primary medium through which the socialization process is enacted. A critical review of existing studies reveals that researchers active in work group dynamics, and those interested primarily in organization socialization, have neglected the process of socialization into work groups. To redress this situation we propose a testable model of work group socialization and conclude the chapter by arguing the need for further research at the group level of analysis.

INTRODUCTION

Researchers in work psychology have long been aware of the important role that socialization procedures play in assimilating newcomers into an organization, its culture and work practices, thus enabling newcomers to carry out their work roles effectively. Despite this widespread acknowledgement of the significance of socialization tactics for newcomer adjustment, relatively little attention has been paid to the role of the newcomer's proximal work group in the socialization process. This is somewhat surprising, since the proximal work group provides the immediate work and socio-cultural environment within which the new recruit must learn to accomplish job tasks and responsibilities; and moreover, it is the proximal group which is likely to be most influenced by the arrival of a new staff member or members (Brim, 1966; Wanous, Reichers & Malik, 1984).

Handbook of Work Group Psychology. Edited by M.A. West.
© 1996 John Wiley & Sons Ltd.

Only a small number of authors have directly compared development or socialization at the work group and organizational levels. Wanous, Reichers & Malik (1984) outline the temporal and conceptual similarities of group development and organizational socialization, in particular, that both of these processes are interpersonal, interactive and occur over time. Louis (1990, p. 93) cites earlier work by Brim (1966, p. 35) on the importance of the proximal work group in socialization, asserting that "... the primary group often is the main agency of socialization with these formal institutions". Moreland & Levine (1984) also discuss the role of the proximal work group in newcomer socialization, specifically referring to co-workers who frequently teach newcomers the informal aspects of what and how things are done (see also Levine & Moreland, 1994). It is therefore perhaps surprising that the whole topic of work group socialization has received comparatively little attention from researchers over the years.

In this chapter we attempt to redress this situation and argue for the consideration of *work group socialization* as a research topic distinct from the wider subject of *organizational socialization*. We also argue that work group socialization should be conceptualized as a bidirectional process: the proximal work group influencing and changing the newcomer and, simultaneously, the newcomer influencing and changing his or her newly encountered work group. This chapter is divided into five sections. First, we argue in greater detail for the utility of research into work group socialization, proposing that the newcomer's proximal work group serves as a focal point for the transmission of the organization's cultural values, group norms and established customs and practices to the newcomer. In particular, given the increasing importance of team working in organizations, we argue that there is a need for researchers to examine processes of proximal work group socialization in addition to wider issues of organization socialization.

Second, we proffer a general definition of work group socialization. Much of the research in this area has either examined organizational strategies and procedures for integrating newcomers or, more recently, has examined the proactive tactics used by newcomers to obtain information relevant to their new work role and their work environment. Relatively little work has considered the work group and so, to delineate work group socialization as a distinct topic area, a guiding definition is put forward.

Third, we review the extant research into group socialization. Particular attention is given to five key issues: sources of socialization; newcomer information acquisition; the psychological contract; the process of newcomer socialization into groups; and the socialization of work groups as newly formed project teams. By necessity, because much of the research reviewed was either conducted originally into organization socialization and newcomer information-seeking behaviours, or evaluated the process of entry into social not working groups, we have extended and extrapolated from these findings to the context of work groups.

Fourth, we develop and expound a processual model of socialization into work groups, drawing from existing models of organization socialization and Moreland & Levine's (1982, 1984) social psychological model of group entry. Subsumed within this model, we propose six testable proposals to guide future work in this neglected area. Fifth, and to conclude, following on from our model of work group socialization, we argue the necessity of further research into work group socialization, and submit a number of directions for future research to address.

WORK GROUP SOCIALIZATION: A RATIONALE

Researchers active in the field of organization socialization have tended to concentrate their efforts at one of two levels of analysis—the *organization* or the *individual*. Empirical studies at the former level have focused upon organizational tactics and procedures for newcomer integration (e.g. Van Maanen & Schein, 1979; Berlew & Hall, 1966), models of the socialization process over time (e.g. Feldman, 1976a, b; Wanous, 1980), and observational case studies of procedures used by both organizations (Louis, Posner & Powell, 1983; Nelson & Quick, 1991) and individuals (Ostroff & Kozlowski, 1992; Morrison, 1993a,b; Smith & Kozlowski, 1994). Such work, at both the organizational and individual levels of analysis, has substantially informed our understanding of the impact of socialization processes.

Despite this quite extensive literature base, there are notably few studies which actually validate organizational socialization procedures. Research at the organizational level remains dogged by a lack of applied empirical studies compared with a proliferation of normative-prescriptive models which undoubtedly have intuitive appeal and superficially appear to offer generalized explanations of organizational socialization tactics and processes. As Feldman (1989) caustically comments, in his recent review of this area, "There has been too much approach, and not enough arrival" (p. 405). This is particularly applicable to socialization at the level of the work group, where the paucity of research in work psychology is particularly marked. Moreover, this shortcoming of existing research will become increasingly apparent as organizations move down the seemingly inexorable path toward team-based methods of work design (see for instance Chapter 10 in this volume). Compounding this shortcoming is the underestimation, common across much of the applied research into work groups, of the rejuvenating impact of new members upon the group. Few studies acknowledge that many organizational groups will be quite changeable and even transient or fixed-term in nature. Higher levels of labour turnover, the creation of new job roles, the formation of fixed duration project teams, task groups and committees are all instances where the socialization of new members is critical to group functioning and performance. In sum, from both vantage points—research into organization socialization and work groups—there is a justifiable case for considerably more research attention to be directed toward the process of work group socialization.

WORK GROUP SOCIALIZATION DEFINED

In attempting to define work group socialization, we turn initially to other researchers' definitions of organizational socialization which are summarized in Figure 17.1. These definitions reflect the changes in conceptions of the socialization process of the past several decades, with these conceptions also having influenced the kinds of research that have been undertaken. The changes in the predominant emphasis of socialization research over time can be crudely classified into four distinct eras:

- 1960s   Coercive integration era.
- 1970s   People-processing era.
- 1980s   Interactive assimilation era.
- Early 1990s   Proactive information acquisition era.

Considering each era briefly, early definitions of organization socialization tended to view this as a process in which the newcomer enters an established bureaucracy, replete with its own rules and regulations, and possessing sufficient power and authority to ensure the newcomer's compliance to this rule structure. From the newcomer's perspective, socialization was portrayed as a process of learning the rules governing task performance and the requisite accepted behaviours for "fitting-in" to this bureaucratic framework (e.g. Caplow, 1964; Brim, 1966).

Conceptions of the socialization process in the 1970s are typified by the definition of Van Maanen in his seminal article, published in 1978, where he used the term "people-processing" to describe the effects of large-scale organization socialization procedures. Van Maanen (1978) and Van Maanen and Schein (1979) focused upon organizational tactics of newcomer socialization, based on the assumption that formal procedures could be designed by organizations, knowledgeable of different combinations of tactics, leading to different outcomes. Thus, again, the newcomer was seen as a passive recipient of "people-processing" strategies. Critical of this stance, researchers in the 1980s, and even more so in the 1990s, have recognized the proactive role that newcomers necessarily take in any organization socialization and entry process, and this change in outlook is reflected by their definitions of this process. Louis (1980), for instance, highlights newcomer proactivity in socialization by defining it as "... the process by which an individual comes to appreciate the values, abilities, expected behaviors, and social knowledge essential for assuming an organizational role...." (p. 230), and similarly Wanous (1992) refers to "... the ways in which newcomers change and adapt to the organization" (p. 187). Nicholson (1984) develops this point of newcomer proactivity more fully, arguing that role innovation is one of the likely outcomes of job change, where the individual experiences personal growth and development as a result of work role transition. We return to this issue of proactivity at several points in this chapter, but would acknowledge here that notably few of these definitions acknowledge the role of the

ERA	EXAMPLE DEFINITIONS
1960s—"Coercive integration" era Organization socialization as: • Learning one's place in the bureaucratic structure • Newcomer compliance with organizational dictates through reward and punishment (Schein, 1968) • An organizationally controlled and directed process—the newcomer as a receptive vessel for "correct" behaviours	"... an organizationally directed process that prepares and qualifies individuals to occupy organizational positions" (Caplow, 1964, p. 16) "... the manner in which an individual learns that behavior appropriate to his position in a group through interaction with others who hold normative beliefs about what his role should be and who reward or punish him for correct or incorrect actions" (Brim, 1966, p. 3)

1970s—"People processing" era
 	
Organization socialization as:
 	
• Organizational tactics and strategies for "people processing" (Van Maanen, 1978)
• Serial processes comprising several distinct phases or stages, each having to be completed before the next is entered. e.g:
   Feldman (1976a, 1976b): *anticipatory socialisation → accommodation → role management*
   Schein (1978): *entry → socialisation → mutual acceptance*
   Wanous (1980): *confrontation → role clarity → location → integration*
	"Organization socialization or 'people processing' refers to the manner in which the experiences of people learning the ropes of a new organizational position, status, or role structured for them by others within the organization" (Van Maanen, 1978, p. 19)
	
	"... the process by which an individual acquires the social knowledge and skills necessary to assume an organizational role" (Van Maanen and Schein, 1979, p. 211)

Early 1980s—"Interactive assimilation" era Organization socialization as: • Acquiring the values and attitudes needed to become assimilated into the organization • Acquiring the knowledge and abilities expected for effective work role performance • The newcomer as active participant in the process rather than as passive subject to it • Assimilation into the work role and organization as the "end point" of the socialization process	"... the process by which an individual comes to appreciate the values, abilities, expected behaviors and social knowledge essential for assuming an organizational role and for participating as an organizational member" (Louis, 1980, p. 230) "Defined globally, organization socialization is the process by which employees are transformed from organization outsiders to participating and effective members" (Feldman, 1981, p. 309)
Late 1980s/Early 1990s—"Proactive information acquisition" era Organization socialization as: • The newcomer as proactive information seeker • The organisation and the newcomer seen as being able to influence outcomes of knowledge acquisition and job role performance • The newcomer obtaining several types of information from multiple sources over time	"Socialization concerns the ways in which newcomers change and adapt to the organization. The types of changes are learning new roles, norms and values. In other words, learning what is "acceptable" behavior" (Wanous, 1992, p. 187) "... the process by which newcomers attempt to comprehend the salient features, processes and events that characterize the new setting, resolve their confusion and uncertainty, and become assimilated into the social and work fabric that defines the organizational and work group context" (Chao et al., 1994, p. 4)

Figure 17.1 A chronology of definitions of organization socialization

immediate work group in socializing new members into the organization (the exceptions are Brim, 1966, and Chao et al., 1994), and this is characteristic of a general neglect of the topic of the proximal work group in newcomer socialization, as noted earlier in this chapter.

No specific definitions of socialization into work groups could be located in the research literature, and so we offer the following:

> Work group socialization is newcomer acquisition of knowledge, abilities and attitudes needed to perform a work role, and the assimilation of the newcomer into the proximal work group via exposure to its norms, psychological climate, rituals and rites de passage, and the concurrent accommodation of the work group to the newcomer over time.

This definition is intended to emphasize two aspects present in any process of socialization. First, that socialization is a *learning process* in that newcomers acquire knowledge, abilities and attitudes necessary for effective job performance. This is, of course, self-evident, but many existing definitions focus solely upon the process of "fitting-in" to the organization and its culture and climate. Further, this learning process extends beyond information acquisition, to include the integration of information into a cognitive schema underlying job performance and the inculcation of appropriate attitudes relevant to the work role (e.g. Ostroff & Kozlowski, 1992; Chao et al., 1994). The degree to which an organization prescreens out and selects in applicants on criteria of attitudes and abilities will of course moderate the need for acquisition and learning during socialization (Schneider, 1987; Chatman, 1991; Anderson & Ostroff, 1996).

Second, the definition notes two inter-dependent *outcomes* in work group socialization: the *assimilation* of the newcomer into the group and the *reciprocal impact* the newcomer has in changing the group's norms, climate and structure. In arguing that newcomer assimilation is only one outcome variable, it is clear that the degree of socialization will vary widely according, on the one hand, to the type of group, its context, its task interdependence and, on the other, to newcomer personality characteristics, beliefs, values and attitudes, and so forth. Extreme forms of assimilation are evident where the newcomer's core values and attitudes are fundamentally changed (e.g. religious cults, special armed services units; e.g. Schein, 1968) or where, for instance, the newcomer demonstrates conformity to the group's behavioural norms by undergoing an unpleasant or degrading initiation ceremony (e.g. street gangs, college fraternities).

Such extreme assimilation, aimed at producing uniformity among group members, is rarely attempted in business organizations. Indeed Schein (1968), in discussing socialization outcomes, proposes that optimal socialization occurs when the newcomer accepts only the essential ("pivotal") values and norms, rejecting all others, producing "creative individualism". Socialization failures lie on either extreme of this, either as "rebellion", in which all values and norms are rejected, or as "conformity", in which they are all accepted. Moreover, Schein (1968) notes the difficulty for the employee of remaining creatively individualistic following promotion or lateral transfers which engender a change of the value system of the proximal work group.

It should be noted that Schein's (1968) paper stems from a time when the focus of socialization research was on the active organization and passive individual (see Figure 17.1). Our definition reflects the more recent recognition that the newcomer is also an active agent capable of affecting others (e.g. Sutton & Louis, 1987). This is highlighted in the final part of our definition, which purposely emphasizes the influence that newcomers often have upon established work groups. Existing definitions have tended to conceive of socialization as a one-way process; the organization influencing and changing the newcomer. However, as Wanous (1992) argues quite justifiably, a simultaneous process of "personalization" is occurring whereby the newcomer is modifying the organization. We extend this point in the definition to suppose that newcomers, particularly if there are several joining the group as a cohort, will influence its norms, climate, structure and patterns of work. However, entering as a cohort with other newcomers can make the socialization process more difficult, since newcomers may provide each other with faulty information or interpretations of events (Sutton & Louis, 1987; Louis, 1990).

SOCIALIZATION RESEARCH

Having noted the need for concentration upon work group socialization, and having propounded a general definition of this process, we come on to critically review existing research in this area. As previously noted, few studies specifically examine work group socialization, but research into organizational socialization more widely and studies of entry into social groups can be extrapolated to the context of work groups. We have sub-divided the existing research into five areas: sources of socialization; newcomer information acquisition; the psychological contract; the process of newcomer socialization into groups; and the socialization of work groups as newly-formed project teams.

Sources of Socialization

As already mentioned, the 1980s saw a change of perspective in socialization research away from organizational procedures to focus on the newcomer's experiences during socialization. Louis, Posner & Powell's (1983) research is one of the earliest studies that adopts this individual-level perspective. A questionnaire was sent to 217 business students from two universities between 6 and 9 months after graduation, containing measures of the availability and helpfulness of ten socialization practices (formal on-site orientations; off-site residential training; business trips; social/recreational activities; and daily interactions with: supervisor; peers; experienced senior co-worker; mentor/sponsor; new recruits; and secretary/support staff) and measures of three socialization outcomes (job satisfaction; commitment; and intentions to stay at the organization). The most available socialization sources were peers, supervisor and senior co-worker relationships, available to 89, 87 and 75% of newcomers respectively. The socialization practice rated as being most helpful, "enabling them to learn the ropes and become effective organizational members" (p. 860), was "daily interactions with peers while working", which was significantly and positively correlated with all three outcome measures. Interactions with senior co-workers and interactions with supervisor were rated as the next two most helpful socialization practices. Furthermore, formal and planned socialization procedures, in the form of on-site orientation and off-site training, were rated as only moderately helpful. Consequently, members of the newcomers' proximal work group were seen as the most useful source of socialization, and more useful than formal organization socialization procedures.

Posner & Powell (1985), in a further analysis of the data from their earlier collaborative work (Louis, Posner & Powell, 1983), compared the socialization experiences of male and female newcomers. In terms of availability, there were two significant differences; females reported mentor/sponsor relationships as having been more available, whilst males reported a greater availability of business trips. There were greater differences in the utility of the various socialization practices, with males rating three of these as significantly more helpful than did females: formal on-site orientation, other new recruits, and first supervisor. From the pattern of sex differences in their results, Posner & Powell suggest that, while there was no evidence for treatment discrimination against women, male newcomers may interpret, respond to, and/or benefit more from certain socialization practices than females. As the only study we could locate comparing sex differences in newcomer experiences in socialization, these findings are important and clearly deserve further research in relation to issues of equal opportunities and women's career possibilities.

A study by Nelson & Quick (1991) has partially replicated this work but, using the same measures of socialization practices, the authors interpreted these scales as measures of social support. A total of 91 newcomers in their ninth month of employment at three separate organizations responded to the questionnaire, which asked about the availability and helpfulness of the ten socialization practices already mentioned, work stressors, job satisfaction, intention to leave, and measured psychological distress symptoms. Performance ratings were obtained from newcomers' supervisors, giving an independent outcome measure. As in Louis, Posner & Powell's (1983) study, peers and supervisors were the most available socialization sources, and these were also rated as the most helpful. Experienced senior co-worker and secretarial/support staff were also given high helpfulness ratings. Considering availability first, the presence or absence of these four socialization aids (peers, supervisors, experienced senior co-worker, and secretary/support staff) did not affect any of the outcome measures, apart from an increase in job satisfaction when senior co-workers were not available. However, there were a number of significant correlations between the helpfulness of these socialization practices and the outcome measures. Supervisors' helpfulness was related to reduced psychological distress symptoms, suggesting that a helpful supervisor was perceived as reducing this potentially stressful job transition (see also Nelson, 1987). Daily interactions with peers was positively related to job satisfaction and negatively correlated with intention to leave, but also negatively with performance, for which a negative correlation was also found with experienced senior co-worker helpfulness. The only positive significant relationships with performance were with helpfulness of peers, experienced senior co-worker, mentor, and other newcomers. Nelson & Quick (1991) suggest that this may be because poor performance leads newcomers to try and form attachments and hence initiate social support, or that organizational insiders will recognize newcomers' performance problems and therefore offer help. The causal direction of these relationships cannot be ascertained by these correlations, of course, but the findings that reduced psychological distress symptoms were associated with the helpfulness of supervisors and other newcomers appear to make sense intuitively.

Taken together, the results from these three studies indicate that newcomers rate peers, supervisors, and senior co-workers as helpful, and that their helpfulness is related to a number of positive socialization outcomes. Moreover, the availability of organizational-level procedures, including formal on-site orientation, off-site residential training, and business trips, are found to have few significant effects on socialization, with only Louis, Posner & Powell (1983) finding such factors to be related significantly to positive socialization outcomes. This indicates that formal socialization activities may be of little benefit to newcomers and reaffirms the importance of the newcomer's proximal work group in this process. Furthermore, it supports our contention that socialization researchers need to shift emphasis from the formal organizational procedures to the group level. We return to the implications stemming from this shift in later sections of this chapter.

Information Acquisition

One area which has witnessed substantial growth in research attention over the last 10 years is that of proactive information acquisition by newcomers during the socialization process. As we noted earlier, a strategic shift in the focus of socialization research occurred during the 1980s, moving attention from formal organizational procedures at the macro-analytical level to the more micro-analytical issues of newcomer information acquisition.

Perhaps the first article to mark this shift in focus was that of Louis (1980), which not only signalled, but was probably causal in, this change from a situational perspective to concentration on the newcomer, and in particular the active role of the newcomer in negotiating his or her new work environment. Louis emphasized the newcomer's need to cope with surprises and make sense of events occurring in the workplace. Hence, newcomer learning is implicit and central to Louis' conception of the socialization process. In more recent research on newcomer learning, the newcomer is seen more explicitly as a proactive agent in his or her own socialization and, in consequence, learning has been conceived of as a process of information acquisition by the newcomer (e.g. Comer, 1991; Ostroff & Kozlowski, 1992; Morrison, 1993a,b). Such research is relevant to work group socialization in that it demonstrates the role and relative importance of members of the work group in newcomer learning.

Comer (1991), for instance, reports two cross-sectional field studies into information acquisitions by newcomers from peers in their immediate work group. In the first study a sample of 30 junior professional staff who had been working in a service organization for 3–4 months were contacted by telephone and a semi-structured interview was conducted. Following Fisher (1986), the interviewer questioned newcomers on the types of information sought during socialization, information sources, and perceptions of the usefulness of different sources of information. Newcomers reported that they acquired both technical and social information from their peers, and used a mixture of actively explicit, passively explicit and implicit tactics to gain such job-relevant data. In Comer's second study, this methodology was extended to include a sample of 15 organizations to whom questionnaires were sent, again covering newcomer information-seeking tactics. A total of 73 questionnaires were returned, and again, newcomers rated peers as useful in providing necessary information on the technical and social aspects of their new job role.

In a carefully constructed study, Ostroff & Kozlowski (1992) looked at the use of different information sources to learn about four domains of learning—task, role, group and organization—using a sample of 151 newcomers. Measures were taken at two time points: within the first few months in their new job and 5 months later. It was found that, generally, observation of others was used most, followed by interpersonal sources (co-workers and supervisors), whilst experimentation was less used, and least use was made of formal organizational literature. Co-workers and supervisors were used to a similar extent for task and organizational information, but supervisors were more used for role-related information whilst co-workers provided more information on the group domain. However, Ostroff & Kozlowski found that the amount of information was not equivalent to its utility. For example, supervisors and co-workers provided equal amounts of information about the organizational domain, but only supervisory information was significantly related to organizational knowledge. This concurs with Louis, Posner & Powell's (1983) finding of non-equivalence between the availability and usefulness of various information sources in socialization, and is corroborated by more recent work reviewed below (Morrison, 1994). Although information from supervisors and co-workers was not always rated as important in gaining knowledge as that from other sources, gaining information from supervisors and co-workers was related to a number of positive attitudinal outcomes such as job satisfaction, commitment and constructive feelings of adjustment. This supports the view that interaction with members of the work group may facilitate integration into the informal social milieu and the establishment of a social support network which can facilitate subsequent adaptation (Fisher, 1986).

As well as showing the centrality of members of newcomers' proximal work groups in the information acquisition process, Ostroff & Kozlowski's (1992) research sheds light on the process by which newcomers actually acquire knowledge during socialization. An examination of knowledge gained in the four different domains over time revealed that knowledge of the group was greatest initially and then remained constant, with knowledge of the task and role increasing over time, whereas organizational knowledge remained relatively low. This shows the fundamental importance of work group socialization as the first forum in and by which the newcomer becomes knowledgeable, as well as again suggesting the precedence of the work group as the primary medium for organizational socialization.

Smith & Kozlowski (1994) investigated newcomers' strategies for information acquisition across two different types of information: functional (how to perform the job) and evaluative (how well they are performing the job), as well as the effects of job characteristics (e.g. task interdependence—the extent to which the newcomer has to coordinate with other group members to accomplish work) and self-efficacy. Newcomers' perceptions of job characteristics were corroborated by a sample of matched co-workers. Their sample comprised 241 newcomers from seven organizations possessing a maximum of 16 months' service in the job. The results for the job characteristic of task interdependence are pertinent to work group socialization. Task interdependence affected the use of most learning strategies involving interaction with, or observation of, others. This is to be expected, since greater task interdependence affords more opportunities for inquiry and observation. However, Smith & Kozlowski also propose that there may have been social pressures encouraging newcomers to take advantage of the opportunity to ask questions. A further finding, contrary to Smith & Kozlowski's original hypothesis, was that task interdependence was positively related to self-evaluation. They suggest that this may have been due to newcomers recognizing the dependence of others on them and reacting by becoming more proactive in evaluating themselves to ensure satisfactory performance. Overall, these findings hint at the important role the proximal work group plays in facilitating certain learning strategies and in encouraging newcomer proactivity, both of which may have positive outcomes for socialization, such as increasing its rate (Reichers, 1987), and positively influencing satisfaction and commitment (Ostroff & Kozlowski, 1992).

Further recent research on information acquisition has been carried out by Morrison (1993a,b, 1994). The first of these (Morrison, 1993a), examined information-seeking in different domains across a sample of accountants in their first, third and sixth months of employment. Although the overall frequency of information-seeking and the patterns of information sought were quite stable over time, changes occurred in the frequency with which certain types of information were sought. Technical information and referent information (relating to role demands and expectations) remained high throughout, although referent and also performance feedback information were sought more over time. Conversely, newcomers sought normative, social feedback and technical information less over time. Since the research only examined newcomers' information-seeking, the results are not directly comparable to research which has looked at the order in which knowledge and task mastery is gained in different domains. However, the overall pattern of information-seeking reflects newcomers' self-perceived needs, and shows that task and role mastery are emphasized throughout; normative and social feedback information were less sought over time, which Morrison (1993a) interpreted as being consistent with Katz's (1980) argument that newcomers' concerns change over time from fitting into the work role to actual job performance levels. An alternative explanation, however, is that newcomers received these types of information from more experienced colleagues in their work group, and were therefore able to reduce their efforts at gaining such information.

In a further publication, Morrison (1993b), presumably analysing the same data set on accountants as used in (1993a), reported that, although information-seeking had a unique effect on socialization, it explained only a modest amount of variance in the measured socialization outcomes of task mastery, role clarity, social integration and acculturation. Hence, although the information acquisition approach has confirmed the proactive role of the newcomer and has shown that newcomers use a variety of informational sources to begin to make sense of their environment, it should be kept in mind that information acquisition is only one element in the complex process of socialization. Moreover, information acquisition cannot imply information integration, and research is sorely needed to shed light upon how newcomers assimilate and integrate the myriad individual pieces of information into a coherent cognitive schema related to effective job performance. In this respect, the work of Wagner & Sternberg (1986, 1991) into "tacit knowledge" and the development of expertise in novice task performers, has been neglected by socialization researchers. In spite of Fisher's optimism in stating that "the study of socialization seems to be on the brink of adopting a whole new approach—that of seeing the newcomer as an active problem solver and agent of his or her own socialization" (1986, p. 138), subsequent research on newcomer socialization has developed a near-myopic focus on newcomer proactive information-seeking. Future research is called for to advance our understanding, not so much of information-seeking, but of information integration and the development of knowledge structures held by newcomers which are paramount in their transition toward becoming effective job performers.

The Psychological Contract

The psychological contract (Schein, 1988; Rousseau, 1989) embodies the exchange relationship that exists between an employee and his or her organization, such that the employee carries out certain actions and behaves in certain ways (e.g. good performance, loyalty) and expects the organization to fulfil its obligations in return (e.g. salary, job security). One role of the psychological contract is to decrease uncertainty and increase the perceived predictability of organizational actions (Herriot, 1984). One "side" of this contract represents an individual's cognitive perception of his or her relationship with the organization, making this part of the psychological contract subjective and private to the individual. Hence, according to McFarlane Shore & Tetrick (1994), the psychological contract is similar to a cognitive schema (Louis, 1980), which individuals develop over time as they have increased experience with the organization. The development of the individual newcomer's psychological contract would thus seem an important aspect of socialization and, since the contract is distinct to the individual and will be based upon events and occurrences in his or her immediate work environment, the newcomer's proximal work group will clearly exert a major impact on the development of the newcomer's psychological contract (see also McLean Parks & Kidder, 1994).

Likewise, the other "side" of the psychological contract, emphasized particularly by Herriot (1984) and Schein (1988), comprises the expectations held by those in the organization of the newcomer. As Herriot (1995, personal correspondence) points out, these expectations are also likely to differ between members of the newcomer's proximal work group and between employees in the wider organization. Hence, conflicting messages are likely to be sent to the newcomer when discrepancies in expectations exist between members of his or her immediate work group. Indeed, here one can imagine that role ambiguity and role conflict will be the highly probable outcomes in such situations. The psychological contract, then, is centrally relevant to the process of work group socialization, both from the viewpoint of differences in expectations held by newcomers themselves and in terms of the different expectations held by existing group members of the newcomer's role and actions at work.

Despite the relevance of the psychological contract, few studies have been conducted which evaluate the impact of the group upon newcomer expectations that are developed into the psychological contract. McFarlane Shore & Tetrick (1994) is one exception, but is discursive rather than empirical in nature, and focuses solely on the individual's psychological contract. The authors argue that the newcomer's supervisor is responsible for carrying out many of the contractual terms, and will therefore be viewed as the principal actor responsible for establishing and maintaining the psychological contract. However, co-workers are proposed to play an informational role, firstly regarding the likelihood that the organization, particularly as embodied by the supervisor, will fulfil its side of the contract, and secondly by providing information which allows the newcomer to compare contractual terms with peers, either directly or indirectly. In addition to the role of the proximal work group proposed by McFarlane Shore & Tetrick (1994), we propose that co-workers will also have a role in maintaining the relational (social) aspects of the psychological contract (Rousseau, 1989), including feelings of trust and interpersonal attachment. Thus, we propose that the newcomer's psychological contract, reflecting his or her relationship with an organization, is a key aspect of socialization, and is principally developed and enacted within the context of the proximal work group. It is unfortunate, then, that applied research in this area is so lacking, although a number of studies in the

UK have found that unmet expectations are a major reason given by university graduates for leaving employers in the first few years of employment (Nicholson & Arnold, 1989; Anderson, 1992).

The Process of Socialization into Groups

In a series of influential articles, now spanning over a decade, Moreland & Levine detail a model of newcomer entry and socialization into social groups (Moreland & Levine, 1982, 1984, 1985, 1988; Levine & Moreland, 1994). In perhaps the most detailed explication of this model, Moreland and Levine (1982) propose a five-stage process of socialization into social groups: *investigation, socialization, maintenance, resocialization* and *remembrance*. Figure 17.2 reproduces this model in full and incorporates the authors' original axes and four role transition points denoted by the asterisks on the commitment scale (EC, AC, DC, and XC), which signify the transition into the next phase of the process.

The *investigation* phase marks the commencement of group membership, at which stage Moreland & Levine describe the newcomer as a "prospective member". Here, the newcomer engages in reconnaissance to search for cues as to the *modus operandi* of the group and whether the group will satisfy his or her wishes for group membership. If both the prospective member and the group decide to extend their relationship, commitment levels rise to meet both parties' "entry criteria" (EC) and the newcomer joins the group as a new member. Clearly, in organizational settings, such entry processes are far more formalized and the recruitment and selection system mediates this process, often allowing existing work group members only a limited role in decision-making (Anderson & Shackleton, 1993; Herriot, 1989).

During the *socialization* phase the newcomer becomes a fully-fledged member of the group and, as Moreland & Levine (1984) argue, "... the group attempts to change the individual so as to maximize his or her contributions to the attainment of group goals; to the extent that the group succeeds, the individual undergoes *assimilation*" (p. 161). Simultaneously, the newcomer will attempt to change the group to maximize the benefits that membership confers on them, so-called "accommodation". This phase ends at the time when the group's and the newcomer's commitment levels rise to their mutually agreeable "*acceptance criteria*" (AC), at which point the individual undergoes a second role transition, becoming a full member of the group.

The third phase in the model, "*maintenance*", is characterized by both parties negotiating roles for their ongoing relationship. Clearly, in a business environment, this process will again be influenced largely by formal methods, especially those of work organization, perhaps the only notable exception being where the group is highly autonomous and can determine its own work methods and practices (see Chapter 10 in this volume). Over time, and if either party's commitment level to the other begins to wane, Moreland & Levine argue that a third role transition can occur. Specifically, if the commitment of either party reduces to the

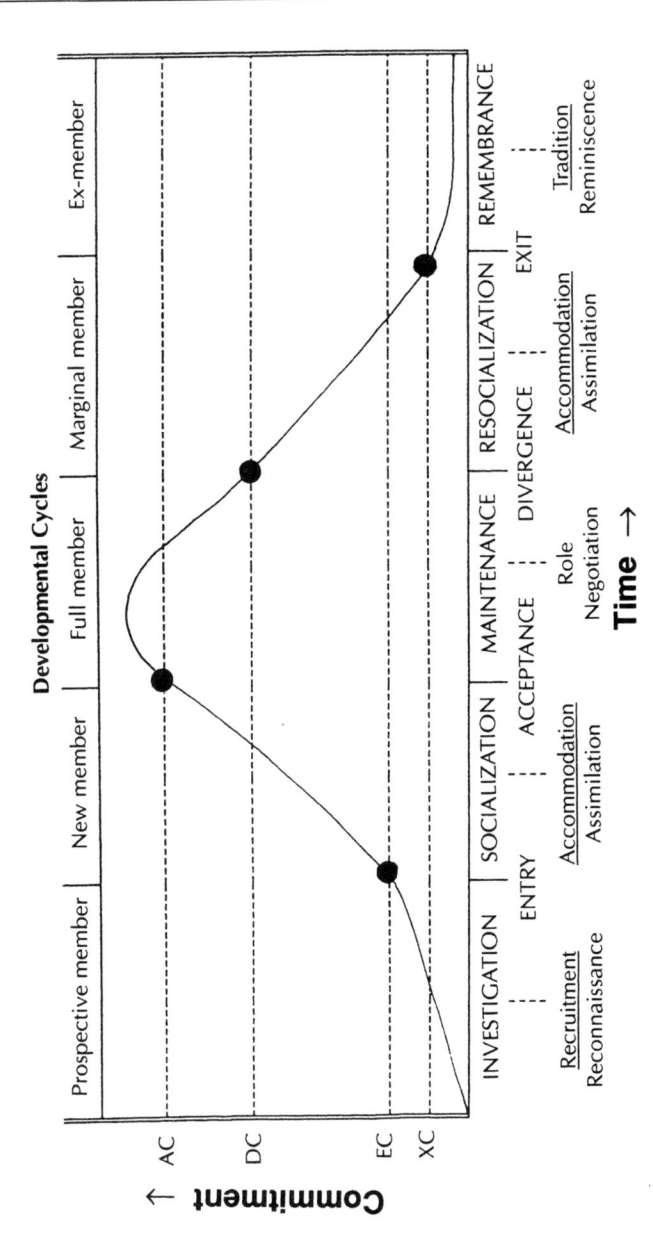

Figure 17.2 Moreland & Levine's (1982) model of group socialization. From Moreland & Levine (1982), with permission

level of *"divergence criteria"* (DC), this marks the point at which commitment to the other no longer warrants full or active group membership. Thus, the individual becomes a "marginal member" and the fourth *"resocialization"* phase of the model is entered. In this phase, the authors assert that both the individual and the group attempt to restore past levels of mutual commitment and perceived rewards through replaying the accommodation and assimilation processes. If this renegotiation fails, and commitment levels continue to fall to either party's *"exit criteria"* (XC), then the final role transition of *"exit"* will occur as the individual leaves the group and the phase of *"remembrance"* commences.

During this final stage, the ex-member will become part of the group's historical *"tradition"*, his or her contributions being remembered more or less favourably. Simultaneously, the individual engages in *"reminiscence"* of the time spent as an active group member, recalling some of the positive and negative psychologically meaningful events which occurred.

Moreland & Levine's five-phase model, incorporating four role transitions, provides a linear-normative model of socialization into social groups, some elements of which are intuitively applicable to work groups (Levine & Moreland, 1994). However, as Moreland & Levine (1984) themselves acknowledge, the model lacks empirical validation and, even in the decade and more since it was originally published, there remain few case studies of organizational socialization which validate this normative model. For example, it is questionable whether the "resocialization" phase of the model, wherein the marginal member and the group will inevitably attempt to restore levels of mutual commitment to previously higher levels, actually occurs in organizational contexts. In work groups, constrained by the wider organization, its formal structures and working practices, it is difficult to imagine this resocialization process actually occurring, particularly if it is the individual who has encouraged this situation through declining commitment to the group. The more likely scenario is that marginality is tolerated for an indefinite period, but is likely to end in exit rather than attempted resocialization.

A further aspect of Moreland & Levine's (1984) model that seems doubtful is the depiction of commitment as typically developing through a curvilinear "n-shaped" trajectory. There are two problems with this. First, as the authors themselves note, situations may exist where there is an imbalance between newcomer commitment to the group, on the one hand, and the group's commitment to the newcomer on the other. Second, it is uncertain that commitment will increase in the early stages of investigation and socialization, reach a peak during the maintenance phase and then tail-off from this point. For example, Vandenberg & Self (1993) investigated newcomers' attitudes in the first 6 months of job role incumbency and found that organizational commitment, organizational identification, and affective and continuance commitment generally declined in magnitude (i.e. alpha changes) over the first 6 months of employment. However, analyses compensating for beta and gamma changes (changes in respondents' perceptions of the measurement scale and the measurement construct respectively) showed reduced levels of change. For affective and continuance commitment,

Vandenberg & Self argue that the reduction in the levels of change were "so dramatic as to render the pattern of mean differences uninterpretable" (p. 557). Conversely, even after partialing out beta and gamma change, there was still a significant decline in newcomer ratings of organizational commitment and organizational identification.

These criticisms noted, the key components of Moreland & Levine's model, based as it is upon the social psychological precepts of mutual commitment and reward, is in principal applicable to the development of processual models of work group socialization. Indeed, Levine & Moreland (1994) discuss the process of newcomer entry into the work group in line with their model, with the third stage of maintenance occurring when the newcomer becomes accepted as a full group member. However, Levine & Moreland do not resolve the problems with the model we have outlined, such as the possibility of inequality between the commitment levels of the group and the newcomer. The strength of Moreland & Levine's model is that it views socialization as a process, occurring over time, which is negotiated between an individual and an established group. A further strength of their model is its simplicity. However, this does have drawbacks of omitting individual, group, and organizational characteristics that affect the socialization process, and which result in specific outcomes. Thus, there is a need for a model of work group socialization which views this as an interactive process occurring over time, and which accounts for individual, group, and organizational factors affecting the input and outcomes of this process; all of these are included in our model of work group socialization (see Figure 17.3).

The Socialization of the Work Group

Our review so far has concentrated upon socialization *into* work groups, the intention being to describe studies which have a bearing upon how newcomers become assimilated into existing work groups. A related, but conceptually distinct, question concerns the socialization of work groups. That is, the socialization of an entirely new group formed to complete a particular project or *ad hoc* task where all group members are newly selected and are thus "newcomers".

Wanous, Reichers & Malik (1984) provide a valuable basis for examining the overlap of work group and organizational levels of socialization. They outline the three situations in which organizational socialization and group development occur simultaneously. The first occurs when an organization uses "collective" tactics (Van Maanen & Schein, 1979) to socialize newcomers, such that they receive their initial training and introduction to the organization as a cohort. Examples of this include military recruits and graduate selection into some corporate organizations. Second, these two processes occur concurrently when a newcomer enters an already established group, necessitating some group redevelopment to re-establish roles, a pecking order, and group norms and climate. Third, Wanous, Reichers & Malik (1984) outline the situation where organizational insiders are placed into new groups, such that group members are, to some

PHASE	NEWCOMER	WORK GROUP
ANTICIPATION	Proposals 1, 2 and 3	

Newcomer Characteristics
- Knowledge, skills and abilities (KSAs)
- Personality
- Interpersonal skills and style
- Values, attitudes and beliefs

Work Group Characteristics
- Structure
- Climate
- Cohesiveness
- Member characteristics
- Norms
- Task performance

Past experience of socialization into work groups

Pre-employment Expectations
- "Anticipatory psychological contract"
- Terms and conditions
- Work role
- Expectations of social contracts and of peers

Expectations of the Newcomer
- Newcomer characteristics
- Degree of conformity to group norms
- Innovativeness of newcomer
- Loyalty and commitment to the group

Organizational socialization procedure, induction training and formal tactics

Expectations created by the organisations selection procedure

Organizational selction procedure – assessment details of newcomer communicated to the work group

ENCOUNTER

Proposals 4 and 5

Socialization Process
- Work group and organizational tactics
- Reactions of the newcomer, including met vs. unmet expectations and unexpected revisions to the psychological contract
- Impact of newcomer upon work group climate, norms and functioning

ADJUSTMENT

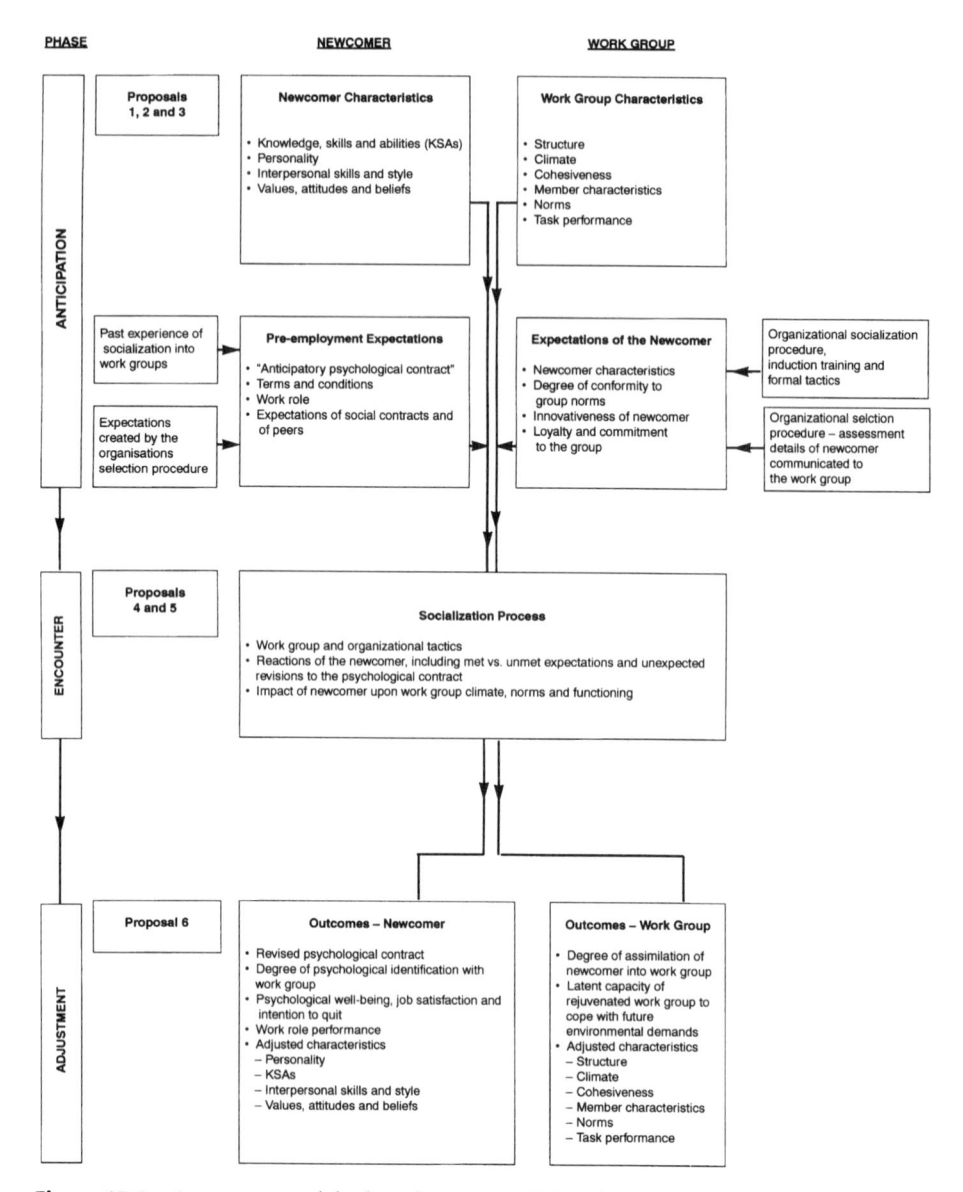

Proposal 6

Outcomes – Newcomer
- Revised psychological contract
- Degree of psychological identification with work group
- Psychological well-being, job satisfaction and intention to quit
- Work role performance
- Adjusted characteristics
  - Personality
  - KSAs
  - Interpersonal skills and style
  - Values, attitudes and beliefs

Outcomes – Work Group
- Degree of assimilation of newcomer into work group
- Latent capacity of rejuvenated work group to cope with future environmental demands
- Adjusted characteristics
  - Structure
  - Climate
  - Cohesiveness
  - Member characteristics
  - Norms
  - Task performance

Figure 17.3 A process model of work group socialization

degree, new to each other; and the group, as an entity, is new to the organization. This third situation is interesting because it contains a wider conception of socialization, enabling veteran insiders to regress to once again become newcomers, and suggesting that the group, as an entity, may have to undergo a process of organizational socialization. Apart from the Wanous, Reichers & Malik (1984) paper, however, a detailed search of the socialization literature revealed no other empirical studies or case studies into the socializtion of work group. Given the increasingly apparent use of such project teams and cross-functional groups in organizations, it is important that future research comes on to explore and chart this process of socializing entire work groups.

Having described the extant resrach in a number of areas which is at least notionally applicable to the field of work group socialization, we move on in the following section to develop and expound a model of work group socialization. Such model development is important, in our view, in the light of the limited attention that socialization at the group level has recevied either from researchers active in organization socialization, or those interested in group processes in organizational settings.

A MODEL OF WORK GROUP SOCIALIZATION

In this section, based upon our preceding review of relevant research and our critical discussion of stage models of organization socialization and social group entry, we posit a model of work group socialization incorporating six testable proposals. Figure 17.3 illustrates our processual model, which highlights the perspective of both the newcomer and the existing group as they interact to produce outcomes for both parties. Outcomes are held to be of two main types—psychological and performance-related. Let us initially consider the structure of the model in overview.

The temporal dimension of socialization—that any socialization process occurs over time and is likely constituted by a series of events which may be clustered into discrete stages—is recognized in many of the existing models of organizational socialization (e.g. Feldman, 1976a,b; Schein, 1978; Wanous, 1992). In the model, we base the three phases of *anticipation*, *encounter* and *adjustment* upon Feldman's (1976a,b) three-stage model of organizational entry—*anticipatory socialization*, *accommodation* and *role management*. However, there are subtle differences in our model in that: (a) we focus specifically upon work group socialization, as opposed to organizational socialization; (b) we highlight the bi-directional impacts of the socialization process upon the newcomer and the group; and (c) we emphasize measurable outcomes for both the individual newcomer and the work group, these being a series of "mutual adjustments" akin to the latter end of Feldman's second stage of "accommodation", moving into the longer-term steady-state phase of "role management".

Phase I: Anticipation

In Feldman's classic model, he used the term "anticipatory socialization" to describe how applicants develop expectations of their new work role prior to organizational entry. Information gleaned from contact with the organization during the selection procedure, contacts with the prospective work group, and the newcomer's past experiences of socialization, are held to affect the nature, type, extent and positiveness of work role expectations. Indeed, Herriot (1989) argues that all selection procedures create mutual expectations between individuals and organizations; the newcomer developing expectations of his or her future work role, conditions of employment and so forth, and the organization developing expectations of the applicant, including job performance standards, loyalty, commitment and, increasingly, flexibility to contribute more generally to team and organizational success via innovation and pro-social organization behaviours (West & Farr, 1990; Anderson & West, in press). Thus we develop our first proposal:

Proposal 1: That newcomers' prior experiences of selection systems and work group socialization will effect their construction of an "anticipatory psychological contract".

Previous studies have found that past experiences of socialization influence newcomers' approaches and reactions to the current socialization process (Feldman & Brett, 1983). We extend these findings to propose that past experience of entry and socialization into teams in the workplace will affect newcomer expectations, attitudes and behaviour during anticipatory socialization. Such past experiences are likely to span a multitude of areas, including information-seeking behaviour, team leader and peer task support, social support within the team, working practices, and so forth. Second, subsumed within this proposal, we assert that newcomer experiences during the selection process will influence expectations. Experiences during interviews, psychometric testing sessions, and especially during multi-day assessment centers, have been found to impact upon candidates quite extensively (Herriot, 1989; Iles & Robertson, 1995; Fletcher, 1991). Here, we develop these findings in selection research to propose that such experiences will affect newcomer attitudes and behaviour during socialization into their work group (see also Anderson & Ostroff, 1996).

Finally, under this proposal, we assert that such experiences will cause the newcomer to generate an "anticipatory psychological contract". This notion is based upon Schein's (1988) original conceptualization of the psychological contract as an exchange relationship, applied to the context of work group socialization. In this situation, the newcomer will develop a naive and imperfect schema, comprising his or her expectations of the group in accordance with the terms and conditions of employment and, more particularly, of anticipated levels of social and task support from work group peers, as well as the newcomer's contribution to the contract in terms of work role expectations, of contributions to both task and social aspects of group functioning, and so forth.

Proposal 2: That newcomer characteristics will mediate individual constructions of the "anticipatory psychological contract".

As a subjective set of perceptions and expectations, the anticipatory psychological contract is clearly open to marked individual differences in form and content. Indeed, this is its very nature. Even where newcomers have progressed as a cohort through standardized selection techniques (e.g. cognitive ability testing, work samples), each individual will construe events differently, leading to the possibility of pronounced differences between individuals in understandings and expectations. Our second proposal, then, is that newcomer characteristics including personality, knowledge, values, interpersonal skills and career motivations, will mediate the construction of the anticipatory psychological contract (e.g. Rousseau, 1990) and the emphasis given to its different aspects (McFarlane Shore & Tetrick, 1994).

> *Proposal 3*: That work group characteristics and selection system information will affect the group's expectations of newcomer behaviour.

From the perspective of the work group, potential newcomers can constitute a threat to established practices, norms and patterns of social interaction between group members. Existing research into work groups and organization socialization has tended to underestimate this point; existing group members may feel particularly apprehensive of the potential newcomer's impact when the group has limited power to influence any selection decision, or where more than one new appointment to the group is being made. We therefore propose that the group will develop a series of unspoken and implicit expectations of newcomer behaviour covering such areas as newcomer loyalty, conformity and innovativeness. We further propose that work group characteristics, including its structure, climate, norms and existing levels of performance, together with information gleaned about the newcomer during the selection process, will affect these expectations.

Phase II: Encounter

In the second phase of the model we consider the initial weeks and months where the newcomer encounters his or her work group and becomes assimilated into its social structure as a valued group member. Here, we develop two further proposals:

> *Proposal 4*: That the newcomer will rely upon his or her proximal work group as the primary source for job-relevant information and reality-testing throughout socialization, and particularly in the initial stages.

Based upon empirical studies reviewed in earlier sections of this chapter, we propose that the proximal work group provides the principal source of information for the newcomer during socialization. Research on information acquisition has found that newcomers rely on strategies of observation and inquiry to gain required knowledge, both of which necessitate the presence of more experienced employees as co-workers and supervisors (e.g. Ostroff & Kozlowski, 1992; Morrison, 1993a,b). Furthermore, Ostroff & Kozlowski's results show that the first area of knowledge in which newcomers feel competent is that relating to their work group, confirming the primacy of this socialization source. As Louis (1990) notes, experienced group members "look at very nearly the same hierarchical and functional slices of the organizational world as does the newcomer" (p. 94), hence they can provide information on aspects of the job such as task performance, as well providing the newcomer with a reference point for reality testing.

Proposal 5: That socialization processes will mutually affect the newcomer and the group.

We hold work group socialization to be quintessentially a bi-directional process, affecting both the individual and the group. That is, that both the newcomer and the group proceed through concurrent processes toward mutual assimilation and acceptance. Although most recent organization socialization studies have focused upon the newcomer, several authors have acknowledged that socialization is likely to affect both parties (Louis, 1980; Chao et al., 1994). Two potential scenarios are apparent in terms of the degrees of change experienced by the newcomer and the group, the second of which can be further divided into two sub-categories. First, *symmetrical development* occurs where both the newcomer and the group undergo a relatively equal degree and type of change during socialization. For example, where a skilled operative joins a small autonomous work group responsible for component assembly, it is likely that both the newcomer and the group will need to develop and modify to a similar extent in order to accommodate the other.

Second, *asymmetrical development* occurs where either the newcomer or, alternatively, the group is forced to undergo considerably more development than the other. In the former case, examples are where a new military recruit joins an active service unit which follows strict in-service rules and regulations or where a new violinist joins the string section of an orchestra. In both of these instances, the onus of change falls more heavily upon the individual newcomer, who is expected to fit in to existing group practices and rule structures. A particularly extreme instance of this asymmetrical individual development is likely to occur where a single newcomer joins an established group suffering from the constrictions of the "groupthink" phenomenon (Janis, 1972). Here, the group is obsessively concerned with maintaining cohesiveness in its decision-making to the extent that they would be expected to be intolerant of newcomer heterogeneity or lack of conformity to group norms. In other circumstances it is the group which is subject to asymmetrical development. In a sporting context, the recruitment of a highly gifted but individualistic player into a team may cause the coach to restructure the whole team around this player. A group is particularly likely to metamorphose when a team leader with a radically different leadership style or orientation is appointed, such as when a new conductor is appointed to an orchestra. Asymmetrical development of the group may occur through the intentional influence strategies of the newcomer (Nicholson, 1984) or through accidental processes, such as minority influence. Minorities can act as models for dissent and resistance of social pressure, modify thought processes, and even stimulate more divergent work role responses (Nemeth, 1986; Mucchi-Faina, Maass & Volpato, 1991). From previous studies, Mucchi-Faina, Maass & Volpato suggest that "minorities not only elicit quantitatively and qualitatively better performance but they also induce more creative and original thinking in majorities" (p. 184) (see Nemeth, this volume, for a review of these issues). The naive newcomer, through questioning members of his or her proximal work group, may influence the group to such an extent as to cause the group to develop and change more than the newcomer does. Equally, the possibility of multiple newcomers unwittingly forming a minority influence in a group should be acknowledged. In these circumstances, the newcomer minority may affect group decision-making through a lack of knowledge of existing procedures or simple mistakes in understanding; a process which may be termed "minority influence via ignorance".

Phase III: Adjustment

The final phase of the model depicted in Figure 17.3 is that of "adjustment"— both the newcomer to the group and the group to the newcomer. Following Feldman (1976a,b), we propose that the socialization process results in a number of measurable outcomes for both parties:

Proposal 6: That socialization processes will result in measurable psychological and performance-related outcomes for both the newcomer and the group.

Previous research in organizational socialization has been criticized for lacking clear or meaningful criteria by which to evaluate the outcomes of this process (Reichers, 1987). We propose that psychological and performance-related outcomes will arise for both the newcomer and the group. For the newcomer, positive psychological outcomes include perceptions of task mastery, self-esteem, personal growth and opportunity for skill use, whilst positive performance-related outcomes clearly include the rate of learning on-the-job, early output levels, establishment of relationships with co-workers which are conducive to acceptable team performance, and so forth. For the group, positive psychological outcomes include maintained or improved team climate and the support of norms conducive to team performance, whilst positive performance-related outcomes include initial improvements in group productivity and the enhancement of the team's productive capacity and ability to respond to changing future and environmental demands. However, it should be noted that the group's performance may temporarily decline during the initial adjustment phase; for example, if new techniques or procedures are introduced, these will need time to be learned and practised before they prove their effectiveness and enable improvements over the group's former outputs. Importantly, such outcomes are measurable at both the individual and group levels and therefore, in principle, can provide useful data allowing post-hoc validation of the socialization process.

To summarize, this processual model with its six related proposals is propounded as a general model of the process of work group socialization, with the caveat that, of course, for different contexts and work groups, the timings of each phase of the socialization process will differ. The six proposals warrant empirical testing in a variety of group and organizational environments, the quintessential component of such study designs being the longitudinal nature of research required to evaluate any specific hypotheses derived from these general theoretical proposals. Our emphasis in the model upon measurable performance-related and psychological outcomes is intentional: researchers in the seemingly disparate fields of work groups and organization socialization need to incorporate such outcome measures into future studies of work group socialization considerably more readily than they have done in the past.

CONCLUSION

In his review of the socialization research at the organizational level of analysis, Feldman (1989), as we quoted earlier in this chapter, concluded acerbically that "... there has been too much approach, and not enough arrival" (Feldman, 1989, p. 405). Having completed this review of the existing research germane to work group socialization, it is tempting to conclude that there has been precious little constructive approach, let alone any signs of arrival. Whereas researchers in socialization have tended to focus at either the organizational or the individual levels of analysis, to the unjustifiable exclusion of studies examining the process of socialization into proximal work groups, researchers studying team-working in organizations can be criticized for neglecting the effects of personnel changes upon work group functioning and performance. The topic of work group socialization appears to have fallen rather unfortunately in the investigative "no man's land" somewhere between these two fields of active research, and has thus remained comparatively unresearched despite its demonstrable and obvious importance to effective team working and to the job performance of individual newcomers into work groups.

Yet, at several points in this chapter the relevance of work group socialization for researchers, practising managers and personnel practitioners has been hinted at. The potential synergistic benefits to be gained from integrative research drawing from existing knowledge and expertise in organizational socialization, on the one hand, and work group processes and performance, on the other, cannot be overstated in relation to future research into work group socialization. The immediate problem faced by researchers intent upon exploring the process of work group socialization, however, will be the sheer volume of possible directions for future investigation, and consequently, of establishing some priority areas for initial attention. For this reason, we have concentrated in the latter sections of this chapter upon developing and explicating a general but testable model of work group socialization. It is our view that there exists an expansive range of potentially fruitful research questions that could be examined in work group socialization. Much of the research reviewed in this chapter is relevant to this topic, but was not originally conducted with the meso-analytical focus of the work group as its primary concern. Early research efforts, specifically investigating work group socialization, therefore need to be preceded by the development of domain-specific theories and operationalizable models capable of further empirical testing in organizational settings.

Returning to our earlier review of the definitions imposed by researchers upon the field of socialization over the last 30 years or so, we would argue that it is now timely for a "fifth era" of definitions to guide future research—the *"bi-directional influence"* era. Newcomers do not merely seek information in an active attempt to fit in to their new work role, they undoubtedly *influence* their role, the existing work group and the wider organization. This influence may be to a greater or lesser extent, and it clearly depends upon a number of complex factors, but nevertheless, the process of newcomer socialization needs to be construed, and thus defined, as a mutually affective process: the organization influencing and changing the newcomer and, simultaneously, the newcomer influencing and changing his or her proximal work group and the organization as a whole.

In conclusion, in this chapter we have attempted to define with some clarity the concept and process of work group socialization, to extrapolate the existing body of research findings in areas tangential but applicable to socialization into and of working groups and, grounded upon this review, to expound a testable model of the process of work group socialization which assumes as unassailable the bi-directional impact of socialization upon both the newcomer and the group. It is our hope that this review and the model as proposed stimulates further research into the so far neglected but undoubtedly important topic of work group socialization.

ACKNOWLEDGEMENT

We thank Michael West and Peter Herriot for their constructive comments on an earlier draft of this chapter.

REFERENCES

Anderson, N.R. (1992). Eight decades of employment interview research: a retrospective meta-review and prospective commentary. *European Work and Organizational Psychologist*, **2**, 1–32.

Anderson, N.R. & Shackleton, V.J. (1993). *Successful Selection Interviewing*. Oxford: Blackwell.

Anderson, N.R. (1995). Graduate organizational socialization and induction training in Britain. In N.R. Anderson & C. Ostroff (Chairs), *The Socialization Process: Organizational Tactics, Individual Differences, Learning and Outcomes.* Symposium conducted at the 10th Annual Conference of the Society for Industrial and Organizational Psychology, Orlando, FL, May 1995.

Anderson, N.R. & Ostroff, C. (1996). Selection as socialization. In N.R. Anderson & P. Herriot (eds), *Assessment and Selection in Organizations*, 2nd Edn. Chichester: Wiley.

Anderson, N.R. & West, M.A. (1996). The team climate inventory: development of the TCI and its application in teambuilding for innovativeness. *European Work and Organizational Psychologist*, in press.

Berlew, D.E. & Hall, D.T. (1966). The socialization of managers: effects of expectations on performance. *Administrative Science Quarterly*, 11, 207–223.

Brim, O.G. Jr (1966). Socialization through the life cycle. In O.G. Brim & S. Wheeler (eds), *Socialization after Childhood: Two Essays*. New York: Wiley.

Caplow, T. (1964). *Principles of Organization*. New York: Harcourt, Brace and World.

Chatman, J.A. (1991). Matching people and organizations: selection and socialization in public accounting firms. *Administrative Science Quarterly*, 36, 459–484.

Chao, G.T., Kozlowski, S.W.J., Major, D.A. & Gardner, P. (1994). The effects of organizational tactics and contextual factors on newcomer socialization and learning outcomes. In S.W.J. Kozlowski (Chair), *Transitions during Organizational Socialization: Newcomer Expectations, Information-seeking, and Learning Outcomes*. Symposium conducted at the 9th Annual Conference of the Society for Industrial and Organizational Psychology, Nashville, TN, April 1994.

Comer, D.R. (1991). Organizational newcomers' acquisition of information from peers. Management Communication Quarterly, 5, 64–89.

Feldman, D.C. (1976a). A contingency theory of socialization. *Administrative Science Quarterly*, 21, 433–452.

Feldman, D.C. (1976b). A practical program for employee socialization. *Organization Dynamics*, **Autumn**, 64–80.

Feldman, D.C. (1989). Socialization, resocialization and training: reframing the research agenda. In Goldstein (ed.), *Training and Development in Organizations*. San Francisco: Jossey-Bass, pp. 376–416.

Feldman, D.C. & Brett, J.M. (1983). Coping with new jobs: a comparative study of new lives and job changers. *Academy of Management, Journal*, 26(2), 258–272.

Fisher, C.D. (1986). Organizational socialization: an integrative review. In K. Roland & G. Feris (eds), *Research in Personnel and Human Resources Management*, Vol. 4. Greenwich, CT: JAI, pp. 101–145.

Fletcher, C. (1991). Candidates' reactions to assessment centres and their outcomes: a longitudinal study. *Journal of Occupational & Organizational Psychology*, 64, 117–127.

Herriot, P. (1984). *Down From The Ivory Tower: Graduates and Their Jobs*. Chichester: Wiley.

Herriot, P. (1989). Selection as a social process. In M. Smith & I.T. Robertson (eds), *Advances in Staff Selection*. Chichester: Wiley.

Iles, P.A. & Robertson, I.T. (1995). The impact of personnel selection procedures on candidates. In N.R. Anderson & P. Herriot (eds), *Assessment and Selection in Organizations*, 2nd Edn. Chichester: Wiley.

Janis, I.L. (1972). *Victims of Groupthink*. Boston, MA: Houghton Mifflin.

Katz, R. (1980). Time and work: toward an integrative perspective. In B.M. Staw & L.L. Cummings (eds), *Research in Organizational Behaviour*, Vol. 2. Greenwich, CT: JAI Press, pp. 81–127.

Levine, J.M. & Moreland, R.L. (1994). Group socialization: theory & research. In W. Stroebe & M. Hewstone (eds), *European Review of Social Psychology*, Vol. 5. Chichester: Wiley.

Louis, M.R. (1980). Surprise and sense making: what newcomers experience in entering unfamiliar organizational settings. *Administrative Science Quarterly*, 25, 226–251.

Louis, M.R. (1990). Acculturation in the workplace: newcomers and lay ethnographers. In B. Schneider (ed.), *Organizational Climate and Culture*. San Francisco, CA: Jossey-Bass.

Louis, M.R., Posner, B.Z. & Powell, G.N. (1983). The availability and helpfulness of socialization practices. *Personnel Psychology*, **36**, 857–866.

McClean Parks, J. & Kidder, D.L. (1994). Till death us do part: changing work relationships in the 1990s. In C.L. Cooper & D.M. Rousseau (eds), *Trends in Organizational Behaviour*, Vol. 1. Chichester: Wiley.

McFarlane Shore, L. & Tetrick, L.E. (1994). The psychological contract as an explanatory framework in the employment relationship. In C.L. Cooper & D.M. Rousseau (eds), *Trends in Organizational Behaviour*, Vol. 1. Chichester: Wiley, pp. 91–109.

Moreland, R.L. & Levine, J.M. (1982). Socialization in small groups: temporal changes in individual–group relations. *Advances in Experimental Social Psychology*, **15**, 137–192.

Moreland, R.L. & Levine, J. (1984). Role transitions in small groups. In V.L. Allen & E. Van de Vliert (eds) *Role Transitions: Explorations and Explanations*. Plenum Press: New York, pp. 181–195.

Moreland, R.L. & Levine, J.M. (1988). Group dynamics over time. In J.E. McGrath (ed.), *The Social Psychology of Time: New Perspectives*. Newbury Park: Sage, pp. 151–181.

Morrison, E.W. (1993a). Longitudinal study of the effects of information seeking on newcomer socialization. *Journal of Applied Psychology*, **78***(2)*, 173–183.

Morrison, E.W. (1993b). Newcomer information seeking: exploring types, modes, sources and outcomes. *Academy of Management Journal*, **36**(3), 557–589.

Morrison, E.W. (1994). Learning the Ropes: Information Acquisition during Socialization. Unpublished manuscript, Stern School of Business, New York University.

Muchhi-Faina, A., Maass, A. & Volpato, C. (1991). Social influence: the role of originality. *European Journal of Social Psychology*, **21**, 183–197.

Nelson, D.L. (1987). Organizational socialization: a stress perspective. *Journal of Occupational Behaviour*, **8**, 311–324.

Nelson, D.L. & Quick, J.C. (1991). Social Support and newcomer adjustment in organizations: attachment theory at work? *Journal of Organizational Behaviour*, **12**, 543–554.

Nemeth, C.J. (1986). Differential contributions of majority and minority influence. *Psychological Review*, **93**(1), 23–32.

Nicholson, N. (1984). A theory of work role transitions. *Administrative Science Quarterly*, **29**, 172–191.

Nicholson, N. & Arnold, J. (1989). Graduate early experience in a multinational corporation, *Personnel Review*, **18**, 3–14.

Ostroff, C. & Kozlowski, S.W.J. (1992). Organizational socialization a learning process: the role of information acquisition. *Personnel Psychology*, **45**, 498–874.

Posner, B. & Powell, G.N. (1985). Female and male socialization experiences: an initial investigation. *Journal of Occupational Psychology*, **58**, 81–85.

Reichers, A.E. (1987). An interactionist perspective on newcomer socialization rates. *Academy of Management Review*, **12**(2), 276–278.

Rousseau, D.M. (1990). New hire perceptions of their own and their employer's obligations: a study of psychological contracts. *Journal of Organizational Behaviour*, **11**, 389–400.

Schein, E.H. (1968). Organizational socialization and the profession of management. *Industrial Management Review*, **9**, 1–16.

Schein, E.H. (1978). Entry into the organizational career. In R.H.J. Hackman, E.E. III Lawler & L.W. Porter (eds), *Perspectives on Behaviour in Organizations*. New York: McGraw-Hill.

Schein, E.H. (1988). *Organizational Psychology*, 3rd Edn. London: Prentice-Hall.

Schneider, B. (1987). The people make the place. *Personnel Psychology*, **40**, 437–453.

Smith, E.M. & Kozlowski, S.W.J. (1994). Socialization and adaptation: individual and contextual influences on social learning strategies. Paper presented at 9th Annual Conference of the Society for Industrial and Organizational Psychology, Nashville, TN, April 1994.

Sutton, R.I. & Louis, M. (1987). How selecting and socializing newcomers influences insiders. *Human Resource Management*, **26**(3), 347–361.

Vandenberg, R.J. & Self, R.M. (1993). Assessing newcomers' changing commitments to the organization during the first six months of work. *Journal of Applied Psychology*, **78**(4), 557–568.

Van Maanen, J. (1978). People processing: strategies of organizational socialization. *Organizational Dynamics*, **14**, 19–36.

Van Maanen, J. & Schein, E. (1979). Toward a theory of organizational socialization. *Research in Organizational Behaviour*, **1**, 209–264.

Wagner, R.K. & Sternberg, R.J. (1986). Tacit knowledge and intelligence in the everyday world. In R.J. Sternberg & R.K. Wagner (eds), *Practical Intelligence: Nature and Origins of Competence in the Everyday World*. New York: Cambridge University Press, pp. 51–83.

Wagner, R.K. & Sternberg, R.J. (1991). Tacit knowledge: its uses in identifying, assessing and developing managerial talent. In. J. Jones, B. Steffy & D. Bray (eds), *Applying Psychology in Business: The Manager's Handbook*. New York: Human Sciences Press, pp. 333–344.

Wanous, J.P. (1980). *Organizational Entry: Recruitment, Selection and Socialization of Newcomers*, 1st Edn. Reading. MA: Addison-Wesley.

Wanous, J.P. (1992). *Organizational Entry: Recruitment, Selection, Orientation and Socialization of Newcomers*, 2nd. Edn. Reading, MA: Addison-Wesley.

Wanous, J.P., Reichers, A.E. & Malik, S.D. (1984). Organizational socialization and group development: towards an integrative perspective. *Academy of Management Review*, **9**(4), 670–683.

West, M.A. & Farr, J.L. (eds) (1990). *Innovation and Creativity at Work: Psychological and Organizational Strategies*. Chichester: John Wiley.

Chapter 18

Approaches to Communication Structure: Applications to the Problem of Information-seeking

J. David Johnson
Department of Communication, Michigan State University, USA

Abstract

This chapter focuses on the problem of information-seeking from the perspective of three different approaches to communication structure, hierarchies, networks and markets. Structure determines what is possible in large organizations since it enables action. Increasingly, information-seeking activity has become a critical determinant of the success of organizational members and of the organization as a whole. There is a persistent dilemma for organizations, the imperative, in part stemming from efficiency needs, to limit the availability of information, and the recognition that structural designs are often flawed and circumstances change, requiring individuals to seek information normally unavailable to them. In this chapter we first examine the traditional perspectives on structure represented by hierarchies, which serve to limit the access of individuals to information. Next, we will consider network analysis which represents an inherently more flexible approach to understanding information-seeking. Then, we will examine more modern conceptions of information-seeking related to the emerging application of market concepts to organizational settings. Finally, we will discuss the interplay of these concepts and ideas in relationship to the critical issue of innovation in organizations.

In a market each element (individual, firm) pursues its own interest and the interaction between elements produces a collective outcome—the market coordinates the separate activities. Coordination by hierarchy is different in that the actions of similar elements (individuals, firms) is to some extent constrained. Hierarchy presupposes an already determined outcome or purpose; the underlying idea of hierarchy is that such an outcome can be broken down into a set of sub-processes. So hierarchy depends upon ideas of organization, task specialization and rationality. (Mitchell, 1991, p. 104).

Organizational communication structure refers to the relatively stable configuration of communication relationships between entities within an organizational context. (Johnson, 1992a, p. 100).

Naturally, for such a central concept in the social sciences, many approaches to structure have been developed in the literature (see Johnson, 1993, for a review). Here we will focus primarily on the increasingly intertwined approaches of hierarchies, networks and markets, referring at times to cultural and gradient (representing spatial forces) approaches as well.

Structure implies some degree of temporal stability or permanence, a relatively enduring set of linkages: "This structure gives regularity and stability to human behavior in a social system; it allows us to predict behavior with some degree of accuracy" (Rogers, 1983, p. 24). This predictability inevitably results in a reduction of uncertainty among organizational members (Rogers & Agarwala-Rogers, 1976). Temporal stability is important in increasing predictability, since organizational relationships that are relatively enduring are also more predictable. Our first choice for information will often be the individuals with whom we have a recurring relationship.

Communication structure determines what is possible in large organizations since it enables action. "Networks make the achievement of output goals (such as production) possible" (Farace, Monge & Russell, 1977, p. 179). Without a predictable pattern of recurring relationships, coordinated activity within the organization would be impossible. The more constraints that exist, the more things occur in known, predictable patterns; the more information people have concerning the organization.

Context, relationships and entities result in a configuration which forms a gestalt of an organization's structure. Following classic discussions of systems (Katz & Kahn, 1978) and contingency perspectives of differentiation and integration (Lawrence & Lorsch, 1967), organizational entities and relationships between them have often been considered the central focus of organizational theory. Organizations, to meet demands from their environment and in order to become more skilled, specialize their labor (Katz & Kahn, 1978). More and more entities emerge within the context of the organization and, in turn, the increased number of groups implies increasingly rich and diverse relationships among these entities, and greater variety in potential sources of information. The nature of these entities ranges from objects to units of a system. How entities are defined determines the level of analysis of communication structure research, an increasingly important issue in management (see Dansereau & Markham, 1987;

Rousseau, 1985 for an exhaustive discussion) and communication research (Berger & Chaffee, 1987; Monge, 1987).

In the classic organizational form, with task specialization, each group is a repository of unique information. How this information is applied to and shared with other groups in ongoing work processes represents a delicate balancing act that is critical to organizational success. If too much is shared, then work teams cannot appropriately specialize. If too little is shared, then there may not be a general understanding of what needs to be done.

Increasingly, information-seeking has become a critical determinant of the success of organizational groups and of the organization as a whole. The comfortable world where one's supervisor provided authoritative directives concerning organizational activities has gradually changed to one where organizational groups must make their own decisions about what goals should be emphasized and how they should be accomplished (Johnson et al., 1995). In this context information-seeking, the purposive acquisition of information from selected information carriers (e.g. messages, sources, and channels), becomes a pivotal force in explaining the development of structures. In turn, structure provides the human framework within which information-seeking can occur within organizations.

Growing interest in information-seeking can be coupled with a renewed interest in ignorance (Kerwin, 1993; LaFollette, 1993; Ravetz, 1993; Smithson, 1993; Stocking & Holstein, 1993). Failures to seek information have numerous consequences. First, ignorance is likely to result in considerable inefficiencies in organizational operations through such impacts as misunderstandings, the duplication of effort, working at cross-purposes, time-delays, etc. (Inman, Olivas & Golen, 1986). Second, ignorance can lead to disastrous outcomes for organizations, such as the Challenger tragedy (Lewis, 1988) or Pinto's exploding gas tanks (Strobel, 1980), where at least some organizational members' knew that these outcomes were likely. Third, these inefficiencies and more dramatic outcomes are likely to have impacts on workers' feelings of stress, tension, burnout and frustration that, in turn, can produce low morale, increased absenteeism and even turnover. Fourth, ignorance can result in a lack of integration of the individual into the group's culture, contributing to a feeling of individual anomie. Fifth, ignorance may be associated with low levels of participation (Marshall & Stohl, 1993) and commitment to organizational change efforts (Miller, Johnson & Grau, 1994) Indeed, a rather a common complaint in organizations is: why doesn't anybody know anything? (Johnson, 1993; Downs, Clampitt & Pfeiffer, 1988).

The information context of the modern organization is rapidly evolving. Information technologies, including databases, new telecommunications systems and software for synthesizing information, make a vast array of information concerning technical problems available to an ever-expanding number of organizational members. Management's exclusive control over information resources is steadily declining, in part because of the downsizing of organizations and the decline of the number of layers in an organizational hierarchy. These trends put increasing responsibility on groups to become active seekers of information, rather than passive recipients, especially for decision support and problem-solving (Rouse & Rouse, 1984). Regrettably, academic approaches to these secular trends have lagged, partly because of traditional focus on management and controls over information (Johnson et al., 1995).

Organizations are specifically designed to encourage ignorance through specialization and rigid segmentation of effort (Kanter, 1983). So there is a constant dilemma for organizations, the imperative, in part stemming from efficiency needs, to limit the availability of information, and the recognition that structural designs are often flawed and circumstances change, requiring groups and their members to seek information normally unavailable to them. However, the design of the formal structure, and the rewards associated with it (e.g. promotion) often are designed specifically to discourage the sharing of information (Powell, 1990). Increasingly, organizations must also structure themselves to promote the gathering and sharing of information. How they resolve these conflicting imperatives is a critical question for the modern organization. Unfortunately, while volumes have been written on formal organizational design, comparatively little is known about the forces which shape information-seeking within organizations (Johnson et al., 1995).

An Example

As an example let us look at the formal and informal communication structures of Conundrum Corporation shown in Figures 18.1 and 18.2. The organizational chart in Figure 18.1 specifies the formal division of groups and the official relationships within this organization. Following the formal organizational chart,

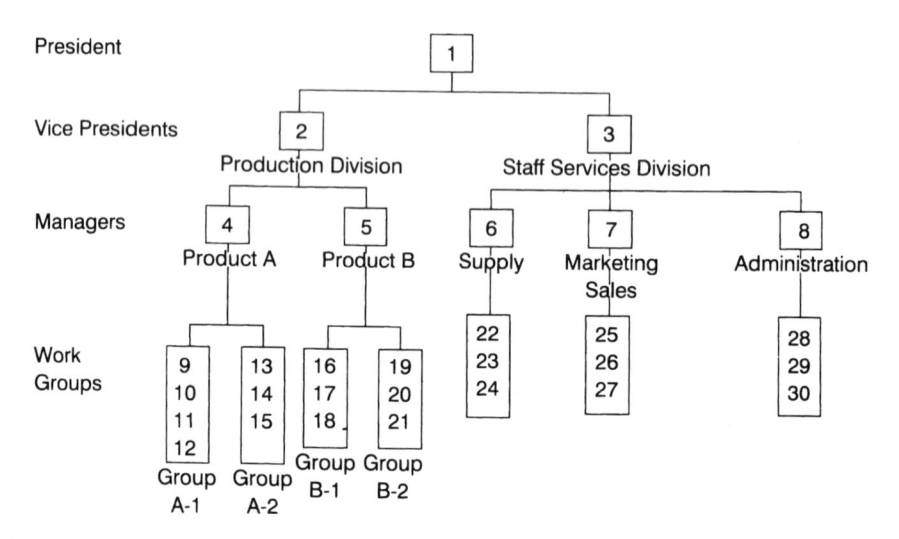

Figure 18.1 Conundrum Corporation organizational chart

APPROACHES TO COMMUNICATION STRUCTURE   455

there are official rules and protocols governing the seeking and giving of information. If the Vice President of Staff Services (3) wants information concerning the morale of formal Group A-2, she/he would know where the information is located and would channel his/her request through managers 1, 2 and 4. Needless to say, this would be cumbersome and time-consuming, and any one of these individuals could gatekeep information, deciding there really wasn't a need for 3 to have this information. In addition, the group members might be reluctant to share this information with an outsider in another division of the organization.

Figure 18.2 represents the network of informal relationships in this organization, portrayed in a communigram, where circles represent individuals and lines indicate relationships between them. Gathering information within a set of informal relationships requires a different approach and set of skills than within a formal structure. Suppose that the President (1) seeks an evaluation of 16 for a possible promotion. Normally, 5 might be somewhat resistant, given that she/he might be losing one of his/her best people. However, because 1 and 5 are both in a relatively cohesive management group, 5 may be more willing to share information. In addition, 1 can obtain information on 16's performance through the back-door channel of 3 and 21.

In contrast to the formal structure, more idiosyncratic sources of information are used in the informal structure, which often require a certain level of experience and history in the work groupings. The rules governing the transmission of information are also different, with informal rather than formal norms governing what is an appropriate target of information-seeking.

These examples illustrate that there can be considerably different approaches to seeking information within different communication structures of the organi-

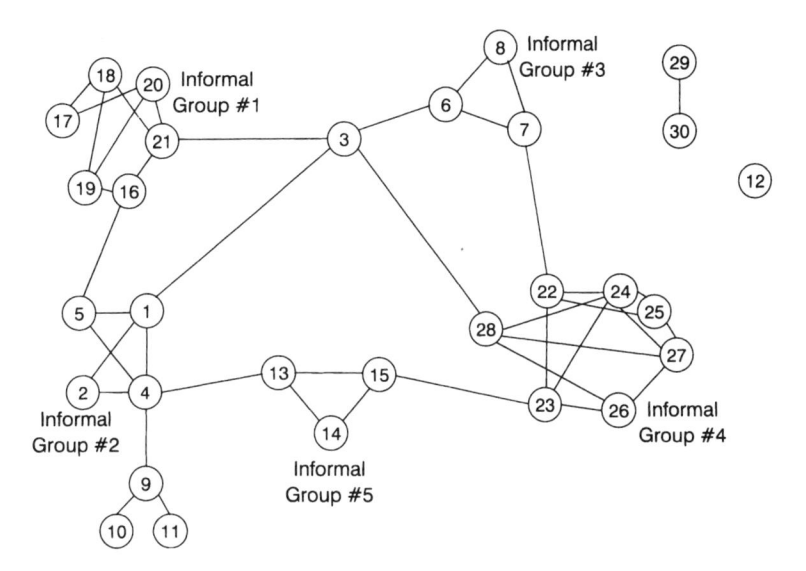

Figure 18.2 Conundrum Corporation communigram of informal network relationships

zation. In this chapter we will explore in more detail the role that structure plays in information-seeking. First, we will examine the traditional perspectives on structure represented by hierarchies or formal approaches. Next, we will consider network analysis, which represents an inherently more flexible approach to understanding information-seeking. Finally, we will examine more modern conceptions of information-seeking related to the emerging application of market concepts to organizational settings.

HIERARCHIES

> If intelligence is lodged at the top, too few officials and experts with too little accurate and relevant information are too far out of touch and too overloaded to cope. On the other hand, if intelligence is scattered in many subordinate units, too many officials and experts with too much specialized information may engage in dysfunctional competition, may delay decisions while they warily consult each other, and may distort information as they pass it up ... (Wilensky, 1968, p. 325).

Early approaches to studying formal communication structure in organizations concentrated on the organizational chart and the flow of messages vertically and horizontally within it. The formal organizational chart is embedded in the assumptions of the classical approach to rational management (Morgan, 1986; Astley & Zajac, 1991). It specifies very clearly who reports to whom and, in effect, constitutes a map for the routing of communication messages and for repositories of key information for those interested in information-seeking (see Figure 18.1).

Hierarchical, or formal, approaches focus on the configurations resulting from the following characteristics of structure: formal authority relationships represented in the organizational hierarchy (Dow, 1988; Jablin, 1987); differentiation of labor into specialized tasks often represented by defined work groups (Dow, 1988; Jablin, 1987); and formal mechanisms for coordination of work among these tasks (Dow, 1988). These characteristics, along with the notion of goal or purpose, have been seen by some to represent the very essence of what an organization is (Schein, 1965). Indeed, hierarchies can be viewed as inevitable features of social organization (Frances et al., 1991), which provide a basic framework for information-seeking. A formal structure specifies who is the official source of particular types of information, and who has officially been defined as representing a group as a seeker and source of information.

One central impetus underlying the development of formal structures, then, is the differentiation of entities into specialized sub-tasks, typically performed by work groups, who depend on each other and therefore must communicate to coordinate their activities (Dow, 1988; Downs, 1967; O'Neill, 1984; Pfeffer, 1978; Thompson, 1967). In general, information load is determined by such factors as size, transmission rules and degree of interdependence (Downs, 1967). Formal structure has often been cast as an information-processing mechanism (e.g. Jablin, 1987), whose primary purpose is to decrease information overload by reducing the possibilities for communication. Structure permits an organization to deal with more information, since a lot of distinct information is processed by means of specialization. This information is then filtered before it is processed by other units. As a result, more information can be processed, since some responsibility is delegated to particular groups, so that everyone does not have to handle the same information. As a result, structure reduces information overload in organizations (Rogers & Agarwala-Rogers, 1976) and thereby increases the efficiency of their operations.

Organizations which severely constrain their structures substantially reduce their level of information load. The more severely constrained the structure, the more the organization is divided into autonomous groups, the less the general distribution of knowledge in an organization. Some have gone so far as to suggest that the classic forms of bureaucracy "are invitations to intelligence and communication failures" (Lee, 1970, p. 101), because of this rigid segmentation of groupings responsible for particular classes of information (Kanter, 1983). Ironically, in reducing information overload, and relatedly information-seeking, a valuable contribution to organizational efficiency, organizations reduce the availability of information, which can reduce organizational effectiveness, particularly in terms of effective decision-making (Johnson, 1993).

The purposive exclusion of groups in the organization from information also deprives them of the information necessary to successfully participate in organization-wide decision-making. So, for example, a common response of management to workers pressing ideas for change is that you do not have all the facts, and if you did you would hold the same position that we do. Thus information is purposively manipulated to maintain the relative power of various groups. Lower-level employees, especially skilled technicians, can also accumulate power by not sharing information with management (Eisenberg & Whetten, 1987).

In fact, planned ignorance is essential to organizational efficiency. By definition, a specialist focuses on a limited domain of knowledge. The broader the domain, the less sophisticated the specialist. Indeed, one way to increase the efficiency of communication is to minimize the need for it by such strategies as coordination by plan, where units concentrate on fulfilling formally assigned tasks that fit into the larger whole (March & Simon, 1958). This design strategy purposely encourages ignorance of the operation of other subunits.

As uncertainty reaches high levels, however, the traditional hierarchical approach runs into difficulty and the organization is confronted with strategies that involve a departure from traditional perspectives of coordination. Essentially, the major choice an organization faces is whether to reduce the need for information-processing or increase its capacity to process information (Galbraith, 1973; March & Simon, 1958). Organizations can be improved not by producing more information, but by reducing the amount any one formal group must handle (Johnson & Rice, 1987). Reduction in need depends primarily on the strategies of creation of slack resources and creation of self-contained tasks, which are both aimed at reducing the need for communication between groups (Galbraith, 1973), and by implication increasing their ignorance of other organizational operations.

Increasing the capacity for information-processing requires investments in vertical information systems, such as computer-based management information systems, and the creation of lateral relations that require a heavy investment in human resources. The creation of lateral resources involves much more personalized integrating mechanisms such as liaisons, task forces and teams, which should result in a greater awareness of organizational members of each other's activities. However, they are extremely costly in terms of communication (Cheng, 1983; Hage, Aiken & Marrett, 1971) and in some contexts may be inefficient (Lawrence & Lorsch, 1967). So, the additional effort put forward in communicating and integrating a work team to solve a problem that might be best confronted by an individual worker detracts from an organization's overall performance.

In fact, there may be a natural tendency for organizations to develop hierarchical communication structures which segment the organization. In reviewing the literature on small group communication network studies, Shaw (1971) found clear evidence of a relationship between effectiveness in the performance of particular types of tasks and the relative degree of centralization of these groups. Shaw (1971) adopts the concept of saturation to explain these findings. For complex problems the most central person quickly becomes overloaded with information and distracted by the burden of relaying information to other group members. When the group is faced with a simple task the volume of communication can be easily handled and there is a benefit to having a central repository of information. However, the independence possible in decentralized groups permits the sharing of the relaying burden of information among group members and also results in a better "match" of individual capabilities to the problems that the group is confronted with.

Guetskow & Simon (1955), in an interesting twist on these experiments, speculated that one of the reasons centralized groups were more efficient was that they had in effect been provided with a plan of action for making decisions. They discovered that if decentralized groups had an opportunity to discuss group organization after they had some experience in the task they became just as efficient as more centralized groups in performing simple tasks. They became more efficient by reducing the number of linkages that were used within the group. Other research studies have also suggested that there is a general trend over time for efficient groups to reduce the number of communication linkages used; in effect, to become more structured or to match their structure to the task at hand (Katz & Kahn, 1978). Indeed, some have argued that these processes can be generalized to a broad range of systems, that hierarchies are inevitable (Krackhardt, 1989).

The context of formal structure lies in the "official world" of the organization. Most often it can be conceived of as embedded in the formal authority structure of the organization, usually associated with bureaucracy. In this context communication is conceived as flowing along the proscribed pathways of the organizational chart, and the content of communication is limited to those production-related matters that concern the organization. While this formal approach constitutes a limited view of the role of communication in organizations, this still may be, especially operationally, the most important role of communication, and certainly one that management must at least try to control. Perhaps most importantly, the traditional view of communication structure reinforces some dangerous assumptions that managers often hold; that messages flow along the conduits represented by the organizational chart without blockage or interruption, that management is in charge, and that messages actually reach their destinations (Axley, 1984). It also suggests that information will be provided to individuals who need to know and that therefore individuals should play a more passive role and not engage in active information-seeking.

So there is a constant dilemma for organizations; the imperative (in part stemming from efficiency needs) to limit the availability of information, and the recognition that structural designs are often flawed and circumstances change, requiring groups to seek information normally unavailable to them. However, formal structure, and the rewards associated with it (e.g. promotion) often are designed specifically to discourage the sharing of information (Powell, 1990). Indeed, some might argue that "... to extract information from those who have it typically requires the bypassing of regular organizational structures" (Wilensky, 1968, p. 324).

NETWORK ANALYSIS

Because of its generality, network analysis has been used by almost every social science to study specific problems and it has been the primary means of studying communication structure in organizations over the last decade (Johnson, 1992a; Johnson, 1993; Monge & Contractor, 1987; Monge & Eisenberg, 1987). Network analysis can be a very systematic and complete means of looking at the overall pattern of communication linkages within an organization. One way this can be accomplished is through graphic representations, such as those found in Figure 2. This form of graphic portrayal is very flexible, since the nodes (circles) can be any type of entity and the linkages represented by the lines can be of any kind (Farace & Mabee, 1980). It is particularly useful for analyzing information-seeking because it can specify the individuals someone turns to for information and, in turn, the sources of information for these individuals. Inherent in the concept of networks is a recognition of the complexity of communication structure and the varied ways in which individuals are enmeshed in structures. Perhaps the most difficult continuing issue in this regard is the identification of cliques and subgroupings within a network (Johnson, 1993; Scott, 1991).

In organizations, partially because of their differentiation into functional groupings, individuals within disparate groups will come to adopt unique perspectives, often associated with their functions (Lawrence & Lorsch, 1967). "As organizations grow, they tend to develop subcultures. This is a result of well defined communication networks in which individuals communicate with a restricted group of people within the organization" (Barnett, 1988, p. 105). Day-to-day social life and the rates of interaction among group members (Homans, 1950) have a strong influence on norms and values of the group (Davis, 1966). Highly cohesive primary group structures exert considerable control over group members (Dunphy, 1963). Thus, as cohesiveness increases, the number of messages exchanged among members also increases (Danowski, 1980). More cohesive groups tend to have greater control over attitudes and actions of group members (Schacter, 1951; Seashore, 1954; Wyer, 1966). Hence, as communication relationships become more cohesive, attitudes within groups begin to conform. In turn, as attitudes become more salient, members are able to arrive at a normative understanding about the costs and benefits which accompany particular behaviors.

It might be expected that if there were enough ties present between groups then the entire network would eventually come to reflect a common position on a particular attitude (Abelson, 1964; French, 1956). The underlying assumptions of this particular perspective have been empirically supported in the work of Albrecht (1979) who found that key communicators were more likely to be cognitively and attitudinally integrated into their organizations. However, recognizing the openness of organizations to communication from other organizations, other institutions within the society (e.g. professional associations), and the mass media, it is unlikely that any organization will be isolated enough or sufficiently long-lived for the entities within them to come to convergence (Taylor, 1968).

The underlying thrust of these ideas are helpful in understanding a number of critical issues related to subgroups and coalitions within cultures and climates and other organizational issues as well (e.g. Abelson, 1979). For example, they may help to explain why technological impacts have always been clearer at the work-unit level (Withey, Daft & Cooper, 1983). Perception of organizational climate has also been found to vary among subgroups within an organization (Drexler, 1977; Jones & James, 1979; Payne & Mansfield, 1973), as well as by positions within networks (Falcione, Sussman & Herden, 1987) with the assertion that collective perceptions of members have a much clearer relationship to such outcome variables as job satisfaction and job performance (Joyce & Slocum, 1984).

Similar arguments can also be advanced in the field of organizational culture. Erickson (1982), while developing arguments from a different conceptual base, especially those related to structural equivalence and related processes of social comparison, has suggested a somewhat similar notion can be found in the development of belief systems in networks. A belief system is an organized diversity of attitudes which can be directly related to notions underlying organizational cultures. She contends that too many ties between groups will result in a commonality of positions, but she offers an interesting twist to the previous arguments. She contends that a moderate amount of ties between divergent groups is likely to result in stronger opposing belief systems, since these groups can now define themselves more clearly in their opposition to other groups.

Her arguments have direct implications for the development of coalitions and subcultures within organizational cultures, particularly in terms of the political processes within organizations, which have been the focus of most work in this area (e.g. Lucas, 1987). According to Stevenson, Pearce & Porter (1985), the following are the defining characteristics of coalitions: interacting group, deliberately constructed, independent of formal organizational structure, lack of formal internal structure, mutual perception of membership, issue-oriented, external focus and concerted member action. Most of these dimensions directly relate to communication structure, particularly concerning the emergence of communication networks. Stevenson, Pearce & Porter (1985) have argued that coalitions are more likely to occur in times of major organizational change, when social comparison indicates one's own position *vis-à-vis* others is unfavorable, when the opportunities for interaction are greater, when members have a fair degree of discretion in carrying out their responsibilities, and with greater visibility of coalitions within the organization. Many of these preconditions for coalitions are dependent on seeking information from outside one's formal grouping.

Subculture-to-subculture relationships form important configurations within the organizations and the manner in which these groupings relate to each other has important consequences for the organization. The existence of multiple cultures and their configuration into coalitions can be taken as a given in most organizations (Morgan, 1986). Perhaps the crucial question relates to whether or not there is a dominant subculture or more of a pluralistic arrangement of subcultures. The emergence of one form or another may be in part dependent on the duality of concerns related to collaboration and to control (Frost, 1987), with the weighting on these dimensions determining the extent of pluralism in an organization: with control associated with the emergence of dominant subcultures and collaboration associated with pluralism.

All of this, of course, has direct implications for structure. If management is the dominant subculture in the organization, then reifications of the power relationships of this subculture, such as the formal organizational chart, take on added significance. Indeed, in some organizations there will be substantial overlaps between formal and cultural approaches, especially when management dominates through bureaucratic structures. Deeper structural elements become reified in the formal structure of the organization, which protects existing power blocks and gives them the cloak of rationality (Mumby, 1987). Similarly coalitions form to reinforce and also to subvert this formal structure and this leads to emergent informal communication networks whose patterns stabilize in part from opposition to the formal structure (Brown & McMillan, 1988). However, if there are in reality multiple, more or less equal subcultures (as in organizations like hospitals and universities), then a formal organizational chart has little real significance for the organization and informal approaches to organizational structure take on more significance (Dow, 1988). While there have been countless studies on how dominant coalitions, particularly management, exert power and influence, there is not a similar wealth of research concerning how roughly equivalent coalitions relate to each other in more pluralistic organizations, particularly at deeper levels.

In recent years a critical issue facing network analysis has been the consequence of an individual's membership in multiple networks of relationships of different kinds, which often determine groupings of various sorts. Multiplexity classically refers to the nature of overlap, or correspondence, between differing networks (e.g. friendship as opposed to work) (Farace & Mabee, 1980; Rogers & Kincaid, 1981). The nature of overlaps between networks is of great pragmatic concern, since it can suggest the inherent capabilities of individual actors within systems, and it also has rich implications for the understanding of social systems generally (Reynolds & Johnson, 1982; Roberts & O'Reilly, 1979). Multiplexity is a network concept that has received increasing attention in recent years (Monge & Eisenberg, 1987). At its heart it refers to the extent to which different types of network relationships overlap: "The relation of one person to another is multiplex to the extent that there is more than one type of relation between the first person and the second" (Burt, 1983, p. 37).

The degree of multiplexity has been related to such issues as the intimacy of relationships (Minor, 1983), temporal stability of relationships (Minor, 1983; Mitchell, 1969; Rogers & Kincaid, 1981), reduction of uncertainty (Albrecht & Ropp, 1984), status (Albrecht & Ropp, 1984), the degree of control of a clique over its members (Rogers & Agarwala-Rogers, 1976), performance (Roberts & O'Reilly, 1979), redundancy of channels (Mitchell, 1969), and the diffusion of information within networks (Minor, 1983). The breadth of someone's linkages also might serve to provide an individual with a variety of information sources, as well as repetition of certain effects, which determine such contagion-related processes as attitude change (Hartman & Johnson, 1989).

The strength of weak ties, which is a special case of multiplexity, is perhaps the most well known concept related to network analysis. It refers to our less developed relationships that are more limited in space, place, time and depth of emotional bonds (Adelman, Parks & Albrecht, 1987; Weimann, 1983), and that can be considered to be more uniplex. This concept has been intimately tied to the flow of information within organizations and by definition is removed from stronger social bonds, such as influence and multiplex relations (Weimann, 1983).

Weak ties notions are derived from the work of Granovetter (1973) on how people acquire information related to potential jobs. It turns out that the most useful information comes from individuals in a person's extended networks; casual acquaintances and friends of friends. This information is the most useful precisely because it comes from infrequent or weak contacts. Strong contacts are likely to be people within subgoupings with whom there is a constant sharing of the same information; as a result, individuals within these groupings have come to have the same information base. However, information from outside this base gives unique perspectives and, in some instances, strategic advantages over competitors in a person's immediate network.

Weak ties are also crucial to integrating larger social systems, especially in terms of the nature of communication linkages between disparate groups (Friedkin, 1980; Friedkin, 1982; Weimann, 1983). Granovetter (1982) has maintained that this bridging function between different groups is a limiting condition necessary for the effects of weak ties to be evidenced. However, weak ties may be discouraged in organizations because of concerns over loyalty to one's immediate work group and questions of control of organizational members. Strong ties may also be preferred because they are more likely to be stable and because, as a result of the depth of their relationship, individuals may be willing to delay immediate gratifications from the other person associated with equity demands (Albrecht & Adelman, 1987). Individuals to whom an individual is strongly tied may also be more readily accessible and more willing to be of assistance (Granovetter, 1982).

Weak ties provide critical informational support because they transcend the limitations of our strong ties, and because, as often happens in organizations, our strong ties can be disrupted or unavailable (Adelman, Parks & Albrecht, 1987). Thus, weak ties may be useful for: discussing things you do not want to reveal to your close work associates; providing a place for an individual to experiment; extending access to information; promoting social comparison; and fostering a sense of community (Adelman, Parks & Albrecht, 1987). Naturally, when individuals have a need for unique, novel information, processes associated with weak ties have great significance.

One way these ideas are operationalized in the network literature is in terms of communication roles that link groups, particularly those of bridges and liaisons. An individual's network communication role is determined by the overall pattern of his/her communication relationships (or linkages) with others. Some individuals, labeled non-participants (e.g. isolates), have relatively few communication contacts with others (e.g. 12, 29, and 30 in Figure 18.2). Participants, on the other hand, form intense patterns that represent communication groups and linkages between these groups (e.g. 5, 15, and 18 in Figure 18.2). Several research studies have found key differences between these two kinds of individuals, with participants being more outgoing, influential, satisfied (Goldhaber et al., 1978) and having more coherent cognitive structures (Albrecht, 1979) and non-participants deliberately withholding information, having lower satisfaction with communication (Roberts & O'Reilly, 1979), reporting less identification, variety, feedback and required interaction (Moch, 1980). Obviously these patterns of findings have interesting implications for the pattern of information-seeking within organizations.

The most important communication role is that of a liaison (3 in Figure 18.2) (see Reynolds & Johnson, 1982 for a review). The liaison links two or more communication groups, while not being a member of any one group. This strategic positioning of liaisons has earned him/her the label of "linking pin", who, through his/her promotion of more positive climates and successful coordination of organizational functions, serves to hold an organization together (Likert, 1967). The role of the liaison in the coordination and control of organizational activities is closely tied to the concepts of integration and differentiation. That is, as the organization divides into more and more groups, greater efforts have to be made at pulling these groups together through integrating mechanisms (Galbraith, 1973; Lawrence & Lorsch, 1967). These integrating mechanisms are crucial to organizational survival, since without them the organization would be a collection of groups each going off in its own direction. Typically, liaisons are the most efficient personal integrating mechanisms because of their strategic positioning. Due to their centrality and their direct linkages with others, liaisons reduce the probability of message distortion, reduce information load, and increase the timeliness of communication (Reynolds & Johnson, 1982). They are also likely to be the most skilled information-seekers within organizations, as well as the primary target of initial information-seeking for others with whom they are linked. Unfortunately, however, liaisons are relatively rare in organizations; this is reflected in the generally low level of communication between diverse groups in organizations (Farace & Johnson, 1974).

Traditionally, control in organizations has been viewed as occurring within the formal communication structure. Roberts & O'Reilly (1979) have argued that effective control in an organization corresponds to the extent to which networks link critical task groups. Increasingly, management functions can be viewed as similar to those of a liaison, a factor reflected in the finding that liaisons tend to be managers (Reynolds & Johnson, 1982). An effective manager must be able to perceive coherent patterns from diverse information inputs and to form clear judgments that can serve as the basis for organizational action. However, only a minority of all managers occupy liaison positions in informal communication networks. Those who are liaisons appear to use persuasion to accomplish their objectives. In fact, many of the characteristics of a liaison (e.g. openness, trust, sensitivity to others and getting a wide array of input) have also been used to specify the characteristics of democratic managers and, more generally, of open communication climates (Reynolds & Johnson, 1982).

Thus, the liaison role points to the convergence of network analysis and formal approaches. It also is a precursor of the growing interests in markets, which makes critical assumptions about the motivations for voluntary interactions and the basic relational qualities necessary for the functioning of social systems.

MARKETS

Recently, yet another view of structure, a market approach, which shares much with both network and formal approaches, and rests on economic and exchange assumptions, has begun to emerge. Markets, through the mechanisms of exchanges, operate to diffuse information rapidly to interested parties (von Hayek, 1989). In focusing on exchanges, this approach provides a compelling theoretical focus for the development of relationships between interactants, who may otherwise lack compelling motives to interact. Indeed, we may seek exchanges with others because they are not like us and they have resources which our group does not possess.

This view also suggests a broader conception of information as something that can be shaped and modified in exchanges, then interpreted in different ways in the collectivity as exchanges proceed. Thus, markets have an inherently dynamic view of information exchanges, with individuals compelled to change their ideas as a result of the reactions of others. This contrasts directly with the view of information in a hierarchical approach as a relatively unchanging commodity that should be passed with minimum transformations from one part of the organization to others (Powell, 1990).

While markets have been seen as occurring outside the context of formal organizations, they have been recognized as containing many authority properties found in organizations, and organizations with complex, multidivisional structures take on market characteristics (Eccles & White, 1988). "The internal operations of real-world firms are controlled by a blend of authority and market-like mechanisms" (McGuinness, 1991, p. 66).

The nature of the relationships is determined by notions inherent in exchange; achieving a fair price for a good or service. In pure market exchange relationships the only thing that may matter is the value of the goods exchanged. In network-based exchanges, normative controls may also be operative in the relationship (Powell, 1990; Lorenz, 1989) and the consequences of untrustworthy behavior may cloud concurrent and future interactions. In fact, for those organizational members who are unscrupulous in their relationships, the possibility of their behavior being sanctioned internally provides a positive incentive to interact outside of the firm (Eccles & White, 1988).

Networks of information exchanges, which also contain market elements, are particularly useful structures for organizations composed of highly skilled work forces who possess knowledge not limited to particular tasks (Powell, 1990). Indeed, more generally it has been argued that knowledge flows may be best accomplished by informal organizational structures because of problems in recognizing the significance of information and communicating it effectively and efficiently (Gupta & Govindarajan, 1991). This form of decentralization often reduces the possibility of information overload within these organizations, and attendant delays and imperfect planning orders. Thus, in organizations like universities it may be better to minimize intrusive formal structures and promote wide-ranging interactions, while providing a framework in which trading relationships can occur.

The availability of information concerning costs and beneficial exchanges is critical to the operation of a pure market (Levacic, 1991). Indeed, inadequate information is one source of market failure (Levacic, 1991). Thus, markets place a premium on information-seeking. Inadequate information can take many forms. One set deals with problems in price and trust that go to the heart of exchange relationships (Levacic, 1991). Opportunistic sellers selectively reveal, distort and withhold information, if they perceive they can do so without penalty (Lorenz, 1989; McGuinness, 1991). Another set of issues deals with uncertainties, especially concerning future (and often unknown) contingencies (Levacic, 1991). Of course, acting in a market (and observation of the actions of others) produces essential feedback and critical information that can be used dynamically to refine future market behavior (Krizner, 1973).

The market approach, especially as it relates to transaction costs, has been used to specify those conditions under which an organization will try to subsume certain relationships under its formal umbrella. Uncertain transactions that recur frequently and require substantial investments of money, time or energy are more likely to occur within a hierarchy. For example, organizations in the USA are increasingly incorporating legal divisions into their formal structures. Increased familiarity with and responsiveness to an organization's idiosyncratic legal problems offset the "costs" of bureaucracy because they provide a means (e.g. formal structure) for adjudicating unforeseen problems in the relationship and the naturally opportunistic impulses of actors (e.g. lawyers in outside firms) are controlled by authority relationships within the organization (Granovetter, 1985; Powell, 1990 discussing the work of Williamson). In this view, organizations are islands of planned coordination relationships, often revealed in intragroup communication, embedded in a sea of market relationships (Powell, 1990).

DISCUSSION

Together these three models (hierarchies, networks and markets) are the major competing explanations for the coordination of all social life, including life within organizations (Frances et al., 1991). Market perspectives essentially argue that coordination between groups occurs automatically because of self-interest, in hierarchies control is consciously and overtly exercised; however, both these approaches neglect the informal forces characteristic of networks of interdependent relationships (Frances et al., 1991).

In many ways hierarchies, markets and networks are idealized concepts that may not exist anywhere in pure form (Bradach & Eccles, 1989). Reflecting this blending, terminology in this area, like all of the social sciences, is sometimes used interchangeably, (e.g. Powell, 1990; Nohria, 1992). With formal structure, a market approach shares a concentration on central rules governing relationships, and, with network analysis, market approaches shares a focus on emergent relationships in a collectivity. In much of the literature on the interrelationship between markets, hierarchies and networks, hierarchies are fairly close to the meaning of formal approaches developed earlier. However, networks have a much more narrow meaning, coming to reflect primarily the more informal trusting relationships that develop in ongoing associations (Thompson et al., 1991). Formal structure can also be encompassed within network conceptions (Monge & Eisenberg, 1987), so both hierarchical and market approaches could be considered to be special cases of networks (Frances et al., 1991).

A recent attempt to systematically compare formal and informal groupings and their impact on the levels of role ambiguity essentially found more similarities than differences between the two types of groupings, and suggested a complex set of contingencies in which one or the other would have the most impact on role ambiguity (Hartman & Johnson, 1990). Somewhat similarly, another recent study found that these two approaches related to such key organizational factors as beliefs, stylistic characteristics and channel usage (Johnson et al., 1994). Much work remains to be done to determine the nature of overlaps and differences between informal and formal views of structure; with some arguing that the views are so divergent it is impractical to simultaneously consider both (Blau, 1974).

Similarly, another issue which needs to be more systematically addressed is the varying levels, individual, group and organizational, at which information-seeking might occur. Organizations inevitably have mixed-level processes (Rousseau, 1985) and the interactions between levels need to be more systematically addressed in information-seeking research. For example, a constant theme of the boundary-spanning literature is the tension an individual group member experiences between the information they acquire and the conventional wisdom of their group. So, while an individual may be charged with seeking information on behalf of the group, group processes may ostracize them if they return with information which is discordant with accepted group norms (Johnson, 1993; O'Reilly & Pondy, 1979), especially under conditions where the group feels threatened by external conditions (Staw, Sandelands & Dutton, 1981). Similarly, very little research has been conducted on the embeddedness of naturally occurring groups in larger social systems (Jablin & Sussman, 1983) and the effects this might have on the sorts of information a group is likely to seek.

Debate over which views of structure are correct and which level should be our focus often clouds the real issue, which is what different types of structures are necessary for different outcomes. For example, at different phases of the innovation process different structures may be emphasized. Formal structures can bar innovativeness within the organization if they are too rigid and confining. Hierarchical structures also interact with a sequential, linear view of innovation processes in organizations to further retard the development of innovations (Bush & Frohman, 1991). Thus more formal organizations do not promote the level of flexibility necessary for groups to initiate innovations and to allow for the collaborative relationships across hierarchical and functional relationships that insure successful completion of projects.

Kanter (1983) has offered compelling arguments that organizations which are segmented into different functional groups with strong barriers, especially with informal rule structures between them, are not going to be capable of generating or diffusing innovations. Differentiation is necessary for the synergy essential to the creation of ideas, but it also makes it difficult to ensure the consensus necessary for their implementation.

A balance must be reached between efficiency, which results from highly constrained systems, and effectiveness. While it is important to reduce information load, for example, it is also important to allow some leakage between groups, so that new ideas and perspectives can be brought to problems. Total segmentation of an organization into isolated work groups may be just as harmful as no segmentation (Kanter, 1983). Zaltman, Duncan & Holbek (1973) have argued that organizations need one type of structure to generate ideas (low formalization, decentralization, and high complexity), which reflects the market-driven forces necessary for informally generated innovations. Markets may be especially useful for more qualitative information exchanges based on expert knowledge or ideas; they also create incentives for learning and the dissemination of information that promotes the quick translation of ideas into action (Powell, 1990). This is also reflected in the work of Aiken & Hage (1971) that suggests that organic organizations, with decentralized decision-making, many occupations, slack resources and a history of innovation, are more likely to be innovative. However, implementation requires high formalization, centralization and low complexity.

Accomplishing both innovation and productivity poses a difficult problem for an organization, since both appear to require different structures (Kanter, 1983). Some organizations choose to emphasize either innovation or productivity, recognizing the inherent difficulties in trying to accomplish both. Another strategy that many organizations adopt is to compartmentalize these processes with very rigid structures in production processes and more flexible ones in R&D labs. This compartmentalization is often coupled with spatial separation, which is directly related to a communication gradient approach to structure (see Johnson, 1988; Johnson, 1992b).

However, although there is little research evidence to speak to this point, the most effective strategy in the long term may be to try to adopt a dynamic synergism between differing structures, which sometimes overlap in messy and troublesome ways. In this regard, organizational incongruence may be related to overall organizational effectiveness, since it may establish the creative tension necessary to move to more productive organizational systems (Fry & Smith, 1987). Indeed, the more market-driven relationships characteristic of the informal approaches to organizational communication structure may be a partial answer to this dilemma. This is an argument that is borne out by the research evidence that suggests individuals in liaison positions in informal networks are more productive (Downs et al., 1988) and also more innovative (Reynolds & Johnson, 1982). Somehow organizations must achieve a balance between stability and flexibility (Weick, 1969); how to strike that balance is still very much open to question.

ACKNOWLEDGEMENTS

I would like to thank Drs Franklin Boster, Vernon Miller and Sally Johnson for reviewing earlier drafts of this chapter.

REFERENCES

Abelson, R.P. (1964). Mathematical models of the distribution of attitudes under controversy. In N. Frederiksen & H. Gulliksen (eds), *Contributions to Mathematical Psychology*. New York: Holt, Rinehart and Winston, pp. 141–160.
Abelson, R.P. (1979). Social clusters and opinion clusters. In P.W. Holland & S. Leinhardt (eds), *Perspectives on Social Network Research*. New York: Academic Press, pp. 239–256.

Adelman, M.B., Parks, M.R. & Albrecht, T.L. (1987). Beyond close relationships: support in weak ties. In T.L. Albrecht & M.B. Adelman (eds), *Communicating Social Support*. Newbury Park, CA: Sage, pp. 126–147.

Aiken, M. & Hage, J. (1971). The organic model and innovation, *Sociology*, **5**, 63–82.

Albrecht, T.L. (1979). The role of communication in perceptions of organizational climate. In D. Nimmo (ed.), *Communication Yearbook 3*. New Brunswick, NJ: Transaction Books, pp. 343–357.

Albrecht, T.L. & Adelman, M.B. (1987). Communicating social support: a theoretical perspective. In T.L. Albrecht & M.B. Adelman (eds), *Communicating Social Support*. Newbury Park, CA: Sage, pp. 18–39.

Albrecht, T.L. & Ropp, V.A. (1984). Communicating about innovation in networks of three U.S. organizations. *Journal of Communication*, **34**, 78–91.

Astley, W.G. & Zajac, E.J. (1991). Intraorganizational power and organizational design: reconciling rational and coalitional models of organization. *Organization Science*, **2**, 399–411.

Axley, S.R. (1984). Managerial and organizational communication in terms of the conduit metaphor. *Academy of Management Review*, **9**, 428–437.

Barnett, G.A. (1988). Communication and organizational culture. In G.M. Goldhaber & G.A. Barnett (eds), *Handbook of Organizational Communication*. Norwood, NJ: Ablex, pp. 101–130.

Berger, C.R. & Chaffee, S.H. (eds) (1987). *Handbook of Communication Science*. Newbury Park, CA: Sage.

Blau, P.M. (1974). A formal theory of differentiation in organizations. In P.M. Blau (ed.), *On the Nature of Organizations*. New York: Wiley, pp. 297–322.

Bradach, J.L. & Eccles, R.G. (1989). Price, authority, and trust: from ideal types to plural forms. *Annual Review of Sociology*, **15**, 97–118.

Brown, M.H. & McMillan, J.J. (1988). Constructions and counterconstructions: organizational power revisited. Paper presented to the Annual Convention of the Speech Communication Association, New Orleans, LA.

Burt, R.S. (1983). A note on inference concerning network subgroups. In R.S. Burt & M.J. Minor (eds), *Applied Network Analysis: A Methodological Introduction*. Beverly Hills, CA: Sage, pp. 283–301.

Bush, J.B. Jr & Frohman, A.L. (1991). Communication in a "network" organization. *Organizational Dynamics*, **19**, 23–36.

Cheng, J.L.C. (1983). Interdependence and coordination in organizations: a role–system analysis. *Academy of Management Journal*, **26**, 156–162.

Danowski, J.A. (1980). Group attitude uniformity and connectivity of organizational communication networks for production, innovation, and maintenance content. *Human Communication Research*, **6**, 299–308.

Dansereau, F. & Markham, S.E. (1987). Superior–subordinate communication: multiple levels of analysis. In F.M. Jablin, L.L. Putnam, K.H. Roberts & L.W. Porter (eds), *Handbook of Organizational Communication: An Interdisciplinary Perspective*. Newbury Park, CA: Sage, pp. 343–388.

Davis, J.A. (1966). Structural balance, mechanical solidarity, and interpersonal relations. In J. Berger, M. Zelditch Jr & B. Anderson (eds), *Sociological Theories in Progress*, Vol. 1, Boston: Houghton-Mifflin, pp. 74–101.

Dow, G.K. (1988). Configurational and coactivational views of organizational structure. *Academy of Management Review*, **13**, 53–64.

Downs, A. (1967). *Inside bureaucracy*. Boston: Little, Brown.

Downs, C.W., Clampitt, P.G. & Pfeiffer, A.L. (1988). Communication and organizational outcomes. In G.M. Goldhaber & G.A. Barnett (eds), *Handbook of Organizational Communication*. Norwood, NJ: Ablex, pp. 171–212.

Drexler, J.A. (1977). Organizational climate: its homogeneity within organizations. *Journal of Applied Psychology*, **62**, 38–42.
Dunphy, D. (1963). The social structure of urban adolescent peer groups. *Sociometry*, **26**, 230–246.
Eccles, R. & White, H. (1988). Price and authority in inter-profit center transactions. *American Journal of Sociology*, **94** (Suppl.), S17–S51.
Eisenberg, E.M. & Whetten, M.G. (1987). Reconsidering openness in organizational communication. *Academy of Management Review*, **12**, 418–426.
Erickson, B.H. (1982). Networks, ideologies, and belief systems. In P.V. Marsden & N. Lin (eds), *Social Structure and Network Analysis*. Beverly Hills, CA: Sage, pp. 159–172.
Falcione, R.L., Sussman, L. & Herden, R.P. (1987). Communication climate in organizations. In F.M. Jablin, L.L. Putnam, K.H. Roberts & L.W. Porter (eds), *Handbook of Organizational Communication: An Interdisciplinary Perspective*. Newbury Park, CA: Sage, pp. 195–227.
Farace, R.V. & Johnson, J.D. (1974). Comparative analysis of human communication networks in selected formal organizations. Paper presented to the International Communication Association Annual Convention, New Orleans, LA.
Farace, R.V. & Mabee, T. (1980). Communication network analysis methods. In P.R. Monge & J.N. Cappella (eds), *Multivariate Techniques in Human Communication Research*. New York: Academic Press, pp. 365–391.
Farace, R.V., Monge, P.R. & Russell, H. (1977). *Communicating and Organizing*. Reading, MA: Addison-Wesley.
Frances, J., Levacic, R., Mitchell, J. & Thompson, G. (1991). Introduction. In G. Thompson, J. Frances, R. Levacic and J. Mitchell (eds), *Markets, Hierarchies & Networks: The Coordination of Social Life*. Newbury Park, CA: Sage, pp. 1–19.
French, J.R.P. (1956). A formal theory of social power. *Psychological Review*, **63**, 181–194.
Friedkin, N. (1980). A test of structural features of Granovetter's strength of weak ties theory. *Social Networks*, **2**, 411–422.
Friedkin, N.E. (1982). Information flow through strong and weak ties in intraorganizational social networks. *Social Networks*, **3**, 273–285.
Frost, P.J. (1987). Power, politics, and influence. In F.M. Jablin, L.L. Putnam, K.H. Roberts & L.W. Porter (eds), *Handbook of Organizational Communication: An Interdisciplinary Perspective*. Newbury Park, CA: Sage, pp. 503–548.
Fry, L.W. & Smith, D.A. (1987). Congruence, contingency, and theory building. *Academy of Management Review*, **12**, 117–132.
Galbraith, J.R. (1973). *Designing Complex Organizations*. Reading, MA: Addison-Wesley.
Goldhaber, G.M., Yates, M.P., Porter, T.D. & Lesniak, R. (1978). Organizational communication: 1978. *Human Communication Research*, **5**, 76–96.
Granovetter, M.S. (1973). The strength of weak ties. *American Journal of Sociology*, **78**, 1360–1380.
Granovetter, M. (1982). The strength of weak ties: a network theory revisited. In P.V. Marsden & N. Lin (eds), *Social Structure in Network Analysis*. Beverly Hills, CA: Sage, pp. 105–130.
Granovetter, M. (1985). Economic action and social structure: the problem of embeddedness. *American Journal of Sociology*, **91**, 481–510.
Guetskow, H. & Simon, H.A. (1955). The impact of certain communication nets upon organization and performance in task-oriented groups. *Management Sicence*, **1**, 233–250.
Gupta, A.K. & Govindarajan, V. (1991). Knowledge flows and the structure of control within multinational organizations. *Academy of Management Review*, **16**, 768–792.
Hage, J., Aiken, M. & Marrett, C.B. (1971). Organization structure and communications. *American Sociological Review*, **36**, 860–871.

Hartman, R.L. & Johnson, J.D. (1989). Social contagion and multiplexity: communication networks as predictors of commitment and role ambiguity. *Human Communication Research*, **15**, 523–548.

Hartman, R.L. & Johnson, J.D. (1990). Formal and informal group communication structures: an examination of their relationship to role ambiguity. *Social Networks*, **12**, 127–151.

Homans, G. (1950). *The Human Group.* New York: Harcourt, Brace, Jovanavich.

Inman, T.H., Olivas, L. & Golen, S.P. (1986). Desirable communication behaviors of managers. *Business Education Forum*, **40**, 27–28.

Jablin, F.M. (1987). Formal organization structure. In F.M. Jablin, L.L. Putnam, K.H. Roberts & L.W. Porter (eds), *Handbook of Organizational Communication: An Interdisciplinary Perspective.* Newbury Park, CA: Sage, pp. 389–419.

Jablin, F.M. & Sussman, L. (1983). Organizational group communication: a review of the literature and model of the process. In H.H. Greenbaum, R.L. Falcione & S.A. Hellweg (eds), *Organizational Communication: Abstracts, Analysis, and Overview.* Beverly Hills, CA: Sage, pp. 11–50.

Johnson, B.M. & Rice, R.E. (1987). *Managing Organizational Innovation: The Evolution of Word Processing to Office Information Systems.* New York: Columbia University Press.

Johnson, J.D. (1988). On the use of communication gradients. In G.M. Goldhaber & G. Barnett (eds), *Handbook of Organizational Communication.* Norwood, NJ: Ablex, pp. 361–383.

Johnson, J.D. (1992a). Approaches to organizational communication structure. *Journal of Business Research*, **25**, 99–113.

Johnson, J.D. (1992b). Technological and spatial factors related to organizational communication structure. *Journal of Managerial Issues*, **IV**, 190–209.

Johnson, J.D. (1993). *Organizational Communication Structure.* Norwood, NJ: Ablex.

Johnson, J.D., Donohue, W.A., Atkin, C.K. & Johnson, S.H. (1994). Differences between formal and informal communication channels. *Journal of Business Communication*, **31**, 111–122.

Johnson, J.D., Donohue, W.A., Atkin, C.K. & Johnson, S.H. (1995). A comprehensive model of information seeking: tests focusing on a technical organization. *Science Communication*, **16**, 274–303.

Jones, A.P. & James, L.R. (1979). Psychological climate: dimensions and relationships of individual and aggregated work environment perceptions. *Organizational Behavior and Human Performance*, **23**, 201–250.

Joyce, W.F. & Slocum, J.W. (1984). Collective climate: agreement as a basis for defining aggregate climates in organizations. *Academy of Management Journal*, **27**, 721–742.

Kanter, R.M. (1983). *The Change Masters: Innovation and Entrepreneurship in the American Corporation.* New York: Simon & Schuster.

Katz, D. & Kahn, R.L. (1978). *The Social Psychology of Organizations.* New York: Wiley.

Kerwin, A. (1993). None to solid: medical ignorance. *Knowledge: Creation, Diffusion, Utilization*, **15**, 166–185.

Krackhardt, D. (1989). Graph theoretical dimensions of informal organizations. Paper presented to the National Meetings of the Academy of Management, Washington, D.C.

Krizner, I.M. (1973). *Competition and Entrepreneurship.* Chicago: University of Chicago Press.

LaFollette, M.C. (1993). Editorial. *Knowledge: Creation, Diffusion, Utilization*, **15**, 131–132.

Lawrence, P.R. & Lorsch, J.W. (1967). *Organization and Environment: Managing Differentiation and Integration.* Boston: Harvard Business School.

Lee, A.M. (1970). *Systems Analysis Frameworks.* London: Macmillan.

Levacic, R. (1991). Markets: introduction. In G. Thompson, J. Frances, R. Levacic & J.

Mitchell (eds), *Markets, Hierarchies and Networks: The Coordination of Social Life*. Newbury Park, CA: Sage, pp. 21–23.

Lewis, R.S. (1988). *Challenger: The Final Voyage*. New York: Columbia University Press.

Likert, R. (1967). *The Human Organization: Its Management and Value*. Highstown, NJ: McGraw-Hill.

Lorenz, E.H. (1989). Neither friends nor strangers: informal networks of subcontracting in French industry. In D. Gambetta (ed.), *Trust: Making and Breaking of Cooperative Relations*. Oxford: Basil Blackwell, pp. 194–210.

Lucas, R. (1987). Political-cultural analysis of organizations. *Academy of Management Review*, **12**, 144–156.

McGuinness, T. (1991). Markets and managerial hierarchies. In G. Thompson, J. Frances, R. Levacic & J. Mitchell (eds), *Markets, Hierarchies, and Networks: The Coordination of Social Life*. Newbury Park, CA: Sage, pp. 66–81.

March, J.G. & Simon, H.A. (1958). *Organizations*. New York: Wiley.

Marshall, A.A. & Stohl, C. (1993). Participating as participation: a network approach. *Communication Monographs*, **60**, 137–157.

Miller, V.D., Johnson, J.R. & Grau, J. (1994). Antecedents to willingness to participate in a planned organizational change. *Journal of Applied Communication Research*, **22**, 59–80.

Minor, M.J. (1983). New directions in multiplexity analysis. In R.S. Burt & M.J. Minor (eds), *Applied Network Analysis: A Methodological Introduction*. Beverly Hills, CA: Sage, pp. 223–244.

Mitchell, J.C. (1969). The concept and use of social networks. In J.C. Mitchell (ed.), *Social Networks in Urban Situations: Analyses of Personal Relationships in Central African Towns*. Manchester: Manchester University Press, pp. 1–50.

Mitchell, J. (1991). Hierarchies: introduction. In G. Thompson, J. Frances, R. Levacic & J. Mitchell (eds), *Markets, Hierarchies & Networks: The Coordination of Social Life*. Newbury Park, CA: Sage, pp. 105–107.

Moch, M.K. (1980). Job involvement, internal motivation, and employees' integration into networks of work relationships. *Organizational Behavior and Human Performance*, **25**, 15–31.

Monge, P.R. (1987). The network level of analysis. In C.R. Berger & S.H. Chaffee (eds), *Handbook of Communication Science*. Newbury Park, CA: Sage.

Monge, P.R. & Contractor, N.S. (1987). Communication networks: measurement techniques. In C.H. Tardy (ed.), *A Handbook for the Study of Human Communication*. Norwood, NJ: Ablex, pp. 107–138.

Monge, P.R. & Eisenberg, E.M. (1987). Emergent communication networks. In F.M. Jablin, L.L. Putnam, K.H. Roberts & L.W. Porter (eds), *Handbook of Organizational Communication: An Interdisciplinary Perspective*. Newbury Park, CA: Sage, pp. 304–342.

Morgan, G. (1986). *Images of Organization*. Beverly Hills, CA: Sage.

Mumby, D.K. (1987). The political function of narrative in organizations. *Communication Monographs*, **54**, 113–127.

Nohria, N. (1992). Introduction: is a network perspective a useful way of studying organizations? In N. Nohria & R.G. Eccles (eds), *Networks and Organizations: Structure, Form, and Action*. Boston: Harvard Business School Press, pp. 1–22.

O'Neill, B. (1984). Structures for non-hierarchical organizations. *Behavioral Science*, **29**, 61–77.

O'Reilly, C.A. III & Pondy, L.R. (1979). Organizational communication. In S. Kerr (ed.), *Organizational Behavior*. Columbus, OH: Grid, pp. 119–150.

Payne, R.L. & Mansfield, R. (1973). Relationships of perceptions of organizational climate to organizational structure, context, and hierarchical position. *Administrative Science Quarterly*, **18**, 515–526.

Pfeffer, J. (1978). *Organizational Design*. Arlington Heights, IL: AHM Publishing.

Powell, W.W. (1990). Neither market nor hierarchy: network forms of organization. In S.B. Bacharach (ed.), *Research in Organizational Behavior*. Norwich, CT: JAI Press, pp. 295–336.
Ravetz, J.R. (1993). The sin of silence: ignorance of ignorance. *Knowledge: Creation, Diffusion, Utilization*, **15**, 157–165.
Reynolds, E.V. & Johnson, J.D. (1982). Liaison emergence: relating theoretical perspectives. *Academy of Management Review*, **7**, 551–559.
Roberts, K.H. & O'Reilly, C.A. III (1979). Some correlations of communication roles in organizations. *Academy of Management Journal*, **4**, 283–293.
Rogers, E.M. (1983). *Diffusion of Innovations*. New York: Free Press.
Rogers, E.M. & Agarwala-Rogers, R. (1976). *Communication in Organizations*. New York: Free Press.
Rogers, E.M. & Kincaid, D.L. (1981). *Communication Networks: Toward a New Paradigm for Research*. New York: Free Press.
Rouse, W.B. & Rouse, S.H. (1984). Human information seeking and design of information systems. *Information Processing and Management*, **20**, 129–138.
Rousseau, D.M. (1985). Issues of level in organizational research: multi-level and cross-level perspectives. In S.B. Bacharach (ed.), *Research in Organizational Behavior*. Norwich, CT: JAI Press, pp. 1–37.
Schacter, S. (1951). Deviation, rejection, and communication. *Journal of Abnormal and Social Psychology*, **46**, 229–238.
Schein, E.H. (1965). *Organizational Psychology*. Englewood Cliffs, NJ: Prentice-Hall.
Scott, J. (1991). *Social Network Analysis: A Handbook*. Newbury Park, CA: Sage.
Seashore, S.E. (1954). *Group Cohesiveness in the Industrial Work Group*. Ann Arbor, MI: Survey Research Center.
Shaw, M.E. (1971). *Group Dynamics: The Psychology of Small Group Behavior*. New York: McGraw-Hill.
Smithson, M. (1993). Ignorance and science: dilemmas, perspectives, and prospects. *Knowledge: Creation, Diffusion, Utilization*, **15**, 133–156.
Staw, B.M., Sandelands, L.E. & Dutton, J.E. (1981). Threat-rigidity effects in organizational behavior: a multilevel analysis. *Administrative Science Quarterly*, **26**, 501–524.
Stevenson, W.B., Pearce, J.L. & Porter, L.W. (1985). The concept of "coalition" in organization theory and research. *Academy of Management Review*, **10**, 256–268.
Stocking, S.H. & Holstein, L.W. (1993). Constructing and reconstructing scientific ignorance: ignorance claims in science and journalism. *Knowledge: Creation, Diffusion, Utilization*, **15**, 186–210.
Strobel, L.P. (1980). *Reckless Homicide? Ford's Pinto Trial*. South Bend, IN: and books.
Taylor, M. (1968). Towards a mathematical theory of influence and attitude change. *Human Relations*, **98**, 121–139.
Thompson, J.D. (1967). *Organizations in Action*. New York: McGraw-Hill.
Thompson, G., Frances, J., Levacic, R. & Mitchell, J. (1991). *Markets, Hierarchies & Networks: The Coordination of Social Life*. Newbury Park, CA: Sage.
von Hayek, F. (1989). Spontaneous ("grown") order and organized ("made") order. In N. Modlovsky (ed.), *Order—With or Without Design*. London: Centre for Research into Communist Economies, pp. 101–123.
Weick, K.E. (1969). *The Social Psychology of Organizing*. Reading, MA: Addison-Wesley.
Weimann, G. (1983). The strength of weak conversational ties in the flow of information and influence. *Social Networks*, **5**, 245–267.
Wilensky, H. (1968). Organizational intelligence. In D.L. Sills (ed.), *The International Encyclopedia of the Social Sciences*. New York: Free Press, pp. 310–334.
Withey, M., Daft, R.L. & Cooper, W.H. (1983). Measures of Perrow's work unit technology: an empirical assessment and a new scale. *Academy of Management Journal*, **26**, 45–63.

Wyer, R. Jr (1966). The effects of incentive to perform well, group attraction, and group acceptance on conformity in a judgmental task. *Journal of Personality and Social Psychology*, **4**, 21–26.

Zaltman, G., Duncan, R. & Holbek, J. (1973). *Innovations and Organizations*. New York: Wiley.

Section VI

Cross-cultural Aspects of Work Group Functioning

Chapter 19

Cultural Differences in Group Processes

Peter B. Smith
University of Sussex and Roffey Park Management Institute, UK
and
Julia Noakes
Sheppard, Moscow Ltd

Abstract

Social psychological research into teams has mostly been conducted in North America, and many of the effects found there do not replicate elsewhere. Cross-cultural researchers have identified Individualism–Collectivism and Power Distance as key dimensions predicting differences between nations in social behaviour patterns. Since the USA is rated very highly on individualistic values, the differences are likely to be greatest in collectivist cultures. Teams in collectivist cultures are more concerned with long-term commitment, more deferent toward authority, and more concerned with in-group harmony, but are just as competitive with out-groups. Experimental studies of multicultural teams within North America have mostly lasted insufficiently long to validly assess team effects. However there is some suggestion that diverse teams surpass monocultural teams on performance criteria over longer time periods. A stage model is presented depicting the dilemmas facing multinational teams over time. In addition to the dilemmas facing monocultural teams, they must initially overcome language problems, difficulties of access and differing understandings of how to get to know one another. Stereotypic expectations may be of some help, but ways must be found of moving beyond them. As the team starts to work together they must resolve differing perspectives on time, on preferred leadership styles and on the functions to be served by meetings. As team development proceeds, alliances of those who share cultural values may form, and these may impede effective decision-making. If these problems are successfully handled, the

Handbook of Work Group Psychology. Edited by M.A. West.
© 1996 John Wiley & Sons Ltd.

team may then capitalize upon diversity rather than be impeded by it. Groupthink may be minimized by drawing upon the diverse perspectives within the team. Ways of training teams to cope with the difficulties they face are considered. Available research studies relevant to all of these issues are reviewed, but it is noted that the area has been insufficiently researched, given its practical importance.

INTRODUCTION

Until recently, much of the research on work teams and other types of small groups was focused upon basic social processes such as social facilitation, conformity, and leadership and relevant performance measures. There is no reason to doubt that these processes are indeed basic, but the manner in which they have been studied has posed two problems concerning the external validity of the results of such studies. Firstly, the great majority of studies has been conducted in North America. This has led to an assumption, usually implicit, that what goes on in teams in North America is also representative of what goes on elsewhere. Secondly, because the thrust of studies has come from that location, so too have many of the concepts and hypotheses employed, even when those studies have been carried out in other parts of the world. Two contemporary trends have revealed this cultural bias more clearly. Firstly, there has developed a much stronger focus upon cultural diversity within present-day North America societies. Secondly, the current steadily increasing internationalization of business has confronted many organizations with the problem of how to manage effectively foreign direct investments and joint ventures that are located in settings which differ markedly from those found in North America.

In this chapter we shall first consider the extent to which cultural differences might be expected to influence team behaviour, and then briefly review currently available models of cultural difference. Having established a framework, we then address three questions in turn. First, do studies of teams from other cultures show different behaviour patterns? Second, what studies are there of multicultural teams within North America? Finally, how do the increasingly widespread multinational teams operate? We conclude by looking in some detail at the stages through which multinational teams are likely to pass and how they may be made more effective.

Cultural Differences in Social Processes

Three examples can illustrate that there are substantial variations in group behaviour between cultures. A great deal of research has been undertaken into the effectiveness of particular work team leadership styles (see Yammarino, this volume). Amongst the various North American theorists, there is a broad consensus that the most effective style of leadership is contingent upon the particular tasks, persons and circumstances facing a work team (Smith & Peterson, 1988; Yukl, 1989). Yet leadership researchers from other parts of the world have had much more success in identifying specific leadership styles which predict team performance, regardless of environmental contingencies. Such results have been obtained, for instance, by Misumi (1985) in Japan, Sinha (1981) in India, Bond & Hwang (1986) in Taiwan and Ayman & Chemers (1983) in Iran.

A second aspect of team working thought to be fundamental by some Western researchers is that of social loafing, whereby the larger a team is, the less effort will be contributed by any one individual (Latane, Williams & Harkins, 1979). Recent studies by Earley (1989) in mainland China and by Earley (1993) in Israel and China showed a reverse effect, whereby team members worked harder than did individuals working on their own, whereas US team members showed the familiar social loafing effect.

Finally, the process of conformity is seen as another basic element within groups and teams. The classic conformity study conducted by Asch (1956) has been replicated more widely than any other social psychological study. A recent meta-analysis of 134 such replications by Bond & Smith (1996) revealed that after variations in experimental design are discounted, the level of conformity found can be predicted from measures of the values espoused within the different nations where the studies were conducted.

There is similar variability of results when other social processes in teams are studied in different countries (Smith & Bond, 1993). What is needed is a conceptual framework which may explain how such variability comes about. The next section outlines our chosen candidate for this role.

How Do Cultures Differ?

The concept of culture has been widely adopted in recent times to describe elements in common among members of teams, of organizations and of whole nations. At this point in our discussion it is the delineation of national cultures which is of primary importance, since we need to understand world-wide variations in the results of studies. The most influential work in this field has been that of Hofstede (1980, 1991), who defined culture as "the collective programming of the mind, which distinguishes the members of one human group from another" (Hofstede, 1980, p. 21).

On the basis of a very large-scale survey of employees of IBM in many countries, Hofstede concluded that respondents' values could be classified along four dimensions. The first of these, Individualism–Collectivism, distinguished societies whose members define their identity in terms of individual choices from societies whose members define their identity in terms of membership in groups, most typically long-lasting ones. The second dimension, Power Distance, separated societies where a respectful distance from superiors is maintained from those with more informal and equal relationships with superiors. The Uncertainty Avoidance dimension distinguished societies which plan ahead and worry about the future from those who do not. The fourth dimension was named Masculinity–Femininity. In Masculine societies achievement and recognition at work are valued highly, whereas in societies identified as Feminine more value is put upon the quality of interpersonal relations at work. Some years after completing his project, Hofstede (1991) accepted that a fifth dimension of cultural variation, identified as Long-term Perspective, is required. This had been identified earlier and named as Confucian Work Dynamism by researchers using a questionnaire based upon traditional Chinese sayings (Chinese Culture Connection, 1987).

Hofstede's procedure was to identify the most typical values endorsed by each nation. Some caution is therefore needed in using his results to interpret the behaviour of specific individuals of teams within a nation. All nations have substantial cultural diversity, and Hofstede cautions against the "ecological fallacy" of assuming that relations between concepts defined at the level of national cultures will also hold for smaller sections within them. His dimensions provide hypotheses as to how teams in different national cultures might behave, rather than asserting that all teams in that culture will behave that way.

Subsequent large-scale surveys have, in general, supported the validity of Hofstede's analysis. While not all surveys have yielded precisely the same five dimensions, it is clear that the specific nature of the IBM sample had no great distorting impact upon the results. Schwartz (1994) classifies values endorsed by students and schoolteachers in 47 nations into seven domains, most of which show similarities to those found by Hofstede. Trompenaars (1993) postulates seven dimensions, also partially overlapping those of Schwartz and Hofstede.

It would be naive to assume that the full complexity of variations in work team behaviour around the world could be explained in terms of variations along a few dimensions, still less one dimension. Despite this, it is the single dimension of Individualism–Collectivism which has attracted the attention of most recent researchers (Kim et al., 1994; Smith & Bond, 1993; Triandis, 1989, 1990). In fact, Hofstede's results showed a strongly inverse relationship between his dimensions of Individualism–Collectivism and Power Distance. Thus, societies which are individualist are mostly also low in Power Distance, while societies which are more collectivist are also high on Power Distance.

There are good reasons why this pair of dimensions may have particular relevance to studies of teams and team-working. According to Hofstede's results, the USA is the most individualist nation of the 53 which were sampled. Thus, the nation within which most research into teams has been undertaken proves to be highly atypical. Furthermore, other nations ranked by Hofstede adjacent to the US scores, namely Australia, UK, The Netherlands and Canada, are those in which many of the remaining studies of teams have been made. Since this section has suggested building our analysis of work teams around cultural variations in Individualism–Collectivism, the next step required is to consider whether the way in which a work team is conceived might be rather different in nations whose values are not so individualist as the USA.

CULTURAL DIFFERENCES IN TEAMWORK

Some of the most detailed analyses of non-Western work teams are provided by the extensive literature on Japanese work organization (Hampden-Turner, 1994; Kashima & Callan, 1994; Smith & Misumi, 1989). Typical attributes of Japanese work teams are said to be high work involvement, long-term time perspective, high organizational commitment, low differentiation of specialist roles, acceptance of hierarchy and collective decision-making.

Japan is widely thought of in the West as a collectivist society. However Hofstede's data give it rank 22 out of 53, suggesting that it is no more than moderately collectivist, at least in comparison with the mostly Latin American societies, which scored highest. Nonetheless, the Japanese work team does appear markedly different from those typically found within Western organizations. Hazama (1978) suggests that some of the essential differences may be captured by thinking of the Japanese work group as a tug-of-war team and the US work group as a baseball team. In the tug-of-war team there is minimal role differentiation and it is very difficult to determine how much each individual is contributing: they win or lose collectively. In the baseball team, roles are individually identified and each player's performance is publicly visible. A team may win while an individual player is dropped for poor performance.

The purpose of comparing Japanese and American work teams is to illustrate the degree to which one's definition of a team is culturally relative, and explicable in terms of Hofstede's concepts. If a team is seen as a group of individuals who each use their skills on a specific part of the task until it is completed, and who would be dropped if their contribution was not adequate, that team probably comes from an individualist culture. If the team comprises employees who vary in seniority but have a long-term commitment to the organization and a shared responsibility for all aspects of its performance, it is more likely to be located in a collectivist, high power distance culture.

Laboratory studies suggest that the long-term commitment found in Japanese work teams is not simply a matter of more collectivist values, but an indication of the different ways in which US and Japanese team members calculate where their interest lies. Yamagishi (1988) compared three-person student teams in the USA and Japan who were working on a task where they could not detect how much the other team members were contributing. Team members had the option of taking an individual reward rather than participating in the team bonus. In the USA the individual reward was popular only where the penalties for taking it were low. In Japan, subjects frequently chose the individual reward even when the penalty for doing so was high. Yamagishi explains this by suggesting that Japanese team members find it difficult to tolerate not knowing what other team members are contributing.

If teams work differently in different cultures, the key question to address is whether this matters. There is growing evidence that it does. First indications of this have long been available. An instance is provided by studies concerning group participation. Coch & French (1948) showed that the introduction of changes in work procedures within a US pyjama factory were best accomplished through group discussion. The subsequent growth of organization development procedures has shown that group participation in the USA does frequently facilitate effective change programmes (Cummings & Worley, 1993). However, attempts to replicate these findings in other countries led to quite different outcomes. French, Israel & As (1960) found that work teams in a Norwegian shoe factory resisted the use of group discussion, which they perceived as an attempt by management to circumvent established agreements with their trade union representatives. Marrow (1964) found that in Puerto Rico the use of group discussion in the introduction of changes led to increased labour turnover. This proved to be because, in the high power distance Hispanic culture of Puerto Rico, employees felt that the use of group discussion indicated that management had run out of ideas, and the firm must be on the brink of bankruptcy. Juralewicz (1974) found that changes were better introduced in Puerto Rico when teams appointed a representative to discuss possible changes with management.

Of course, not all attempts to replicate results cross-culturally fail. Where two nations are relatively similar, one may predict effects more reliably. For instance, West (1990) found that UK work teams high on vision, participation, task orientation and support for innovation would score higher on objective indices of innovation. Agrell & Gustafson (1994) obtained similar results with Swedish teams.

The contrast between the results from the USA and elsewhere indicates that employees within individualist nations have most often responded more positively to group participation than have employees in more collectivist, high power distance cultures. Other more recent developments in the USA and elsewhere, such as the growing popularity of self-managed work teams (Manz, 1992), are consistent with this. However, there are many other personal and organizational factors which can determine where participation is most favoured (Locke & Schweiger, 1979). It is likely that positive response to participation by US workers is related to how much more control over their work it gives them. Both this and the argument that under some circumstances the need for leadership can be eliminated can be seen as characteristic of a low power distance culture.

In contrast, within more collectivist cultures, participation may restrict one's freedom of choice but enhance social motivation to perform well. We have noted already Earley's (1989, 1993) studies of the reversal of social loafing in Chinese and Israeli work teams. The success of quality circles in Japan and their relative failure in Western countries (van Fleet & Griffin, 1989) provide a further instance. Erez & Earley (1987) compared the effects of different goal-setting procedures among groups of US and Israeli students. The Israelis reacted much more negatively to assigned goals and much more positively to group participation. These effects were particularly strong for kibbutz members and for those who endorsed collectivist values. This study provides an advance over those cited earlier because it showed that cross-national differences in team performance could be explained by the contrasting values held by the research participants.

These illustrations indicate that the meanings of team behaviours, such as participation and the obligations of team membership, do vary by cultural location. For this reason, it is appropriate to consider separately the various types of studies of multicultural teams. We consider first teams located within organizations in Western, individualist nations and comprising members of varying ethnic background, who are nonetheless permanently resident in that country. Because our primary focus is upon national cultures and their impact upon team performance, we shall address ethnic diversity, rather than other aspects of diversity such as age or gender. Our intention in referring to selected single-country studies in this area here is to link their outcomes to the more general themes of this chapter. In subsequent sections, we consider more fully issues relating to teams with expatriate members.

THE CULTURALLY DIVERSE TEAM

The notion that North American societies function as a cultural "melting pot" has recently come under sustained scrutiny (Triandis, Kurowski & Gelfand, 1994; Jackson et al., 1992). Controlled laboratory experiments have shown that the type and amount of contribution to teams is to some extent related to the ethnic background of team members. At the same time, field studies have confirmed that demographic effects are not restricted to short-term laboratory settings. However, most of the studies considered in this section are based upon short-term studies of student groups. A willingness to rely upon this type of research can itself be considered as representative of distinctive cultural values. Members of collectivist, high power distance societies will give more credence to the longer-term context of social actions.

Ruhe & Eatman (1977) compared productivity in two-person US student groups. Groups were all black, all white or mixed. White productivity was unaffected by team composition, whereas blacks did better in mixed teams. Zamarripa & Krueger (1983) compared interaction within three homogeneous and three heterogeneous seven-person US student teams over a 30-minute period. Heterogeneous teams had French and Arab members in addition to Americans. Orientations toward the type of leadership perferred were more diverse in the heterogeneous groups.

Kirchmeyer & Cohen (1992) constructed four-person student discussion groups in Canada, where each group contained one ethnic minority member. Most of the ethnic minority members were described as oriental and gender balance was controlled. Minority members' contributions were rated lower than those of majority members. Members' ratings of the quality of the group's decision were positively related to ratings of the presence of constructive conflict. Furthermore, minority members' contributions were rated higher where constructive conflict was present, whereas majority members' contributions were rated lower where constructive conflict was present.

Watson, Kumar & Michaelsen (1993) studied US student groups varying in cultural homogeneity over a more extended time period, namely 17 weeks. The homogeneous groups had all white Americans, while the heterogeneous groups had one white American, one black American, one or two Hispanic Americans and one or two foreign nationals. Their heterogeneous groups were thus much more diverse than those studied by Kirchmeyer and her associates. The teams worked on business case studies at four different times. After each case the group submitted a written account of their analysis. Initially, the homogeneous groups scored higher on all the ratings made by independent judges. However, the performance of the heterogeneous teams improved over time and by the end of the 17 weeks they were judged superior on range of perspectives and alternative solutions generated, there being no significant difference on the two remaining criteria.

These studies of student teams all agree that cultural heterogeneity enhances the likelihood of there being diverse viewpoints. However, in Kirchmeyer's studies, the minority view was mostly not heard, either because it was the view of a single person, or because time was not available to allow diverse views to be heard. In the Watson, Kumar & Michaelsen (1993) study, the diverse teams were able over time to benefit from their diverse composition.

A further possible explanation as to why the views of minority members were not heard in the Canadian study is that minority members may not endorse the value of putting forth conflicting views. This possibility was investigated by Kirchmeyer (1993), who used a design similar to her earlier study, to examine correlates of low-rated contribution by minority members. Low contribution was associated with low self-rated communication competence, and with femininity rather than masculinity as rated by the Bem Sex Role Inventory (Bem, 1974). In a similar way, Cox, Lobel & McLeod (1991) asked homogeneous and heterogeneous four-person teams of US students to participate in a two-party Prisoner's Dilemma experiment. The homogeneous teams were all Anglo, while the heterogeneous teams contained Anglo, Asian, Black and Hispanic Americans. The heterogeneous team members favoured more cooperative choices than the homogeneous Anglo teams. Kim, Park & Suzuki (1990) asked students how they would distribute rewards among a small group of fellow students. Students from Korea, where collectivist values prevail, favoured the most equal distribution, whereas the Japanese and the Americans were in favour of differentiating on the basis of individual contribution.

One should not conclude from these three studies that team members from collectivist cultures always favour cooperative or non-assertive behaviours. Numerous studies indicate that whether a member of a collectivist culture favours cooperation or competition depends upon their relationship with the other party (Smith & Bond, 1993). Cooperation and the preservation of harmony are high priorities within the in-group, but competition with adversaries may be even more intense than that favoured by members of individualist cultures. A team may or may not be perceived as an in-group, depending on how it has been constructed. The time required for the creation of in-group cohesion and trust is a likely explanation for the gradual improvement in performance of Watson, Kumar & Michaelsen's (1993) heterogeneous teams. Other teams may acquire in-group status simply on the basis of how they were created. Yamagishi & Sato (1986) compared five-person Japanese student teams, composed of either friends or strangers. Team members were asked whether they were willing to make individual contributions to a team bonus. If the bonus was to be at the level of the lowest individual contribution or at the level of the average contribution, friends volunteered more than did strangers.

All of these studies of student teams were of rather short duration and there is room for doubt as to whether the effects reported would also occur in longer-term work teams. Leiba & Ondrack (1994) report an evaluation of a Canadian MBA programme within which students are required to work in multicultural teams throughout their first year of study. They found greater dissatisfaction than among comparison groups of non-diverse teams. However, they hypothesize later positive effects within their ongoing study, particularly when students encounter diversity-related issues within work organizations after graduation.

The effects of cultural diversity within non-student teams in North American work organizations has been extensively examined through the studies of "organizational demography" (Pfeffer, 1983), but most studies have focused upon similarities in variables such as age, organizational tenure and gender rather than ethnicity. Studies not including ethnicity as a variable are presented in detail by Jackson (this volume). These studies consistently show that similarity enhances the likelihood that a team will remain together over time, communicate more with one another and become more cohesive.

The only studies of this type which do include an ethnicity variable are focused upon superior–subordinate relations rather than the behaviour of teams (Kraiger & Ford, 1985). For instance, Tsui & O'Reilly (1989) compared performance ratings within homogeneous and heterogeneous superior–subordinate dyads in a US corporation. No effect of ethnicity on performance ratings was found, and there was a trend in the data suggesting that working in mixed-race dyads was preferred. Objective measures such as labour turnover may be required in future studies, in order to test more definitely whether ethnic heterogeneity does really have quite different long-term effects on group performance than do other aspects of organizational demography.

THE MULTINATIONAL TEAM

The escalating number of international business partnerships and strategic alliances has faced organizations, teams and individuals with the need to work within culturally less familiar environments (De Wit & Meyer, 1994; Lane & Beamish, 1990). Although many companies do report success (Moran, Braaten & Walsh, 1994), the evidence suggests that international ventures are frequently beset with difficulties that lead to their failure (Franck, 1990). The notion that effective cross-cultural interpersonal processes are a key factor in international business success has been explored by a number of writers (Adler, 1991; Choi, Lynskey & Scott, 1993; Swierczek & Hirsch, 1994). This can be most clearly understood at the level of the team, the forum within which interpersonal dynamics are most directly played out.

This section considers group processes within multinational work teams and the way in which values may affect group functioning, learning and ultimately performance. The central aim is to understand how team effectiveness can develop over time. Whilst task-specific problems, such as the need to design a new product or achieve company targets may be similar, the way in which these problems are handled can vary enormously across cultures. For instance, the collectivist emphasis on maintaining team harmony and consensus contrasts with the emphasis in individualist cultures upon open discussion of conflicting views as a valued and sought-after aspect of team work. Numerous other differences in relevant norms were found in a comparison between Japan, Hong Kong, Italy and UK (Argyle et al., 1986). The central question is thus *how* group members with different value orientations can work together effectively and achieve organizational ends when their team, task and interpersonal orientations differ significantly. We consider first some structural aspects of team composition and then explore the development of teams toward effective operation.

Structural Aspects

The organizational context within which a team operates determines a number of fixed points, such as the status and positions that people occupy. Several of these aspects are unlikely to change greatly over time. These include the task assignment of the team, for instance whether it is a project team, an established department or a quality circle, as well as its life-span. Airline flightdeck crews provide an example who come together for rather short periods, are bounded by marked role differentiation, but whose effectiveness is nonetheless constrained by cultural differences in team members' expectations as to appropriate leader and team member behaviours. Substantial differences were found by Merritt & Helmreich (1996), who studied US, Taiwanese and Filipino crews. The Asian respondents favoured greater deference to authority, loyalty and harmony, while the US crews gave more emphasis to self-reliance and personal responsibility for success or failure.

A key factor is the basis upon which team membership is defined and implemented. One relatively fixed point concerns how team members communicate, be it through face-to-face meetings, computer conferencing or videoconferencing. A team which rarely meets face to face has distinctive problems to overcome. A further problem is that increasing numbers of management teams are composed multiprofessionally as well as multinationally, which makes the utilization of each member's contribution essential, even though cultural differences within the team make that more difficult. There is also the matter of whether or not members can choose to join a team. In a field study of teams in mainland China, Putai (1993) found a higher level of motivation in voluntarily formed multinational teams than in non-voluntarily formed teams.

The culture of an organization provides the setting within which company norms, values and implicit rules of behaviour are established (Schein, 1985) and these play a crucial role in determining how cultural diversity is handled (Adler, 1983, 1991). For instance, if the organizational culture values the "melting-pot" view of integration, whereby competing differences are assimilated into the generally accepted way of doing things, then minority influence is likely to be limited. This view of integration is probably more attractive to majority group members and less appealing to minority group members. Stacey (1993) argues strongly against the melting-pot model, asserting instead that the goal should be to develop pockets of difference and competing values within the organization in order to harness development, new mind-sets and innovation. The most frequent responses of organizations to cultural diversity are shown below in Table 19.1.

A further structural aspect of multinational teams is whether a team member's own nation is also a key stakeholder in the business, thereby providing some members with an implicitly privileged status that may manifest itself in inequality of power and influence. Trevor (1983), for instance, found that within some Japanese-owned plants in Britain, Japanese managers relied upon the characteristically Japanese participative decision-making technique of *ringi-seido*, which involves extensive circulation of written proposals for change. However they did not include UK team members in this procedure, on the grounds that they would not understand it.

A final factor is the actual team membership. Bi-national teams often result from two-country mergers and acquisitions, while multinational organizations more often create teams with three or more nationalities represented. While the first of these runs the particular risk of polarized win/lose conflicts between the

Table 19.1 Organizational orientations toward ethnic diversity

Orientation	Perception	Strategy
Parochial "One best and only way"	Cultural diversity seen as having no impact	Ignores impact on the organization
Ethnocentric "Our way is the best"	Cultural diversity has negative impact	Minimizes source and impact of diversity
Synergistic Creative combinations of harnessing both "our way" and "their way"	Cultural diversity leads to both problems and advantages for the organization	Manages differences

Adapted from Adler (1983).

two parties, teams with multiple national memberships are faced with an unfolding series of logistical and procedural problems, which we now consider.

Team Development

Multinational teams evolve over time, just as do other types of team. Figure 19.1 presents a model of this process, which draws upon the early formulation by Tuckman (1965), as well as contemporary versions (McGrath & O'Connor, this volume). The top right segment identifies four phases of team formation, which have some similarity with the Tuckman stages of "forming, storming, norming and performing". We have chosen to give these stages different names because although there may be some universality to the themes which emerge in teams, these themes will be handled in different ways depending upon cultural values.

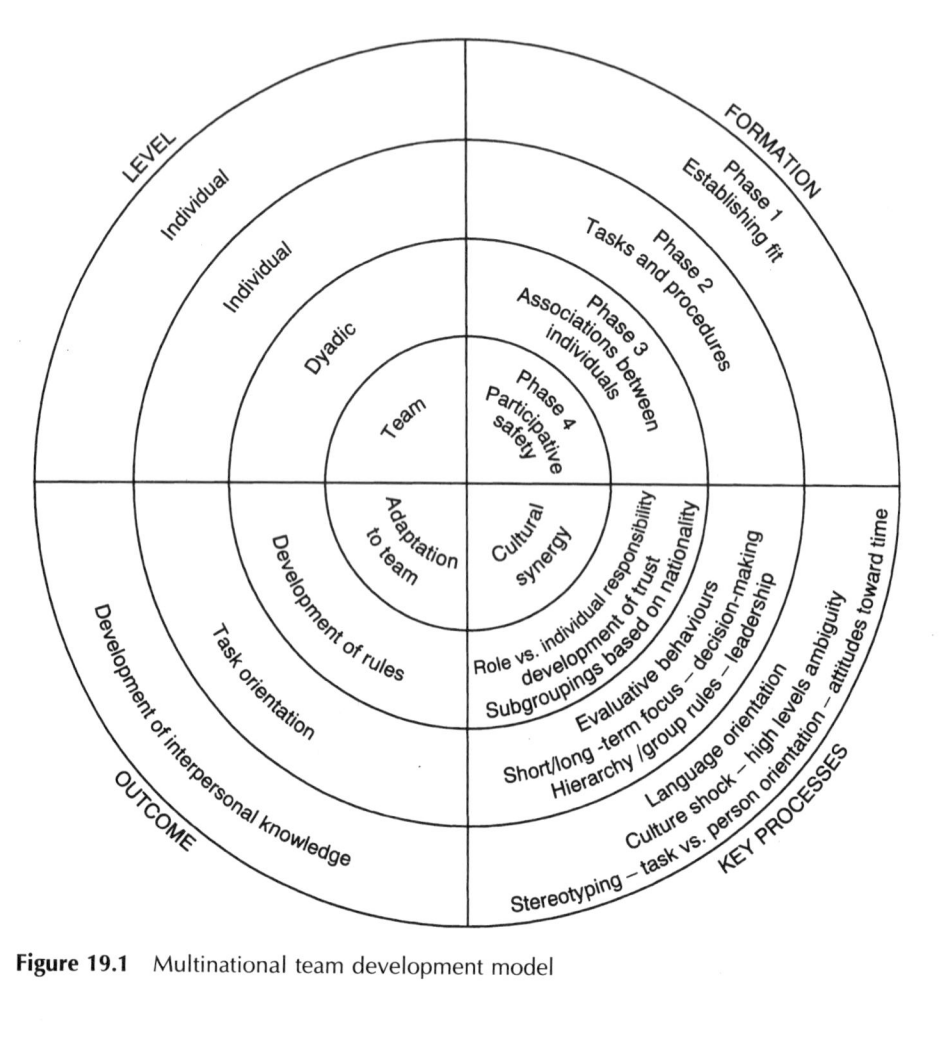

Figure 19.1 Multinational team development model

For instance, control issues may well predominate in Phase 2, but overt expressions of "storming" will only occur within cultures where open expression of differences is positively valued. We prefer the more general title of "tasks and procedures" in this case. Similarly, we prefer to refer to Phase 4 as "participative safety", since this underlines more precisely the way in which members of a Phase 4 team can safely assume that their participation in the team will be valued and utilized without regard to cultural difference.

Process stages in teams are of course not discrete, but signify change and movement over time and can provide a framework for understanding particularly salient behaviours. The upper left segment indicates the likely level of involvement of team members at each of these stages. The lower segments focus upon different aspects of team process associated with each stage. The lower left segment identifies outcomes likely to predominate as the team develops. The lower right segment emphasizes issues facing the team as an entity.

Phase 1—Establishing Fit

It is likely that the need to establish an adequate level of trust within a team is universal, but the way in which this is accomplished may vary across cultures. Although there is much debate concerning the value of the stage approach to groups (McGrath & O'Connor, this volume), studies of groups in Western settings indicate that this early phase in a team's life is the one which poses many difficulties. One of the principal reasons for this is that team members have very limited information about one another.

For multinational teams an immediate issue is which language the team will use. Although most multinational organizations have a corporate national language in which to communicate, when the composition of a team is heavily weighted towards a different preferred language, attempts to challenge the headquarters rule are likely to emerge. The primacy of language issues is well-illustrated by Fiedler's (1964) attempt to test his well-known contingency theory of leadership. Teams of Belgian naval ratings were composed either homogeneously or heterogeneously from the Flemish and Walloon communities within Belgium. The impact of the contingencies specified by Fiedler's theory was completely overshadowed by disputes in the heterogeneous groups as to whether to speak in Flemish or French.

While ethnic identity is not so intensely linked to language in all parts of the world, agreeing to speak to other team members in one's second or third language, while they are speaking their native language, does have consequences for both parties. Impressions of the task competence of second language speakers may erroneously be based upon their linguistic fluency (Wible & Hui, 1985). Native language speakers will need to accommodate to the situation by speaking more slowly and less idiomatically (Pierson & Bond, 1982), and if they do not they are likely to be seen as arrogant or incomprehensible.

During this initial phase of group formation the most significantly different value orientation will be in terms of the way in which group members attempt to

> **Box 19.1   The European management team of EUROSYS**
>
> EUROSYS, the Association of European Office Systems Wholesalers, is a coalition of eight national market-leader companies from Switzerland, UK, Denmark, Germany, Greece, Turkey, Spain and The Netherlands. The aim of the coalition is to enhance members' profitability on an international level by sharing information and management expertise.
>
> The management team encountered several difficulties. Initially, they used simultaneous translators to communicate with one another, but this was found to hinder discussion and communication. The shift to English as the team's official language proved equally problematic, due to the variance in language competency. The key cross-cultural issues for the group concerned national differences in management style, relationships between the older and younger members of the team and between the company owners and managers.
>
> The underlying problem facing team members was their resistance to sacrificing national independence in order to achieve international cooperation. At the same time there was some agreement that there was a need for greater cooperation and that the conflicting styles were obstacles. An international management consultant was asked to conduct a series of interventions to enhance collaboration. The intervention enabled the majority of members to see the futility of attempting to change one another and enabled the team to use their energies instead to work more effectively toward joint goals.
>
> From Moran, Kerschen, Rosier & Wagner (1994), with permission

establish trust. This may range from attempts to focus on sharing task-related issues to attempts at personal disclosure or discussing non-work-related issues, as a way of building relationships and establishing common ground. Won-Doornink (1985) reviewed studies of communication style and concluded that self-disclosure is more highly valued in individualist cultures. In collectivist societies it is more important to be know what is the other person's standing, affiliations and context. Such differences in approach will surface within a multinational team, and may lead to high levels of ambiguity, mistrust, miscommunication and inaccurate evaluations of one another.

For instance, a case study of a German–American venture found that procedures for relationship-building varied enormously between the two countries (Meyer, 1993). Whereas the American mode of transition was characterized by instant conversations of an informal and personal nature, for the German team members, developing interpersonal trust within the work team was much more gradual, with discussions emphasizing technical and procedural aspects of the tasks in hand. Meyer concludes that the German mode of relating to others is characterized by "distrust until reason to trust" and the American mode as "trust unless reason to distrust" (p. 98). These results show close parallels with the characterization of German–American differences first outlined by Lewin (1936).

Reliance on stereotyped expectations will be strongest during the initial stage of team development and, given members' lack of alternative sources of information about one another, can have some positive value. Knowing the "kernel of truth" (Mackie, 1973) as to what values and patterns of behaviour are favoured in some other part of the world provides an initial basis for contributing to team development.

Ratiu (1983) found that among a culturally very diverse sample of managers attending the INSEAD business school in France, those ranked by their peers as "most internationally effective" were able to modify their stereotypic expectations to fit the actual persons with whom they were dealing, whereas managers ranked "least internationally effective" maintained their stereotypes even in the face of contrary information. Achieving "international" effectiveness thus requires moving beyond thinking in terms of national categories and using the actual information which is available concerning both the person and the situation.

This process of adjustment will be impeded if some team members experience their national status as privileged over others, thereby determining whose opinions are sought and acted upon. Inequalities can arise from colonial history, historical antagonisms, economic dependence of some countries on others, or company-specific reasons such as the location of headquarters or commercial considerations that have geographic implications (Bartlett & Ghoshal, 1987; Ohmae, 1990). Intergroup polarization of this type appears to be widespread. Laurent (1983) compared the values of managers in France working in multinationals with the values of managers who were not. The values of those working in multinationals were closer to the stereotypic average for each national group represented than were those not in multinationals. Everett & Stening (1987) found mutual stereotyping of Japanese, British and American managers working in Hong Kong and Singapore.

Stereotypic images also abound in foreign direct investments and joint ventures involving less developed countries. Everett, Krishnan & Stening (1984) reported mutual stereotyping of Japanese managers and their South East Asian counterparts. Thais and Indonesians were particularly negative about the Japanese. While adversity may encourage negative mutual stereotyping in teams, it appears that members of multicultural teams do very often maintain stereotypes of one another, and that these are not always negative.

For a manager arriving in a foreign culture, particularly for the first time, the process of establishing membership in a work team will merely be one element in their overall experience of "culture shock" (Furnham & Bochner, 1986). While it is beyond the scope of this chapter to explore fully how adaptation to new situations is best accomplished, one element in this process is clarification of how the team is to conduct its business.

Phase 2—Tasks and Procedures

Once an intercultural team has been established it will quickly experience the need for clarity as to where and when it is to meet, what is the purpose of its meetings and how they are to be conducted. In other words, what control systems can best guide it toward task accomplishment?

Cultural attitudes toward time vary substantially, and these variations have immediate relevance to the work of the team. The time at which it is appropriate to arrive for a meeting, and the degree of lateness which is sufficient to give offence both vary substantially. Levine, West & Reis (1980) obtained ratings of persons who habitually arrived early or late for meetings. In Brazil, the latecomer was perceived as more likeable and successful, whereas the US results showed the reverse effect.

Variations in time perspective will also affect expectations as to how far ahead a team is looking in defining whether or not it is achieving its goals. The values of Confucian Work Dynamism (Chinese Culture Connection, 1987) are built around a long-term future time perspective, and team members from several Pacific Rim cultures will have difficulty assimilating Western emphases upon short-term results. A key feature in joint venture failures between Europeans and East Asia has been differences in time expectations and a European emphasis upon short-term advantage rather than long-term growth(Swierczek & Hirsch, 1994).

There are also considerable cultural differences in the perceived purpose of meetings. In Anglo cultures, meetings are often seen as the occasion for differing opinions to be expressed, leading to some type of group decision. Openness and directness are emphasized in individualist, low power distance cultures. In France and Japan, on the other hand, it is more frequently the case that differences of opinion will be resolved in advance of a meeting: the purpose of the meeting will be for the senior figure to announce the decision which has been made. In Germany, conduct of a meeting will often be structured around the assembling and interpretation of technical data.

Meetings involving cross-cultural teams thus face difficulties as to what is to be said and what is to be left unsaid. A study in progress by the second author examined teams of British and French managers in a joint-venture organization. It was found that the French preferred to negotiate prior to team meetings, gathering and gaining support for ideas outside, so that team meetings functioned as a confirmation of previously discussed ideas. The British experienced frustration with these procedures. Pre-meeting consultations are also a preference in the case of team members with a more collectivist orientation, who favour negotiation and conflict resolution in private rather than public, lest the overt expression of alternative views causes loss of face. The Japanese practice of *nemawashi* involves extensive pre-meeting consultations of this type (Smith & Misumi, 1989; Kashima & Callan, 1994).

The conduct of team business is intimately related to leader behaviour. Variability across cultures in effective leader style has already been noted. Part of the explanation for this may rest upon the fact that similar behaviours convey different meanings depending upon the cultural context in which they are enacted. Smith et al. (1989) compared responses of assembly-line work teams to leader-

> **Box 19.2** *"C'est trop Anglais, Monsieur"*
>
> A representative of a major British transport organization sought to negotiate a deal with an equivalent French organization. Pleased that he spoke sufficiently fluent French to negotiate in that language, he made a series of increasingly successful visits to meet a group of representatives of the French organization in Paris. Having reached agreement to purchase, he returned to Britain and had lawyers draw up a draft contract. Returning to Paris he was dismayed to be told that the contract was "too English" and that the deal could not go through.
>
> Subsequent discussions with cross-cultural consultants in Britain led him to understand the ways in which he had failed to take account of British–French differences in ways of reaching agreement. His choice to negotiate as an individual had conveyed to the French side that he was of low status, which was confirmed by his failure to invite the French team to meet his UK colleagues, and his failure to understand the need to socialize over good food in order to develop requisite trust. His draft contract was also far too imprecise for the French, and suggested that he was not a serious partner for future collaboration.
>
> Having understood these difficulties, he was able to retrieve the situation and to complete negotiation of a mutually fruitful contract.
>
> From Harper & Cormeraie (1992), with permission

ship behaviours in UK, USA, Hong Kong and Japan. They found that behaviours such as eating lunch with one's team or discussing individuals with others in the team were given different meanings in each culture.

Many procedures used by Western leaders to enhance team effectiveness have implicitly individualist assumptions, which generate problems if these procedures are employed in collectivist or high power distance settings. For instance, Child et al. (1990) studied joint ventures in China. Procedures for selection, appraisal and promotion favoured by American partners proved particularly problematic, since they generated decisions incongruent with existing status differences among the high power distance Chinese. A further study by Child & Markoczy (1993) found that among joint ventures in Hungary, American partners experienced much less difficulty, even though they were equally insistent upon implementing human resource policies stemming from US practice. In contrast, Japanese joint ventures in Hungary were found to experience many more problems than in China, with Hungarian managers and staff resisting the Japanese emphasis upon team work. Child & Markoczy interpret these differences in terms of shared individualist values between USA and Hungary, and shared collectivist values between Japan and China.

Wang & Satow (1994) also found positive evaluations by Chinese team members of various aspects of team performance within Japanese joint ventures in China. However, shared collectivist values do not necessarily always lead to greater satisfaction. Sonoda (1994) found Chinese members of joint ventures with Japan less satisfied with their pay than Chinese members of joint ventures with other nations. Sonoda suggests that because the Japanese ventures were seen as successful, Chinese members felt entitled to a more equal share of the profits.

Phase 3—Associations Between Individuals

An indication of the development of trust within a team is the way in which individual group members begin to form dyadic or subgroup alliances. Given that individuals tend to be drawn to similar others, national groupings within a team may emerge, particularly in the case of company mergers. This will often be based on an exaggeration of one's resemblance to the positions of fellow nationals. These subgroups may set limits to alternative suggestions offered by others, supporting instead their own subgroup proposals (Brislin, 1981). This ethnocentrism, or regard for one's own in-group as more correct than the outgroup, leads to polarization outside meetings with members actively seeking support from others "on the side-lines".

The extent to which the team polarizes into national camps may partially depend on the degree of cultural dissimilarity represented within it. However it is also possible for organizations to transcend polarization through careful planning. Graen & Wakabayashi (1994) studied the development of teams within Japanese plants in the USA. Training of US team leaders in Japan, allied with a "buddy system" of US–Japanese paired leadership, was said to achieve the creation of a work team climate which integrated both US individualism and Japanese team spirit. In due course such teams have only US membership. No studies have been reported of the degree to which they retain their initial culture.

Phase 4—Participative Safety

Teams operating within Phase 4 have overcome many of the problems outlined above, so we need say less about them. They can be said to have arrived at Phase 4 when the team's diversity is seen as a strength rather than a weakness. Potentially, the major strength of mixed national teams is that they provide a limit on "groupthink", a syndrome defined by Janis (1982) as occurring when group members' need to reach agreement outweighs their desire to satisfactorily assess different strategies of action. In teams characterized by groupthink, high cohesion and strong leadership foster poor decision-making, whereas in a culturally diverse team, the availability of competing and minority views make this less likely to occur. The nature of the balance of nationalities within the team is important. Minority influence is important not necessarily for its correctness, but in fostering "... the kinds of attention and thought processes that, on balance, permit the detection of new truths and raise the quality of group decision-making and performance" (Nemeth, 1992, p. 100). The experimental study by Watson, Kumar & Michaelsen (1993), which we discussed earlier, provides evidence that this can in fact occur.

Swierczek & Hirsch (1994) review joint ventures between Asian, European and American firms. They hypothesize a potential for convergence of management styles towards "multicultural management", because contemporary multinational teams need both entrepreneurship and team orientation, and these can be provided by members coming from individualist and collectivist cultures. Studies are required to establish how often this is accomplished.

In this section we have described some of the dilemmas faced by team members at each phase in the development of a hypothetical team. Whether a team ever arrives at the later stages specified in our model of course depends upon how well the earlier stages are handled. The most numerous and the most basic problems are those encountered in Phase 1 and we have given them proportionately more attention. Ensuring the successful development of teams is the primary responsibility of management, with or without the assistance of external consultants (see Bouwen, this volume). In the case of multinational teams, those providing external assistance need also to take account of relevant cultural issues and we close this chapter by considering what these issues are.

Creating Effective Cross-cultural Teams

The central aim of any intervention in multinational team process is both to maximize advantages such as multiple perspectives, creativity and innovation and to reduce weaknesses such as ambiguity, mistrust and miscommunication. To accomplish this, two emphases are required. The first is an appreciation of the cultural relativity of management conceptions, styles and practices, while the second is a sensitivity at the level of the individual and the group, sometimes referred to as "valuing difference".

Cross-cultural training for managers ranges from briefings on approaches to business in different cultures to cultural awareness and diversity training programmes, which give greater emphasis to interpersonal processes and one's own impact on others. The more didactic approach relies on the international work value dimensions described earlier (e.g. Hofstede, 1991; Trompenaars, 1993), cases and team exercises concerning international business scenarios. Experiential approaches favour more direct involvement with aspects of cultural difference, either simulated or real. Earley (1987) compared didactic and experiential training as preparation for US managers who were to work in Korea. Both forms of training had positive effects. Managers subsequently rated as working most effectively in Korea were those who had received both forms of training. In a similar way, Hammer & Martin (1992) found that both cognitive and experiential approaches had value in training US managers within American–Japanese joint ventures.

When working with a mixed national group it is important that culturally appropriate training methods are used (Pun, 1993). Trainers need to consider how Western methods such as role plays, group discussion and simulations will be received by members of non-Western cultures. Preferred methods of training are related to underlying learning expectations. For instance, Hofstede (1983) emphasized that the Chinese value harmony in learning situations, whereas in the West learning of a more participative or confronting nature is preferred. In a study of team training for negotiation skills with students in Hong Kong, Kirkbride, Durcan & Tang (1990) found that the Chinese valued formal methods with the trainer as expert teacher. Both students and Chinese trainers were resistant to participating in open debate. Similarly, Rigby (1987) reported that teams from high power distance cultures valued less confronting learning methods. Earley (1994) showed that while US managers responded better to a training programme which was focused upon themselves as individuals, Chinese managers responded more to a programme which provided feedback on team performance.

Training initiatives need to tackle not only the "why" of cultural differences in managerial attitudes and assumptions but "how" this knowledge can be usefully applied cross-culturally. The weakness of cultural briefings is that they often focus on stereotyped cross-cultural solutions to particular dilemmas. Such training gives no help in understanding how to adapt to ongoing experiences within a team. More effective interventions will be those that enable team members to see how to tackle the specific dilemmas they are confronted with. To achieve this more specific approach, trainers and consultants need to consider carefully the desired outcome of the training, the level of international competence within the team and the nature of the organization's international role.

The challenge of training for a new team is to enable members to move beyond reliance on stereotyped expectations. Enabling individuals to become more aware of their own and one another's managerial assumptions has been found to be a useful "ice-breaker" activity (Laurent, 1983), providing these are not too readily interpreted or evaluated (Adler, 1991). Team members can then use such activities to understand the way in which other members think and act. Similarly, activities that enable members to share their experiences of encounters with culturally different others allow them to compare experiences of "culture-shock" (Furnham & Bochner, 1986).

With teams that have progressed to later stages, external interventions will need to address whatever difficulties have led the team to request external intervention. The most important guideline for such interventions is that they should not exacerbate or collude with the cultural issues that the team faces. For instance, in situations where there is polarization between members of two cultural groups, an external consultant from each of the parties' cultural groups will be required.

CONCLUSION

In this chapter we have examined some of the difficulties facing multicultural and multinational work teams. Much more extensive empirical investigation is needed to clarify how these difficulties are being handled in practice. Our phase model recognizes that teams are not static entities, but develop and change over time. As has been the case in other areas of social psychology, experimental studies have addressed samples who were brought together for very short periods. Consequently they have little chance of aiding understanding of naturalistic work teams. Future research should focus on both the objective and subjective elements in the development of naturalistic teams. If we consider the current influence in the world of multinational teams, not just within business ventures, but in United Nations organizations, the European Union, diplomacy, development agencies, military alliances and the full range of organizations within ethnically diverse societies, it is quite remarkable how neglected have been the processes occurring within them. Two principal reasons may be advanced for this state of affairs, both of them usually expressed implicitly rather than explicitly, and neither of which will stand scrutiny when examined closely. Firstly, the "melting-pot" myth has been widely endorsed: the view that it is the obligation of minorities within a team (or a society) to learn how the majority operate and find ways of joining in. Secondly, the individualistic values endorsed within Western societies favour individualistic explanations of behaviour. Thus if a team fails to operate effectively it is frequently attributed to deficiencies in the personality or skills of one or more team members.

Both of these alibis for failure rationalize but do not excuse the loss of opportunity which cultural diversity provides. Studies should now consider both how multicultural teams may best capitalize upon their diversity and the degree to which participation in them itself leads to changes in values and behaviour. The lessons to be learned from such studies should prove relevant also to the management of difference within monocultural teams.

REFERENCES

Adler, N.J. (1983). Organizational development in a multicultural environment. *Journal of Applied Behavioral Science*, **19**, 349–365.

Adler, N.J. (1991). *International Dimensions of Organizational Behavior*. Boston, MA: Kent Publishing.

Agrell, A. & Gustafson, R. (1994). The Team Climate Inventory (TCI) and group innovation: a psychometric test on a Swedish sample of work groups. *Journal of Occupational and Organizational Psychology*, **67**, 143–152.

Argyle, M., Henderson, M., Bond, M.H., Iizuka, Y. & Contarello, A. (1986). Cross-cultural variations in relationship rules. *International Journal of Psychology*, **21**, 287–315.

Asch, S. (1956). Studies of independence and conformity: a minority of one against a unanimous majority. *Psychological Monographs*, **70**(9) (whole number 416).

Ayman, R. & Chemers, M.M. (1983). Relationship of supervisory behavior ratings to work group effectiveness and subordinate satisfaction among Iranian managers. *Journal of Applied Psychology*, **68**, 338–341.

Bartlett, C.A. & Ghoshal S. (1987). *Managing Across Borders: The Trans-national Solution*. Boston, MA: Harvard Business School Press.

Bem, S. (1974). The measurement of psychological androgyny. *Journal of Consulting and Clinical Psychology*, **42**, 155–162.

Bond, M.H. & Hwang, K.K. (1986). The social psychology of Chinese people. In M.H. Bond (ed.), *The Psychology of the Chinese People.* Hong Kong: Oxford University Press, pp. 213–266.

Bond, R. & Smith, P.B. (1996). Culture and conformity: a meta-analysis of studies using the Asch line judgement task. *Psychological Bulletin,* **119,** January.

Brislin, R. (1981). *Cross-Cultural Encounters: Face to Face Interation.* Oxford: Pergamon.

Child, J., Boisot, M., Ireland, J., Li, Z. & Watts, J. (1990). *The Management of Equity Joint Ventures in China.* Beijing: China–EC Management Institute.

Child, J. & Markoczy, L. (1993). Host country managerial behaviour and learning in Chinese and Hungarian joint ventures. *Journal of management Studies,* **30,** 611–632.

Chinese Culture Connection (1987). Chinese values and the search for culture-free dimensions of culture. *Journal of Cross-Cultural Psychology,* **18,** 143–164.

Choi, C., Lynskey, M. & Scott, M. (1993). European opportunities in Asia: images, misinformation and cultural barriers. Templeton College, Oxford: *Management Research Papers.*

Coch, L. & French, J.R.P. (1948). Overcoming resistance to change. *Human Relations,* **1,** 512–532.

Cox, T.H., Lobel, S. & McLeod, P.L. (1991). Effects of ethnic group cultural differences on cooperative and competitive behavior on a group task. *Academy of Management Journal,* **34,** 827–847.

Cummings, T.G. & Worley, C.G. (1993). *Organization Development and Change.* St. Paul, MN: West.

De Wit, B. & Meyer, R. (1994). *Strategy, Process, Content, Context: An International Perspective.* St. Paul, MN: West.

Earley, P.C. (1987). Intercultural training for managers: a comparison of documentary and interpersonal methods. *Academy of Management Journal,* **30,** 685–698.

Earley, P.C. (1989). Social loafing and collectivism: a comparison of the United States and the People's Republic of China. *Administrative Science Quarterly,* **34,** 565–581.

Earley, P.C. (1993). East meets West meets Mid-east: further explorations of collectivistic and individualistic work groups. *Academy of Management Journal,* **36,** 319–348.

Earley, P.C. (1994). Self or group? Cultural effects of training on self-efficacy and performance. *Administrative Science Quarterly,* **39,** 89–117.

Erez, M. & Earley, P.C. (1987). Comparative analysis of goal-setting strategies across cultures. *Journal of Applied Psychology,* **72,** 658–665.

Everett, J.E., Krishnan, A.R. & Stening, B.W. (1984). *Through a Glass Darkly—South-East Asian Managers: Mutual Perceptions of Japanese and local counterparts.* Singapore: Eastern Universities Press.

Everett, J.E. & Stening, B.W. (1987). Stereotyping in American, British, and Japanese corporations in Hong Kong and Singapore. *Journal of Social Psychology,* **127,** 445–460.

Fiedler, F.E. (1964). A contingency model of leadership effectiveness. In L. Berkowitz (ed.), *Advances in Experimental Social Psychology,* **1,** 149–190.

Franck, G. (1990). Mergers and acquisitions: competitive advantages and cultural fit. *European Management Journal,* **8,** 40–44.

French, J.R.P., Israel, J. & As, D. (1960). An experiment on participation in a Norwegian factory: interpersonal dimensions of decision-making. *Human Relations,* **13,** 3–19.

Furnham, A. & Bochner, S. (1986). *Culture Shock: Psychological Reactions to Unfamiliar Environments.* London: Methuen.

Graen, G.B. & Wakabayashi, M. (1994). Cross-cultural leadership making: bridging American and Japanese diversity for team advantage. In H.C. Triandis, M.D. Dunnette & L.M. Hough (eds), *Handbood of Industrial and Organizational Psychology,* Vol. 4. Palo Alto, CA: Consulting Psychologists' Press, pp. 415–446.

Hammer, M.R. & Martin, J.N. (1992). The effects of cross-cultural training on American managers in a Japanese–American joint venture. *Journal of Applied Communication Research,* **20,** 161–182.

Hampden-Turner, C. (1994). *The Seven Cultures of Capitalism*. New York: Doubleday.
Harper, J. & Cormeraie, S. (1992). "C'est trop Anglais, Monsieur": a case study of an Anglo-French cross-cultural misunderstanding. University of Sussex and Roffey Park Management Institute: *CRICCOM Papers*, 2.
Hazama, H. (1978). Characteristics of Japanese-style management. *Japanese Economic Studies*, **6**, 110–173.
Hofstede, G. (1980). *Culture's Consequences: International Differences in Work-Related Values*, Beverly Hills, CA: Sage.
Hofstede, G. (1983). The cultural relativity of organizational practices and theories. *Journal of International Business Studies*, **14**, 31–46.
Hofstede, G. (1991). *Cultures and Organizations: Software of the Mind*. London: McGraw Hill.
Jackson, S.E. and Associates (1992). *Diversity in the Workplace: Human Resource Initiatives*. New York: Guilford Press.
Janis, I. (1982). *Groupthink: Psychological Studies of Policy Decisions and Fiascos*. Boston, MA: Houghton Mifflin.
Juralewicz, R.S. (1974). An experiment in participation in a Latin-American factory. *Human Relations*, **27**, 627–637.
Kashima, Y. & Callan, V. (1994). The Japanese work group. In H.C. Triandis, M.D. Dunnette & L.M. Hough (eds), *Handbook of Industrial and Organizational Psychology*, Vol. 4. Palo Alto, CA: Consulting Psychologists' Press, pp. 609–646.
Kim, K.I., Park, H.J. & Suzuki, N. (1990). Reward allocations in the United States, Japan and Korea: a comparison of individualistic and collectivistic cultures. *Academy of Management Journal*, **33**, 188–198.
Kim, U., Triandis, H.C., Kagitcibasi, C., Choi, S.C. & Yoon, G. (eds) (1994). *Individualism and Collectivism: Theory, Method and Applications*. Thousand Oaks, CA: Sage.
Kirchmeyer, C. & Cohen, A. (1992). Multicultural groups: their performance and reactions with constructive conflict. *Group and Organization Management*, **17**, 153–170.
Kirchmeyer, C. (1993). Multicultural task groups: an account of the low contribution level of minorities. *Small Group Research*, **24**, 127–148.
Kirkbride, P.S., Durcan, J. & Tang, S. (1990). The possibilities and limits of team training in South East Asia. *Journal of Management Development*, **9**, 41–50.
Kraiger, K. & Ford, J.K. (1985). A meta-analysis of ratee race effects in performance ratings. *Journal of Applied Psychology*, **70**, 56–65.
Lane, H. & Beamish, P. (1990). Cross-cultural cooperative behavior in joint ventures in LDSC. *Management International Review*, **30**, 87–102.
Latane, B., Williams, K. & Harkins, S. (1979). Many hands make light the work: causes and consequences of social loafing. *Journal of Personality and Social Psychology*, **37**, 822–832.
Laurent, A. (1983). The cultural diversity of Western conceptions of management. *International Studies of Management and Organization*, **13**, 75–96.
Leiba, S. & Ondrack, D. (1994). Assessment of a multi-cultural training programme in the University of Toronto's full-time MBA programme. Paper given at workshop on Cross-Cultural Perspectives on Comparative Management, European Association for Advanced Studies in Management, Henley College, UK.
Levine, R.V., West, L.J. & Reis, H.T. (1980). Perceptions of time and punctuality in the US and Brazil. *Journal of Personality and Social Psychology*, **38**, 541–550.
Lewin, K. (1936). Some social psychological differences between the United States and Germany, *Character and Personality*, **4**, 265–293.
Locke, E. & Schweiger, D.M. (1979). Participation in decision-making: one more look. In B.M. Staw & L.L. Cummings (eds), *Research in Organizational Behavior*, **1**, 265–339.
Manz, C.C. (1992). Self-leading work teams: moving beyond self-management myths. *Human Relations*, **45**, 1119–1140.

Mackie, M. (1973). Arriving at the "truth" by definition: the case of stereotype inaccuracy. *Social Problems*, **20**, 431–447.

Marrow, A.J. (1964). Risks and uncertainties in action research. *Journal of Social Issues*, **20**, 5–20.

Merritt, A.C. & Helmreich, R.L. (1996). Human factors on the flightdeck: the influence of national culture. *Journal of Cross-Cultural Psychology*, (in press).

Meyer, H-D. (1993). The cultural gap in long-term international work groups: A German-American case study. *European Management Journal*, **11**, 93–101.

Misumi, J. (1985). *The Behavioral Science of Leadership: An Interdisciplinary Japanese Research Program*. Ann Arbor, MI: University of Michigan Press.

Moran, R.T., Braaten, D.O. & Walsh, J.O. (eds) (1994). *International Business Case Studies For the Multicultural Marketplace*, Houston, TX: Gulf.

Moran, R.T., Kerschen, J., Rosier, G. & Wagner, J. (1994). Cross-cultural collaboration at EUROSYS. In R.T. Moran, D.O. Braaten & J.E. Walsh (eds), *International Business Case Studies for the Multicultural Marketplace*. Houston, TX: Gulf, pp. 264–278.

Nemeth, C.J. (1992). Minority dissent as a stimulant to group performance. In S. Worchel, W. Wood & J.A. Simpson (eds), *Group Process and Productivity*. London: Sage, pp. 95–111.

Ohmae, K. (1990). *The Borderless World*. New York: Harper Business.

Pfeffer, J. (1983). Organization demography. In L.L. Cummings & B.M. Staw (eds), *Research in Organizational Behavior*, Vol. 5. Greenwich, CT: JAI Press, pp. 299–357.

Pierson, H.D. & Bond, M.H. (1982). How do Chinese bilinguals respond to variations in interviewer language and ethnicity? *Journal of Language and Social Psychology*, **1**, 123–139.

Pun, A. (1993). Managing the cultural differences in learning. *Journal of Management Development*, **9**, 35–40.

Putai, J. (1993). Work motivation and productivity in voluntarily formed work teams: a field study. *Organizational Behavior and Human Decision Processes*, **54**, 133–154.

Ratiu, I. (1983). Thinking internationally: a comparison of how international executives learn. *International Studies of Management and Organization*, **13**, 139–150.

Rigby, M. (1987). The challenge of multinational team development. *Journal of Management Development*, **6**, 65–72.

Ruhe, J. & Eatman, J. (1977). Effects of racial composition on small work groups. *Small Group Behavior*, **8**, 479–486.

Schein, E.H. (1985). *Organizational Culture and Leadership*. San Francisco: Jossey-Bass.

Schwartz, S.H. (1994). Cultural dimensions of values: towards an understanding of national differences. In U. Kim, H.C. Triandis, C. Kagitcibasi, S.C. Choi & G. Yoon (eds), *Individualism and Collectivism: Theory, Method and Applications*. Thousand Oaks, CA: Sage, pp. 85–119.

Sinha, J.B.P. (1981). *The Nurturant Task Manager: A Model of The Effective Executive*. Atlantic Highlands, NJ: Humanities Press.

Smith, P.B. & Bond, M.H. (1993). *Social Psychology Across Cultures: Analysis and Perspectives*, Hemel Hempstead: Prentice-Hall–Harvester Wheatsheaf.

Smith, P.B. & Misumi, J. (1989). Japanese management: a sun rising in the West? In C.L. Cooper & I. Robertson (eds), *International Review of Industrial and Organizational Psychology*, Vol. 4. Chichester: Wiley, pp. 330–369.

Smith, P.B. & Peterson, M.F. (1988). *Leadership, Organizations and Culture*, London: Sage.

Smith, P.B., Peterson, M.F., Misumi, J., Tayeb, M.H. & Bond (1989). On the generality of leadership styles across cultures. *Journal of Occupational Psychology*, **62**, 97–110.

Sonoda, S. (1994). Japanese management in Chinese context: a tentative analysis of acculturation process in Sino-Japanese joint ventures. In Institute of Social Sciences, Chuo University (ed.), *Market Economy and Social Justice*. Tokyo: Chuo University, pp. 277–291.

Stacey, R. (1993). *Strategic Management and Organizational Dynamics*. London: Pitman.
Swierczek, F. & Hirsch, G. (1994). Joint ventures in Asia and multicultural management. *European Management Journal*, **12**, 197–209.
Trevor, M. (1983). *Japan's Reluctant Multinationals*. London: Pinter.
Triandis, H.C. (1989). The self and social behaviour in different cultural contexts. *Psychological Review*, **96**, 506–520.
Triandis, H.C. (1990). Cross-cultural studies of individualism and collectivism. In J.J. Berman (ed.), *Nebraska Symposium on Motivation, 1989*, **37**, 41–133.
Triandis, H.C., Kurowski, L.L. & Gelfand, M. (1994). Workplace diversity. In H.C. Triandis, M.D. Dunnette & L.M. Hough (eds), *Handbook of Industrial and Organizational Psychology*, Vol. 4. Palo Alto, CA: Consulting Psychologists' Press, pp. 769–827.
Trompenaars, F. (1993). *Riding the Waves of Culture*, London: Brealey.
Tsui, A. & O'Reilly, C.A. (1989). Beyond simple demographic effects: the importance of relational demography in superior–subordinate dyads. *Academy of Management Journal*, **32**, 402–423.
Tuckman, B.W. (1965). Developmental sequences in small groups. *Psychological Bulletin*, **63**, 384–399.
van Fleet, D.D. & Griffin, R.W. (1989). Quality circles: a review and suggested future directions. In C.L. Cooper & I. Robertson (eds), *International Review of Industrial and Organizational Psychology*, Vol. 4. Chichester: Wiley, pp. 213–233.
Wang, Z.M. & Satow, T. (1994). Leadership styles and organizational effectiveness in Chinese–Japanese joint ventures. *Journal of Managerial Psychology*, **9**, 31–36.
Watson, W.E., Kumar, K. & Michaelsen, L.K. (1993). Cultural diversity's impact on interaction process and performance: comparing homogeneous and diverse task groups. *Academy of Management Journal*, **36**, 590–602.
West, M.A. (1990). The social psychology of innovation in groups. In M.A. West & J.L. Farr (eds) *Innovation and Creativity at Work: Psychological and Organizational Strategies*. Chichester: Wiley, pp. 309–333.
Wible, D.S. & Hui, C.H. (1985). Perceived language proficiency and person perception. *Journal of Cross-Cultural Psychology*, **16**, 206–222.
Won-Doornink, M. (1985). Self-disclosure and reciprocity in conversation: a cross-national study. *Social Psychology Quarterly*, **48**, 97–107.
Yamagishi, T. (1988). Exit from the group as an individualistic solution to free rider problem in the United States and Japan. *Journal of Experimental Social Psychology*, **24**, 530–542.
Yamagishi, T. & Sato, K. (1986). Motivational basis of the public goods problem. *Journal of Personality and Social Psychology*, **50**, 67–73.
Yukl, G. (1989). *Leadership in Organizations*. Englewood Cliffs, NJ: Prentice-Hall.
Zamarripa, P.O. & Krueger, D.L. (1983). Implicit contracts regulating small group leadership: the influence of culture. *Small Group Behavior*, **14**, 187–210.

Chapter 20

Promoting Team Effectiveness*

Scott I. Tannenbaum
Eduardo Salas**
and
Janis A. Cannon-Bowers**
State University of New York at Albany and **Naval Air Warfare Center, Training Systems Division, USA

Abstract

Organizations increasingly rely on the effectiveness of teams to attain organizational goals. Yet most teams do not operate at peak effectiveness. Therefore, this chapter addresses a key question: "What can be done to promote team effectiveness?". First, the chapter summarizes a model of team effectiveness. The model highlights where breakdowns can occur and where interventions may be appropriate. Five categories of team interventions are then examined: team-member selection, team building, team training, leadership development, and work redesign/restructuring. Based on theoretical and empirical developments, the chapter explains why each intervention should work and what the current state of knowledge is regarding its actual efficacy. On the basis of this review, recommendations for research and practice are provided.

---

*The views expressed in this chapter are those of the authors and should not be construed as an official position or policy of their respective organizations.

Handbook of Work Group Psychology. Edited by M.A. West.
© 1996 John Wiley & Sons Ltd.

INTRODUCTION

Teams are becoming increasingly prevalent in the work environment (Hackman, 1990; Nahavandi & Aranda, 1994). At their best, teams are ideal structures for generating and sharing knowledge, enhancing performance and improving satisfaction. Unfortunately, teams do not always operate "at their best". In fact, although the demand for teams and teamwork is increasing, teams often suffer problems and setbacks that inhibit their usefulness. This trend is confirmed by a recent Towers Perrin/IBM study of 3000 managers and executives from 12 different countries. They reported that the use of teams is a highly important action for gaining competitive advantage in the coming years. Teamwork was rated among the highest business priorities for the year 2000. Unfortunately, although business leaders view teams as an increasingly important factor in business success, their current satisfaction with teamwork is quite low (Towers Perin/IBM, 1993).

Given the growing use and importance of teams, and the reality that most teams are not operating at peak performance, the question becomes "what can be done to promote team effectiveness?" Addressing that question is the purpose of this chapter.

The chapter is organized as follows. First, we define and explicitly state our assumptions about team effectiveness. Second, we present a model of team effectiveness. The model identifies the key factors that influence team effectiveness and helps highlight where team problems can occur. Next, we examine a few possible interventions for enhancing team effectiveness. For each we describe why it should work and note which variables in the model the intervention is designed to affect. We also present a brief review of the research regarding the effectiveness of the intervention, and provide some recommendations for research and practice.

This chapter is not intended as a comprehensive review of all team interventions. Rather, it is a selective review of prevalent or promising options.

SETTING THE STAGE—"ENHANCING TEAM EFFECTIVENESS"

The purpose of the chapter is to examine what can be done to promote team effectiveness. To establish a common frame of reference, first we clarify what we mean by the terms "team" and "effectiveness".

For the purposes of this chapter we have adopted a fairly broad definition of a team. We use the term *team* to refer to a distinguishable set of two or more people who interact dynamically, interdependently and adaptively and who share at least some common goals or purpose. Thus, a wide range of teams fall into our domain, including some that are temporary in nature and some for which the team's task may not be the primary responsibility of the team members (e.g. project teams). This definition is intentionally broad, because we believe the interventions described in this chapter are applicable to a wide variety of teams (cf. Salas et al., 1992; Tannenbaum, Beard & Salas, 1992).

We use the term *effectiveness* to refer to how well a team accomplishes its purpose or mission. Although effectiveness may be operationalized differently for each team, it most directly refers to a team's performance, including the quality and quantity of the products it produces and the services it provides. However, we also use the term to refer to a team's ability to reverse the forces of entropy, to remain vital and "alive" and to grow and regenerate itself. This enables a team to sustain its performance and accomplish its mission over a period of time.

Before proceeding, we want to make explicit a few of our assumptions about team effectiveness. These assumptions describe prerequisites for team success. They pertain to the context in which a team operates. If these prerequisites are not met, then most of the interventions we discuss in this chapter can have only limited efficacy.

Assumptions

1. *The use of teams, as defined above, makes sense.* If the situation does not call for the use of a team, for example, if there are no inherent interdependencies or an individual could perform the task better, then developing a team is a waste of time. "Teamwork asks more of employees..." (Beer, Eisenstat & Spector, 1990)—so there must be a logical reason to use a team.
2. *Management shows they support the team.* Top management, project sponsors, or direct supervisors are examples of management stakeholders that can demonstrate support, apathy or even distrust of teams. The extent to which they show their support makes a difference. For example, Tang, Tollison & Whiteside (1991) studied 47 quality circle teams over a 3-year period. They found that upper management and middle management behaviors were related to team member attendance and quality circle performance. Another study of 10 task groups from several organizations found that the commitment of the project sponsor was positively related to team performance (Bushe & Johnson, 1989). Support can be symbolic but it also must be reflected in resource allocations, which leads to our third assumption.
3. *The team's resource needs are met or being met.* Even the best functioning team can fail if they lack the necessary resources to complete the task. Team members need time to work on the team's tasks (Bushe & Johnson, 1989) and access to information necessary for task completion (Magjuka & Baldwin, 1991). Resource deficiencies, such as lack of equipment and personnel, act as prohibitive situational constraints. Factors such as organizational policies can also inhibit team effectiveness. An investigation of airplane crews found that 15 of 23 fatal accidents were adversely influenced by policy factors (e.g. stressing on-time performance over safety) (Bruggink, 1985).

Goodman, Ravlin & Schminke (1987) reported that 60% of the variance in group output across several different companies could be predicted on the basis of machine and labor availability and exogenous support. Situational constraints can also have a long-term impact on team effectiveness because they can inhibit the development of self-efficacy and skill acquisition (Mathieu, Martineau & Tannenbaum, 1993).

Assuming that the situation calls for the use of a team, the team is being supported, and its resource needs are at least minimally met, then there is a good opportunity to enhance team effectiveness. However, for this to occur our fourth assumption must also be met.

4. *The team's needs are appropriately diagnosed.* Different types of teams have different requirements for success. Moreover, a given team will exhibit different needs at different stages in its development. There are no interventions that will work in all situations. A team that lacks technical skills requires a different intervention than one that has communication problems or exhibits role conflict. One cannot choose an appropriate intervention before identifying a team's needs. Unfortunately, some change agents rely on one predominant intervention for use with all teams. Accurate diagnosis is critical for selecting the right tool or intervention. Moreover, it is important to be familiar with a full range of options for enhancing team effectiveness.

If these four assumptions are met, then a wide range of interventions become available for developing, improving and maintaining team effectiveness. These interventions promote team effectiveness by enhancing relevant competencies, improving team processes and work flow, refining team interactions and modifying team structure. In the next section we present a model of team effectiveness. The model depicts many of the factors that influence team performance—in a sense it suggests how and why the interventions described in this chapter should promote team effectiveness.

MODEL OF TEAM EFFECTIVENESS

To improve team *effectiveness*, one must first identify the critical factors that influence team effectiveness. Interventions can then be targeted to improve those factors in need of change. Several models of team effectiveness have been presented in the literature (e.g. Gladstein, 1984; Hackman, 1987; Guzzo & Shea, 1992; Tannenbaum, Beard & Salas, 1992). It is beyond the scope of this chapter to review these models (see Salas et al., 1992). However, it is safe to say that although each model makes a unique contribution, there is a reasonable amount of commonality between them (Campion, Medsker & Higgs, 1993). Thus, we will use the Tannenbaum, Beard & Salas (1992) model as the framework for thinking about the interventions described in this chapter. This model has been used as a general conceptual framework to guide team performance and team training research (e.g. Salas, Cannon-Bowers & Blickensderfer, 1993). The model is depicted in Figure 20.1.

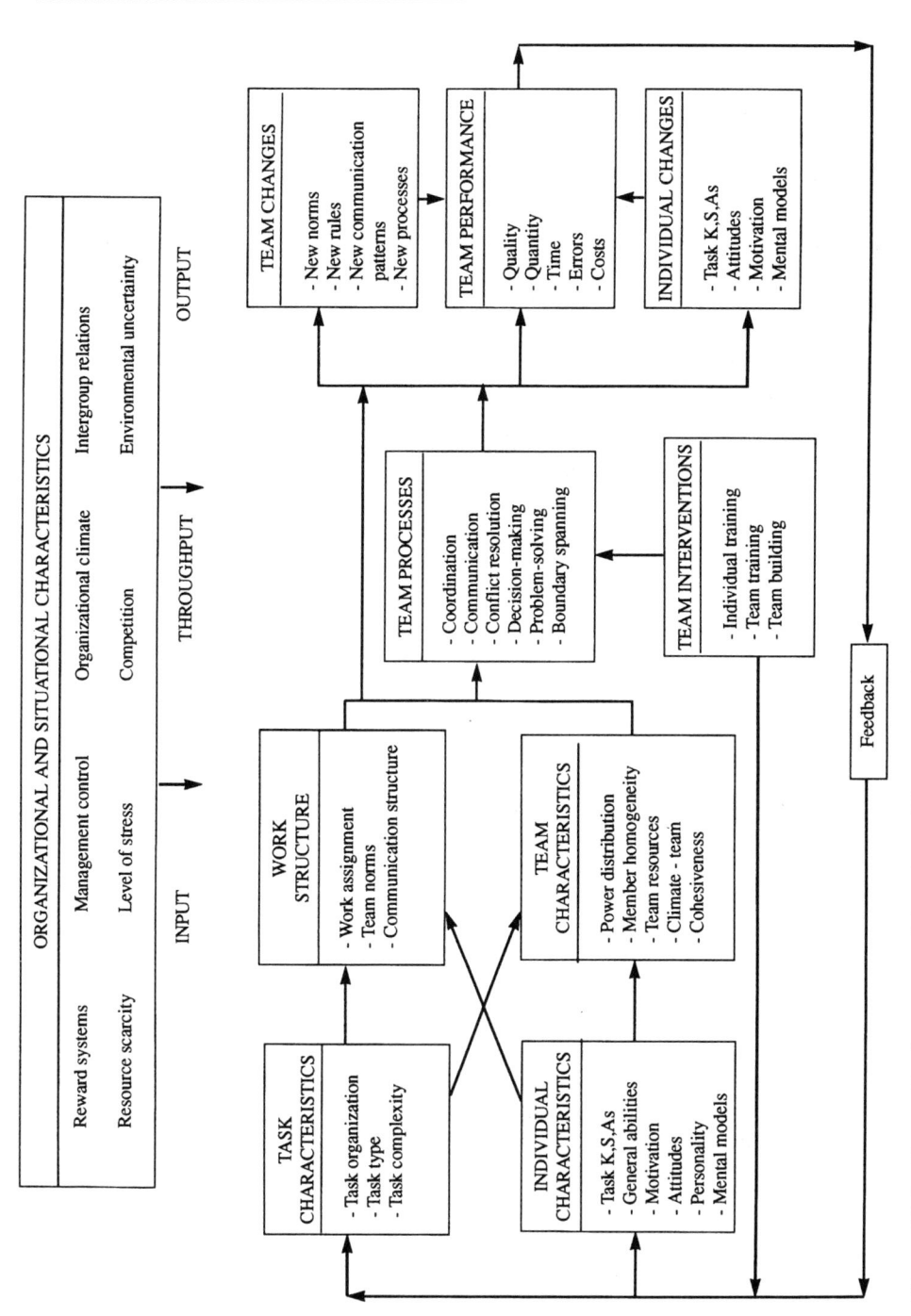

Figure 20.1 Team effectiveness model. (Adapted from Tannenbaum, Beard and Salas (1992))

As this model has been described elsewhere (Tannenbaum, Beard & Salas, 1992; Salas et al., 1992) we will only provide a brief overview of it here. The framework shown in Figure 20.1 is an input, throughput, output model. The major categories of variables are task characteristics, work structure, individual characteristics, team characteristics, team processes, team interventions, team changes, team performance and individual changes. Specific variables are noted as bullets within each box. These variables are meant to be representative of the broader categories and are not an exhaustive list. At the top of the figure is a box labeled "organizational and situational characteristics". These describe the context within which the team operates, and reflect some of the assumptions noted above (e.g. resource scarcity).

Team inputs include individual characteristics (e.g. individual task proficiency, attitudes), team characteristics (e.g. cohesiveness, heterogeneity), the characteristics of the task(s) on which the team is working (e.g. task complexity), and the way in which the work is structured (e.g. work assignment). The throughputs are the way the team interacts over time. They are the processes through which the team communicates, resolves conflict, makes decisions, spans boundaries, solves problems and coordinates with one another. They are also the way the team converts its inputs into outputs.

The outputs, are the indicators of team effectiveness we described earlier. These include primary indicators of team performance, such as quality and quantity of products produced and services provided. However, the outputs also reflect individual and team changes—for example, improvements in individual skills and new group norms—that should help perpetuate team performance over time and help reverse entropy (Katz & Kahn, 1978).

The model also highlights three team interventions, individual training, team training and team building. In this chapter we discuss several other interventions that can influence a variety of factors described in the model.

Where Can Things Go Wrong?

By definition, an intervention is "a state of coming or being between" or "any interference in the affairs of others" (Webster's New Twentieth Century Dictionary, 1983). It is logical that one should only intervene or "interfere" in a team's affairs if there are problems or concerns. Unfortunately, the plethora of problems described in the literature suggests that this state is not uncommon (e.g. see Hackman, 1990). Moreover, our personal experience with many teams suggests that at some point in time most teams have problems worthy of some form of intervention.

Team performance trends often serve as triggering mechanisms for interventions (e.g. service quality or productivity is down, errors are up), but other factors such as declining morale or poor adjustments to new roles may also trigger interventions. Why do these problems occur? The model of team effectiveness discussed earlier suggests a number of possible causes of team problems. Table

Table 20.1 Some causes of team problems

Category of variables	Symptoms	Specific variable at root of problem
Task characteristics	The task is overly complex or poorly understood	Task complexity
	The organization of the task is sub-optimal	Task organization
Work structure	Work is assigned suboptimally or by the wrong people	Work assignment
	Team norms regarding work are inconsistent with organization culture	Team norms
Individual characteristics	Team members or team leader lacks necessary skills or abilities	Task KSAs; general abilities
	Team members do not clearly understand their own or other's role	Mental models
	Team members have poor motivation or attitudes	Motivation; attitude
Team characteristics	Skill/experience/attitude mix of team is sub-optimal	Member heterogeneity
	Team lacks cohesiveness	Cohesiveness
Team processes	Team handles conflicts poorly	Conflict resolution
	Team makes decisions or solves problems poorly	Decision-making; problem-solving

20.1 lists some of the common causes of team problems, with specific variables from the model identified as well.

Naturally, these are only a few of the areas where team performance can break down. Often multiple problems occur concurrently. Moreover, the appropriate intervention for one underlying problem may be totally inappropriate for addressing a different problem. All this suggests that a careful diagnosis is called for to determine if an intervention is needed and, if so, what problems (or more optimistically, what "opportunities") exist that should be addressed. It also suggests that to enhance team effectiveness one must be capable of employing different types of interventions. As the old adage says, "To a person with only a hammer, everything looks like a nail". A full tool kit of interventions is needed. Some of these are described in subsequent sections.

What Types of Interventions Are Available to Promote Team Effectiveness?

A number of methods have been used in an attempt to improve team effectiveness. Table 20.2 notes prevalent or promising categories of interventions. For each category, the table lists sample intervention methods, information about the

Table 20.2 Interventions to promote team effectiveness

Intervention	Sample methods	Primary variables influenced by intervention	Resources/references
Team-member selection	Competency-based selection interviews Assessment center exercises	All individual characteristics including traditional ones such as task KSAs, as well as team-related attitudes and skills Member heterogeneity	Schmitt et al. (1993)
Team building	Role/goal clarification Interpersonal approach/conflict resolution Problem-solving approach	Team norms Attitudes Power distribution Climate—team Cohesiveness Team processes (in particular, communication, conflict resolution, and problem-solving)	Tannenbaum, Beard & Salas (1992)
Team training	Training shared mental models Team coordination training	Coordination Communication Decision-making Mental models	Swezey & Salas (1992)
Leadership development	Leadership training Coaching 360° feedback Briefing skills	Individual characteristics (of team leader) Individual characteristics of other team members Work assignment Team characteristics	Yukl & Van Fleet (1992); Bass (1990)
Work redesign/Restructuring	Autonomous and semi-autonomous work groups Process re-engineering Restructuring	Task organization Work assignment Power distribution Team processes	Campion, Medsker & Higgs (1993); Hammer (1990)

variables each intervention is most likely to affect, and a few key references. The remaining sections of this chapter describe these interventions.

First we discuss promoting team effectiveness through improved team member selection. Next, we discuss the development of team members through team building and team training interventions. We then address leadership development as a method of enhancing overall team performance; and modifying the way the team performs their work through work re-design/re-structuring interventions.

Team Member Selection

Selection interventions refer to a variety of systematic assessment methods designed to identify the best person for a job. Extending this to the team environment, selection interventions can be used to identify the best people to become team members. Our experience has been that even those organizations that use sophisticated methods for selecting employees for jobs often use fairly unsystematic methods of selecting or assigning people to teams. The increased use of work teams places new demands on selection systems (Offerman & Gowing, 1993).

There are three reasons why selection interventions should, at least theoretically, improve team effectiveness. First, systematic selection methods can help identify individuals with greater individual skill levels. There is strong evidence that, all else being equal, a team composed of better skilled and more highly motivated personnel will outperform other teams. For example, in two studies of three-man tank crews, Tziner found that individual abilities and motivation levels were predictive of group performance (Tziner & Eden, 1985; Tziner, 1988).

The selection/assessment literature is replete with methods for selecting people for individual jobs (Schmidt et al., 1993). Research examining these methods shows that the payoffs of improved selection decisions are usually quite large (Kopelman, 1986; Schmidt et al., 1986). Using selection methods to staff teams with individuals who possess greater task competence should enhance team effectiveness.

The second reason why selection interventions could improve team effectiveness is because of their influence on the mix or heterogeneity of team members. Increased heterogeneity is often recommended because it increases the range of competencies in the group (Gladstein, 1984). Although there are mixed opinions about the importance of heterogeneity (Jackson, 1992; and this volume), a number of studies have shown that heterogeneity can influence team performance (e.g. Magjuka & Baldwin, 1991). For example, Wiersema & Bantel (1991) found that the demographic make-up of top management teams was related to organizations' propensity to change corporate strategy. Bantel & Jackson (1989) studied 199 top management teams in the banking industry. They found that more innovative banks were managed by teams who were diverse with respect to their functional expertise. While increased heterogeneity may not always be called for, Bantel's research suggests at a minimum, the potential value of considering the existing skill and experience mix of the team when selecting new or replacement team members.

Finally, selection interventions may help team performance by identifying those individuals who will work best in a team environment. Historically, selection methods have focused on predicting performance within a narrowly defined criterion domain. That domain was defined by the specific tasks associated with an individual job. Borman & Motowidlo (1993) argue that the criterion domain should be expanded to include things that go beyond one's individual job, including factors such as helping and cooperating with others. Team assignments rely on individuals who are not only capable of performing their own task but who also possess skills and attitudes that support their team. In fact, a recent taxonomy of job performance includes "facilitating peer and team performance" as one of the eight most prevalent performance components (Campbell et al., 1993).

"Traditional methods of individual performance prediction must be expanded to include skills such as supporting and building on the work of others, getting along with others, and managing conflict" (Offerman & Gowing, 1993, p. 396). One recent line of research has examined competency requirements for various jobs (Spencer & Spencer, 1993). A competency is "an underlying characteristic of an individual that is causally related to a criterion-referenced effective and/or superior performer in a job or situation" (Spencer & Spencer, 1993, p. 9). In other words, competencies are the knowledges, skills, attitudes, traits, etc. that are related to success in a given context. An examination of this research reveals that team-related competency requirements emerge consistently across a variety of occupations. For example, Spencer & Spencer reported that "teamwork and cooperation" was among the core competencies for such diverse occupations as technical professionals, sales people, helping and human services professionals, and managers. In fact, "teamwork and cooperation" was the most often mentioned managerial competency (p. 204).

Cannon-Bowers et al. (1995a) described many of the competency requirements for team-related performance. They identified over 50 knowledges, skills and abilities that may contribute to team effectiveness. They clustered these competencies into four categories:

1. *Context-driven*—specific to both the team members one is working with and the task being performed.
2. *Team-contingent*—specific to the team but applicable to any task that team might perform.
3. *Task-contingent*—applicable to any team performing a specific task.
4. *Transportable*—applicable to any team working on any task.

Given the prevailing trend towards increased teamwork, the demand for these competencies is likely to increase. Yet almost no research has been directed towards examining selection methods to predict team-related competencies.

One selection method that is beginning to be applied in some organizations is the competency-based interview (Spencer & Spencer, 1993). In this approach, research is conducted to determine the competencies possessed by successful individuals. During the selection interview, applicants are asked questions designed to elicit information about those critical competencies (e.g. "Tell me about a time you helped a co-worker acquire a new skill"). This approach could be used to examine how individuals have handled team-related experiences and whether they possess the competencies that successful team members usually possess.

Another method that may be useful for examining team-related competencies are some of the leaderless group exercises often included in assessment centers. Particular attention could be paid to how candidates interact, facilitate and support others. For example, SEFCU, a financial institution in New York State, presented small groups of "quality forum" candidates (a form of TQM team) with a series of problems to solve. Senior managers observed and rated candidates on their individual problem-solving skills and on how well they worked with others—including how they handled disagreements. These ratings were then used to select individuals for the team assignment. Interestingly, many companies that rely heavily on teamwork skills, such as Motorola, Saturn and Hewlett-Packard also invest heavily in the development of assessment centers (Snow & Snell, 1993).

Recommendations

Although the payoffs from improved selection are usually quite high, only limited attention has been given to the systematic selection of team members. There is a need to begin applying some of the traditional selection methods to improve the overall competency levels of teams. We currently know enough about those methods (e.g. interviewing, assessment center exercises, biodata, etc.) to improve the way we select someone to fill a team-based assignment. While these selection methods are often used to hire someone to join the organization, the process of selecting among internal candidates for team assignments is often less systematic.

While we know a great deal about selecting individuals to fit jobs, research is needed that examines how to select a new team member while considering current team member competencies. Currently, we know little about how to select individuals with complementary skills or whether doing so will increase utility beyond selecting the person with the best individual skills. We know little about selecting individuals to improve the "mix" of competencies within a team.

Finally, there is a need for research that examines methods for predicting an individual's "team competencies". Much has been written and said about the need to act as a "team player". Research has begun to define what that means (e.g. Campbell et al., 1993; Cannon-Bowers et al., 1995a) but little has been done to determine: (a) how to predict whether someone will act that way; (b) which methods are best suited to select individuals with team competencies and; (c) whether selection based on those attributes improves team performance. Ideally, team member selection should consider both individual task competencies plus a candidate's team-related competencies.

Team Building

Team building refers to a variety of interventions that typically focus on team interactions or processes. Team building shares elements with team training in that both interventions are designed to enhance team functioning. However, they are different:

> ... (Team) training is a systematic effort to facilitate the development of job-related knowledge, skills, and attitudes (KSA's). The specific KSA's to be developed are determined and learning objectives are established prior to the start of training... Team building is more of a "process intervention" (Beer, 1980). A process intervention is a set of activities which is aimed at helping individuals and groups examine and act upon their behavior and relationships (Schein, 1969). Although the general framework of a team building intervention may be established up front, the content of the intervention will in part be determined by the discussions among team members (Tannenbaum, Beard & Salas, 1992, p. 126).

Thus, while team training and team building often focus on similar issues (e.g. communication, coordination) their approaches to addressing those issues are different.

Different team building interventions emphasize different factors and methods (Beer, 1980; Dyer, 1987). Some focus on role or goal clarification (e.g. Paul & Gross, 1981), some on interpersonal or conflict resolution issues (e.g. Boss & McConkie, 1981), and others take more of a general problem solving approach (see Buller & Bell, 1986).

In theory, team building can affect many of the variables described in the team effectiveness model. Team norms, attitudes, climate, power distribution and cohesiveness could be affected by any of the team building approaches. Many team processes, including communication, conflict resolution and problem-solving are often direct targets of team building interventions.

Role conflict, ambiguity and overload can have an adverse impact on individual motivation and team performance (Roos & Starke, 1981; Kahn et al., 1964). Team building interventions that include role clarification exercises are designed to address these issues. One common exercise involves the use of a responsibility analysis matrix (RAM). In a typical RAM exercise, actions (i.e. tasks and decisions) are listed down the first column and individuals or sub-groups who may be responsible for performing or approving the actions are listed across the top row. The team works to fill in the cells by noting which individuals or sub-groups are responsible for each action. For example, the board of directors at a mid-sized financial institution was having difficulty with role ambiguity. There were questions about the roles of the chairman, the committees, the president and individual board members. We used a RAM exercise to identify perceived overlaps and gaps in roles. Tasks/decisions examined included who is responsible for: approval of budgets; appointment of board committees; authorization of new services; selection/approval of branch locations; research, negotiation and approval of acquisitions/mergers; and overseeing/evaluating the CEO. In this case, they identified almost 90 tasks/decisions for consideration.

Each Board member completed the matrix individually and then we discussed their perceptions collectively. The group discussions clarified gaps and perceived role overlaps and led to agreements regarding role definitions. Re-administration of a diagnostic survey over 1 year after the intervention, showed improvements in role clarity among board members (mean rating 3.9 prior to intervention and 5.1 after the intervention, based on a 7-point scale).

Cohesiveness has been shown to be related to team performance. For example, Keller's (1986) study of 32 project groups from a large R&D organization found that group cohesiveness was related to project performance. However, Greene (1989) found that cohesiveness was only related to team performance if the team had accepted the organization's goals. This suggests that team building interventions that help clarify team and individual goals and align them with organizational goals should enhance team effectiveness.

Conflict can adversely affect cohesiveness and may reduce team effectiveness (O'Connor, Gruenfeld & McGrath, 1993). However, avoiding conflict is not the solution; some conflict is inevitable and some tension is desirable (Pascale, 1990). The key is how conflict is handled (Wall & Nolan, 1987). For example, Murnighan & Conlon (1991) found that successful string quartets use different conflict resolution strategies than less successful quartets. Teams can be taught conflict resolution tactics as part of a team training intervention. Alternatively, teams can address sources of conflict and develop methods of dealing with conflict through team building interventions as well.

Do team building interventions work? Several reviews have examined the efficacy of team building interventions (DeMeuse & Liebowitz, 1981; Sundstrom, DeMeuse & Futrell, 1990; Tannenbaum, Beard & Salas, 1992). It is impossible to conclude that any one team building method works better than others on a consistent basis, and there is a trend towards combining multiple approaches into a broader problem-solving approach (Tannenbaum, Beard & Salas, 1992). However, the cumulative evidence suggests that team building interventions can have a positive impact on individual perceptions and attitudes. There are also examples in the literature of team building interventions that demonstrated positive behavioral results (e.g. Eden, 1986), but overall the results regarding behavioral outcomes are more equivocal.

It is logical that team building interventions would show a stronger effect on attitudes and perceptions than performance. As noted in the model, team performance is a function of many factors, some of which are well beyond the scope of most team building interventions. The further removed the dependent variable is from the immediate control of the team, the less likely it is that the team building intervention will demonstrate improvements. Moreover, it is possible that in some studies the time-lag between the intervention and the collection of team performance data was too short to allow process improvements to translate into performance improvements (e.g. Woodman & Sherwood, 1980b).

Recommendations

While the quality of team building studies has improved, there is still a need for research that employs at least quasi-experimental designs to assess effectiveness. Unfortunately, it is often difficult to tell whether appropriate diagnostic work was done prior to the intervention. More detailed reporting about why the intervention was conducted and why the method used was selected would help future readers interpret study results.

Similar to the developments in the field of training research, future team building studies need to go beyond the question of "whether" team building works and should begin to address "why" team building works. This will require the collection of both team process and team outcome measures, and will require an examination of multiple time-lags between them.

The stage of a team's development should logically influence the efficacy of various team building interventions. Yet, little research has examined how team building interventions work at different points in the team life-cycle. There is also a need to examine the potential interaction of team building and other interventions.

On the practical side, it appears that team building interventions can be fairly effective, particularly for addressing perceptions and attitudes. However, we need to have realistic expectations about what a team building intervention can accomplish. The results about performance change are equivocal. It may be unrealistic to rely on team building as the sole mechanism for improving team performance. Instead team building should best be considered part of a larger improvement strategy—with other interventions dictated by the specific needs of the team.

One area where team building interventions may be useful is with secondary teams—teams whose purpose is not the primary task of its members (e.g. project teams, task forces, quality action groups). Organizations are using secondary teams more frequently. While having multiple roles can be beneficial for need fulfillment (Cummings & ElSalmi, 1970), there are some unique team building needs in secondary teams. Secondary team members can have conflicting role identity—they represent their permanent team/department and they represent the secondary team. Team members may also suffer from overload as they often maintain membership in both teams. Team building interventions which clarify team member roles and which explicitly address members' dual team identify and potential overload could prove beneficial.

Team Training

Team training can be characterized as a set of instructional strategies and tools aimed at enhancing teamwork knowledge, skills, processes and performance. These strategies and tools are similar to those used to train individuals. However, the focus tends to be on teamwork, and the targeted audience is a team rather than individuals. Moreover, the unique aspects of the team context (e.g. task interdependence) present different challenges and opportunities than those which exist when training individuals (see Cannon-Bowers et al., 1995a). Team training strategies and tools are designed to enhance team effectiveness through their effect on individual characteristics (i.e. individual skills, attitudes and mental models related to team performance) and team processes (e.g. coordination, communication, decision-making).

In general, team training research is beginning to receive more attention (Tannenbaum & Yukl, 1992). Recent developments have included advancements in collective task analysis (Bowers, Baker & Salas, 1994); in identification of the required knowledge, skills and attitudes for effective team functioning (Cannon-Bowers et al., 1995a); in development of team performance measurement tools (Brannick et al., in press; Fowlkes et al., 1994; Baker & Salas, 1992); in the elaboration of specific instructional strategies (Salas, Cannon-Bowers & Johnston, in press) and in guidelines for designing team training interventions or systems (Swezey & Salas, 1992; Salas, Cannon-Bowers & Blickensderfer, in press).

Given recent effort, it is now appropriate to ask: does team training improve team effectiveness? Also, how do recent advancements help improve the usefulness of team training? Two bodies of research pertinent to these questions are reviewed: training shared mental models and team coordination training.

Training Shared Mental Models

Shared mental model theory is a framework guiding much of the research in this area, and helps to explain why team training should enhance team effectiveness (Cannon-Bowers, Salas & Converse, 1993). Specifically, the team mental model construct seems to be useful in understanding how teams are able to coordinate behavior and select task strategies in the absence of explicit coordination activities (e.g. communication). Under conditions of high workload, time pressure and other kinds of stress (which most teams experience at some time), such implicit coordination (i.e. performing without overtly communicating) appears to be critical (Orasanu, 1990).

Recently, Cannon-Bowers, Salas & Converse (1993) argued that effective team performance can occur when team members have a shared understanding of the task, their team-mates' roles and expertise, as well as the context in which they operate. Shared mental model theory, as an explanatory mechanism, argues that members of effective teams must have accurate knowledge structures (or mental models). These are necessary so that team members can generate predictions and expectations about their team-mates, the task demands and the environment in which they are operating. It is the ability to anticipate and predict fellow team members' information and coordination demands that allows a team to coordinate effectively. Therefore, the overriding goal of training is to foster a shared understanding of the task structures, team members' roles, and the process by which the team coordinates.

A team training strategy consistent with shared mental model theory that has been employed and researched recently is cross-training. Specifically, a potentially useful strategy to train shared expectations in team members is to cross-train members on team-mates' tasks that are related to their own task. This is an intervention designed to provide information regarding the structures of the team and task, the interrelationships among team member positions, and the roles and responsibilities of each team member. This intervention is hypothesized to improve team performance by enhancing common task and team expectations. Such training is beneficial to the extent that it helps team members to learn what their other team-mate's task responsibilities and coordination requirements are (i.e. in terms of resources, information and assistance). That is, by exposing team members to, and providing practice on each member's tasks, team effectiveness should improve.

Cannon-Bowers et al. (1995b) tested the effects of cross-training on team processes and performance on two-person teams performing in a simulated task. They found that teams who were informed about and received practice on tasks relating to their team-mate's job, out-performed those who did not receive such information (dependent variables included task coordination, communication and performance). Similar results have been found by Duncan et al. (1995). They tested the impact of a PC-based device designed to cross-train individual members of a five-person naval command-and-control team. Duncan et al. (1995) concluded that the cross-training group significantly improved their team communication as scored by trained raters, and their shared understanding of the task (i.e. interpositional knowledge) determined by a set of probe questions presented after the training.

Team Coordination Training

A second team training strategy of interest is team coordination training. This is a strategy designed to enhance (or maintain under stress) teamwork skills, team processes and communications. The targeted teamwork skills, among others, include decision-making, assertiveness, team leadership, adaptability, back-up behaviors, planning and situational awareness (see Cannon-Bowers et al., 1995a).

The theoretical bases underlying this strategy vary by application. Some are based on shared mental model theory (e.g. Salas, Cannon-Bowers & Johnston, in press); others are based on the small group literature (e.g. Helmreich & Foushee, 1993); while others use the team performance literature or a skills-based approach (e.g. Prince & Salas, 1993). However, the objectives of training are essentially the same—to demonstrate effective (and ineffective) teamwork skills in a particular context, and create opportunities to practice these skills and provide task-relevant feedback. A variety of delivery systems are used to fulfil these training objectives. These include lectures, video demonstration, role-playing and simulations of varying degrees of fidelity.

There has been extensive research in this area primarily from the commercial and military aviation community. For example, Prince & Salas (1993) have specified the skills and instructional strategies appropriate for military team coordination training. Cannon-Bowers et al. (1995a) has delineated the team competencies required for effective team effectiveness and have outlined specific practical propositions for how to select team training strategies. Leedom & Simon (1995) have evaluated the efficiency of a behavioral-based coordination training program in the Army. They found performance improvements due to the training. Similar results have been shown in other environments (e.g. Fowlkes et al., 1994; Weiner, Kanki & Helmreich, 1993).

In sum, teamwork can be promoted through team training by providing relevant and meaningful information (interpositional knowledge) about other team-mates' tasks and responsibilities; demonstrating effective and ineffective teamwork behavior and creating opportunities to practice (via role-playing, simulation or on-the-job) in a relevant context and providing feedback regarding critical aspects of team functioning. The tools and methods that can be used to promote team effectiveness have started to emerge.

Recommendations

The science and practice of team training is alive and well. From an applied perspective, recent theoretical and empirical developments lend greater confidence to the practitioner wishing to use a team training intervention. In particular, skills-oriented team training and cross-training interventions appear to enhance team performance.

From a research perspective, additional work needs to be done. For example, we need to know more about how to train the team leader. While countless studies of leadership have been conducted, we are only beginning to uncover what the role of the leader is in the team training context (Kozlowski et al., in press). We also need research that tests specific instructional strategies aimed at enhancing the team leader's ability to fulfil the instructional role. We discuss this further in a subsequent section of this chapter.

Team membership is becoming more dynamic. This has important implications for team training. Organizations are using many temporary types of teams, such as project teams and task forces. Individuals are often members of multiple teams. This makes it difficult to train intact teams and creates a need for "transportable" competencies. In theory, there are a number of team competencies that can be taught to people individually or in an environment with other individuals who are not team members (e.g. conflict resolution skills). These skills should be transportable, so that individuals can apply them in any team environment in which they perform (Cannon-Bowers et al., 1995a). For example, individuals throughout the organizations could be trained to elect a time-keeper and a scribe for all project team or task force meetings. When a new team is formed, all members should have a common understanding of these roles even though they were not trained together. While Cannon-Bowers et al. (1995a) have advanced a number of propositions about transportable (and task- and team-contingent) competencies, this is an area where additional research is clearly needed.

Decision-making is centrally important for effective team functioning. We need to design and develop team training interventions that allow team members to practice how to use task-relevant information (i.e. cues) for effective team decision-making. This is particularly critical for teams that perform under rapidly evolving situations where information ambiguity and stakes are high.

Finally, we are witnessing an explosion in computer-based technology. Team training could be enhanced by this technology, especially the application of multi-media presentation formats. In this regard, we need answers to questions such as: how do we use multi-media techniques (e.g. animation, simulation, video) to impart team training? What principles can emerge to guide the design of computer-based team training?

Leadership Development

Leadership development refers to a variety of methods for enhancing a leader's capabilities. In a team environment the leader role may be a relatively permanent designation, or it may be more of an emergent, shared or dynamic role. Recently, team leaders in many organizations have been asked to change from a traditional supervisor-type role to more of a facilitator/coach-type role. The new relationship is less of a hierarchical, top-down arrangement and more of a collaborative one, where the team leader removes obstacles, facilitates team processes and helps team members build competencies.

There is a great deal of evidence that team leaders make a difference in team performance (e.g. Brewer, Wilson & Beck, 1994; Komaki, Desselles & Bowman, 1989). Team leader decisions and behaviors can influence almost every variable in the team effectiveness model. Team leaders bring individual task expertise and their own abilities and attitudes to the team. Moreover, through their monitoring, feedback, coaching and influencing behaviors, they also play a central role in the development of the other team members' competencies (McIntyre & Salas, 1995; Kozlowski et al., in press). Even in the most democratic of teams, the team leader often has the greatest influence of any team member in defining work structure (e.g. by determining work assignments) and modifying team characteristics such as member heterogeneity (e.g. through hiring decisions) and team climate (e.g. through their leadership style). Moreover, they are influential factors in determining team processes such as communication, decision-making and problem-solving. This is evidenced by the resulting changes in team processes when leadership changes occur (Kozlowski et al., in press).

For these reasons, interventions that enhance the team leader's effectiveness will often improve the team (Yukl, 1989). The leadership literature is voluminous. Many interventions exist including leadership training (Tetrault, Schrieschiem & Neider, 1988), coaching (Koonce, 1994), and 360° feedback (O'Reilly, 1994). It is beyond the scope of this chapter to review the leadership development literature. Fortunately, a number of excellent reviews and resources exist (see Bass, 1990; Yukl & Van Fleet, 1992, for detailed reviews). We will, however, describe one potential intervention because of its importance in developing other team members' competencies.

It is well-established that people need feedback in order to learn and improve. Team leaders can serve as an important source of feedback, both directly and indirectly by facilitating feedback between team members. We observed newly commissioned Navy crews during their first 2 weeks of team training. In this context, the commanding officer ("team leader") and his combat information center team perform a series of simulated battle engagements. Prior to each simulation the team conducts a pre-brief, and after each simulation the team conducts a de-brief. Several interesting observations emerged from watching these teams in action: (a) different team leaders exhibited very different ways of providing feedback; (b) the team leader's behavior during the first few de-briefs appeared to affect how well the team learned throughout the 2 weeks (e.g. whether team leaders critiqued themselves early in the process); (c) effective team leaders involved team members more during de-briefs, focused attention on both team processes and team outcomes, and created an environment where team members were comfortable critiquing themselves and others.

On the basis of these observations we developed a training program for team leaders and are conducting experiments on its effectiveness. Preliminary results reveal that teams led by individuals who have been trained to conduct effective team briefings perform significantly better on a series of simulated battle engagements than did teams with untrained leaders. Although this application was specific to the military environment, there are a number of parallels to other team environments. Most teams have the opportunity to go through a briefing–performance–briefing cycle, but rarely do so in a systematic manner. Team leaders can be trained to: conduct "pre-briefs" (where they clarify team action plans and priorities, and jointly establish goals); monitor and observe team performance (both processes and outcomes); conduct periodic "de-brief" sessions (where they encourage team members to share observations about team performance). Coupled with more traditional team leader training on how to give one-on-one coaching and development, this type of intervention could help team leaders fulfil one of their primary obligations—developing their team's competencies and stimulating team learning.

Recommendations

In many organizations the role of team leaders is changing from one of a supervisor to more of a facilitator/coach. There is ample evidence that the team leader plays an influential role in team performance—so it is critical that team leaders effectively make this transition. Unfortunately, the transition is not easy. Any organization that relies on their team leaders to facilitate and develop their teams must provide them with the necessary training and tools to fulfil their new role. A variety of methods are available including leadership training and upward feedback. Organizations cannot expect team leaders to develop the skills they need by chance, but instead need to develop a meaningful process of training, practice and feedback to build team leader skills.

One area where additional research would be beneficial is in examining the team leader's role in team learning. Numerous studies of leadership have been conducted, but we know little about the role of the team leader in enhancing team learning. The preliminary research we conducted observing team leaders suggests that different team leader behaviors can have significantly different effects on team learning. Future research should help uncover what team leaders need to do to maximize their team's learning in both training and experiential environments.

Work Redesign/Restructuring

Another category of interventions attempts to modify or restructure the way work is performed—how work flows through the team, how it is assigned, how the task is organized, and the amount of flexibility and autonomy team members have in performing tasks and making decisions. While job design qualities have been extensively studied at the individual level, there is an increasing recognition that team tasks have job design qualities too (Campion, Medsker & Higgs, 1993). Teams can be structured to have different levels of participation, task variety, task significance, autonomy, etc.

Work re-structuring affects several variables in the team performance model. Task characteristics such as task organization and task complexity can be directly affected, as can work assignment. Less directly, most restructuring efforts also affect the power distribution of the team and various team processes (e.g. coordination and communication). Theoretically, these variables are related to overall team performance.

One of the most prevalent restructuring approaches is referred to as "process re-engineering" (Hammer, 1990). This approach diagnoses and modifies work and information flow in an attempt to reduce inefficiencies, streamline operations and improve performance. Re-engineering has been applied extensively throughout many organizations, but it does not specifically target team tasks and peformance. However, there is no reason why the tools and methods associated with process re-engineering could not be applied to examining work and information flow within teams.

Two related work structure issues that have been examined in team environments are increased team autonomy (e.g. self-managing teams) and greater structural flexibility (i.e. more organic/fluid team structures).

Team Autonomy

There is some evidence that greater participation and autonomy in work decisions can increase performance and productivity (Cotton et al., 1988; Pearson, 1987). Many organizations have been increasing the extent to which teams control work related decisions. Examples of this are seen in the application of self-managing, semi-autonomous or autonomous work groups (see Cordery, this volume). Self-managing teams are "groups of individuals who can self-regulate work on their interdependent tasks (Goodman, Devadas & Griffith-Hughson, 1988, p. 296)". The terms "autonomous team" and "self-managing team" seem to be used interchangeably. The term "semi-autonomous team" tends to be used to describe a team that is responsible for managing and executing a more limited number of tasks. However, not all organizations or authors use these terms identically. In some cases, self-managing or autonomous teams do not have an "officially-sanctioned" leader (Wall et al., 1986). In other cases, a designated team leader or supervisor is appointed or elected by the team. A recent visit to a Motorola factory showed that even within a single company, different structural models can be in effect.

Does the shift to a more participative/autonomous structure improve team performance? There is some evidence that performance improvements are possible. Macy et al.'s meta-analysis (1986) showed improved productivity but the results appeared variable over time. Beekun's (1989) meta-analysis of sociotechnical interventions found stronger effects for teams that had complete autonomy over their work scheduling, work partners, and work techniques (i.e. truly autonomous teams), than either semi-autonomous or non-autonomous teams. Wall et al. (1986) studied autonomous groups that could influence the pace of their work and task distribution, and that participated in team member recruitment and training. They reported an increase in intrinsic job satisfaction but no significant change in motivation or performance.

It is not easy to change team structure. For example, at one food-processing plant, team leaders were chosen strictly to serve as a communication link with others outside the team. The team, as a team, was supposed to perform the traditional management functions of planning and scheduling. However, once selected, the team leaders tended to revert to a more traditional team leader role (Stayer, 1990).

Moving to an autonomous team structure, if done properly, is not a superficial change—it is a riskier intervention than most others and must be consistent with the overall culture and direction of the organization. A great deal of consideration must be given as to whether to change and, if so, how to change. Some positive outcomes have been exhibited as a result of increasing team autonomy, but the results are not universal. The process of change is likely to be as important as the shape of the new structure.

Structural Flexibility

A number of authors have encouraged greater fluidity and flexibility in team structure (Nahavandi & Aranda, 1994). Greater fluidity means that role changing and even role overlap may be acceptable—work assignments and task strategies are dynamic. This is consistent with a trend towards focusing more on the work to be performed and less on specific job tasks (Business Week, 1994; Fortune, 1994). The rationale behind this shift is that business and customer needs are changing rapidly; so individuals, teams and organizations must have greater flexibility to respond quickly. Traditional structures, with carefully delineated boundaries between jobs, are less capable of responding to rapid change.

Campion, Medsmer & Higgs (1993) found that teams with greater flexibility were rated as more effective by managers. Some teams have been granted "role-making" flexibility (Haga, Graen & Dansereau, 1974). These teams are not limited by assigned roles but instead can change member roles dynamically without outside approval.

In apparent contrast to the call for greater "fluidity", the team building, mental model and role literatures emphasize the importance of role clarity and the need to avoid role conflict. This implies a need for greater structure and less role overlap. How structured and unambiguous should team roles be? Given the growing emphasis on flexible, organic organizational structures and multiple team memberships, should there be tight hierarchical team roles in those environments?

Despite the apparent conflict within the literatures, there may be a consistent answer to these questions. In environments where teams are dealing with dynamic, ambiguous team tasks, and team members have the competencies they need to assume multiple roles, it may be desirable or even inevitable that the team structure be more fluid. Role changing and overlap, although occasionally inefficient, may be necessary. However, this does not necessarily mean that role conflict is inevitable or desirable. Teams in this environment need to have a shared understanding that role fluidity is acceptable and should be aware of the boundaries to that fluidity. Structural flexibility and role clarity can co-exist, if role clarity is attained by ensuring that all team members understand how their roles can change and what are the acceptable limits to role fluidity.

Recommendations

There is a need for additional research on the effect of changing team structures. Research should continue to examine autonomous and semi-autonomous teams, in particular examining the processes by which teams make the transition from a traditional hierarchical structure to one with greater autonomy and flexibility. For these interventions to work there is a need to better understand *when and how* to convert teams to a more participative style. Research that examines job design characteristics at the team level (e.g. Campion et al., 1993) can be helpful in enhancing our understanding of how to change team structure to improve team effectiveness.

The trend towards greater flexibility in organizational structure will probably continue. Organizations should consider granting teams that deal with dynamic tasks greater role-making authority and greater role fluidity. However, for this type of intervention to work it probably needs to be coupled with other interventions such as team building (to ensure understanding of new, flexible roles) and cross-training (to provide individuals with the competencies to assume multiple roles). Researchers should consider examining the effects of combined interventions.

We would also encourage the application of process re-engineering methods to enhance team effectiveness. These methods can be used to modify the nature and structure of the team task and can also have an impact on team processes. We are not aware of any empirical research that has specifically examined re-engineering of team organization and work flow.

Structural changes are riskier interventions than most others. They often involve fundamental changes. For this reason it is essential that structural interventions have the full support of senior management and that careful diagnostic work has been conducted prior to committing to the change.

SUMMARY

In this chapter we addressed the question, "What can be done to enhance team effectiveness?" We examined five categories of team interventions, each of which, in theory, should influence one or more factors identified in the team effectiveness model. Clearly these are not the only possible interventions to enhance team effectiveness. For example, team-based reward systems and team-based feedback systems are other possible interventions. But each of the five types of interventions described in this chapter demonstrate potential for enhancing team effectiveness, if the assumptions we described at the beginning of the chapter are met (e.g. the team's needs are appropriately diagnosed). The research suggests that some optimism is acceptable.

While each method holds potential, questions remain about them as well. Research that addresses these questions should advance our general understanding about team effectiveness, while providing valuable information to practitioners who are responsible for enhancing team effectiveness. Given the increasing reliance on teams, and the increasing expectations for teamwork in the work environment, we encourage additional sharing of information about the application of team interventions in various environments. For the foreseeable future, the question, "What can be done to enhance team effectiveness?" can only increase in importance.

REFERENCES

Baker, D.P. & Salas, E. (1992). Principles for measuring teamwork skills. *Human Factors*, **34**, 469–475.
Bantel, K.A. & Jackson, S.E. (1989). Top management and innovations in banking: does the composition of the top team make a difference? *Strategic Management Journal*, **10**, 107–124.
Bass, B.M. (1990). *Bass & Stodgill's Handbook of leadership: Theory, Research and Managerial Applications*, 3rd Edn. New York: Free Press.
Beekun, R.I. (1989). Assessing the effectiveness of sociotechical interventions: antidote or fad? *Human Relations*, **42**, 877–897.
Beer, M. (1980). *Organization Change and Development: A Systems View*. Glenview, IL: Scott, Foresman & Co.
Beer, M., Eisenstat, R.A. & Spector, B. (1990). Why change programs don't produce change. *Harvard Business Review*, **68**, 158–166.

Borman, W.C. & Motowidlo, S.J. (1993). Expanding the criterion domain to include elements of contextual performance. In N. Schmitt, W.C. Borman & Associates, *Personnel Selection in Organizations*. San Francisco: Jossey-Bass, pp. 71–98.

Boss, R.W. & McConkie, M.L. (1981). The destructive impact of a positive team-building intervention. *Group and Organization Studies*, **6**, 45–56.

Bowers, C., Baker, D.P. & Salas, E. (1994). Measuring the importance of teamwork: the reliability and validity of job/task analysis indices for team-training design. *Military Psychology*, **4**, 205–214.

Brannick, M.T., Prince, A., Prince, C. & Salas, E. (in press). The measurement of team process. *Human Factors*.

Brewer, N., Wilson, C. & Beck, K. (1994). Supervisory behavior and team performance amongst police patrol sergeants. *Occupational and Organizational Psychology*, **67**, 69–78.

Bruggink, G.M. (1985). Uncovering the policy factor in accidents. *Air Line Pilot*, 22–25.

Buller, P.F. & Bell, C.H. (1986). Effects of team building and goal setting on productivity: a field experiment. *Academy of Management Journal*, **29**, 305–328.

Bushe, G.R. & Johnson, A.L. (1989). Contextual and internal variables affecting task group outcomes in organizations. *Group and Organization Studies*, **14**, 462–482.

Business Week (1994). Rethinking work, October 17, pp. 74–87.

Campbell, J.P., McCloy, R.A., Oppler, S.H. & Sager, C.E. (1993). A theory of performance. In N. Schmitt & W.C. Borman (eds), Personnel Selection in Organizations. San Francisco, CA: Jossey-Bass, pp. 35–70.

Campion, M.A., Medsker, G.J. & Higgs, A.C. (1993). Relations between work group characteristics and effectiveness: implications for designing effective work groups. *Personnel Psychology*, **46**, 823–850.

Cannon-Bowers, J.A., Salas, E., Blickenrdesfer, E.L. & Travillian, K. (1995). Cross-training and Team Effectiveness. Unpublished manuscript. Naval Air Warfare Center Training Systems Division, Orlando, FL.

Cannon-Bowers, J.A., Salas, E. & Converse, S.A. (1993). Shared mental models in expert team decision making. In N.J. Castellan Jr (ed.), *Current Issues in Individual and Group Decision-making*. Hillsdale, NJ: Lawrence Erlbaum, pp. 221–246.

Cannon-Bowers, J.A., Tannenbaum, S.I., Salas, E. & Volpe, C.E. (1995a). Defining team competencies and establishing team training requirements. In R. Guzzo & E. Salas (eds), Team Effectiveness and Decision-making in Organizations. San Francisco, CA: Jossey-Bass, pp. 333–380.

Cotton, J.L., Vollrath, P.P., Froggett, K.L., Lengnick-Hall, M.C. & Jennings, K.R. (1988). Employee participation: diverse forms and different outcomes. *Academy of Management Review*, **13**, 8–22.

Cummings, L.L. & ElSalmi, A.M. (1970). The impact of role diversity, job level, and organizational size on managerial satisfaction. *Administrative Science Quarterly*, **15**, 1–10.

DeMeuse, K.P. & Liebowitz, S.J. (1981). An empirical analysis of team-building research. *Group and Organization Studies*, **6**, 357–378.

Duncan, P.C., Cannon-Bowers, J.A., Johnston, J. & Salas, E. (1995). Using a simulated team to model teamwork skills: the team model trainer. Paper presented at the World Conference on Educational Multimedia and Hypermedia, Graz, Austria.

Dyer, W.G. (1987). *Team Building: Issues and alternatives*, 2nd. Edn. Reading, MA: Addison-Wesley.

Eden, D. (1986). Team development: quasi-experimental confirmation among companies. *Group and Organization Studies*, **11**, 133–146.

Fortune (1994). The End of the Job, September **19**, 62–74.

Fowlkes, J.E., Lane, N.E., Salas, E., Franz, T. & Oser, R. (1994). Improving the measure-

ment of team performance: the TARGETs Methodology. *Military Psychology*, **6**, 47–61.
Gladstein, D. (1984). Groups in context: a model of task group effectiveness. *Administrative Science Quarterly*, **29**, 499–517.
Goodman, P.S., Devadas, R. & Griffith-Hughson, T.L. (1988). Groups and productivity: analyzing the effectiveness of self-managing teams. In J.P. Campbell R.S. Campbell & Associates, *Productivity in Organizations*. San Francisco, CA: Jossey-Bass.
Goodman, P.S., Ravlin, E.C. & Schminke, M. (1987). Understanding groups in organizations. In B.M. Staw & L.L. Cummings (eds), *Designing Effective Work Groups*. San Francisco, CA: Jossey-Bass, pp. 1–27.
Greene, C.N. (1989). Cohesion and productivity in work groups. *Small Group Behavior*, **20**, 70–86.
Guzzo, R.A. & Shea, G.P. (1992). Group performance and intergroup relations in organizations. In M.D. Dunnette & L.M. Hough (eds), *Handbook of Industrial and Organizational Psychology*. Chicago: Rand-McNally, pp. 269–313.
Hackman, J.R. (1987). The design of work teams. In J. Lorsch (ed.), *Handbook of Organizational Behavior*. New York: Prentice-Hall, pp. 315–342.
Hackman, J.R. (1990). *Groups That Work (and Those That Don't)*. San Francisco, CA: Jossey-Bass.
Haga, W.J., Graen, G. & Dansereau, F. (1974). Professionalism and role making in a service organization: a longitudinal investigation. *American Sociological Review*, **39**, 122–133.
Hammer, M. (1990). Reengineering work: don't automate, obliterate. *Harvard Business Review*, **68** (4), 104–113.
Helmreich, R.I. & Foushee, H.C. (1993). Why crew resource management? Empirical and theoretical bases of human factors training in aviation. In E.L. Weiner, B.B. Kanki & R.L. Helmreich (eds), *Cockpit Resource Management*. San Diego, CA: Academic Press, pp. 3–45.
Jackson, S.E. (1992). Team composition in organizational settings: issues in managing an increasingly diverse work force. In S. Worchel, W. Wood & J.A. Simpson (eds), *Group Process and Productivity*. Newbury Park, CA: Sage, pp. 138–176.
Kahn, R.L., Wolfe, D.M., Quinn, R.P., Snoek, D.J. & Rosenthal, R.A. (1964). *Organizational Stress*. New York: Wiley.
Katz, D. & Kahn, R.L. (1978). *The social psychology of organizations*, 2nd Edn. New York: Wiley.
Keller, R.T. (1986). Predictors of the performance of project groups in research and development organizations. *Academy of Management Journal*, **29**, 715–726.
Komaki, J.L., Desselles, M.L. & Bowman, E.D. (1989). Definitely not a breeze: extending an operant model of effective supervision to teams. *Journal of Applied Psychology*, **74**, 522–529.
Koonce, R. (1994). One on one. *Training and Development*, **48**, 34–40.
Kopelman, R.E. (1986). Managing Productivity in Organizations. New York: McGraw-Hill.
Kozlowski, S.W.J., Gully, S.M., McHugh, P.P., Salas, E. & Cannon-Bowers, J.A. (in press). A dynamic theory of leadership and team effectiveness: developmental and task contingent leader roles. In G.R. Ferris (ed.), *Research in Personnel and Human Resource Management*, Vol. 15. Greenwich, CT: JAI Press.
Leedom, D. & Simon, R. (1995). Improving team coordination: a case for behavior-based training. *Military Psychology*, **7**, 109–122.
Macy, B.A. et al. (1986). Meta-analysis of United States empirical organizational change and work innovation field experiments: methodology and preliminary results. Paper presented at the 46th annual meeting of the National Academy of Management, Chicago, August.

Magjuka, R.J. & Baldwin, T.T. (1991). Team-based employee involvement programs: effects of design and administration. *Personnel Psychology*, **44**, 793–812.

Mathieu, J.E., Martineau, J.W. & Tannenbaum, S.I. (1993). Individual and situational influences on the development of self-efficacy: implications for training effectiveness. *Personnel Psychology*, **46**, 125–147.

McIntyre, R.M. & Salas, E. (1995). Measuring and managing for team performance: lessons from complex environments. In R. Guzzo & E. Salas (eds), *Team Effectiveness and Decision-making in Organizations*. San Francisco, CA: Jossey-Bass, pp. 9–45.

Murnighan, J.K. & Conlon, D.E. (1991). The dynamics of intense work groups: a study of British string quartets. *Administrative Science Quarterly*, **36**, 165–186.

Nahavandi, A. & Aranda, E. (1994). Restructuring teams for the re-engineered organization. *Academy of Management Executive*, **8**, 58–68.

O'Connor, K.M., Gruenfeld, D.H. & McGrath, J. (1993). The experience and effects of conflict in continuing work groups. *Small Group Research*, **24**, 362–382.

O'Reilly, B. (1994). 360° feedback can change your life. *Fortune*, **130**, 93–100.

Offerman, L.R. & Gowing, M.K. (1993). Personnel selection in the future: the impact of changing demographics and the nature of work. In N. Schmitt, W.C. Borman & Associates (eds), *Personnel Selection in Organizations*. San Francisco, CA: Jossey-Bass, pp. 385–417.

Orasanu, J. (1990). Shared mental models and crew decision making. Paper presented at the 12th Annual Conference of the Cognitive Science Society, Cambridge, MA.

Pascale, R.T. (1990). *Managing on the Edge*. New York: Touchstone, Simon & Schuster.

Paul, C.F. & Gross, A.C. (1981). Increasing productivity and morale in a municipality: effects of organization development. *Journal of Applied Behavioral Science*, **17**, 59–78.

Pearson, C.A.L. (1987). Participative goal setting as a strategy for improving performance and job satisfaction: a longitudinal evaluation with railway track maintenance groups. *Human Relations*, **40**, 473–488.

Prince, C. & Salas, E. (1993). Training and research for teamwork in the military aircrew. In E.L. Wiener, B.B. Kanki & R.L. Helmreich (eds), *Cockpit Resource Management*. San Diego, CA: Academic Press, pp. 337–366.

Roos, L.L. & Starke, F.A. (1981). Organizational roles. In P.C. Nystrom & W.H. Starbuck (eds), *Handbook of Organizational Design*, Vol. 3. London: Oxford.

Rouse, W.B., Cannon-Bowers, J.A. & Salas, E. (1993). The role of mental models in team performance in complex systems. *IEEE Transactions on Systems, Man*, and Cybernetics, **22**, 1296–1308.

Salas, E., Cannon-Bowers, J.A. & Blickensderfer, E.L. (1993). Team performance and training research: emerging principles. *Journal of the Washington Academy of Sciences*, **83**(2), 81–106.

Salas, E., Cannon-Bowers, J.A. & Johnston, J. (in press). How can you turn a team of experts into an expert team? Emerging training strategies. To appear in C. Zsambok & G. Klein (eds), *Naturalistic Decision-making*. Hillsdale, NJ: Erlbaum.

Salas, E., Dickinson, T.L., Converse, S.A. & Tannenbaum, S.I. (1992). Toward an understanding of team performance and training. In R.W. Swezey & E. Salas (eds), *Teams: Their Training and Performance*. Norwood, NJ: Ablex, pp. 3–29.

Schein, E.H. (1969). *Process Consultation: Its Role in Organization Development*. Reading, MA: Addison-Wesley.

Schmidt, F.L., Hunter, J.E., Outerbridge, A.N. & Trattner, M.H. (1986). The economic impact of job selection methods on size, productivity, and payroll costs of the federal workforce: an empirically-based demonstration. *Personnel Psychology*, **39**, 1–29.

Schmitt, N., Borman, W.C. & Associates, (1993). *Personnel Selection in Organizations*. San Francisco, CA: Jossey-Bass.

Snow, C.C. & Snell, S.A. (1993). Staffing as strategy. In N. Schmitt, W.C. Borman & Associates (eds), *Personnel Selection in Organizations*. San Francisco, CA: Jossey-Bass, pp. 448–480.

Spencer, L.M. & Spencer, S.M. (1993). *Competence at Work: Models for Superior Performance.* New York: Wiley.

Stayer, R. (1990). How I learned to let my workers lead. *Harvard Business Review,* **68,** 66–83.

Sundstrom, E., De Meuse, K.P. & Futrell, D. (1990). Work teams: applications and effectiveness. *American Psychologist,* **45,** 120–133.

Swezey, R.W. & Salas, E. (1992). Guidelines for use in team-training development. In R.W. Swezey & E. Salas (eds), Teams: Their Training and Performance. Norwood, NJ: Ablex, pp. 219–245.

Tang, T.L., Tollison, P. & Whiteside, H.D. (1991). Managers' attendance and the effectiveness of small work groups: the case of quality circles. *Journal of Social Psychology,* **131,** 335–344.

Tannenbaum, S. & Yukl, G. (1992). Training and development in work organizations. *Annual Review of Psychology,* **43,** 399–441.

Tannenbaum, S.I., Beard, R.L. & Salas, E. (1992). Team building and its influence on team effectiveness: an examination of conceptual and empirical developments. In K. Kelley (ed.), *Issues, Theory, and Research in Industrial/Organizational Psychology.* Amsterdam: Elsevier Science Publishers B.V.

Tetrault, L.A., Schriesheim, C.A. & Neider, L.L. (1988). Leadership training interventions: a review. *Organization Development Journal,* **6,** 77–83.

Towers Perrin/IBM (1993). *Priorities for Competitive Advantage.* New York: Towers Perrin.

Tziner, A. & Eden, D. (1985). Effects of crew composition on crew performance: does the whole equal the sum of its parts? *Journal of Applied Psychology,* **70,** 85–93.

Tziner, A.E. (1988). Effects of team composition on ranked team effectiveness. *Small Group Behavior,* **19,** 363–378.

Wall, T.D., Kemp, N.J., Jackson, P.R. & Clegg, C.W. (1986). Outcomes of autonomous workgroups: a long-term field experiment. *Academy of Management Journal,* **29,** 281–304.

Wall, V.D. & Nolan, L.L. (1987). Small group conflict: a look at equity, satisfaction and styles of conflict management. *Small Group Behavior,* **18,** 188–211.

Webster's (1983). Webster's New Twentieth Century Dictionary (2nd Edn). New York: Dorset & Baber.

Wiener, E.L., Kanki, B.B. & Helmreich, R.L. (eds) (1993). *Cockpit Resource Management.* San Diego, CA: Academic Press.

Wiersema, M.F. & Bantel, K.A. (1991). Top management team demography and corporate strategic change. *Academy of Management Journal,* **35,** 91–121.

Woodman, R.W. & Sherwood, J.J. (1980a). The role of team development in organizational effectiveness: a critical review. *Psychological Bulletin,* **88,** 166–186.

Woodman, R.W. & Sherwood, J.J. (1980b). Effects of team development intervention: a field experiment. *Journal of Applied Behavioral Science,* **16,** 211–227.

Yukl, G. (1989). Managerial leadership: a review of theory and research. *Journal of Management,* **15,** 251–289.

Yukl, G. & Van Fleet, D. (1992). Theory and research on leadership in organizations. In M.D. Dunnette & L.M. Hough (eds), *Handbook of industrial and organizational psychology,* Vol. 3, Chicago: Rand-McNally, pp. 147–197.

Chapter 21

Facilitating Group Development: Interventions for a Relational and Contextual Construction

René Bouwen
and
Ron Fry*
University of Leuven, Belgium and
*Case Western Reserve University, Cleveland, USA

Abstract

Although groups and teamwork are mentioned again and again as the forceful promise for new forms of organization, groups' efforts often fall short of the potential that is available through the group composition. Groups, like all social meaning systems, grow and develop over time through a process of "concrescence" among all the parties involved. The status of practice and research poses serious questions about our ways of seeking, discovering and sharing knowledge about group research. This chapter offers a social constructionist reinterpretation of our thinking about group effectiveness and group development. Three dominant constructions in the study of evolving small group systems can be distinguished from the literature: the group development construction, the functional effectiveness construction and the group-in-context construction. Groups can potentially be several things at once but the focus of attention, resulting from the interacting parties, will direct the evolvement of a group system. A vocabulary and a conceptual framework for the three dominant constructions is developed and discussed. In the group-for-effectiveness construction the most common descriptive indicators are: goals, roles procedures and interper-

Handbook of Work Group Psychology. Edited by M.A. West.
© 1996 John Wiley & Sons Ltd.

sonal relations. In the group-in-context construction the descriptive concepts are the patterns of interaction with stakeholders in the environment. The group-development construct gives an account of how participants and facilitators mutually negotiate relationship in consecutive phases. From our premise that groups operate according to a dominant or shared social construction, it follows that interventions to change or facilitate a group are, in essence, acts to clarify or create the groups dominant construction of itself. Interventions can be considered as interruptive actions to alter conversations in such a way as to create new or renewed commitment to some construction or meaning about the group itself. Life in groups is embedded in conversation and language is the essential and unique carrier of meaning-in-the-making. Intervening can be seen as an act of co-authoring a history or narrative, that can create new generative "conversations for possibilities" and new listening in others.

Groups often fall short of the potential that is available through composition of the group. Groups also do not always live up to the expectations of the group members. Nevertheless, in organizational life groups and teamwork are mentioned again and again as the forceful promise for new forms of organization in a fast changing and turbulent environment. Indeed, as this volume indicates, the search continues for relevant theory and action to realize this promise of effective groups. Yet the more consensus there appears to be about the instrumentality of work groups or teams as necessary forms of organizing, the less there actually appears to be concern for nurture, sustenance and development of these living social systems. In theory as well as in practice, the process of group development is very often overlooked as a crucial phenomenon in the life of groups.

We want to document the position that work groups, like all social meaning systems, grow and develop over time through a "concrescence" (Whitehead, 1978) process; they cannot be engineered from an outsiders' expert position. There is, nevertheless, a wide range of possibilities for the social construction of different forms of group life, depending on the dominant frames in use and the extent of cooperation within those frames by all parties involved. Groups can be constructed as instruments for task accomplishment or as living environments for experiencing close relationships. But the architecture of the group will only actualize group potential to the extent that it is a social construction of a shared meaning, and this process requires interaction, development and shared ownership. Groups form the elements of larger social units. The turbulence and demands for creativity in larger social entities, such as organizations, put a heavy emphasis on the actualization of this group potential. High expectations are put on work groups at all levels of organizations—some organizations move even towards a virtual structure of groups or network of cells. Yet observers in the field see a lot of failures and frustrations related to so many efforts to build viable work groups in organizations (Cordery, Mueller & Smith, 1991). The aim of this chapter is to raise the awareness of the social construction quality of such viable groups and to suggest some frames to help conceptualize and intervene to support the "concrescence" of group processes.

THE RE-EMERGENCE OF "TEAM-AWARENESS"

It is commonplace to ascertain that attention to teams and teamwork has received a definitive revival over the past few years. New books on teams are appearing at an unprecedented rate and get even bestseller recognition (Katzenbach & Smith, 1993) on the current management books market. "Teams" are frequently stated as the core concept of several "organizational improvement or transformation" efforts. Whether creating "competitive advantage" (Porter, 1985), employee involvement or quality improvement programs (Lawler, 1992), or even strategic reorientation efforts, all put a core emphasis on the crucial role of effective teamwork. In large manufacturing firms, the "lean organization", as well as the implementation of team-wise assembly methods, relies on the critical contribution of well functioning teams and teamleaders. Also in the "learning organization", as propagandized by Senge (1990), "team learning" is considered to be one of the five critical disciplines and processes to actualize the learning potential of an organization. Upon closer examination of this new wave of attention on groups, one could discover that "nothing new" is pointed out here. Senge is building on Argyris' life-long work on double loop learning in groups and social interactive contexts. Schein's (1969) classic book on "process consultation" is re-edited and extended by the author himself. Employee involvement programs and the implementation of the team concept is based on writings and insights from the 1960s (e.g. Likert, 1961) and 1970s (e.g. Lawler, 1971).

Nevertheless, there has been a drastic change in the local and international socio-economic and business context. Through technological developments, internationalization of markets and redistribution of work across the world, the emphasis in organized group work has been changed from "participation" for quality of working life reasons to "effectiveness through quality and customer orientation". The leverage for this new form of organization is alignment among actors at the various operational levels in the organization. Therefore, group processes have again become the focus of attention of many improvement programs.

A main cross-cultural impetus to look into processes of alignment on the micro level in organizations came from Japanese and other Asian methods of organized group work. Here the groupwise organization was interpreted largely as a "cultural construction", which is very difficult to transfer as such to other cultural contexts. The growing awareness of context dependency led into research into contextual elements influencing group processes (Gladstein, 1984; Guzzo, this volume). From this development one can draw the following lessons: little progress has been made in the understanding of internal group alignment and the research shift is towards contextual factors in a continued hope of finding the "determinants" of effective group processes.

Practitioners go on developing their own action theories of groups; they write "bestselling" books on how to deal with groups without even experiencing the necessity to refer to the results of years of research efforts in small group research and organizational work forms. These books report common sense wisdom about best practices in groups. One could say they repeat the field observations made by seminal authors such as Kurt Lewin and his co-workers, who "invented" the T-group in a concrete training context (Marrow, 1969). Some authors on group processes, mainly in the field of group practices, still refer to the original first works on group dynamics by the pioneers in the field such as Bion, Homans, Slater and other, while many current authors have no awareness of these influences. It is as if results of rigorous research do not help to support work in the field, or as if practitioners are unable, or even do not feel a need, to apply the discoveries made from this research. Levine & Moreland (1990) conclude a recent overview of research on small groups with the conclusion, "Groups are alive and well, but living elsewhere"; they intend to say, "outside of social psychology". They go on, concluding, "... Ivan Steiner (1974) once wrote an optimistic analysis of the future of group dynamics, arguing that the zeitgeist was favorable for a resurgunce of interest in this important but neglected topic. Steiner (1986) more recently concluded that this analysis was wrong. With the benefit of hindsight, he argued that social psychology is wedded to theories and research methods inimical to the study of small groups" (Levine & Moreland, 1990, p. 620). And their conclusion finishes by stating, "There is nothing so good as a practical theory".

From a group member's or manager's perspective, this search for a "practical theory" appears frustrating, at best. Universal theory or models that appeal in their logical consistency and predictive promise fail miserably in embracing the complexity, contrariness and uniqueness of the social situation. Thickly descriptive and contextually bounded "stories from the real world", on the other hand, fail to lend the predictive, unequivocal direction that practitioners seek to help them design and implement their unique, complex and seemingly equivocal group experiences. It is as if practitioners and theorists are colluding to accept *as given* a state where the theory of group dynamics or team development is similar to Einstein's often quoted characterization of mathematics: "Insofar as the propositions of mathematics give an account of reality, they are not certain; and insofar as they are certain, they do not describe reality". We view this situation as an unsteady state that poses serious questions about the status of research and practice in groups and, perhaps more importantly, about our ways of seeking, sharing and making knowledge about group research and experiences from the past.

Although research and practice do not seem to influence each other very much at present, there is nevertheless a growing interest and need for adequate understanding of group processes in organizational life. Groups are not only the core of all improvement programs, they are also the vital context for organizational creation and socialisation. Groups continue to be the microcosm of societal life in all work and life contexts. But maybe we need another way of framing our knowledge about group processes and how we can disseminate this "knowledge" in a usable way. Therefore, this chapter tries to offer a reinterpretation of our thinking about group effectiveness and group development through a social constructionist perspective.

DOMINANT CONSTRUCTIONS OF GROUP LIFE

Looking into the group literature one can observe a large variety of theories to describe "development" in groups. In the footsteps of Bales and Bion, Tuckman (1965) documented about 60 different theories before developing his four-phase model (forming, storming, norming, performing). Banet (1976) mentions that Hill, who was once a specialist in group development, stopped practicing his hobby when he arrived at more than 100 different theories. Two streams of literature can be distinguished on the basis of the emphasis put on task development or on relational development within the group. The attention to group evolvement over time can be described in terms of the group's decision effectiveness and task accomplishment (Hackman, 1989) or development of internal group processes and relationship patterns (Smith & Berg, 1987).

Two dominant contexts in which groups were studied have delivered two dominant constructions of evolved group systems or group development. Leaderless learning groups have often been documented in the context of training, therapy and organization development: the framing was mostly made then in terms of the development of relational processes. These groups changed over time in terms of openess in communication, building of thrust, developing of cohesion, establishing feedback mechanisms and reshaping of influence structures. Task groups in organizations, on the other hand, have been studied mainly in terms of effectiveness or functionality in relation to their external environment and goal attainment. The framing of dominant issues has been in terms of utilization of resources, role of leadership, effectiveness in decision-making and group output and goal attainment. In this sense one can speak about two dominant "constructions" of group life.

During the past few years a third dominant stream, or social construct, of groups-in-context has emerged (Gladstein, 1984). Internal relational development and task oriented constructions are more and more treated in a context of alignment with the larger, organizational task of quality and customer orientation. Groups seem to be "constructed" from inside out (members) as well as from outside-in (management, customer, etc.). The negotiation of an activity space within the group's environment and the boundary management with outside actors constitutes the group's identity purpose and in close interaction and continuous interfacing with stakeholders in the organizational context.

"Whose construction is it?" one could ask. In the first place it is the construction of the authors and the researchers. They were often involved in action research contexts and their particular focus of research was directed by the attention given by the trainers, facilitators and participants in that setting. But this focus of attention is also negotiated with the participants and a process of consensual validation will have developed around the central focus of attention. In that sense a dominant social construction directs the attention of group members, leaders and researchers. In task orientation the instrumental focus is dominant; in relational orientation the development focus is dominant. In the context orientation the organizational milieu is the focus. All knowledge is perspectivistic and each particular focus will deliver different kinds of knowledge. In this chapter we will develop the idea that any intervention into group life is focusing on a particular perspective and is fostering a particular focus. Groups can potentially be several things at once and the focus of attention will direct the evolvement of a group system. We will document the social construction for effectiveness, the social construction for development and the social construction for context and try to relate those approaches to each other. Groups are in this sense the result of the joint effort of the participants involved and the dominant focus of attention will guide the direction of evolvement.

An Effectiveness Construction of Groups and Teams

A dominant focus in a lot of the work in groups and in the related literature is the social construction of groups-for-effectiveness. This perspective is pervasive in the actual team concept literature (Katzenbach, 1993). Teams are expected to perform interdependent tasks, which can not be done as effectively by individuals or by installing procedures or rules. Resource allocation tasks, control tasks, maintenance tasks and other boundary management tasks are attributed to teams. This focus in the social construction of work groups has a long tradition. The seminal work of Ivan D. Steiner (1972), more than 20 years ago, developed and illustrated the concept of "process loss" in task groups. Given the tasks' demands and the resources, the group will achieve a certain actual level of productivity, which equals the potential productivity minus the losses due to faulty processes, the so called "process loss". This is a measure to indicate to what extent the group is actualizing the potential resources of the indivual group members. Steiner documents extensively how most groups stay largely below their theoretical level of potential: the group outcome is much below the sum of the individual outcomes. There is little, if any, possibility of a synergy effect, which would be going beyond the sum of the individual contributions. Steiner relates internal process to task characteristics, such as unitary and divisible tasks, to group size and to group composition. An important emphasis is given to rewards to influence motivation. To characterize the process he uses Bales' categorization scheme (Bales & Strodtbeck, 1953).

In 1978 Hackman & Morris (1978) published an overview of the research following this effectiveness paradigm. Group composition, task design and group norms were considered as imputs for a group interaction process that led to group productivity dimensions. The group interaction process could not be differentiated further than into three summary variables: utilization of knowledge and skills, utilization of task strategies and coordination of member's effort. One can distinguish here a content level, a procedural level and a process or relational level.

This effectiveness construction by researchers is closely related to the main categories of the team-building model developed by Fry, Rubin & Plovnick (1981). They start from the constructions of team participants, who are asked to inventorize indicators of good or poor functioning in work groups. These descriptive indicators can easily be grouped under the following constructs: goals, roles, a procedures and interpersonal relations. In variety of group contexts these four categories can be identified by the participants and they can use these concepts to co-construct and communicate with each other about critical aspects to improve and to agree upon. "Goals" refer to what the team is trying to achieve. What are its tasks? "Roles" refer to *who*—which resources of people or skills—is required to accomplish the task. "Procedures" refer to *how* people should work together in performing their roles. "Interpersonal relations" refer to how goals, roles, procedures and relations affect people's emotions and feelings.

Goal issues are perhaps the most complex concerns problems faced by work groups and teams in an organizational context. Groups have to mediate between the goals and expectations of individuals and the mission and goals of the organization. The work team or work group is the most direct natural environment—the individual has to deal with the always present social dilemma of taking care for oneself and taking care for the other(s). This interindividual goal alignment has to be negotiated constantly, or at least on a regular basis with external parties, other groups in the organization, the structural arrangements of the larger organization and influences from the environment, such as customer demands, social groups and the local environment of family and community. In the goal negotiation of the work group, careers, task requirements, expectations of others, organizational demands and demands from the environment have to be mediated. The first question about goals is that of goal clarity. Do we really know and understand the different demands coming from the different constituencies? The next question is to come to a shared goal base, which is large enough to agree upon the concrete next step to be taken. Then an operationalization of these goals is possible in concrete, attainable and motivating targets. Under these conditions team members can experience ownership of the task and feel empowered to engage in action.

Role negotiation follows directly from agreement on goals. Role ambiguity is especially present when forms of interdisciplinary work are to be executed, when multi-skilled jobs have to be performed or when non-routine work is being coordinated. In the team concept organization there is less and less reliance on job descriptions. The team forms a continuous base for distribution and rotation of task assignments. Often team members have multiple memberships and a specific team serves as the interfacing device at the boundary of departments or disciplines. Some, maybe only temporary, clarity of roles is desirable. The ability of the group to negotiate and reconstruct shared role definition seems critical. The role definition of the leadership role in a team is usually a very critical one. In the new organizational forms this role is often left undefined or without clear authority intending to engage as many team members as possible in a shared task of team coordination. This can put a very high pressure on team members, who are used to classical role definitions.

Procedures refer to task strategies to coordinate activities. How are we going to make decisions? How do we collect and share information? Which arrangements in time and place do we have for mutual consultation? How do we deal with conflicts? How do we structure work and which rules and regulations are we going to agree upon? This can be a very large domain of tasks to agree upon and some roles—such as a facilitator—can be assigned to deal continuously with these procedural issues. Groups are also linked via procedures to the wider organizational arrangements for rewards and resource allocation. Procedures always have an interfacing quality with the environment.

Interpersonal relations concern the distribution of personal energy to tasks and relationships. How do people wish to relate in order to achieve necessary collaboration in the team? This includes the group culture or the set of norms and values, implicit and explicit, that make the group work. Group cohesion or climate can be another indicator. Mutual perceptions of team members and their contribution to the team can exchanged through more or less explicit giving and receiving of feedback.

The SGRPI model (System–Goal–Role–Procedure–Interpersonal) also emphasizes the system issues surrounding team functioning. Are we working within a system that allows for real teamwork to exist. Fry and colleagues stress the mirroring quality of system characteristics on team functioning. Reward systems, information systems and personnel policies, and all other rules and regulations of the organization as a larger system, are shadowing their influence on internal team processes and products. Resources, input, output and all interactions with the environment of the organization and even the larger environment are mediated through system characteristics. An organization is built on interrelated groups and teams, connected by link-pins in the roles of leaders and representatives. It is this embeddedness into a higher layer of the system that is becoming more and more a part of the effectiveness construction in the recent literature (Gladstein, 1984; Gurly & Fry, 1993).

This awareness of the context surrounding a group as a very important constraint on the functioning of groups and teams has gradually become a major research topic during the last years. Guzzo, for example (this volume) is focusing on context characteristics to understand group functioning. The work of Gladstein (1984) on sales teams in organizations stresses the role of boundary management between the team and context demands and opportunities. Self-reported effectiveness and team satisfaction are related to internal group processes, such as communication and mutual support. Effectiveness measured by outside performance criteria did not relate to internal functioning, but rather to the way the groups dealt with the requirements of the environment. This led Gladstein (publications now under the name of Ancona) (Ancona & Caldwell, 1992) to develop a theory of an external perspective. Groups mediate their relation with the context through three groups of interfacing activities. "Ambassador" activities include both buffering and representation. This means protecting the team and absorbing outside pressure. "Representational" activities include persuading others to support the team and lobbying for resources. "Task coordinator" activities are aimed at coordinating technical and design issues; this means discussing design problems with others, obtaining feedback negotiating with outsiders and other forms of lateral interaction. "Scout" activities involve general scanning for ideas and information about the competition, the market and the larger environment. K. Gurley & R. Fry (1993), in their study of cross-functional teams in a R&D environment, also document the "fit" between distinctively different customer environments and the internal processes of cross-functional product development. They propose a general model of help managers and team members in designing and developing teams as integrating mechanisms. Three patterns of team–context interaction are described: coordinators, expediters and owners. Different teams develop typical patterns of interaction with the environment and those patterns are related to performance evaluations by the environment.

We see here that the task-oriented effectiveness construction of groups is also leading into the contextual construction. Groups not only react to their environment. They also enact and select their environment; they construct or co-construct the environment they live in. On this dimension of being able to "react" to the environment, groups will differ a lot and this difference will be related to performance and to development, as we will see in the next section.

The task-oriented construction of groups has become very popular during recent years, but most writings still put their major emphasis on internal task construction of the work group. The third edition of Dyer's (1995) team-building book talks mainly about internal design issues, emphasizing clarity in design and implementation, and working on the internal climate of trust and openess. West (1994) also puts effectiveness in the title of his practical guide, but he emphasizes the innovative or creative aspect of the output and introduces the concept of team reflexivity as way of learning and self-development of the team. The emphasis on team support and open relationships introduces a relational construction into the conceptualization. The strong interconnectedness between task and relational construction becomes more and more evident.

A "Developmental" Construction of Groups and Teams

Another family of literatures about group evolvement talks about a development construction of groups. It documents mainly internal group processes and relationship patterns and stems from studies of therapy groups, and was studied further and expanded in the T-group practice (Benne, 1964).

There is a very large variety of group development theories and some authors even question the idea of group development itself. Even Kenneth Benne (1964), who was one of the pioneers of T-group theory development, suggests the possiblity of a "self-fulfilling prophecy" effect. That is how the influence of expectations on future events is phrased at a given moment in time. Expectations and theories about group development could be responsible for creating or eliciting the process. We want to replace this *entitative* way of thinking about development by a social constructionist way of thinking and acknowledge fully the development process as a co-construction.

The goals of the participants in a T-group are indeed to "learn about group processes" and to "learn how to learn about groups". The goal of the trainer is to foster this learning among the participants. Development of relationships and learning about this process can indeed be the shared concerns in a group. The group can therefore organize itself in the desired direction. This position of Benne comes close to what is currently considered to be a social constructionist standpoint. It is through mutual influence and the exchange of expectations that a new social reality is created. The purpose of a T-group is in fact the building in the "here and now" of a group context by continuously enacting relationships and reflecting on them. The sharing of goals and the exchange of efforts to reach those goals are sufficient reasons to understand why people engage in developing relationships. This illustrates also that this development is not a blind or unintended process. It is a joint process, that cannot be steered from the outside. Participants and facilitators together can engage in an enterprise of joint relational development. It becomes self-evident, then, that a development construction is going to be the dominant group concern. Belonging to the social system, exerting influence, opening up communication and feedback, overcoming dependency and evolving towards interdependency, open confrontation and sharing of information and competencies are the dominant and consecutive concerns of the parties involved in the social entreprise. Bennis & Shepard (1956) and Srivastva, Obert & Neilsen (1977), among many others, have built their "group development" models on this set of relational concerns. Their context was the self-learning leaderless group, reflecting on and enacting its own relational evolution: members in relation with each other and with the group facilitator. In the context of therapy groups or self-learning groups (e.g. encounter groups) the relationship with the therapist and self-defensive mechanisms are often in the foreground. This is different again with groups where the task process is central. A group working for a short period on a task will go through: (a) an orientation phase; (b) an evaluation phase, based on available information; and then (c) a control phase, where the emergence of the decision is central.

Group development theories differ along several key points: the task, the structure, relations with the leader, the mutual relations of the members and the attitude towards the context. These aspects can be grouped under the three classical group features: the task or content, the procedures or structures and the process or relationships. The purpose of this chapter is not to give an overview of all the development theories, but to point out the underlying themes and forces as they are enacted throughout group processes. We want to identify some of the key mechanisms underlying the social construction of groups as developmental entities.

Banet (1976) gives an overview of group development theories by distinguishing three kinds of models: the linear model, the spiral model and the polarity model. Recently Gersick (1988) added the "punctuated equilibrium model".

In *linear models*, group development is conceptualized as an orderly succession of consecutive phases following a predefined sequence. The line of development is comparable to the individual growth and development models in developmental psychology. Some models, like the Schutz (1958) model (inclusion, control and affection) have been applied also to individual development. Group development is then a secondary socialization, which follows the same developmental steps as the primary socialization of the young individual. Other examples of a linear concept of development are Bennis & Shepard (1956), Srivastva, Obert & Neilsen (1977) for relational development, and Tuckman (1965) and Bales (1958) for task development in decision-making processes (orientation, evaluation and control).

To further understand whether, in fact, group members carried such "developmental" constructions of their group experiences with them, the authors used the Srivastva, Obert & Neilsen (1977) model to develop a Likert-type self-scoring attitude scale, to have group members score themselves for their experiences of concerns at different moments during the existence of the group. For each phase 12 items are scored and this scoring should allow definition of where the dominant concerns of the group can be situated at a particular moment of group life. Therefore, we want to discuss this model more closely. Five phases are distinguished: the three phases of Schutz (inclusion, control, affection) are separated by two intermediary phases of transition:

- The first phase concerns are mainly about inclusion. It is the "each-for-himself" mode of interaction. Being accepted as a member steers the participation. It is activity for activity's sake, following closely the instructions of the leader, which are expected to be structured and well defined. The environment is seen as inimical and the mutual relationships among the members are rather superficial.
- The second phase is a transition between inclusion concerns and influence concerns. Dyadic relationships are being formed and similarities and differences are explored in "we" and "they" terms For the Srivastva, Obert & Neilsen (1977) model, the authors have been working with different characteristics. The relationship towards authority shifts towards counter-dependency, the goal of the task is being questioned and hostility towards the environment is openly expressed.
- The third phase is the open testing of influence in the group. Gaining recognition and acceptance in the group at large is at stake. Different subgroups strive for power to secure newly formed identities. Also, authority is challenged and questioned openly. The task gets redefined and renegotiated, also in relation to the environment. Gradually the members take up more responsibility for interdependent tasks, which makes the move to further development possible.
- Phase four is again a transition phase between influence concerns and inti-

macy concerns. The conflict of the previous phase is resolved by establishing a shared pattern of mutual influence and task interdependency. The shared concern becomes, "Who are we in the context of this group space?". Inclusive interpersonal networks encompass the entire group. There is a high degree of emphathetic listening and the relationships become as important as the joint task accomplishment. Some euphoric "group feelings" can be expressed.

- Phase five is a kind of ideal maturity phase. Full interdependency between members and authority can be established. Members take complemantary roles, they are task-oriented without "playing games" further on. They share goal commitment, communicate in an open and confrontative way and can adapt towards environmental demands without defensiveness.

The authors applied the 60-item instrument in nine "unstructured self-experiential learning groups", at the beginning (end of first day) and at the end of a week-long training program. The groups usually consisted of 10–14 participants and one or two group facilitators. This week-long program was also the start of a 2-year program on consultancy in organizational change or human resources. The participants were in their thirties and forties and all were involved in some kind of internal or external change agent role in their home organization. In each group a similar pattern emerged.

In the first measurement of the starting group, there was no difference between the scores on the five subscales. All concerns were equally represented and no differentiation was possible. At the end of the week a clear picture emerged with the dominant concerns in the fourth and fifth phases. There was a clear differentiation. When we applied the instrument after 2 days in one of these groups, the highest score was at the third and fourth phases. All the differences observed were significant and could be interpreted within the framework of group phases discussed above.

When we looked into the individual scores, some clear differences could be observed. These scores were fed back to the group members for "consensual validation". At the end of the week-long program, those individuals with lower scores on the fourth and fifth phase subscales acknowledged some problems they had in "fitting in" with the group and mentioned "that they had some more work to do".

We also applied this instrument to existing work groups in organizations. In eight research teams of an engineering firm, no differentiation among the phases could be observed. In three staff groups of a personel department, the highest score was on the fourth and fifth phase subscales. Functional groups do not seem to follow, in the majority of the cases, the differentiation of concerns over the phases. A subscale on "contextual characteristics" (Srivastva, Obert & Neilsen, 1977), defining task space through task structure, reactivity space and learning space, could be related to the extent of differentiation among the phases. In general we can conclude for the work groups that high scores for context autonomy (high activity space perceived) are related to high scores on the fourth and fifth phase subscales. This can be interpreted in this way: when group members experience a large group space for activity and reaction, then they experience the concerns of a "more developed" group. In the analysis at individual level in the training groups we could make the same observation. Those individuals that perceive a large activity space in the group, express concerns of the fourth and fifth phases. We do not want to interpret these findings in a causality paradigm, but as parallel experiences of group members at a certain moment in time. We believe these data illustrate the joint focal construction of group concerns at a given moment. These concerns shift during the time spent together and in different contexts. Also there is a support for the co-existence of an internal relational construction and the external activity space construction.

Following the for observations made with the instrument, which we want to consider not as an "objective instrument to measure" but rather as an instrument for self-reflection, we are inclined to state that experiences of a joint shift in concerns among the members of groups can be documented. There is a shift in relational, task-related and context-related concerns. It is much more difficult to argue what is causing this shift. Like Bennis & Shepard, and some other authors, who question the possibility of group development, one can interpret these data as the result of a joint self-fulfilling prophecy or as a "joint learning of the theory". The social construction of mutual concerns nevertheless seems to shift and even evolve over a period of time and also in relation to the experience of the activity space in the context.

Up to now we have been referring mainly to so-called linear models. Several authors have conceptualized the evolvement of the members' concerns following a *spiral model*. The development is conceived as a circular process, that is repeating the same concerns after a while, but then on a "higher level". Linear models, such as those of Srivastva or Bennis, can easily be conceived as spiral movements, repeating the main concerns on a different group theme. Bion (1961), Slater (1966) and Whitaker & Lieberman (1964) can be mentioned as typical examples of spiral models. They have been working mainly with therapy groups and their inspiration from psycho-dynamic thinking is therefore understandable. Not taking into account the specificities of these different models, one can observe a general emphasis on shift between "explicit" and "implicit" themes or issues. Groups seem to shift from one dominant, explicit theme (e.g. participation) to another theme at the moment that a new, rather implicit or conflicting theme is emerging (e.g. dependency) and is getting support in the group. Groups seem to develop through spirals of repeated general themes, which are described in more detail in the different models.

It is clear that we are not far away here from the *polarity model* of group development. In the polarity models group development is conceived as a continuous field of tensions between opposing or equilibrating forces such as "individuality" vs. "sociability" or "dependency" vs. "independency", etc. Maybe the most elaborated of these models is the recent work of Smith & Berg (1987). They describe the life of groups as a continuous dealing with ten opposite forces, which they call dilemmas. These tensions will never be resolved but choices have to be made at each moment, and each actor and group has to situate itself somewhere on the continuum between these opposing forces. The energy for involvement and interaction stems from the confrontation of the developmental dilemmas a group has to struggle through. As examples of other polarity models, the work of Pages (1968) ("amour et separation") can be mentioned. In these models polarities are situated mainly at the individual level.

Recently there has been growing interest in the "punctuated equilibrium model", stimulated by the original work of Gersick (1988). Development is conceived here mainly as a temporal issue. It is the awareness of past and future time, which guides development through periods of continuity and transition. Transitions are enacted under the awareness of time pressure. When time becomes the dominant concern it can facilitate the necessary shifts in concerns to move ahead and to get reorganized around shared group goals.

The different theories reveiwed here, have been conceived from a rather rationalist-positivist point of view: "That's the way it is; and this is the best way to look at group development". If we look to group development as a process among all parties involved that cannot be engineered from an outside expert position, but as a socially constructed process, resulting from the interaction, then all those frames get a new meaning and can also be integrated or at least related to each other.

The core consideration for the group is at any time: where is the shared energy and focal awareness of this group at a given moment? Different vocabularies can be used to phrase these concerns. Benne (1964), talking about the T-group process, already referred to the importance of vocabularies in framing ongoing concerns in a consensual and jointly understandable way. "The T-group constructs a basis of security and community in commonly acceptable ways of treating 'experimentally' the concrete empirical 'realities' of its here-and-now situation." (Benne, 1964, p. 241). The language, which is often expressed through metaphors—have not all theories been treated as metaphors in their own way— is the carrier for the development of a community of understanding of what is going on. Some language is offered or introduced by the direct and indirect comments of the facilitators and other participants. Time, task-related themes, individual concerns, group interaction themes or common experience themes can serve as the common language base to phrase group developmental concerns relating to time or task development or polarities or spiral or linear phases or even group dilemmas. The joint construction of a vocabulary to phrase experiences seems to be a overall concern. It is as if the group learns to speak with a common voice.

An Integrative Matrix: Towards a Generative Construction

The matrix model of Figure 21.1 is a conceptual integration of task effectiveness and the relational development construction on the background of a parallel contextual construciton. Task and relation are pictured as two dimensions, while context is the third integrating dimension. We want to present this matrix not as a theory representing an outside reality but rather as examples of intelligible

FACILITATING GROUP DEVELOPMENT 545

PHASES IN GROUP DEVELOPMENT

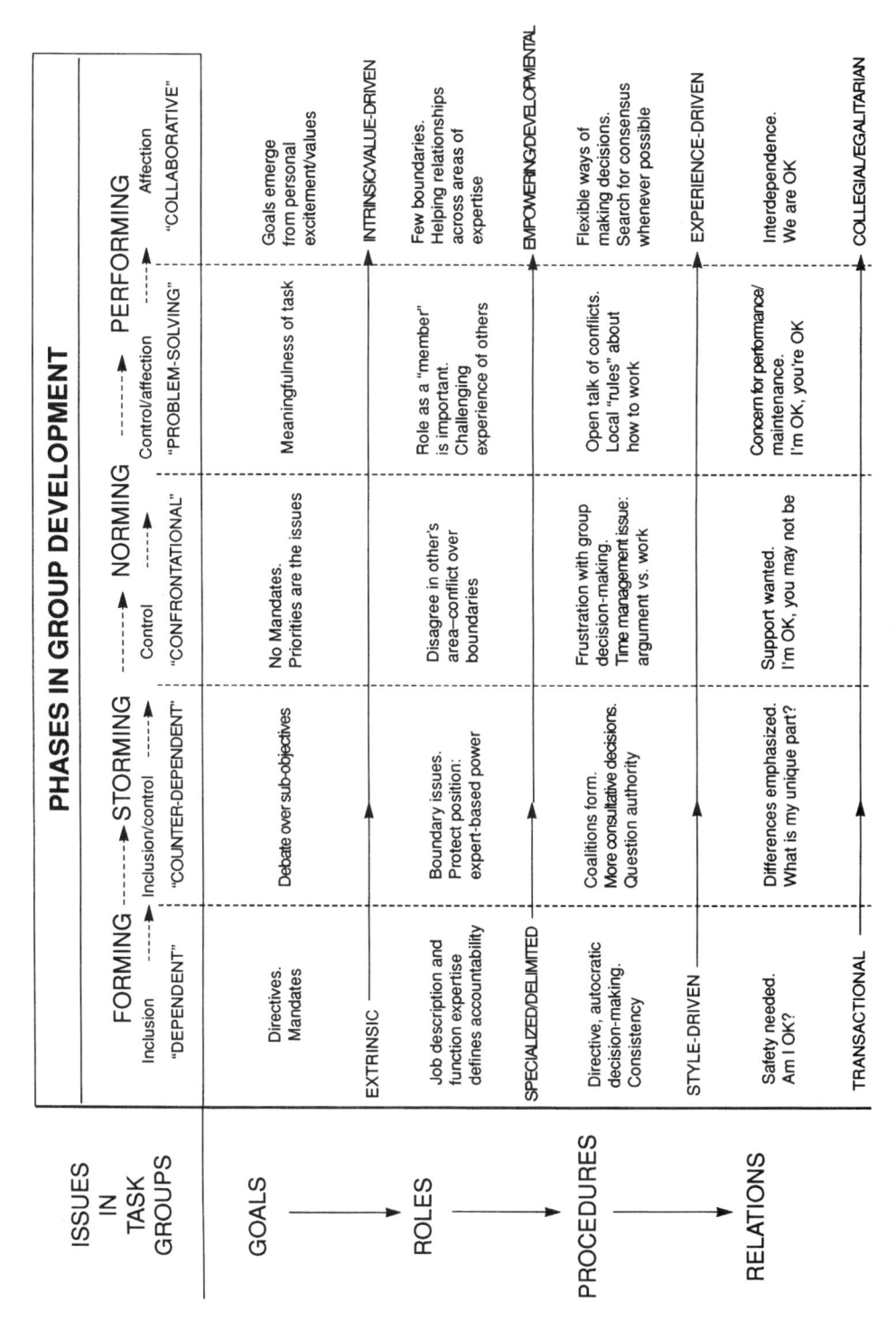

ISSUES IN TASK GROUPS	FORMING Inclusion "DEPENDENT"	STORMING Inclusion/control "COUNTER-DEPENDENT"	NORMING Control "CONFRONTATIONAL"	PERFORMING Control/affection "PROBLEM-SOLVING"	Affection "COLLABORATIVE"
GOALS	Directives. Mandates	Debate over sub-objectives	No Mandates. Priorities are the issues	Meaningfulness of task	Goals emerge from personal excitement/values
	EXTRINSIC				INTRINSIC/VALUE-DRIVEN
ROLES	Job description and function expertise defines accountability	Boundary issues. Protect position: expert-based power	Disagree in other's area–conflict over boundaries	Role as a "member" is important. Challenging experience of others	Few boundaries. Helping relationships across areas of expertise
	SPECIALIZED/DELIMITED				EMPOWERING/DEVELOPMENTAL
PROCEDURES	Directive, autocratic decision-making. Consistency	Coalitions form. More consultative decisions. Question authority	Frustration with group decision-making. Time management issue: argument vs. work	Open talk of conflicts. Local "rules" about how to work	Flexible ways of making decisions. Search for consensus whenever possible
	STYLE-DRIVEN				EXPERIENCE-DRIVEN
RELATIONS	Safety needed. Am I OK?	Differences emphasized. What is my unique part?	Support wanted. I'm OK, you may not be	Concern for performance/ maintenance. I'm OK, you're OK	Interdependence. We are OK
	TRANSACTIONAL				COLLEGIAL/EGALITARIAN

Figure 21.1 Matrix of phases in group development and themes of effectiveness

formulations of what is often experienced as a chaotic welter of impressions (Shotter, 1993).

The horizontal dimension of Figure 21.1 shows the developmental construction modes. Tuckman (1965) was using the forming–storming–norming–performing vocabulary. Srivastva, Obert & Neilsen (1977), following Schutz, are speaking in inclusion–control–affection terms, and Bennis & Shepard (1956) talk in terms of dependency–confrontation–collaboration. The five vertical columns describe group concerns following the vocabulary of Srivastva, Obert & Neilsen (1977). This vocabulary was presented in the discussion of the developmental construction above. In the matrix the vocabulary of the phases is expressed in the "language expressions" that these different effectiveness criteria can take in the interactions of a group member having concerns for the development of the group concerns.

The vertical dimension is formed by the concepts from the effectiveness construction: goals–roles–procedures–relations. By combination we arrive at a 4 × 5 matrix. Goals are phrased as evolving from extrinsically imposed or mandated clear goals over priority debates about goals, towards the emergence of intrinsic or value-driven goals. It is self-evident that each task–relation construction is encompassed and aligned with a contextual construction, which is not made explicit here. The interaction with the outside stakeholders will also influence the form this construction is taking. In a task-oriented group this interaction is more constrained by the organizational context. In leaderless training groups there is very loose and undefined context constraint and the internal construction has more "room" then, up to a certain point of group ending or transfer limitations. Roles can develop from specialized to flexible and self-defined. Procedures also can be constructed as predetermined system conditions or an experience-drive jointly defined arrangement. Relations especially develop from "me"-concerned, via looking for support, towards egalitarian and interdependent relationships.

This matrix shows a variety of possible co-constructions of task and relational concerns. This scheme can help practitioners to orient themselves in ongoing group dialogues to acknowledge moments of joint or conflictual group construction. It can be a vocabulary members can use to continue ongoing negotiation for common ground in process terms. In training contexts these process constructions can be made explicit to move in a direction of more group reflexivity and more shared group awareness. In organizational group contexts the construction process will be implicit to a large extent. But the more group members and facilitators have a common language, the more one can expect that all constituencies will be involved in group interaction. We hope that this matrix can serve as a generative device to make the social negotiation process more fruitful.

TOWARDS A NEW PERSPECTIVE ON GROUP INTERVENTION

From our premise that a group operates according to a dominant or shared social construction (either tacit or explicit) about its purpose, intern, desire and process, ect., it follows that interventions to change, facilitate or maintain group life are, in essence, acts taken to clarify, understand, or create the group's dominant construction of itself. In this section we wish to explore this proposition more fully. Specifically, "intervention" will be examined as an interruptive act to alter conversations in such a way as to create new or renewed commitment to some construction or meaning about the group, itself. From this conversational perspective, the listening, reframing, and commitment to some actions that can result from an intervention will be explored as conversation-for-possibility (vs. Productivity, or sensitivity). Intervening to create such conversations thus becomes a form of co-authoring a history or group narrative. This role or function of group interventions will be discussed in contrast to instrumental or purely interpretive interjections into group dialogue. Finally, the "generative potential" of interventions is discussed in relation to the main premise of this chapter: that the apparent dominant constructions of group life we see in current literature and practice are insufficient in meeting the complex, practical demands put on groups in today's social systems. The call for new "dominant constructions" of group life becomes, in essence, a call for interventions to create generative "conversations-for-possibilities".

Life in groups is embedded in conversation. Nothing happens without language. From our discussion above, the dominant conversations in groups appear to be either conversations-for-action (instrumental, task-oriented productivity issues) or conversations-for-relation (interpersonal, developmental issues). Schein's (1988) classic distinction of "process' and "content" levels of work in groups mirrors these two realms of conversation and has guided an entire field of group interventions known as "process consultation". Assuming that group process leads to effectiveness (McGrath, 1984), process has been viewed as either maintenance behavior (Bales, 1958; Benne & Sheats, 1948) that builds, stengthens, and regulates group life through attention to relationships or relating in the group, or task behavior that enables the group to accomplish tasks and solve the objective problem to which the group is committed (Philip & Dunphy, 1959). Gladstein (1984) notes that the focus on maintenance behaviors in groups had been characterized by a normative approach that encourages openness and smooth interpersonal relations in order to improve effectiveness. It is this *instrumental* orientation to intervening in groups that is important to his discussion. While "process interventions" are often intended to educate or illustrate patterns or trends in a group's dynamics, it is also often the case that such interruptions are intended to fit a science or theory to a particular situation in order to influence those dynamics toward some end (e.g. increased trust, openness, cohesion, etc.). Similarly, with task functions in groups interventions are "aimed" at behaviors that have been scientifically hypothesized to aid group performance in various areas, such as novel problem analysis, intergroup alliance, boundary management, boundary spanners, autonomy workgroups and leader roles. In sum, the practice of interventions into group life is primarily driven by the "... predict[ion] that groups that exhibit maintenance behaviors, good decision-making skills, and communication with external groups with which they are interdependent, will be more effective" (Gladstein, 1984, p. 501).

The choice we are illuminating here is that between using group theory-as-tool to engineer, direct or facilitate a process toward some ideal or theoretically hypothesized state, and theory-as-story of an intelligible formulation amidst what others may be experiencing as "a chaotic welter of impressions" (Shotter, 1993). To refer to a systematic theory when facing a crisis in human conduct, or the rich and detailed account of primordial emotions and complexity of Bion's (1961) classic study of groups, or the widely varied task-groups in Hackman & Morris (1978) study, ect., is to treat groups as if they were a certain, already-known state of affairs. Schon (1983) sees this as a particularly inappropriate epistemology. Such technical rationailty, as he calls it, emphasizing the putting of theory into practice; of applying science to the situation from the position of a solitary thinker attempting to choose between theoretical alternatives to *solve* a problem. Morgan (1986) posits that this mode of intervention disempowers actors in the situation. They are made to feel that possibilities are predetermined; that some logic of the system is in command. This is absolutely the antithesis of our position that groups are continuously enacted by their participants through the social construction process. The challenge, therefore, is how to intervene in a way that is theoretically informal, but does not create a passive stance by actors toward their situation. As Shotter states:

> The task is not one of choosing but of generating a clear and adequate formulation of what the problem situation is, of creating from a set of incoherent and disorderly events a coherent "structure" within which both current actualities and future possibilities can be given an intelligible "place"—and doing all this, not alone, but in continual conversation which all the others who are involved . . . (Shotter, 1993. p. 152).

Shotter goes on to differentiate the act (of managers) to "do science" from the act of actually being involved "in making of history". We see the act of intervening in group life to be that of *co-authoring* a history or narrative: a dominant, shared and temporal construction of group life that involves the participants in co-inquiry and co-visioning with the intervenor(s).

To author a narrative or construction that is generative (vs. passive) and justifiable (vs. fictitious), intervention into group life need to be theoretically informed *and* grounded or rooted to the context at hand. Novelty or provocativeness is a source of interest, curiosity and engagement. Theoretical propositions and findings can help reframe the situation in new ways. For example, the earlier matrix to suggest a possible way of simultaneously viewing the dominant task-oriented and developmental constructions of groups could enable one to offer a "framing" of a group situation as a struggle to resolve attractive group goals that were less externally driven and more intrinsically connected to members' values. Likewise, the recent research on groups-in-context could provide novel language through metaphors of ambassador, scout, expeditor, owner, etc., with which to provide possible new meaning to a situation in question. At the same time, theoretically informed interruptions must go beyond clever, if not logically sound, reading or interpretation of a situation. To be justified in their authoring of an ongoing narrative, interveners need to provide sharable, linguistic formulation to already shared feelings arising from, group circumstances (Shotter, 1993). Authoring a justifiable account or narrative is similar to Argyris' (1970) criterion for effective interventions, where he maintains they should be based on "valid information". Interventions from a constructionist perspective need to be consensually validated in order that tacit and partial "constructions" or meanings carried by individual members can be made explicit and shared. Searching for meaning via a conceptual fit of theory to practice is no longer sufficient or useful. *Making* meaning through conversation about the understanding members take from their past and intended future group experience is what provides possibilities for generative acts in and on the group. In this regard, metaphors and metaphorical language may be particularly useful ways to interrupt group conversations-for-action or -development and initiate conversations-for-possibilities grounded in hope, affirmation and equifinality (Morgan, 1986; Srivastva & Barrett, 1988).

One reason metaphors provide exciting possibilities as a source or even style of intervention is that they are expressed through language in time and space that purposely intends to create a "new listening" in others. From a social constructionist perspective, whatever is overtly spoken and listened to at any moment rests on a background or totality of listening that makes the current conversation possible. There is, at the same time, listening-back (a learned, habitual, or "thrown" way of hearing and perceiving) and a potential to listen-ahead (consider new possibilities and actions through words). The "act" of intervening rests on framing an interruption with language that: (a) shifts a conversation-for-action or -relation to a conversation-for-possibility; and (b) produces (or seduces) the listening we wish. The "measure" of an intervention in therefore not in whether it is true or false, but in what kinds of commitments are generated for the speaker and listener by the speech acts generated by the interruption, and how these commitments generate the space for possible action (Winograd & Flores, 1986).

In summary, the constructionist perspective of group life suggests that interventions in groups are potentially "conversation starters" to open up possible action from discovering new, shared understanding about what members expect and wish the group to be(come). The role of theory and research is to inform the linguistic framing of an intervention: to help ground it in the contextual situation of a particular group and its member relations and, at the same time, to help produce in others a space for hearing the idea, image, proposition or description in a way that leads to more questions, willingness to discuss further, wish to amend, and so on. As winograd & Flores assert for managers, we see the same for practitioners intervening in groups: "The essential responsibility ... can be characterized as participation in conversations-for-possibilities that open new backgrounds for conversations-for-action" (Winograd & Flores, 1986, p. 151).

The following propositions emerge from this constructionist view of interventions into group life:

- The generative power of an intervention is in the language used and how it causes "hearers" to listen and consider things in new ways.
- Interventions that enable the group are co-authored or consensually validated formulations of complex impressions already existing about the situation.
- Theory informs interventions in order to add novel possibilities to existing constructions being enacted by the group.
- Interventions interrupt the dominant conversations-for-action (task-related) or conversations-for-cohesion (development-related) to open up space for conversations-for-possibilities.
- Interventions that seek to "fit" theory to an observation of a group's dynamics will often disable the group by fostering passivity, dependance and acquiescence to some external determinism.
- Interventions that seek to make new meaning out of conversations about various constructions being enacted in the same context will often enable the group to make new declarations, requests and promises to each other.

CONCLUSIONS AND IMPLICATIONS FOR INQUIRY (PRACTICE AND RESEARCH)

The actual practice and discourse about teams and the widespread efforts to implement team concepts are not at all paralleled by an equal intensity of research in group dynamics. The body of small group theory is not offering new perspectives (Levine & Moreland, 1990), because of its concentration on minimal and atomic social interaction situations in controlled experiments. We have sought to advocal here a renewed need for research on group-development-in-context. It is a call for both a new focus in small group research and for new methods of inquiry.

The focus of inquiry into small groups needs to combine and align the study of internal group processes (task-oriented and maintenance-oriented perspectives) with the study of the groups' external orientation to boundary issues and management. This linking of the group dynamics perspectives to the organization or contextual perspectives is believed to be more naturally or organically in concert with those images and notions (social constructions) that group members, leaders and key constituents actually embody. Such research on organizational groups requires longitudinal inquiries, in depth, over a period of time. From the social constructionist perspective, this research also needs to embrace methodologists that: (a) seek to create histories; (b) are embedded in dialogue or conversation; and (c) actively engage the inquirer as co-author rather than as an observer or interpretor. The role of leaders, facilitators and key actors in the surrounding context of the group in this social construction deserves special attention. How do they co-construct common or uncommon meaning about the group experience taking into account the three domains discussed above: internal relational processes; internal task requirements, and external boundary management? One can reasonably expect group members to simultaneously carry with them partially shared understandings or "constructions" about activities, intentions and issues in each of these domains. How a group actually comes to align, sequence or alternate actions in these three domains with a sense of "shared reality" about what they are doing demands attention. Interventions informed by this type of research can help managers, facilitators, group members and related key figures to articulate, envision and meet alignment activities that are collectively expected or desired. This enhancement of the group reflexivity in the relational and contextual domain will be especially important to increase that group's adaptability and, hence, its actual *development*.

REFERENCES

Argyris, C. (1970). *Intervention Theory and Method*. Reading, MA: Addison-Wesley.
Ancona, D. & Caldwell, D. (1992). Bridging the boundary: external activity and performance in organizational teams. *Administratise Science Quarterly*, **37**, 634–665.
Bales, R.F. (1958). Task roles and social roles in problem-solving groups. In E. Maccoby, M. Newcomb & E. Hartley (eds), *Social Psychology*, 3rd Edn. New York: Holt, Rinehard & Winston, pp. 437–447.
Bales, R.F. & Strodtbeck, F.L. (1953). Phases in group problem solving. *Journal of Abnormal Social Psychology*, **46**, 485–495.
Banet, A.G. (1976). Yin/yang: a perspective on theories of group development. In J.W. Pfeiffer & J.E. Jones (eds), *The 1976 Annual for Group Facilitators*. La Jolla, CA: University Associates.
Barrett, F. & Srivastva, S. (1990). Metaphor. In S. Srivastva & D.L. Cooperrider (eds), *Appreciative Management and Leadership*. San Francisco: Jossey-Bass.
Benne, K. (1964). *T-Group Theory and Laboratory Method. Innovation in Re-education*. New York: Wiley.
Benne, K.D. & Sheats, P. (1948). Functional roles of group members. *Journal of Social Issues*, **2**, 42–47.
Bennis, W.G. & Shepard, H.A. (1956). A theory of group development. *Human Relations*, **9**, 415–437.
Bion, W.R. (1961). *Experiences in Groups*. London: Tavistock.
Cordery, J.L., Mueller, W.S. & Smith, L.M. (1991). Attitudinal and behavioral effects of autonomous group working: a longitudinal field study. *Academy of Management Journal*, **34**, 464–476.
Dyer, W.G. (1995). *Team Building. Current Issues and New Alternatives*, 3rd Edn. Reading, MA: Addison-Wesley.
Fry, R., Rubin, I. & Plovnick, M. (1981). Dynamics of groups that execute or manage policy. In R. Payne & C. Cooper (eds), *Groups at Work*. New York: Wiley, pp. 41–57.
Gersick, C.J. (1988). Time and transition in work teams: toward a new model of group development. *Academy of Management Journal*, **31**, 9–41.
Gladstein, D. (1984). Groups in context: a model of task group effectiveness. *Administrative Science Quarterly*, **29**, 499–517.
Gurley, K. & Fry, R. (1993). From coordinators to expeditors to owners: a study of cross-functional teams as integrating mechanisms. *Journal of High Technology Management*, **4**, 1.
Hackman, J.R. (1989). *Groups That Work (and Those That Don't): Creating Conditions for Effective Teamwork*. San Francisco: Jossey Bass.
Hackman, J.R. & Morris, C. (1978). Group tasks, group interaction process, and group performance: a review and proposed action. In L. Berkowitz (ed.), *Group Processes: Papers from Advances in Experimental Social Psychology*. New York: Academic Press.

Katzenbach, J.R. & Smith, D.K. (1993). *The Wisdom of Teams: Creating the High-performance Organization*. Boston, MA: Harvard Business School Press.
Likert, R. (1961). *New Patterns of Management*. New York: McGraw-Hill.
Lawler, E.E. (1971). *Pay and Organizational Effectiveness: A Psychological View*. New York: McGraw-Hill.
Lawler, E.E. III (1992). *The Ultimate Advantage. Creating the High-involvement Organization*. San Francisco: Jossey-Bass.
Levine, J.M. & Moreland, R.L. (1990). Progress in small group research. *Annual Review of Psychology*, **41**, 585–634.
Marrow, A. (1969). *The Practical Theorist. The Life and Work of Kurt Lewin*. New York: Basic Books.
McGrath, J.E. (1984). *Groups: Interaction and Performance*. Englewood Cliffs, NJ: Prentice Hall.
Morgan, G. (1986). *Images of Organization*. London: Sage.
Philip, H. & Dunphy, D. (1959). Developmental trends in small groups. *Sociometry*, **22**, 162–174.
Pages, M. (1968). *La Vie Affective des Groupes. Esquisse d'une Theorie de la Relation Humaine*. Paris: Dunod.
Porter, M.E. (1985). *The Competitive Advantage*. New York: Free press.
Schein, E. (1969). *Process Consultation: Its role in Organization Development*. Reading, MA: Addison-Wesley.
Schein, E. (1988). *Process Consultation*. Reading, MA: Addison-Wesley.
Schon, D. (1983). *The Reflective Practitioner*. London: Maurice Temple Smith.
Schutz, W.C. (1958). *Firo: A Three-dimensional Theory of Interpersonal Behavior*. New York: Holt.
Senge, P. (1990). *The Fifth Discipline. The Art and Practice of the Learning Organization*. New York: Doubleday Currency.
Shotter, J. (1993). *Conversational Realities*. London: Sage.
Slater, P.E. (1966). *Microcosm; Structural, Psychological and Religious Evolution in Groups*. New York: Wiley.
Smith, K.K. & Berg, D.N. (1987). *Paradoxes of Group Life: Understanding Conflict, Paralysis and Movement in Group Dynamics*. San Francisco: Jossey-Bass.
Srivastva, S. & Barrett, F.J. (1988). The transforming nature of metaphors in group development: a study in theory. *Human Relations*, **41**, 31–64.
Srivastva, S., Obert, S.L. & Neilsen, E.H. (1977). Organizational analysis through group processes: a theoretical perspective for organizational development. In C. Cooper (ed.), *Organizational Development in the UK and the USA: a Joint Evaluation*. London: Macmillan.
Steiner, I.D. (1972). *Group Processes sand Productivity*. New York: Academic Press.
Steiner, I.D. (1974). Whatever happened to the group in social psychology? *Journal of Experimental Social Psychology*, **10**, 94–108.
Steiner, I.D. (1986). Paradigms and groups. *Adances in Experimental Social Psychology*, **19**, 251–289.
Tuckman, B.W. (1965). Developmental sequences in small groups. *Psychology Bulletin*, **63**, 384–399.
Tuckman, B.W. & Jensen, M.C. (1977). Stages of small group development revisited. *Group and Organizational Studies*, **December**, 419–427.
West, M. (1994). *Effective Teamwork*. Leicester: British Psychological Society.
Winograd, T. & Flores, F. (1986). *Understanding Computers and Cognitions*. New York: Ablex.
Whitaker, D.S. & Lieberman, M.A. (1964). *Psychotherapy Through the Group Process*. New York: Atherton Press.
Whitehead, A.M. (1978). *Process and Reality: An Essay in Cosmology*. New York: Free Press.

Section VII

Conceptual Integration

Chapter 22

Reflexivity and Work Group Effectiveness: a Conceptual Integration

Michael A. West
Institute of Work Psychology, University of Sheffield, UK

The rich conceptual analyses offered in preceding chapters explore the complexities and processes involved in group collaboration. It would be misguided to attempt an overarching integration and coherent theoretical representation of these analyses. Nevertheless, an editor has the advantage of repeatedly reading about and dwelling on the ideas articulated by the contributors and is thus in a privileged position from which to discern common themes. I believe there are such common themes in this volume and below I try to draw them within a bounded frame which offers a limited conceptual integration.

In this chapter I describe a model of group effectiveness which focuses on a specific class of groups, because it seems clear that the diversity of work group types requires such specific approaches. Complex decision-making groups, in particular, are becoming increasingly common in modern organizations and so demand high priority in the theorizing of organizational psychologists. This chapter proposes that such groups will be effective to the extent that they reflect upon their objectives, strategies, processes and environments, and adapt these aspects of their task-functional worlds accordingly. The approach described here builds on earlier models and, in order to explore the value of existing approaches to understanding group effectiveness, three representative models will be referred to.

Handbook of Work Group Psychology. Edited by M.A. West.
© 1996 John Wiley & Sons Ltd.

A CRITIQUE OF EXISTING MODELS OF GROUP EFFECTIVENESS

The thinking of most researchers in the area of work group effectiveness in the last 20 years has been influenced by an important review by Hackman & Morris (1975). They described models of work group effectiveness based on relationships between inputs, processes and outputs. Inputs included factors such as group composition, group norms and task design. Group processes included use of member skills, appropriate task performance strategies and level of member effort. Hackman (1983) later distinguished three dimensions of outcomes: group performance in organizational terms; long-term viability of the group; and the well-being of group members. This model has been examined subsequently in multiple case studies of work group performance (see Hackman, 1990).

Gladstein (1984) also offers an input–process–output model of group performance, with inputs including group composition, group structure, available resources and organizational structure. Interaction processes then impact upon group effectiveness depending upon the characteristics of the group's task, including task complexity or interdependence amongst group members. Environmental uncertainty also plays a moderating role in the group process–group outcome relationship.

Sundstrom, De Meuse & Futrell (1990) construct an "ecological" framework for understanding work group performance. They describe three types of factors influencing team effectiveness: the organizational context, group boundaries and group development. Context includes task design, organizational culture, mission clarity, group autonomy, feedback, reward systems, physical environment, training and support. Boundaries differentiate teams while team development refers to temporal patterns in team processes (see McGrath & O'Connor, this volume, Chapter 3).

These approaches represent a generation of descriptive structures which helped a great deal in clarifying what broad classes of variables researchers and theoreticians should consider. However, although useful descriptively, these models embody problematic limitations. The first is that each presents a generalized description of work group effectiveness which, as Hackman & Morris (1975) suggested, may be inappropriate: "... no single theory can encompass and deal simultaneously with the complexity of factors that can affect group task effectiveness". Even this may be understating the difficulty. The variety of forms of work groups is rich and growing. They include, for example, senior management teams of large hospitals, teams in long-wall mining, autonomous work groups, assembly line teams, professional sports teams, cockpit crews, surgical teams, police crowd control teams, orchestras, military groups and research teams. The aim of developing a generalized model to account for group outcomes across such diverse setting seems now naively optimistic (though I am as guilty as others of such naiveté—see West, 1990).

The second limitation of these models is the lack of the parsimony we expect in elegant theory. Perhaps because of the attempt to make them applicable across diverse work groups, the models depict conceptual structures characterized by high complexity, evidenced in the large numbers of variables included. For example, Sundstrom et al. include 17 variables; Gladstein over 20 variables; and Hackman 14. To investigate empirically the representational validity of these models is therefore very challenging for researchers (although an example of some success is the cross-sectional study conducted by Campion, Medsker & Higgs, 1993).

The most important criticism, however, is that the models do not make testable predictions or generate hypotheses. Existing models are largely descriptive of broad classes of variables which may influence effectiveness (e.g. organizational rewards and appropriate group member skill use). Consequently their theoretical status is limited and they have largely failed to stimulate vigorous research endeavour and further theoretical development. This is disappointing given the huge effort in group psychology and the demand from students and practitioners for clear evidence and understanding about factors determining work group effectiveness.

For these reasons, therefore, it would seem helpful to abandon the search for an overall theory of work group effectiveness in favour of more focused and context-specific theoretical approaches.

EFFECTIVENESS IN COMPLEX DECISION-MAKING (CDM) GROUPS

The approach of psychologists to understanding work groups has traditionally reflected what might be termed a "technical-rational" perspective (Schön, 1983). Yet the complexity of teams and their environments suggests that such an orientation is unlikely to produce valid and powerful explanatory frameworks. As Schön (1994) suggests, technical-rational orientations to understanding work groups are based on the notion that mechanical manipulations of elements of work group design and functioning can be undertaken in order to effect particular consequences, e.g. clarifying goals for groups will, in most circumstances, lead to greater effectiveness. However, such formulations ignore the fact that groups and their environments change over time (McGrath & O'Connor, this volume, Chapter 3) and that goals are likely to be multiple and competing (Brodbeck, this volume, Chapter 13). In some circumstances it is necessary for groups to be unclear about their objectives. A hospital management team which has to begin generating income rather than relying on central government funding will require a period of goal orientation characterized by consideration and uncertainty. In such circumstances, goal clarity might be premature and contribute to ineffectiveness rather than effectiveness. Moreover, this concept of effectiveness itself is political rather than empirical (or technical-rational) in the sense that there are multiple constituents of most complex decision-making teams in modern organizations. Effectiveness in relation to one stakeholder group will spell ineffectiveness for another (e.g. saving money for a local health organization may not be in the best interests of patients who want the best quality of care) (cf. Brodbeck, this volume, Chapter 13; Poulton & West, 1993, 1994).

According to technical-rational orientations, professional activity consists in instrumental problem-solving made rigorous by the application of scientific theory and technique. Schön describes an alternative approach, which he terms:

> ... reflection-in-action ... both ordinary people and professional practitioners often think about what they are doing, sometimes even while doing it. Stimulated by surprise, they turn thought back on action and on the knowing which is implicit in action (Schön, 1983, p. 50).

He goes on:

> It is this entire process of reflection-in-action which is central to the "art" by which practitioners sometimes deal with situations of uncertainty, instability, uniqueness and value conflict (Schön, 1983, p. 50).

In the approach described below I adopt this reflection-in-action orientation to understanding complex decision-making (CDM) group effectiveness, which is referred to as "reflexivity".

This has led me to distinguish between CDM and simple decision-making (SDM) groups. There appears a clear qualitative difference between groups operating with relatively low control and discretion (SDM groups—for example in a shop floor environment which is relatively certain and predictable) and those with high autonomy, in unpredictable environments, where the picture of appropriate job performance for achieving desired outputs is relatively complex and unclear (CDM groups). Examples of CDM groups are: top management teams; primary health care teams; social service teams; community psychiatric teams; project teams in commercial settings; nursing teams; and research teams. Characteristic of these groups is that:

- They operate in uncertain, unpredictable environments.
- They often work with complex and unpredictable technology.
- Task performance requirements can change daily.
- They have high team member interdependence.
- They have autonomy over their day to day work.
- The nature of the tasks they are required to perform is complex, i.e. there are multiple elements and multiple interactions between elements
- The components of effectiveness are multiple and the team is responsible to multiple constituents.

CDM groups differ from laboratory groups "as greatest doth least", in the sense that the complexity and multiplicity of task, effectiveness and environment elements are at the opposite extreme of the scale from the laboratory groups social psychologists have traditionally studied. Such groups are particularly interesting theoretically because they represent an extreme of people with different skills, attempting to combine them in demanding task environments.

Existing models of group performance also tend to represent static rather than dynamic processes. Group variables such as participation are assumed to have a consistent relationship with productivity. However, it is questionable whether such models are appropriate for CDM groups of professionals from diverse backgrounds (an increasingly common form) working in challenging and changing environments.

Moreover groups themselves often change rapidly as a result of experience (e.g. McGrath & O'Connor, this volume, Chapter 3; Gersick, 1988, 1989) and member turnover. Such changes require processes of adaptation. Finally, groups often change their environments as a result of their own work via processes of innovation (e.g. Bunce & West, 1995; West & Anderson, 1992), political pressure or simply their own effectiveness. Consequently, for a team to be effective it must respond to these changing circumstances appropriately. The conceptual approach offered here focuses on group processes and outcomes, and proposes that what may best predict group effectiveness is an overarching factor which potentially will influence all aspects of group performance—group task reflexivity.

The approach proposes that:

1. Group task reflexivity will have a direct positive impact upon group task effectiveness in complex decision-making (CDM) groups.
2. Group task reflexivity will have an indirect effect upon group member mental health via group task effectiveness.
3. Non-task group social processes will have a direct positive impact upon member mental health, but will not influence group task processes or outcomes in any direct way.
4. Group task reflexivity will have a direct impact upon group (non-task) social processes, but not *vice versa*.

GROUP TASK REFLEXIVITY

> Group task reflexivity is defined as the extent to which group members overtly reflect upon the group's objectives, strategies and processes, and adapt them to current or anticipated endogenous or environmental circumstances.

There are two central elements to the concept of reflexivity (the root of which is to "bend back")—reflection and adaptation. Rennie (1992) describes reflexivity in the following way:

> Throughout the history of philosophy and psychology, this quality has been described as *consciousness, will, thinking, reason, judgement, reflection, agency, self-*

monitoring, recursion, meta cognition, and reflexivity among others (pp. 224–225, italics in original).

Reflexivity has also been described as "a turning back on the self" and can encompass both self-awareness and agency. The reflection component of group task reflexivity parallels Kahn's (1992) concept of psychological presence, but at the group level. Non-reflexivity, according to Rennie (1992), is "... the state of acting ... without awareness of the action". The group is not aware of doing, just doing. A reflexive model of group processes incorporates the idea that group task processes are "circular" or "spiralling". The group's reality is continually renegotiated during group interactions. Understandings negotiated in one exchange between group members may be drawn upon in a variety of ways in order to inform subsequent discussions, and offer the possibility of helpful and creative transformations in meaning. The meanings of particular representations of the group's circumstances are not stable, but depend on context of use and group members' reactions to them (see Bouwen & Fry, this volume, Chapter 22). Reflection involves behaviours such as questioning, planning, exploratory learning, analysis, diversive exploration, making use of knowledge explicity, planfulness, learning at a meta level, reviewing past events with self-awareness, digestion, and coming to terms over time with a new awareness.

How does reflection change into action or adaptation? It is through reflection that intentions are formed and the potential for carrying them out is built up. During reflection, courses of action can be contemplated and decisions may be reached about contemplated actions. Subsequently a decision may be converted into action. During reflection there is indeterminacy and the group has choices and hence the possibility of control over change. Some groups may reflect without subsequently taking action while others may adapt (appropriately or inappropriately) without reflection. The proposition does not require the actions of reflexive groups to be "right", "appropriate" or "adaptive", since group actions will lead to new information, further reflection and action, continuing in a spiral until group members are satisfied with the outcome (similar to Miller, Galanter & Pribram's test–operate–test–exit model, 1960). The result of continuous cycles of reflection and action will be group task effectiveness.

Indicators of Group Task Reflexivity

What are the domains of reflection and action which characterize reflexive groups? Broadly reflexive groups are likely to focus upon and effect change in relation to objectives, strategies, processes and environments. Reflection might therefore be upon:

- *Group objectives,* e.g. their appropriateness, clarity, value and the group's commitment to them.

- *Group strategies or plans for achieving goals*, e.g. their detailedness, clarity, value, alternatives, time-span, effectiveness.
- *Group processes*, e.g. decision-making, communication, interaction frequency, controversy, monitoring, feedback, self-appraisal, support for innovation, effectiveness.
- *Environment*, e.g. impact of technology, reward systems, inter-group relations, organizational objectives, wider social impact (e.g. ecological issues).

Non-reflexive groups can be identified by their failure to articulate consideration of objectives, strategies, processes and environments, and by a tendency to react to the situation that exists at the moment. This is contrast to reflexive groups which plan strategies ahead and actively structure the situation, including potential feedback (cf. Hacker, 1986). Reflexive groups will have a more comprehensive and penetrating intellectual representation of their work, a longer timeframe, a larger inventory of environmental cues to which they respond, a better knowledge and anticipation of errors and a more active orientation towards their work. Non-reflexive groups will exhibit defensiveness against awareness of group processes, strategy planning and change, and be recalcitrant in their willingness to review and reflect on their experience and objectives.

Between reflection or awareness and action will be some degree of group planning, and action theory (see Tschan & von Cranach, this volume, Chapter 6; and Frese & Zapf, 1994) provides a very helpful deconstruction of planning or action programming. Frese & Zapf (1994) describe four dimensions of plans, which can be used to gauge the extent of reflexivity. *Detailedness* is simply the extent to which a plan is worked out in detail before, as opposed to being worked out during, action. *Inclusiveness of potential problems* refers to the extent to which a group develops alternative plans in case of inadvertent circumstances. *A priori hierarchical ordering of plans* is the extent to which plans are broken up into sub-plans before actions are commenced. *Long- vs. short-range plans* is self-evident, although in uncertain environments both may be necessary to sustain effectiveness. *Ceteris paribus*, high reflexivity will exist when group planning is characterized by greater detail, inclusive of potential problems, hierarchical ordering of plans, and long- as well as short-range planning.

How a group reacts to and seeks feedback is also an indicator of reflexivity. Groups which process performance feedback in a self-serving manner rather than reflecting on performances issues are likely to be low in reflexivity (and consequently low in performance—cf. Dörner, 1989). Feedback search rate is another useful indicator of reflexivity, since it suggests that a group is sufficiently open in its interpretation of its world and functioning to value external feedback.

In relation to the wider organizational environment, such non-reflexive groups will tend to comply unquestioningly with organizational demands and expectancies; accept organizations limitations; fail to challenge organizational incompetence; communicate indebtedness and dependence on the organization; and rely heavily on organizational direction and reassurance. Reflexive groups, in contrast, will be more likely to reflect on the relationship with the organization and other organizational groups, and be prepared to challenge the appropriateness of organizational objectives. They are more likely to be minority influence groups (see Nemeth & Owens, this volume, Chapter 7) within the organization, generating conflict and innovation.

But is reflexivity a group level phenomenon or simply an attribute of individuals within the group? Undoubtedly, it can be accepted as an individual property of both cognition and behaviour—I think about whether I still have the energy to write clearly and creatively; decide not and pack my bag to go home. But here it is proposed that, although reflexivity is a property of individual group members (and that the aggregated reflexivity of individuals may well contribute to group reflexivity), group task reflexivity should be conceptualized as a group level phenomenon. Larson & Christensen (1993) have argued that social cognition (such as group reflection) can be applied usefully at the group level of analysis to refer to those social processes:

> ...that relate to the acquisition, storage, transmission, manipulation and use of information for the purpose of creating a group-level intellective product. In this context, social cognition is not merely cognition "about", it is cognition "by", with the word "social" referring to the way in which cognition is accomplished. At the group level of analysis, cognition *is* a social phenomenon (p. 6).

In the same vein, the reflection component of group task reflexivity is seen as a manifestation of social cognition. Within groups, individuals will communicate their perceptions and reflections, which interact to produce some degree of common perception or understanding (cf. Johnson, this volume, Chapter 19).

EMPIRICAL SUPPORT FOR THE REFLEXIVITY–EFFECTIVENESS RELATIONSHIP

There is good support for the proposition that task reflexivity will predict group task effectiveness in both social psychological and organizational research. Hackman & Morris (1975) found that in 100 laboratory groups (three persons per group, working on a 15-minute task) only 142 comments were made about the performance strategy of the group (less than 2 comments per group). However, process discussions following these comments turned out to facilitate group performance. The judged creativity of group products was related to the number of comments made about performance strategy. Previous work also suggests that task orientation (a conceptually similar factor) is associated with team innovation and effectiveness (see Ulich & Weber, this volume, Chapter 12; West & Anderson, 1995; Anderson, Hardy & West, 1990). Tjosvold (1990) describes constructive controversy within groups as the extent of exploration of opposing opinions. He argues for a direct causal relationship with effectiveness and offers empirical support for this proposition (Tjosvold 1985). Similar notions, though not well developed, have been proposed by Shiflett (1979) in relation to groups and, at the organizational level, Argyris (1993) proposed the idea of "double-loop learning" in organizations as an indication of members' ability to recognize and modify underlying assumptions about organizational functioning.

At the individual level, Dörner (1981, 1987) found that self-reflection was an important prerequisite in problem-solving. Those high in self-reflection solved problems better than those low in self-reflection. Furthermore, the number of self-reflections was decreased under conditions of failure. In a study of "superworkers", Dörner et al. (1983) used complex computer simulations where subjects were required to take the role of a city mayor:

> Successful subjects had more precise goals, asked more questions, particularly more "why" and more abstract questions... they also developed more hypotheses and tested their hypotheses... and did not "act out of the moment"... they were more self-reflective and they thought more actively about changing things rather than just describing them (Frese & Zapf, 1994, p. 44).

At the group level, evidence suggests that group problem-solving, especially early on, is significantly improved when members examine the way in which they have defined the situation and considered whether or not they are solving the "right" problem (see for example Bottger & Yetton, 1987; Hirokawa, 1990; Landsberger, 1955; Maier, 1970; Schwenk, 1988). Evidence has been accumulated in this area as a result of the coherent and major body of research developed by Maier and colleagues. Maier's work suggested that cognitive stimulation in groups may produce novel ideas, a unique combination of sub-ideas, or a complex solution whose total value is "greater than the sum of its parts". The group product might be improved, Maier found, if groups were encouraged to be "problem-minded" rather than "solution-minded" (Maier & Solem, 1962), i.e. to question its current approach or to consider other aspects of the problem (see also Maier, 1950, 1970). Maier also found that group productivity was improved when the group analysed problem facets as sub-tasks, and if members separated and recombined problem-solving strategies (Maier, 1952; Maier & Hoffman, 1960; Maier & Maier, 1957). Similar effects on productivity were found when groups were encouraged to produce two different solutions to a problem, so that the better of the two might be adopted (Maier, 1970). Particularly for CDM groups, more planning enhances group performance (Hackman, Brousseau & Weiss, 1976; Smith, Locke & Barry, 1990).

Another line of supportive findings for this general proposition comes from research on problem identification by groups (Moreland & Levine, 1992). For example, a group that detects problems too slowly or misdiagnoses them will probably fail, whatever solutions it develops for those (D'Zurilla & Goldfried, 1971; Mitroff & Featheringham, 1974). Indeed, misdiagnosis of problems is a major threat to group effectiveness. Attributing problems to the wrong causes, or not thinking through potential consequences, are common failings which can undermine group effectiveness, especially when group members refuse to reflect on the possibility of error (cf. Jervis, 1976; Schwenk, 1984; Staw & Ross, 1988). A major factor determining group task effectiveness is group norms regarding problem-solving. Non-reflexive groups regard problems as threats to morale and discourage identification of problems by their members (Janis, 1982; Miceli & Near, 1985; Smircich, 1983). Those who become aware of problems in such groups are reluctant to talk about them because they expect to be censured. When problems are brought into the awareness of non-reflexive groups, the tension produced can prevent appropriate planning and action (cf. Lyles, 1981; Schwenk & Thomas, 1983). Reflexive groups that engage in more extensive scanning of their environments are also better than non-reflexive groups at identifying problems (Ancona & Caldwell, 1988; Main, 1989; Billings, Milburn & Schaalman, 1980). Moreover, as the environment of groups becomes more uncertain, problem identification becomes more difficult (Hedburg, Nystrom & Starbuck, 1976; Kiesler & Sproull, 1982). Non-reflexive groups will tend to deny, distort or hide problems and wait and watch to see what occurs with them (Stein, this volume, Chapter 8; Moreland & Levine, 1992). In non-reflexive groups, identifying a problem is more likely to be seen as harmful, by threatening morale or creating conflict over such issues as who caused the problem and who should solve it (cf. Ancona, 1987; Leary & Forsythe, 1987; Lyles & Mitroff, 1980; Tesser & Rosen, 1975; Watson, 1976).

Research designed to improve group decision-making also provides further support for the general position adopted here. For example, Rogelberg, Barnes-Farrell & Lowe (1992) had groups use a technique of structured decision-making to solve complex and novel problems, which produced higher quality decisions than groups using conventional methods. The "stepladder" technique employed by Rogelberg, Barnes-Farrell & Lowe, involved each group member presenting his or her perceptions of the problem and potential solutions to the group in turn, without having heard the input of other members. One consequence was the constant reiteration and verbalization of group members' ideas in discussion, leading to the types of processes the model would predict in highly reflexive groups. Because each group member had an opportunity to present his or her views there was less pressure to conform, which may have enabled groups to freely evaluate ideas rather than actively avoiding disagreements and promoting conformity. Group members also tended to work very hard and to fully understand the group outcome. The stepladder groups were in effect continually re-making their decisions.

Other research on the remaking of group decisions has indicated beneficial effects on group output (Maier & Hoffman, 1960). For complex tasks, a higher rate of communication is clearly and positively related to group performance (Foushee, 1984; Williges, Johnson & Briggs, 1966). Moreover, the act of communication itself reveals knowledge so that the most knowledgeable members on particular issues in stepladder groups could reveal their knowledge to the group, thus making individual expertise known. Better ideas were more likely to be expressed, and were more likely to be attended to and recognized as better.

Johnson & Johnson (1987) also showed that verbalization and reiteration increased comprehension, understanding and retention of information within groups, which together are likely to promote greater effectiveness. Rogelberg, Barnes-Farrell & Lowe comment that:

> An entering member maybe acted as a consultant or reviewer with all other members curious and active listeners. It was a common anecdotal report by participants that, while an entering member was presenting options the core group would constantly ask "why do you say that"? This questioning of views may have led to more viable and effective information, which the group could use when making a final decision" (p. 736).

Van Offenbeek & Koopman's analysis of interaction and decision-making in groups (this volume, Chapter 9) also suggests that non-reflexive teams will make decisions primarily at the operational level. Unlike reflexive and "stepladder" groups, they will neglect tactical and strategic decisions.

What Initiates Task-reflexive Processes?

When groups "turn back on themselves" and examine their objectives, group processes, strategies and their environments, it is likely that discrepancies between actual and desired circumstances are revealed and that this may be aversive. "Every symptom embodies a contrast between realism and idealism; members realize that conditions within the group are not what they ought to be" (Moreland & Levine, 1992, p. 19). Similar propositions about problem identification and group arousal have been put forward by Cowan (1986), Pounds (1969) and Smith (1989). As a consequence of reflection or problem identification, the group experiences anxiety and uncertainty, members become increasingly aroused, and thus the motivation to reflect may be reduced (although above a certain threshold of arousal, problem-solving activity will take place—see Billings, Milburn & Schaalman, 1980; Lyles, 1981; Turner, 1976; Yarrow et al., 1955). Because reflection often involves recognizing discrepancies between real and ideal circumstances, it is unlikely to arise spontaneously within the group. Moreover, reflection may demand change in action and much organizational and psychological research has indicated that individuals in organizations are chronically resistant to change (French & Bell, 1978).

Reflecting or turning back on oneself can be aversive for individuals also. The work of Duval & Wickland (1972), for example, shows that when we monitor ourselves (by listening to a tape recording of our voices, looking at ourselves in the mirror, or seeing ourselves on video) we experience aversive consequences, since the discrepancy between how we see ourselves and how we would like to be is revealed (see also Buss, 1980; Carver & Scheier, 1982; Scheier & Carver, 1977; West, 1982). Therefore, group task reflexivity is unlikely to arise naturally (it is argued), but would have to be induced by events.

The kinds of factors which are likely to induce reflexivity are *interruptions* and particularly conflicts, crises, shocks, surprises, obstacles, and changes. When *intragroup task conflicts* occur, groups characterized by high levels of task reflexivity are more likely to respond by reflecting on the underlying processes associated with the conflict as well as the causes of them. Similarly, *interruptions to the group's work* by senior managers or other groups are likely to lead to reflection and action. *Unpredictable outside events* could interfere with the group's functioning and offer another opportunity for reflection. *Technical interruptions* due to machine breakdown or malfunction, and organizational problems such as lack of supplies, provide further opportunities for reflection. *Errors and failures* in group functioning in particular can stimulate groups to reflect on the processes or assumptions which led to them. Task-reflexive groups are more likely to respond to errors, failures and crises by reflecting upon underlying assumptions as well as strategies and processes. Non-reflexive groups in contrast will tend to deny errors or give up on long-term planning and fall back upon short-term strategies at times of crises (cf. Schultz, 1980).

Group member changes are another example of interruptions which provide an opportunity for reflection (Anderson & Thomas, this volume, Chapter 18). As Katz (1982) has argued, project newcomers represent a novelty-enhancing condition, challenging and improving the scope of existing methods and accumulated knowledge. Interestingly, the longer groups have been together, the less they communicate with key information sources, scan the environment and communicate within the group and with other organizational divisions and external professions. Group longevity is associated with a tendency to ignore and become increasingly isolated from sources that provide the most critical kinds of feedback, evaluation and information (Katz, 1982). This suggests that without optimal changes in membership and function, groups may become less reflexive over time.

Difficulties over time allocation and *synchronization of time use* present further opportunities for reflection (see McGrath & O'Connor, this volume, Chapter 3). Gersick's (1988, 1989) notion of punctuated equilibrium suggests that there are critical temporal points in the lives of teams which also have the potential to stimulate reflection and action. Other examples include *group successes*—non-reflexive groups are likely to accept successes unquestioningly; groups high in reflexivity are more likely to analyse and consider the causes of success. Similarly, *organizational change* can trigger a group to consider its objectives, strategies, processes, its organizational environment and its relationship with the wider social environment.

Other factors which may impact upon the group's propensity to reflect or take action and adapt include the characteristics of team members. Jackson's review (this volume, Chapter 4) of work on the composition of work groups suggests that group heterogeneity or diversity may stimulate many opportunities for reflexivity, while in homogeneous groups such opportunities would be rare. Group cultural heterogeneity may operate in a similar way (Smith & Noakes, this volume, Chapter 20). However, Susan Jackson's analysis suggests that diversity in status and power would decrease reflexivity.

George's chapter indirectly suggests reflexivity will be moderated by the affective tone of the group. Groups which are interested, excited, strong, enthusiastic, proud, alert, inspired, determined, attentive and active—in short, those with positive affective tone—will enable members to be:

> more cognitively flexible, more able to make associations, to see dimensions and to see potential relations among stimuli.

Positive affective tone thus fosters both group task reflexivity and creativity. Another important influencing factor is the group's relationship with the wider organization (Guzzo, this volume, Chapter 2). Attachment theory (Ainsworth, 1982) offers a possible framework for how relationships between the group and senior managers might be conceptualized—relationships could be characterized by secure, avoidant or ambivalent attachment, with consequent impacts upon group reflexivity. For example, groups which have a relatively secure relationship with the organization, feeling that their work is valued, appreciated and supported would be more likely to be reflexive in their orientation towards the organization itself and the wider environment. They would be more prepared to challenge organizational goals and to seek additional resources from the organization than non-reflexive groups. The latter are apt to adopt an avoidant position towards organizations, finding their interactions with senior management so aversive or negative that they avoid interaction with them as much as possible, preferring instead to immerse themselves in their day-to-day work without considering or attempting to alter relationships with the wider organization. Other non-reflexive groups are ambivalent, being unsure of the extent to which they are securely supported by the organization. Consequently, they may consistently need reassurance and clarity of direction, and exhibit a reluctance to criticize or challenge organizational policies or objectives.

So far this chapter has focused upon the notion of group task reflexivity and its relationship with group effectiveness. Group effectiveness, for example, has been discussed as if it were a single and simple construct. Now, we shall turn to examine group task effectiveness in more detail along with two other principal elements in conceptualizations of work group functioning: non-task social processes and member well-being.

GROUP TASK EFFECTIVENESS

Traditional approaches to conceptualizing group effectiveness either have tended to adopt an organizational productivity notion (for example, Guzzo, 1988; Pritchard & Watson, 1992) or have extended this to include notions of team viability over time (Hackman, 1990) and member well-being (see for example Sonnentag, this volume, Chapter 15).

Here, task effectiveness is distinguished from member well-being and group viability. Indeed, group member well-being is described as quite separate from, though affected by group task effectiveness. In the first place, it is an individual level variable and should not be misconstrued as a group level outcome. Second, combining the quite different domains of well-being and task effectiveness into a catch-all concept of group effectiveness is likely to hamper rather than aid understanding. At the same time a more elaborated concept of team task effectiveness than a single productivity dimension is proposed (even one as sophisticated as that developed by Pritchard—see Brodbeck, this volume, Chapter 13; Pritchard & Watson, 1992).

Group task effectiveness is framed within a constituency model (Connolly, Conlon & Deutsch, 1980).

> Effectiveness is defined as the extent to which the group successfully meets the competing criteria of task effectiveness held by interested stakeholders, but based on group members' appraisals of the relative importance of those criteria (Poulton & West, 1993, 1994).

To illustrate, the effectiveness of a primary health care team (doctors, nurses, physiotherapists, counsellors, receptionists) would be judged along differing dimensions by those stakeholders with an interest in the team's functioning. These would include patients and their relatives, carers, the employing organization which funds members of the team, drug companies, national health policy makers, the wider community and, of course, the team members themselves. Group task effectiveness, for the purposes of this theory, is best defined as the extent to which the group satisfies these varied (and often competing) criteria, *based on the group's rating of the importance of each criterion to its own perceptions of effectiveness*. Thus, the drug company representative may rate prescribing many expensive drugs as an indication of the team's effectiveness. National health policy-makers may take an opposite view. If group members leaned more towards the latter position, then this criterion (not prescribing expensive drugs) would receive much more weight in measuring the group's effectiveness (for an operationalization of this approach, see Poulton & West, 1993, 1994; Slater, West & Kellett, 1996).

This approach to group effectiveness seems appropriate for the particular case of CDM groups, which tend to operate in situations where multiple stakeholders attempt to influence their work in competing directions. Moreover, because such groups tend to require a high degree of autonomy to function, relying heavily on group ratings of the importance of various criteria seems more appropriate than using imposed organizational (or research-defined) metrics of task effectiveness. It also reflects the fact that such groups are likely to be measured along multiple effectiveness dimensions (e.g. quality, quantity, innovation, "customer" responsiveness) rather than any single dimension.

Non-task Social Processes

This social element of group functioning may be described by four social process factors: social support; methods of conflict resolution; support for group member growth and development; and management of group climate.

These social processes, it is proposed, will directly predict member job-related well-being. There are good reasons for arguing this. With regard to the first, we know that social support has an important buffering and possibly direct impact upon the well-being of individuals at work (Sonnentag, this volume, Chapter 15; Cohen & Wills, 1985; Kahn & Byosiere, 1992), so the social support provided by one's immediate work group(s) is likely to impact upon job-related individual well-being. CDM groups often operate in relatively unpredictable environments, so social support is likely to be important.

Research has demonstrated that the quality of relationships at work can be a powerful determinant of job-related well-being (see Sonnentag, this volume, Chapter 15; Warr, 1987) and effective methods of interpersonal conflict resolution (the second category of social processes) are therefore likely to have a significant impact. Where groups are able to resolve conflicts without enduring hostility, tension or resentment, it is likely that the job related well-being of team members will be relatively good. CDM groups often include professionals from diverse disciplinary backgrounds and, as Jackson (this volume, Chapter 4) indicates, although such diversity may stimulate innovation, it can also produce higher levels of conflict and threaten group viability. Developing effective conflict resolution strategies in such groups is therefore particularly important.

The third type of social process is support for growth and development. Growth and development opportunities are important aspects of people's experience at work and directly contribute to well-being and stress (Nicholson & West, 1988; Warr, 1987; West, Nicholson & Rees, 1990). To the extent that group members provide support for individual member growth and development, then job-related well-being of individual group members is likely to be better. Particularly in CDM groups, where skill variety and challenge are likely to be high, the needs to develop new skills and experiences and learn from colleagues probably will be strongly felt. Therefore, the supportiveness of colleagues in enabling these needs to be met will be important.

Finally, with regard to the fourth social determinant of well-being, in groups which provide a warm, friendly, pleasant environment, team member job-related well-being will tend to be good (cf. George's work on positive affect in groups, this volume, Chapter 5). The links from social functioning to group member job related well-being therefore are relatively uncontroversial.

The third proposition is that group task reflexivity will impact upon these non-task social processes. When a group develops patterns of task-related reflection and adaptation, it is argued that these will generalize to social functioning also. Social learning theory (Bandura, 1971) would support a direct link between the ability to manage constructive task-related controversy, and the ability to manage non-task-based social conflicts effectively. Moreover, since part of task-based reflexivity may involve reviewing member interdependence and mutual task-based support, it is argued that this will generalize to consideration of non-task-based social support during times of difficulty and crisis. Similarly, since task reflexivity is likely to produce a climate of task excellence (West, 1990) this will also influence social climate. Finally, task reflexivity will stimulate members to explore new challenges and develop skills appropriate to meeting them, which will encourage group members to provide support for skill development of others within the group, in order to increase the likelihood of goal achievement.

However, these descriptions of links between group task reflexivity and non-task social functioning offer a mechanistic view of the relationships. The task processes established in reflexive groups involve components such as group reflection, awareness, and attention which (it is proposed) will spill over into non-task-related group functioning—patterns of interaction will replicate across domains. If such social cognitions develop in relation to task functioning, it is argued they will inevitably be embodied in group functioning not directly related to task functioning. Awareness of the need to support and maintain a positive social climate in the group will be a natural consequence in reflexive groups, encouraging prosocial behaviour (cf. George, this volume, Chapter 5). The preparedness to give up time to support the learning and understanding of another group member will mirror the awareness and action involved in enabling more effective task functioning by another member of the group. There is a strong argument for suggesting that it is through acting in the world together that people develop and sustain good relationships. Within family groupings, much of the development of loving relationships occurs through the shared management of children, household tasks and dealing with difficult life events. Similarly, within work groups, it is argued that social relationships are likely to be developed and improved as a consequence of task-reflexive ways of working, since this will deepen understanding and acceptance by group members of their respective orientations and positions within the team.

The direction of causality is proposed to be from task reflexivity to social functioning rather than *vice versa*. While extremes of social functioning may interfere with task performance, it is unlikely that social functioning within the normal range will affect the organizational imperatives of day-to-day task performance. There are a number of indications in the literature to support this assertion. For example, a review by Mullen & Copper (1994) suggests that although there is a significant relationship between cohesiveness and performance, the direction appears to be from performance to cohesiveness, rather than *vice versa*. Reviews of the literature on team-building interventions designed to improve social interaction processes and thereby group task effectiveness (Sundstrom, De Meuse & Futrell, 1990; Tannenbaum and colleagues, this volume, Chapter 21) conclude that such interventions have reliably positive effects upon member attitudes and perceptions, but have no reliable impact on task effectiveness. In particular, interventions designed to improve the interpersonal processes in groups are least likely to effect any changes in group performance. Finally, as Ulich & Weber (this volume, Chapter 12) indicate, work groups based mainly on socio-emotional relationships are less stable than those characterized by a common task orientation. However, the team task training which Tannenbaum et al. describe is highly likely to impact upon task reflexivity, requiring, as it does, group members to see others' perspectives, learn their roles and reflect on task and team functioning issues (with hypothesized consequent positive effects upon non-task social processes).

In summary, it is argued that it is through enabling group members to work reflexively and actively together, thereby achieving effective change in their work environments, that people come closer together in mutual understanding, caring and support.

Group Member Well-being

Finally, it is proposed that team task effectiveness will impact upon group member well-being. High levels of group task effectiveness will affect individuals' sense of job competence and thereby reduce work-related anxiety or depression. Moreover, job aspirations will be met and raised, giving individuals a sense of accomplishment and commitment (Warr, 1987), with consequent benefits for well-being. It is proposed that team task effectiveness will have an impact upon well-being but that this relationship will not be reciprocal. There is also little theoretical or empirical basis for assuming that aggregated, individual, job-related well-being will predict group task effectiveness. Although one study (Wright, Bonett & Sweeney, 1993) has demonstrated a positive relationship between individual mental health and subsequent individual work performance, the causal link has not been established. Overall, it is concluded that there is no clear empirical support in the literature for a causal relationship from group member well-being to group task effectiveness.

Research Methods

The concept of group task reflexivity refers to a broad category of group behaviour, subsuming two major components (reflection and action), and a wide variety of manifestations, as described earlier. Studying reflexivity, therefore, demands methodologies and empirical approaches which can gauge the depth and richness of the concept. Clearly, conceptual development is of limited value if there are not research methods and designs which enable the concepts to be operationalized and propositions examined. Below are described methods which can be used to achieve this. One strategy is to use *audio recordings of group meetings* to determine the extent of reflexive behaviour in groups (cf. West & Anderson, 1995; Kuk et al., 1994). Generally, at least six sessions should be recorded to give an adequate time-sampling frame. The definition and descriptions of reflexivity should be exploited to enable precise categorizations of verbal interactions and patterns of discussions. An advantage of such a procedure is that categorizations of group processes rather than individual responses about group processes are studied. Questionnaire designs suffer from the disadvantage that inferences about group level variables are made on the basis of individual level data.

Critical incident techniques offer a particularly useful method for determining how work groups respond to interruptions, surprises and crises. By asking group members to report (collectively or individually) on how the group responded to interruptions in its work, rich data on patterns of group behaviour can be gathered.

Focus group discussions which examine group behaviour over time also enable group level data to be gathered which provide information specifically about reflection and action, non-task social processes and task performance. They can also be used to generate weighted effectiveness criteria for groups.

Longitudinal studies in which researchers deliberately intervene in group functioning enable more precise conclusions to be drawn about relationships between group responses to interruptions and outcomes such as task effectiveness. The introduction of autonomous group working (see Cordery, this volume, Chapter 11) or the use of team training interventions (Tannenbaum et al., this volume, Chapter 21) are examples of such interventions.

More traditional questionnaire studies of group processes can be employed with large numbers of groups, but they should always be augmented by the types of data gathering described above, given the nature of the concepts being explored in this research. A questionnaire measure of group task reflexivity and non-task social processes, with reliable scales and a sound factor structure has been developed (Slater, West & Kellett, 1995), but this remains a crude, and at best partial, way of accessing reflexivity, which is considered a rich or "thick" aspect of group behaviour.

Contingencies

The propositions about reflexivity are based on the notion that CDM groups have a relatively high degree of autonomy and operate in complex situations; where there is a multiplicity of factors to take into account in the decision-making process; where the outcomes of group functioning are multiple and varied; and where the group is responsible to multiple constituents. Overall, however, one contingency is considered to be particularly important, and that is environmental uncertainty. Environmental uncertainty refers primarily to the static–dynamic quality (speed and unpredictability of change) of the environment (see Duncan, 1972), but also to the simple–complex dimension, i.e. the number of significant influencing factors (cf. the concept of problem analysability—Perrow, 1967). It is proposed that if the group's environment is uncertain, high reflexivity will lead to greater effectiveness. In other words, where factors within the work group's environment change swiftly and unpredictably, reflexivity is all the more important. The group needs to reflect and act to change its objectives, strategies or processes in response to its rapidly changing environment. It is proposed that the "fit" between actions and environment is not an issue—as long as groups reflect and act in a continuous "cycle" or "spiral", closer approximations of "fit" are generally likely to result. Where the environment is relatively static, less reflexivity will be required. This contingent argument, therefore, makes further propositions that in circumstances of low environmental uncertainty and complexity, reflexivity will be a relatively weak predictor of effectiveness, whereas in circumstances of high environmental uncertainty, reflexivity will be a strong predictor of effectiveness. However, it is proposed that reflexivity will always positively predict effectiveness in CDM groups to a greater or a lesser extent.

CONCLUSIONS

The propositions (relating group task reflexivity, task effectiveness, non-task social processes, and group member well-being) described above are represented in Figure 22.1. However, it is important to stress that the propositions are not meant simply to describe the current pattern of group processes in organizational settings. Many "groups" in organizations do not have sufficient member interdependence, clear objectives, and appropriate group task performance feedback necessary for minimally effective CDM group performance. Indeed, group or team functioning in a wide variety of organizational settings appears to be rather

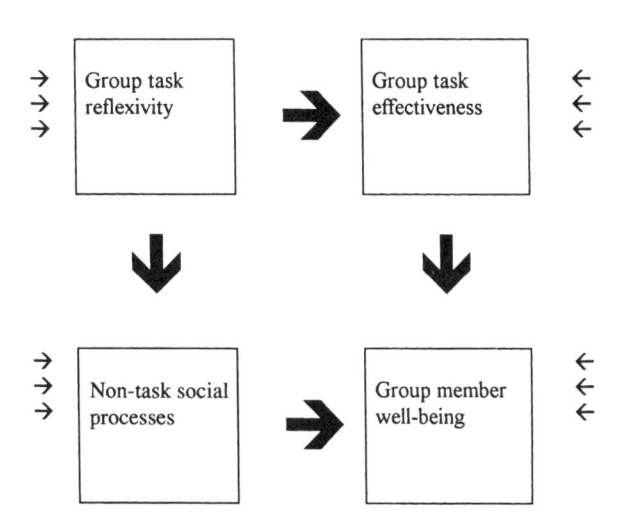

Figure 22.1 Reflexivity, group effectiveness and member well-being. Large arrows = relationships between principal variables; small arrows = extrinsic factors affecting principal variables

primitive. Consequently, it is suggested that processes of task reflexivity in group functioning require considerable practical development if the potential of work groups is to be realized.

For example, in relation to reflexivity towards wider organizational and social environments, teams in modern organizations seem generally non-reflexive. Group members behave as though organizational objectives and wider social issues are givens and not for consideration (cf. Allen, this volume, Chapter 16). However, it is argued that group members display high reflexivity not just when they focus on group objectives, strategies and processes, but also when they consider the appropriateness of their organization's objectives in the wider society. Such a reflexive group, working within a chemical-producing organization, might take a position contrary to the organization, demanding that it produce chemicals which are not environmentally damaging (see Hartley, this volume, Chapter 17). Groups high in reflexivity might thus become whistle-blowers and are certainly more likely to be minority influence groups within organizational settings (see Nemeth & Owens, this volume, Chapter 7) than non-reflexive groups.

However, even in relation to reflexivity on group objectives, strategies and processes, only rarely do groups possess a high degree of reflexivity. This is not to argue that the propositions described above are not generalizable. The fact that group functioning in many organizational settings is somewhat primitive is no reason for abandoning the propositions. Rather, they can provide a stimulus for those involved in working with groups to consider how levels of reflexivity could be raised and maintained.

These ideas about reflexivity challenge researchers and practitioners to reflect on, and change, how we work with groups, because (according to the propositions) so few are functioning optimally. Some implications of the position adopted here are that interventions and group leadership in CDM groups should be based on enabling groups and individuals to be reflexive over time (cf. Yammarino, this volume, Chapter 10), rather than on static technical-rational fixes of group processes. Indeed, it is suggested that practitioners should be giving processes of team self-development and functioning away—reflexivity interventions involve enabling group members themselves to nuture reflexivity over time, so that it is truly group development rather than indoctrination. Group task reflexivity also encourages group members to examine the role of the team in the wider organization and the role of the organization in society, so it is explicity a pluralist rather than a unitarist view of groups within organizations. Significantly, it is proposed that practitioners should focus principally on task processes in efforts to enhance group task effectiveness. Group social functioning, member well-being and team viability, will all consequently be developed.

In this chapter, a number of propositions have been offered and challenges remain to further refine the ideas presented and to determine their boundary conditions. One view of social science is that it should offer alternative views to the *status quo* and in this chapter alternative conceptions to existing models within group research are offered, drawing upon the expertise and ideas of the authors of the preceding chapters. The content will hopefully stimulate some agreement, some cognitive conflict and some disagreement in order that new avenues for vigorous constructive debate within the field can be followed to meet the challenges of integrating diverse disciplinary perspectives and promoting effective group work within organizations.

ACKNOWLEDGEMENTS

I would like to acknowledge useful comments from a number of colleagues about the ideas articulated in this chapter, particularly Chris Clegg, Michael Frese, Robert Roe and Toby Wall. Gillian Hardy has helped enormously in clarifying my thinking, and I owe her most thanks.

REFERENCES

Ainsworth, M.D.S. (1982). Attachment: retrospect and prospect. In C.M. Parkes & J. Stevenson-Hinde (eds), *The Place of Attachment in Human Behavior*. New York: Basic Books, pp. 3–30.
Ancona, D.G. (1987). Groups in organizations: extending laboratory models. In C. Hendrick (ed.), *Group Processes and Intergroup Relations*. Newbury Park, California: Sage, pp. 207–230.
Ancona, D.G. & Caldwell, D.F. (1988). Beyond task and maintenance: defining external functions in groups. *Group and Organization Studies*, **13**, 468–494.
Anderson, N.R., Hardy, G.E. & West, M.A. (1990). Innovative teams at work. *Personnel Management*, **September**, 48–53.
Argyris, C. (1993). On the nature of actionable knowledge. *The Psychologist*, **6**, 29–32.
Bandura, A. (1971). *Social Learning Theory*. Morristown, NJ: General Learning Press.
Billings, R.S., Milburn, T.W. & Schaalman, M.L. (1980). A model of crisis perception: a theoretical and empirical analysis. *Administrative Science Quarterly*, **25**, 300–316.
Bottger, P.C. & Yetton, P.W. (1987). Improving group performance by training in individual problem solving. *Journal of Applied Psychology*, **72**, 651–657.
Bunce, D. & West, M.A. (1995). Changing work environments: innovative coping responses to occupational stress. *Work and Stress*, **8**, 319–331.
Burningham, C. & West, M.A. (1995). Individual, climate and group interaction processes as predictors of work team innovation. *Small Group Research*, **26**, 106–117.
Buss, A.H. (1980). *Self-consciousness and Social Anxiety*. San Francisco: Freeman.
Campion, M.A., Medsker, G.J. & Higgs, A.C. (1993). Relations between work group characteristics and effectiveness: implications for designing work groups. *Personnel Psychology*, **46**, 823–850.
Carver, C.S. & Scheier, M.F. (1982). Self-awareness and the self-regulation of behaviour. In G. Underwood (ed.), *Aspects of Consciousness*, Vol. 3 *Awareness and Self-awareness*. London: Academic Press, pp. 235–266.
Cohen, S. & Wills, T.A. (1985). Stress, social support and the buffering hypothesis. *Psychological Bulletin*, **98**, 310–357.
Connolly, T., Conlon, E.J. & Deutsch, S.J. (1980). Organizational effectiveness: a multiple-constituency approach. *Academy of Management Review*, **5**, 211–217.
Cowan, D.A. (1986). Developing a process model of problem recognition. *Academy of Management Review*, **11**, 763–776.

Dörner, D. (1981). Über die Schwierigkeiten menschlichen Umgangs mit Komplexität. *Psychologische Rundschau (Sonderdruck)*, **31**, 163–179.

Dörner, D. (1987). *Von der Logik misslingens: Denken, Planen und Entscheiden in Unbestimmtheit und Komplexität.* Bonn–Bad Godesberg: Lehrstuhl Psychologie II, Universität Hamburg, Projekt, "Mikroanalyse", DFG 200/5-7, No. 54.

Dörner, D. (1989). *Die Logik des Misslingens.* Hamburg: Rowohlt.

Dörner, D., Kreuzig, H.W., Reither, F. & Stäudel, T. (1983). *Lohhausen-Vom Umgang mit Unbestimmtheit und Komplexität.* Bern: Huber.

Duncan, R.D. (1972). Characteristics of organizational environments and perceived environmental uncertainty. *Administrative Science Quarterly*, **17**, 313–327.

Duval, S. & Wicklund, R.A. (1972). *A Theory of Objective Self-awareness.* New York: Academic Press.

D'Zurilla, T.J. & Goldfried, M.R. (1971). Problem solving and behavior modification. *Journal of Abnormal Psychology*, **78**, 107–126.

Foushee, M.C. (1984). Dyads and triads at 35000 feet: factors affecting group process and aircrew performance. *American Psychologist*, **39**, 885–893.

French, W.L. & Bell, C.H. (1978). *Organization Development: Behavioral Science Interventions for Organization Improvement*, 2nd Edn. Englewood Cliffs, NJ: Prentice-Hall.

Frese, M. & Zapf, D. (1994). Action as the core of work psychology: a German approach. In H.C. Triandis, M.D. Dunnette & L.M. Hough (eds), *Handbood of Industrial and Organizational Psychology*, Vol. 4, 2nd Edn. Palo Alto, CA: Consulting Psychologists Press, pp. 271–340.

Gersick, C.J.G. (1988). Time and transition in work teams: toward a new model of group development. *Academy of Management Journal*, **31**, 9–41.

Gersick, C.J.G. (1989). Marking time: predictable transitions in task groups. *Academy of Management Journal*, **32**, 274–309.

Gladstein, D. (1984). Groups in context: a model of task group effectiveness. *Administrative Science Quarterly*, **29**, 499–517.

Guzzo, R.A. (1988). Productivity research: reviewing psychological and economic perspectives. In J.P. Campbell & R.J. Campbell (eds), *Productivity in Organizations.* San Francisco: Jossey Bass, pp. 63–81.

Hacker, W. (1986). *Arbeitpsychologie.* Bern: Huber.

Hackman, J.R. (1983). The design of work teams. In J.W. Lorsch (ed.), *Handbook of Organizational Behavior*, Englewood Cliffs, NJ: Prentice-Hall, pp. 315–342.

Hackman, J.R. (ed.) (1990). *Groups That Work (and Those That Don't): Creating Conditions for Effective Teamwork.* San Francisco: Jossey Bass.

Hackman, J.R., Brousseau, K. & Weiss, J.A. (1976). The interaction of task design and group performance strategies in determining group effectiveness. *Organizational Behavior and Human Performance*, **16**, 350–365.

Hackman, J.R. & Morris, C.G. (1975). Group tasks, group interaction process, and group performance effectiveness: a review and proposed integration. In L. Berkowitz (ed.), *Advances in Experimental Social Psychology*, Vol. 8. New York: Academic Press, pp. 47–97.

Hedburg, B.L.T., Nystrom, P.C. & Starbuck W.H. (1976). Camping on seesaws: prescriptions for a self-designing organization. *Administrative Science Quarterly*, **21**, 41–65.

Hirokawa, R.Y. (1990). The role of communication in group decision-making efficacy: a task-contingency perspective. *Small Group Research*, **21**, 190–204.

Janis, I.L. (1982). *Groupthink: Psychological Studies of Policy Decisions and Fiascos.* Boston: Houghton Mifflen.

Jervis, I.L. (1976). *Perception and Misperception in International Politics.* Princeton, NJ: Princeton University Press.

Johnson, D. & Johnson, F. (1987). *Joining Together: Group Theory and Group Skills.* Englewood Cliffs, NJ: Prentice-Hall.

Kahn, R.L. & Byosiere, P. (1992). Stress in organizations. In M.D. Dunnette & L.M. Hough (eds), *Handbook of Industrial and Organizational Psychology*, Vol. 3, 2nd Edn. Palo Alto, California: Consulting Psychologists Press, pp. 571–650.

Kahn, W.A. (1992). To be fully there: psychological presence at work. *Human Relations*, **45**, 321–349.

Katz, R. (1982). The effects of group longevity on project communication and performance. *Administrative Science Quarterly*, **27**, 81–104.

Kiesler, S. & Sproull, L. (1982). Managerial responses to changing environments: perspectives on problem sensing from social cognition. *Administrative Science Quarterly*, **27**, 548–570.

Kuk, G., Wood, D., Anderson, N. & West, M.A. (1994). The relationship between types of interruption and chair intervention styles in incidents of conflict. Paper presented at 23rd International Congress of Applied Psychology, Madrid.

Landsberger, H.A. (1955). Interaction process analysis of the mediation of labor–management disputes. *Journal of Abnormal and Social Psychology*, **51**, 202–228.

Larson, J.R. & Christensen, C. (1993). Groups as problem-solving units: towards a new meaning of social cognition. *British Journal of Social Psychology*, **32**, 5–30.

Leary, M.R. & Forsythe, D.R. (1987). Attributions of responsibility for collective endeavors. In C. Hendrick (ed.), *Review of Personality and Social Psychology*, Vol. 8. Newbury Park, CA: Sage, pp. 167–188.

Lyles, M.A. & Mitroff, I.I. (1980). Organizational problem formulation: biases and assumptions embedded in alternative decision-making models. *Journal of Management Studies*, **25**, 131–145.

Lyles, M.A. (1981). Formulating strategic problems: empirical analysis and problem development. *Strategic Management Journal*, **2**, 61–75.

Maier, N.R.F. (1950). The quality of group decisions as influenced by the discussion leader. *Human Relations*, **3**, 155–174.

Maier, N.R.F. (1952). *Principles of Human Relations*. New York: Wiley.

Maier, N.R.F. (1970). *Problem-solving and Creativity in Individuals and Groups*. Belmont, CA: Brooks/Cole.

Maier, N.R.F. & Hoffman, L.R. (1960). Quality of first and second solutions in group problem-solving. *Journal of Applied Psychology*, **44**, 278–283.

Maier, N.R.F. & Maier, R.A. (1957). An experimental test of the effects of "developmental" vs. "free" discussions on the quality of group decisions. *Journal of Applied Psychology*, **41**, 320–323.

Maier, N.R.F. & Solem, A.R. (1962). Improving solutions by turning choice situations into problems. *Personnel Psychology*, **15**, 151–157.

Main, J. (1989). At last, software CEOs can use. *Fortune*, March 13, 77–83.

Miceli, M.P. & Near, J.P. (1985). Characteristics of organizational climate and perceived wrong-doing associated with whistle-blowing decisions. *Personnel Psychology*, **38**, 525–544.

Miller, G.A., Galanter, E. & Pribram, K.H. (1960). *Plans and the Structure of Behaviour*. London: Holt.

Mitroff, I.I. & Featheringham, T.R. (1974). On systematic problem solving and the error of the third kind. *Behavioral Science*, **19**, 383–393.

Moreland, R.L. & Levine, J.M. (1992). Problem identification by groups. In S. Worchel, W. Wood & J.A. Simpson (eds), *Group Process and Productivity*. Newbury Park, CA: Sage, pp. 17–47.

Mullen, B. & Copper, C. (1994). The relation between group cohesiveness and performance: an integration. *Psychological Bulletin*, **115**, 210–227.

Nicholson, N. & West, M.A. (1988). *Managerial job change: men and women in transition*. Cambridge: Cambridge University Press.

Perrow, C. (1967). A framework for the comparative analysis of organizations. *American Sociological Review*, **32**, 194–208.

Poulton, B.C. & West, M.A. (1993). Effective multidisciplinary teamwork in primary health care. *Journal of Advanced Nursing*, **18**, 918-925.
Poulton, B.C. & West, M.A. (1994). Primary health care team effectiveness: developing a constituency approach. *Health and Social Care*, **2**, 77–84.
Pounds, W.F. (1969). The process of problem finding. *Industrial Management Review*, **11**, 1–19.
Pritchard, R.D. & Watson, M.D. (1992). Understanding and measuring group productivity. In S. Worchel, W. Wood & J.A. Simpson (eds), *Group Process and Productivity*. London: Sage, pp. 251–275.
Rennie, D.L. (1992). Qualitative analysis of the client's experience of psychotherapy. In S.G. Toukmanian & D.L. Rennie (eds), *Psychotherapy Process Research*. Newbury Park, CA: Sage, pp. 211–234.
Rogelberg, S.G., Barnes-Farrell, J.L. & Lowe, C.A. (1992). The stepladder technique: an alternative group structure facilitating effective group decision-making. *Journal of Applied Psychology*, **77**, 730–737.
Scheier, M.F. & Carver, C.S. (1977). Self-focused attention and the experience of emotion: attention, repulsion, elation and depression. *Journal of Personality and Social Psychology*, **35**, 625–636.
Schön, D.A. (1983). *The Reflective Practitioner: How Professionals Think in Action*. New York: Basic Books.
Schön, D.A. (1994). Teaching artistry through reflection-in-action. In H. Tsoukas (ed.), *New Thinking in Organizational Behaviour*. Oxford: Butterworth-Heinemann, pp. 235–249.
Schulz, P. (1980). Regulation und Feldregulation in Verhalten, V: Die wechselseitige Beeinflussung von mentaler und emotionaler Beanspruchung. *Psychologische Beiträge*, **22**, 633–656.
Schwenk, C.R. (1984). Cognitive simplification processes in strategic decision-making. *Strategic Management Journal*, **5**, 111–128.
Schwenk, C.R. (1988). *The Essence of Strategic Decision-making*. Massachusetts: D.C. Heath.
Schwenk, C.R. & Thomas, H. (1983). Formulating the mess: the role of decision aids in problem formulation. *Omega*, **11**, 239–252.
Shiflett, S. (1979). Towards a general model of small group productivity. *Psychological Bulletin*, **86**, 67–79.
Slater, J.A., West, M.A. & Kellett, S. (1995). Developing experience in newly created workgroups. Unpublished manuscript, Institute of Work Psychology, University of Sheffield, UK.
Smircich, L. (1983). Organization as shared meanings. In L.R. Pondy, P. Frost, G. Morgan & T. Dandridge (eds), *Organizational Symbolism*. Greenwich, CT: JAI Press, pp. 55–65.
Smith, G.F. (1989). Defining managerial problems: a framework for prescriptive theorizing. *Management Science*, **35**, 963–981.
Smith, K.G., Locke, E.A. & Barry, D. (1990). Goal setting, planning and organizational performance: an experimental simulation. *Organizational Behavior and Human Decison Process*, **46**, 118–134.
Staw, B.M. & Ross, J. (1989). Understanding behavior in escalation situations. *Science*, **246**, 216–220.
Sundstrom, E., DeMeuse, K.P. & Futrell D. (1990). Work-teams: applications and effectiveness. *American Psychologist*, **45**, 120–133.
Tesser, A. & Rosen, S. (1975). The reluctance to transmit bad news. In L. Berkowitz (ed.), *Advances in Experimental Social Psychology*, Vol. 8. New York: Academc Press, pp. 194–232.
Tjosvold, D. (1985). Implications of controversy research for management. *Journal of Management*, **11**, 21–37.

Tjosvold, D. (1990). *Team Organization: An Enduring Competitive Advantage.* Chichester: Wiley.
Turner, B. (1976). The organizational and interorganizational development of disasters. *Administrative Science Quarterly,* **21**, 378–397.
Warr, P.B.W. (1987). *Work, Unemployment and Mental Health.* Oxford: Oxford University Press.
Watson, C.E. (1976). The problems of problem-solving. *Business Horizons,* **19**, 88–94.
West, M.A. (1982). Meditation and self-awareness: physiological and phenomenological approaches. In G. Underwood (ed.), *Aspects of Consciousness,* Vol. 3, *Awareness and Self-awareness.* London: Academic Press, pp. 201–234.
West, M.A. (1990). The social psychology of innovation in groups. In M.A. West & J.L. Farr (eds), *Innovation and Creativity at Work: Psychological and Organizational Strategies.* Chichester: Wiley, pp. 309–333.
West, M.A. & Anderson, N. (1992). Innovation, cultural values, and the management of change in British hospitals. *Work & Stress,* **6**, 293–310.
West, M.A. & Anderson, N.R. (1995). Innovation in top management teams. Unpublished manuscript. Institute of Work Psychology, University of Sheffield, UK.
West, M.A., Nicholson, N. & Rees, A. (1990). The outcomes of downward managerial mobility. *Journal of Organizational Behaviour,* **11**, 119–134.
West, M.A. & Wallace, M. (1991). Innovation in health care teams. *European Journal of Social Psychology,* **21**, 303–315.
Williges, R.C., Johnston, W.A. & Briggs, G.E. (1966). Role of verbal communication in teamwork. *Journal of Applied Psychology,* **50**, 473–478.
Wright, T.A., Bonett, D.G. & Sweeney, D.A. (1993). Mental health and work performance: results of a longitudinal field study. *Journal of Occupational and Organizational Psychology,* **66**, 277–284.
Yarrow, M.R., Schwartz, C.G., Murphy H.S. & Deasy, L.L. (1955). The psychological meaning of mental illness in the family. *Journal of Social issues,* **11**, 12–24.

Author Index

Aavids, K. 246
Abbey, A. 334, 340
Abelson, R.P. 460, 468
Abrams, D. 402, 404, 408, 409, 417, 419
Ackerman, P.L. 178, 185
Adam, E.E. 228–9, 241
Adams, J.R. 295, 310
Adams, J.S. 195, 196, 203, 204, 207, 208, 219
Adelman, M.B. 462, 463, 469
Adeney, M. 414, 417
Adler, N.J. 486, 487, 496, 497
Agarwala-Rogers, R. 452, 457, 462, 473
Agrell, A. xxx, 326, 340, 482, 497, 567
Aiken, M. 458, 468, 469, 470
Ainsworth, M.D.S. 567, 575
Aitkenhead, M. 410, 420
Albrecht, T.L. 460, 462, 463, 469
Alderfer, C.P. xxxi, 15, 17, 19, 398, 399, 400, 401, 405, 408, 410, 411, 412, 417
Alexander, R.A. 228, 229, 242
Algera, J.A. 170, 172, 174, 182, 185, 187
Alioth, A. 248, 249, 251, 253, 257, 258, 259, 278
Allen, N.J. xxx, 373, 375, 376, 394, 395, 574
Allen, P.T. 408, 417
Allen, T.J. 295, 310
Allen, V.L. 61, 64, 70, 127, 128, 138
Altman, I. 10, 20, 36, 49, 127, 138
Alutto, J.A. 190, 192, 193, 194, 196, 197, 199, 200, 203, 204, 207, 208, 209, 211, 214, 216, 217, 220
Amabile, T.M. 136, 138, 319, 331, 340
Amman, R. 103, 120
Ancona, D.L. (*see also* Gladstein, D.L. and Gladstein-Ancona, D.L.) 10, 19, 64, 65, 70, 71, 324, 325, 340, 388–9, 394, 538–9, 551, 564, 575
Anderson, L.R. 113, 117

Anderson, N.R. xxxi, 235, 241, 326, 333, 340, 351, 364, 436, 442, 447, 448, 559, 562, 566, 571, 575, 579
Andrews, F.M. 324, 340
Andrews, S.B. 381, 395
Angle, H.L. 376, 394
Antoni, C. 255, 262, 278, 354, 362
Applebaum, E. 12, 13, 17, 19
Aranda, E. 385, 395, 504, 523, 528
Argote, L. 26, 40, 43, 48, 49, 50, 51, 287, 294, 296, 310, 311, 350, 363
Argyle, M. 80, 90, 486, 497
Argyris, C. 160, 177, 182, 320, 321, 328, 329, 338, 340, 533, 549, 551, 563, 575
Armstrong, D.J. 56, 71
Arnold, J. 168, 178, 179, 182, 436, 449
Aronson, E. 127, 138
Arrow, H. 27, 42, 43, 44, 45, 47, 48, 50, 58, 65, 67, 68, 73
Arundale, R.B. 47, 48
Arvonen, J. 333, 340
As, D. 482, 498
Asch, S.E. 60, 61, 64, 71, 127, 128, 130, 138, 250, 278, 479, 497
Ashforth, B.E. 377, 394, 411, 414, 416, 417
Ashmos, D.P. 173, 174, 175, 176, 182
Ashton, N. 66, 74
Astley, W.G. 456, 469
Atkin, R.S. 113, 116
Atsumi, T. 135–6, 138
Atwater, L.E. 200, 217, 219, 220
Austin, 178
Austin, J.T. 286, 297, 310
Austin, W. 399, 417
Avolio, B.J. 200, 202, 203, 204, 209, 210, 211, 212, 216, 220, 223
Axelson, R. 162, 182
Axley, S.R. 459, 469
Ayman, R. 199, 202, 203, 205, 208, 220, 479, 497
Azumi, K. 229–30, 246

AUTHOR INDEX

Baal, T. 379, 395
Bacharach, S.B. 169, 182
Back, K. 64, 72
Badke-Schaub, P. 103, 110, 116
Baker, D.P. 517, 525, 526
Baker, M.R. 374, 396
Baldwin, T.T. 505, 511, 528
Bales, R.F. 5, 19, 28, 38, 48, 108, 116, 535, 536, 541, 547, 551
Balke, W.M. 399, 417
Bamforth, K.W. 233, 246, 248, 257, 258, 259, 281, 349, 352, 366
Bandura, A. 106, 116, 178, 179, 183, 235, 241, 246, 319, 320, 328, 340, 569–70, 575
Banet, A.G. 535, 540–1, 551
Bantel, K.A. 67, 71, 132, 138, 320, 325, 343, 511, 525, 529
Barker, J.R. 237, 241
Barley, S.R. 36, 48
Barling, J. 346, 364
Barnd, S.E. 295, 310
Barnes-Farrell, J.L. 564, 565, 578
Barnett, G.A. 459, 469
Barnett, W.P. 63, 67, 73
Baron, R.A. 64, 72, 86, 87, 92
Barratt, F.J. 180, 183, 549, 551, 552
Barrett, G.V. 125, 138
Barrick, M.R. 228, 229, 242
Barron, F. 136, 138, 320, 340
Barry, D. 106, 111, 120, 563, 578
Bartlett, C.A. 491, 497
Bartunek, J.M. 406, 419
Bass, B.M. 126, 138, 190, 191, 198, 199, 200, 201, 202, 203, 204, 208, 209, 210, 211, 212, 213, 215, 216, 220, 223, 224, 510, 520, 525
Bateman, T.S. 228, 246
Batstone, E. 411, 412
Batt, R. 12, 13, 17, 19
Beamish, P. 485, 499
Beard, R.L. 350, 366, 505, 506–8, 510, 514, 515, 529
Beaumont, P.B. 237, 242
Beck, K. 520, 526
Becker, A.S. 231, 242
Becker, T.E. 373, 374, 376, 394
Beckmann, J. 103, 116
Bedeian, A.G. 355, 357, 360, 365
Beehr, T.A. 358, 360, 362, 364
Beekun, R.I. 6, 19, 236, 242, 353, 362, 523, 525
Beer, M. 505, 514, 525
Begley, T.A. 375, 394

Bell, C.H. 176, 184, 514, 526, 565, 570
Bem, S. 484, 497
Benington, J. 400, 419
Benne, K.D. 539–40, 544, 547, 551
Bennis, W.G. 540, 541, 543, 546, 551
Berdahl, J.L. 44, 45, 47, 50, 58, 65, 68, 73
Berg, D.N. 535, 543–4, 552
Berger, C.R. 453, 469
Berger, J. 58, 59, 61, 71
Berggren, C. 353, 362
Berlew, D.E. 425, 448
Berry, P.C. 132, 140
Berscheid, E. 63, 71, 196, 204, 208, 220
Bertalanffy, L.V. 248, 278
Bettenhausen, K.L. 41, 48, 89, 91, 226, 242, 294, 310
Bexton, W.H. 147, 152, 158
Beyer, J.M. 399, 421
Bellig, M. 405, 417
Billings, R.S. 373, 376, 394, 564, 565, 575
Bion, W.R. xxix, 6, 19, 28, 38, 48, 144, 145, 150–1, 153, 158, 329, 340, 398, 399, 417, 534, 535, 543, 548, 551
Bitz, D.S. 66, 73
Blackler, F.H.M. 170, 175, 183
Blake, R.R. 129, 138, 409, 413, 417, 418
Blake, R.P. 408, 418
Blaney, P.H. 86, 90
Blau, P.M. 467, 469
Blickensderfer, E.L. 506–7, 517, 528
Block, C.H. 132, 140
Blood, M.R. 240, 244
Bluen, S.D. 407, 418
Blumberg, M. 232, 234, 242, 249, 263, 274–6, 278
Bobko, 178
Bochner, S. 491, 496, 498
Bodenhausen, G.V. 34, 48
Bond, M.H. 479, 480, 484, 489, 498, 500
Bond, R. 480, 484, 498
Bonett, D.G. 571, 579
Booth, P. 384, 386–7, 394
Borastone, I. 412, 417
Borman, W.C. 286, 287, 291, 297, 300, 305, 307, 310, 512, 526, 528
Boss, R.W. 514, 526
Botman, H.I. 356, 365
Bottger, P.C. 563, 575
Bourgeois, L.J. 70, 71
Bourhis, R.Y. 413, 418, 420
Bouwen, R. xxxii, 177, 183, 495, 560
Bowers, C. 517, 526
Bowers, K.S. 80, 90
Bowman, E.D. 520, 527

Braaten, D.O. 485, 500
Bradach, J.L. 466, 469
Brady, G.F. 232, 242
Bramel, D. 229, 242
Brannick, M.T. 517, 526
Brass, D.J. 63, 64, 71
Bray, R.M. 113, 116
Breaugh, J.A. 231, 242
Brett, J.M. 404, 411, 418, 442, 448
Brewer, M.B. 69, 71, 402, 404, 418
Brewer, N. 520, 526
Bridger 154
Brief, A.P. 81, 83, 84, 89, 90, 91, 346, 362
Briggs, G.E. 104, 121, 564, 579
Brilhart, J.K. 109, 116
Brim, O.G., Jr. 423, 424, 426, 427, 428, 448
Brislin, R. 494, 498
Brockner, J. 228, 242
Brodbeck, F.C. xxx, 295, 310, 345, 557, 558, 568
Broedling, L. 239, 244
Brousseau, K.R. 103, 111, 118, 274, 278, 563, 570
Brown, C. 170, 175, 183
Brown, G.R. 353, 366
Brown, M.H. 461, 469
Brown, R. 113, 116, 240, 242, 402, 404, 408, 409, 413, 418, 419
Brownell, J. 160, 184
Browning, L.D. 182, 187
Bruggemann, A. 272, 278, 346, 362
Bruggink, G.M. 505, 526
Bruning, N.S. 229, 242, 356, 366
Bryne, D. 81, 90
Buch, K. 229, 242
Bucklow, M. 233, 242
Buller, P.F. 514, 526
Bullinger, H.J. 262, 278
Bunce, D. 559, 575
Bungard, W. 255, 262, 278
Bunning, R.L. 28, 48
Burke, M.J. 83, 90
Burke, P.J. 81, 90
Burke, R.J. 359, 361, 366, 402, 418
Burningham, C. 567, 575
Burns, J.M. 199, 200, 202, 203, 209, 211, 220
Burns, R.N. 162, 183
Burns, T. 399, 404, 418
Burnstein, E. 135–6, 138
Burt, R.S. 462, 469
Bush, J.B. 467, 469
Bushe, G.R. 505, 526

Buss, A.H. 565, 575
Byham, W.C. 231, 232, 246
Byosiere, P. 358, 364, 569, 577
Byrne, D. 63, 71, 195, 196, 203, 207, 220

Caldwell, D.F. 10, 19, 63, 65, 67, 71, 73, 324, 325, 340, 388–9, 394, 538–9, 551, 564, 575
Callan, V. 481, 492, 499
Callus, R. 226, 242
Campbell, A. 347, 362
Campbell, D.T. 130, 138, 349, 362
Campbell, J.P. 132, 138, 286, 287, 289, 290, 298, 300, 307, 310, 512, 513, 526
Campbell, R.J. 286, 287, 289, 290, 298, 300, 307
Campion, M.A. 10, 11, 19, 236, 237, 238, 242, 245, 348, 351, 352, 354, 357, 358, 361, 363, 366, 381, 383, 394, 396, 510, 522, 524, 526, 557, 575
Canon-Bowers, J.A. xxxii, 18, 19, 86, 90, 506, 512, 513, 516, 517, 518, 519, 526, 528
Canter, D. 103, 121
Caplow, T. 426, 427, 448
Cappella, J.N. 34, 48
Carnall, C.A. 179, 183, 231, 239, 242
Carnevale, P.J. 64, 71
Carson, R.C. 80, 90
Carver, C.S. 565, 575, 578
Cashman, J.F. 199, 221
Castore, C. 351, 366
Catano, V.M. 356, 361
Chaffe, S.H. 453, 469
Chao, G.T. 427, 428, 444, 448
Chapple, E.D. 34, 48
Chase, R. 234, 245
Chatman, J.A. 382, 394, 428, 448
Checkland, P. 167, 183
Chemers, M.M. 199, 202, 203, 205, 208, 220, 479, 497
Cheng, J.L.C. 458, 469
Cheraskin, L. 381, 394
Cherns, A.B. 236, 242, 251, 278
Child, D. 319, 340
Child, J. 170, 183, 493, 498
Chiles, C. 134–5, 140
Choi, C. 486, 498
Christensen, C. 101, 103, 118, 562, 577
Church, A.T. 81, 90
Ciborra, C.U. 175, 176, 183
Cissna, K.N. 28, 48
Clampitt, P.G. 453, 469
Clarke, K.E. 190, 198, 201, 220

Clark, L.A. 79, 83, 85, 91, 93
Clark, M.B. 190, 198, 201, 220
Clark, M.S. 79, 83, 86, 89, 90, 91
Clark, R.D. III. 67, 75
Clauss, A. 102, 117
Clegg, C.W. 173, 183, 239, 242, 257, 258, 259, 281, 353, 354, 367
Clegg, S. 398, 418
Clement, D.E. 62, 71
Cobb, L. 34, 49
Coch, L. 481–2, 498
Cogslier, C.C. 205, 208, 216, 217, 223
Cohen, A. 375, 394, 483, 499
Cohen, B.P. 61, 62, 71, 74
Cohen, J.M. 63, 71
Cohen, S.G. 6, 19, 20, 231, 235, 236, 237, 239, 242, 358, 363, 569, 575
Cole, P. 56, 71
Cole, R.E. 7, 19
Collins, E.B. 5, 19
Colman, A.D. 147, 152, 153, 158
Comer, D.R. 432, 448
Condor, S. 403, 418
Conlon, D.E. 515, 528
Conlon, E.J. 301, 310, 568, 575
Conolly, T. 178, 183, 301, 310, 568, 575
Contractor, N.S. 459, 472
Converse, P.E. 31, 51
Converse, S.A. 517, 526
Cook, R.L. 70, 71
Coons, A.E. 199, 202, 205, 223
Cooper, C.L. 160, 168, 178, 179, 182, 186, 294, 295, 313, 339, 342, 355, 365, 373, 395, 570, 577
Cooper, R. 233, 242
Cooper, W.H. 460, 473
Cooperrider, D.L. 180, 183
Coopey, J.G. 319, 341
Coovert, M.D. 18, 19
Cordery, J.L. xxix, 6, 19, 231, 232, 234, 235, 236, 237, 238, 239, 241, 243, 353, 354, 363, 532, 551, 572
Cordingley, P. 400, 419
Cormeraie, S. 493, 499
Cosier, R.A. 63, 70, 71, 131, 138
Costa, P.T. 78, 79, 91
Cotton, J.L. 13, 19, 351, 363, 522, 526
Cowan, D.A. 60, 71, 565, 575
Cox, 68
Cox, T.H. 484, 498
Coutant-Sassic, D. 28, 52
Craiger, J.P. 18, 19
Cressey, P. 174, 176, 183
Crutchfield, J.H. 62, 74

Cummings, L.L. 516, 526
Cummings, T.G. 90, 91, 239, 243, 257, 258, 263, 274–6, 278, 287, 288, 291, 293, 300, 301, 303, 311, 352, 363, 482, 498
Curphy, G.J. 190, 198, 201, 222
Czajka, J.M. 375, 394

Daft, R.L. 181, 183, 460, 473
Damon, W. 87, 91
D'Andrea Tyson, L. 13, 20
Danowski, J.A. 460, 469
Dansereau, F. 190, 191, 192, 193, 194, 196, 197, 199, 200, 202, 203, 204, 206, 207, 208, 209, 211, 214, 216, 217, 220, 222, 452, 469, 524, 527
Das, T.K. 31, 48, 49
Daubman, K.A. 87, 92
Davids, K. 234, 246
Davidson, M. 402, 418
Davis, G.A. 132, 139
Davis, G.B. 162, 171, 176, 183, 186
Davis, J.A. 460, 469
Davis, J.H. 40, 49
Davis, L.E. 7, 19
de Board, R. 152, 158
de Chalendar, J. 31, 48
Deci, E.L. 136, 138
De Dreu, C.K.W. 133, 138
Deighton, J. 88, 93
Demaree, L.R. 304, 312
Demaree, R.G. 83, 92
De Meuse, K.P. 11, 14, 17, 21, 226, 231, 245, 286, 287, 288, 290, 291, 293, 298, 302, 314, 334, 338, 343, 350, 352, 359–60, 363, 366, 515, 526, 529, 556, 570, 578
Deming, W.E. 9, 19
Demmer, B. 256, 279
De Ninno, J.A. 351, 366
De Nisi, A.S. 305–6, 311
Denison, D.R. 239, 243
Dennis, A.R. 162, 183
De Sanctis, G. 41, 51
Desselles, M.L. 520, 527
Deutsch, M. 128, 130, 138, 376, 394
Deutsch, S.J. 301, 310, 568, 575
Devadas, R. 6, 19, 43, 49, 236, 243, 272, 273, 279, 352, 363, 522, 527
De Vader, C.L. 191, 222
Devine, P.G. 58, 71
de Vries, N.K. 133, 138
Dewar, D.L. 227, 243
Dewey, J. 109, 116

De Wit, B. 485, 498
Diamant, E. 355, 361, 365
Dickson, J.J. 398, 420
Dickson, J.W. 334, 340
Dickson, M.D. 7, 19
Dickson, W.J. 4, 20, 349, 366
Diederiks, J. 352, 366
Diehl, M. 292, 311
Diener, E. 346, 347, 363
Digman, J.M. 81, 91
Dion, K.L. 355, 363
Dobbins, G.H. 356, 367, 374, 396
Dodson, J.D. 133, 140
Dollard, J. 407, 418
Donaldson, 413, 420
Donnellon, 239, 244
Donnellon, A. 402, 407, 418
Dorner, D. 99, 116, 561, 563, 576
Dougherty, D. 132, 138, 324, 341
Dow, G.K. 456, 461, 469
Downs, A. 456, 468, 469
Downs, C.W. 453, 469
Drago, R. 230, 243
Drapeau, R. 227, 245
Drexler, J.A. 460, 470
Dubin, R. 406, 419
Dubinsky, AJ. 191, 193, 194, 195, 196, 197, 199, 200, 203, 204, 207, 208, 209, 210, 211, 212, 216, 224
Duchon, D. 173, 174, 175, 176, 182
Duff, A.R. 179, 183
Duncan, P.C. 518, 526
Duncan, R.D. 335, 343, 467, 473, 572, 576
Dunnette, M.D. 132, 138
Dunphy, D. 460, 470, 547, 552
Durcan, J. 496, 499
Dutton, J.E. 88, 93, 467, 473
Duval, 565, 576
Dwyer, D.J. 359, 366
Dyer, W.G. 359, 363, 514, 526, 539, 551
Dyer-Smith, M.B.A. 149–50, 158
D'Zurilla, T.J. 563, 576

Earley, P.C. 111, 116, 177, 178, 183, 479, 482, 495, 496, 498
Easterbrook, J.A. 133, 136, 138
Eatman, J. 483, 500
Eccles, R.G. 465, 466, 469, 470
Eden, D. 191, 220, 511, 515, 526, 529
Edwards, J.E. 360, 365
Edwards, J.R. 346, 363
Edwards, P.K. 411, 412, 418
Edwards, S.A. 319, 342
Eflal, B. 409, 412, 421

Egan, T.D. 58, 74
Egri, C.P. 330, 341
Ehrlich, S.P. 191, 222
Eils, L.C. 109, 116
Eisenberg, E.M. 457, 459, 462, 466, 470, 472
Eisenhard, K.M. 169, 183
Eisenstat, R.A. 505, 525
Ekegren, G. 178, 183
Ekvall, G. 333, 341
Elchardus, M. 31, 49
ElSalmi, A.M. 516, 526
Emery, F.E. 250, 251, 253, 254, 257, 258, 259, 279
Emery, M. 251, 257, 258, 259, 279
Emler, N. 403, 418
Emmett, D.C. 160, 187
Endler, N.S. 80, 91
Endres, E. 255, 279
Episkopou, D.M. 162, 183
Epple, D. 294, 310
Erber, R. 40, 52
Erez, M. 174, 177, 183, 482, 498
Erffmeyer, R.C. 102, 109, 116
Erickson, B.H. 460, 470
Evans, C.R. 355, 363
Evans, M.G. 199, 203, 206, 220
Everett, J.E. 491, 498
Ewen, R.B. 60, 67, 74

Fabi, B. 230, 243
Fahey, L. 86, 88, 93
Falcione, R.L. 460, 470
Fandt, P.M. 354, 363
Fantasia, R. 414, 418
Farace, R.V. 355, 367
Farace, R.V. 452, 459, 462, 464, 470
Farr, J.L. 178, 183, 286, 305, 312, 320, 328, 338, 341, 343, 319, 442, 450
Farr, R.M. 403, 418
Farsides, T. 413, 418
Featheringham, T.R. 563, 577
Feldman, D.C. 425, 427, 441–2, 445, 446, 448
Feldstein, S. 34, 50
Fenelon, J.R. 62, 72
Fennema, E. 57, 72
Festinger, L. 64, 72, 106, 116
Fiedler, F.E. 162, 184, 198, 199, 202, 203, 205, 208, 220, 221, 333, 341, 489, 498
Filley, A.C. 67, 72
Firestein, R.L. 102, 117
Fisher, C.D. 82, 91, 432, 448
Fisher, R.J. 401, 418

Fiske, D.W. 349, 362
Fiske, J.T. 86, 90
Fiske, S.T. 137, 140
Flanders, A. 276, 279
Flatt, S. 324, 342
Fleischman, E.A. 287, 288, 290, 303, 313, 333, 341
Fletcher, C. 442, 448
Flood, R.L. 173, 184
Ford, C.M. 320, 328, 338, 341
Ford, J.K. 485, 499
Flores, F. 549, 552
Forsythe, D.R. 564, 577
Foster, L.W. 129, 139
Foster, M. 233, 242
Foti, R.J. 191, 222
Foucault, M. 403, 419
Foushee, A.C. 103, 104, 115, 118
Foushee, H.C. 518, 527
Foushee, M.C. 104, 117, 564, 570
Fowlkes, J.E. 517, 519, 526
Frances, J. 456, 466, 470
Franck, 486, 498
Frank, A. 160, 184
Frank, F. 113, 117
Freedman, E.G. 103, 117
French, J.R.J. Jr. 358, 365
French, J.R.P. 460, 470, 481–2, 498
French, W.L. 176, 184, 565, 570
Frenkel, S. 412, 417
Frese, M. 100, 101, 104, 107, 117, 119, 250, 279, 293, 310, 311, 345, 350, 352, 363, 561, 563, 576
Freud, S. 145, 147, 158, 407–8, 419
Frey, D. 135, 139
Friedkin, N.E. 409, 419, 462, 470
Friedman, R. 415, 416, 419
Friend, R. 229, 242
Frohman, A.L. 467, 469
Frone, M.R. 356, 357, 363
Frost, P.J. 200, 202, 209, 222, 330, 341, 399, 419, 461, 470
Fry, L.W. 468, 470
Fry, R. xxxii, 177, 183, 537–8, 539, 551, 560
Fulbright, J.W. 137, 139
Fullerton, T.D. 356, 365
Furnham, A. 491, 496, 498
Futoran, G.C. 34, 35, 50, 106, 112, 117, 118
Futrell, D. 11, 14, 17, 20, 226, 231, 245, 286, 287, 288, 290, 291, 293, 298, 302, 314, 334, 338, 343, 350, 352, 359–60, 366, 515, 529, 556, 570, 578

Gaebler, T. 398, 420
Gaines, J. 356, 363
Galanter, E. 560, 577
Galbraith, J.R. 162, 184, 399, 419, 457, 463, 470
Galanter, E. 100, 107, 119
Gamst, F.C. 47, 49
Ganster, D.C. 102, 117
Garber, S. 384, 394
Garcia, J.E. 199, 202, 205, 221
Gasser, L. 233, 244
Gelfand, M. 483, 501
Geller, M.H. 147, 153, 158
Gemmill, G. 44, 51
George, J.M. xxviii, xxix, 78, 79, 80, 81, 82, 83, 84, 88, 89, 90, 91, 304, 311, 351, 360, 363, 567, 569, 570
Gerard, H.B. 128, 130, 138
Gersick, C.J.G. 35, 40, 46, 49, 102, 103, 104, 106, 114, 117, 294, 311, 387, 391, 392, 394, 541, 544, 551, 559, 566, 576
Geshka, H. 323, 341
Ghiselli, E.E. 67, 72, 308, 311
Ghoshal, S. 491, 497
Gibertini, M. 115, 119
Giddens, A. 182, 184, 411, 419
Gilbreth 144
Giles, H. 399, 421
Gilfallen, D.P. 42, 52
Ginnett, R.C. 190, 198, 201, 222, 391, 394
Ginsberg, A. 70, 72
Gladstein, D.L. (*see also* Ancona, D.L.) 10, 19, 287, 288, 289–290, 292, 302, 303, 306, 311, 345, 350, 351, 353, 354, 363, 506, 511, 527, 533, 535, 538–9, 547, 551, 556, 557, 576
Glick, W.H. 304, 311
Globerson, S. 229, 245
Glorieux, I. 31, 49
Godkin, L. 227, 245
Goedvolk, J.G. 177, 184
Gohde, H.E. 255, 279, 280
Goldfried, M.R. 563, 570
Goldhaber, G.M. 463, 470
Goldstein, S.G. 227, 243
Golen, S.P. 453, 471
Gollob, H.F. 304, 311
Gomez-Mejia, L.R. 191, 221
Gonzalez-Roma, V. 355, 365
Goodenow, C. 356, 365
Goodman, P.S. 6, 19, 97, 98, 117, 160, 184, 236, 243, 272, 273, 279, 287, 288, 290, 292, 295, 297, 298, 300, 302, 311,

345, 350, 352, 363, 373, 376, 384, 394, 505–6, 522, 527
Gollwitzer, P.M.   103, 116
Gorman, M.W.   103, 117
Gordon, J.   7, 15, 19
Gottman, J.M.   34, 49
Govindarajan, V.   465, 470
Gowing, M.K.   511, 512, 528
Graen, G.B.   194, 199, 202, 206, 210, 220, 221, 494, 498, 524, 527
Graf, O.   255, 279
Graham, J.W.   200, 202, 209, 221
Grandori, A.   162, 184
Granovetter, M.S.   462, 463, 466, 470
Grau, J.   453, 472
Gray, J.A.   85, 91
Greenberg, C.I.   254, 279
Greene, C.N.   515, 527
Greiner, B.   268, 279
Greller, M.M.   350, 355–6, 363
Griffin, R.W.   227, 228, 229, 243, 246, 482, 501
Griffith-Hughson, T.L.   522, 527
Griffitt, W.   81, 90, 92
Grob, R.   260, 279
Groskurth, P.   272, 278, 346, 362
Gross, A.C.   514, 528
Grossman, M.   28, 52
Gruenfeld, D.H.   40, 49, 50, 515, 528
Guest, D.E.   240, 243
Guetzkow, H.   5, 19, 132, 139, 458, 470
Guilford, J.P.   136, 139, 319, 341
Gulowsen, J.A.   232, 243, 247, 256, 260, 262, 263, 264, 279, 293, 311
Gupta, A.K.   328, 341, 465, 470
Gurly, K.   538, 539, 551
Gustafson, R.   xxx, 326, 340, 482, 497, 567
Guzzo, R.A.   xxviii, xxxi, 4, 5, 7, 11, 13, 18, 19, 21, 98, 117, 160, 184, 236, 240, 243, 286, 287, 288, 291, 293, 300, 301, 306, 311, 312, 313, 314, 328, 331, 338, 341, 345, 350, 352, 354, 355, 364, 366, 373, 394, 398, 419, 506, 527, 533, 538, 567, 576
Gyllenhammer, P.G.   7, 19
Gyr, J.   132, 139

Hacker, K.I.   103, 117
Hacker, W.   100, 101, 102, 104, 106, 107, 117, 249, 251, 253, 268, 279, 293, 312, 350, 364, 366, 561, 576
Hackman, J.R.   5, 8, 10, 11, 19, 20, 40, 49, 90, 92, 96, 97, 98, 102, 103, 104, 105, 111, 106, 114, 117, 118, 237, 239, 132,

133, 139, 160–1, 162, 172, 184, 186, 226, 235, 238, 239, 240, 243, 251, 257, 258, 259, 273–4, 279, 280, 287, 288, 289, 290, 291, 292, 293, 294, 296, 297, 300, 301, 302, 303, 305, 306, 311, 312, 337, 338, 341, 345, 347, 349, 350, 351, 352, 354, 355, 364, 387, 391, 392, 394, 395, 504, 508, 527, 535, 536, 548, 551, 556, 557, 562, 563, 568, 576
Haga, W.J.   194, 199, 202, 220, 524, 527
Hage, J.   458, 468, 469, 470
Hales, C.   398, 404, 419
Hall, D.F.   129, 139
Hall, D.T.   425, 448
Hall, E.R.   60, 67, 74
Hall, F.S.   129, 139
Hall, R.J.   195, 196, 203, 204, 207, 208, 217, 221, 222
Halton, W.   145–6, 158
Hambrick, D.C.   57, 59, 72
Hammer, M.R.   495, 498, 510, 522, 527
Hammond, K.R.   70, 71, 399, 417
Hampden-Turner, C.   481, 498
Handfinger, R.   28, 49
Hanlon, S.C.   386, 395
Hanna, C.   40, 51
Harburg, E.   67, 72, 332, 341
Hardy, G.E.   562, 575
Hare, A.P.   27, 28, 38, 49
Harkins, S.   292, 312, 479, 499
Harmon, J.   40, 49
Harper, J.   493, 499
Harrington, D.M.   320, 340
Harris, D.H.   11, 20
Harris, E.F.   333, 341
Hart, P.M.   355, 364
Hartley, J.F.   xxxi, 400, 406, 407, 409, 412, 414, 415, 419, 574
Hartley, S.W.   216, 224
Hartman, R.L.   462, 466, 471
Hartwig, R.   169, 184
Hattem, E.   229, 245
Hattrup, K.   304, 312
Havelin, A.   63, 75
Hay, M.   31, 49
Hayes, D.P.   34, 49
Haythorn, W.W.   60, 72
Hazama, H.   481, 499
Head, T.C.   229, 243
Hedburg, B.L.T.   564, 576
Heemstra, F.J.   172, 184
Heider, F.   195, 203, 207, 221
Heinen, J.S.   28, 49
Heller, F.A.   162, 173, 174, 180, 184

AUTHOR INDEX

Hellpach, W.   253, 280
Helmreich, R.L.   486, 500, 518, 519, 527, 529
Helson, H.   322, 341
Henderson, C.M.   88, 93
Henry   151
Herbst, P.G.   233, 243, 258, 259, 280
Herden, R.P.   460, 470
Hermann, C.F.   9, 20
Herriot, P.   435, 436, 442, 448
Hesketh, B.   298, 299, 306, 312
Hess, T.   228, 242
Hesse, B.W.   36, 49
Hewstone, M.   400, 408, 419
Hickson, D.J.   162, 184
Higgs, A.C.   10, 11, 19, 236, 237, 242, 348, 351, 352, 357, 358, 361, 363, 510, 522, 524, 526, 557, 575
Hill, G.W.   5, 20, 61, 72, 292, 303, 312
Hill, K.D.   239, 244
Hill, S.   227, 229, 243
Hiller, E.   412, 414, 419
Hinkin, T.   191, 221
Hirokawa, R.Y.   109, 110, 118, 563, 576
Hirsch, G.   486, 492, 495, 501
Hinshelwood, R.D.   145, 152, 158
Hirschheim, R.   177, 184
Hirschhorn, L.   147, 158
Hirschman, A.O.   388, 395
Hirschman, C.   61, 73
Hinsz, V.   40, 49
Hochschild, A.R.   144, 158
Hodson, R.   237, 243
Hoffman, E.   64, 72
Hoffman, L.R.   60, 67, 72, 109, 118, 132, 139, 332, 341, 342, 563, 564, 577
Hofman, D.A.   178, 183
Hofstede, G.   479–80, 481, 495, 496, 499
Hogg, M.A.   402, 404, 408, 409, 417, 419
Holbeck, J.   335, 343, 467, 473
Holland, J.L.   80, 92
Hollander, E.P.   190, 194, 195, 196, 198, 199, 200, 201, 202, 203, 204, 206, 207, 208, 212–13, 221
Hollingshead, A.B.   10, 15, 20, 36, 37, 40, 45, 49, 50, 51
Holstein, L.W.   453, 473
Hom, P.W.   199, 206, 222
Homans, G.H.   6, 20, 199, 203, 206, 221, 399, 419, 459, 471, 534
Hopkins,   403, 418
Horwitz, L.   146, 158
Horwitz, M.   401–2, 404, 420
Hosking, D.   403, 419

Hotz-Hart, B.   276, 280
House, J.S.   350, 358, 364, 365
House, R.J.   67, 72, 179, 184, 198, 199, 200, 202, 203, 204, 206, 209, 210, 211, 212, 221, 222
Hovland, C.   128, 139
Howard, H.   60, 74
Howell, J.M.   200, 202, 209, 222
Hughes, R.L.   190, 198, 201, 222
Hughson, T.L.G.   6, 19, 352, 363
Hughson, T.G.   236, 243
Hughson, T.L.   272, 273, 279
Hui, C.H.   489, 501
Hulbert, L.   41, 49
Hulin, C.L.   177, 183, 240, 244, 346, 364
Hull, F.   229–230, 246
Hunt, D.   80
Hunt, J.G.   191, 222
Hunt, S.D.   374, 395
Hunter, J.E.   304, 314
Hwang, K.K.   479, 498
Hyde, J.S.   57, 72

Ibarra, H.   63, 64, 72, 381, 395
Iles, P.A.   442, 448
Ilgen, D.R.   97, 98, 100, 105, 115, 118, 119, 298, 313
Inman, T.H.   453, 471
Innami, I.   86, 88, 92
Insko, C.A.   42, 50
Isaacs, S.   145, 158
Isen, A.M.   64, 71, 72, 86, 87, 89, 91, 92
Israel, J.   482, 498
Ives, B.   168, 174, 175, 176, 177, 184
Izumi, H.   12, 13, 20

Jaastad, K.   132, 138
Jablin, F.M.   64, 73, 456, 467, 471
Jackofsky, E.F.   355, 364
Jackson, J.W.   409, 419
Jackson, M.C.   173, 184
Jackson, P.R.   234, 237, 283, 240, 246
Jackson, S.E.   xxviii, 57, 59, 66, 67, 68, 69, 71, 72, 126, 132, 138, 139, 324, 341, 351, 356, 364, 365, 483, 485, 499, 511, 525, 527, 566, 567, 569
Jacobs, T.O.   199, 203, 206, 222
Jacobsen, A.   127
Jacobson, E.   28, 49
Jaeggi, C.   112, 114, 118, 120
Jaffe, J.   34, 50
Jaffe, M.P.   61, 72
Jago, A.G.   169, 174, 175, 176, 180, 187, 199, 202, 205, 206, 223

James, L.R. 80, 83, 84, 91, 92, 304, 311, 312, 349, 364, 460, 471
Janis, I.L. 63, 73, 103, 104, 109, 118, 128, 130, 131, 139, 170, 184, 328, 341, 376, 395, 444, 448, 494, 499, 564, 576
Jaques, E. 146, 148–9, 158, 250, 280
Javian, S. 232, 242
Jehn, K.A. 106, 120
Jensen, M.A.C. 28, 46, 52, 294, 314, 331, 343, 552
Jenish, D. 383, 395
Jermier, J.M. 191, 222, 356, 363
Jervis, I.L. 564, 576
Jessup, L.M. 36, 50
Jette, R.D. 13, 19, 236, 243, 299, 311
Jex, S.M. 359, 366
Jick, T.D. 126, 139
Jochem, L.M. 109, 116
John, R.S. 109, 116
Johns, G. 376, 395
Johnson, A.L. 505, 526
Johnson, B.M. 457, 471
Johnson, D. xxxi, 562, 565, 576
Johnson, F. 565, 576
Johnston, J. 517, 518, 528
Johnson, J.D. 452, 453, 454, 457, 459, 462, 463, 464, 467, 466, 468, 470, 471, 473
Johnson, J.R. 453, 472
Johnston, W.A. 104, 121, 564, 579
Johnston, W.B. 61, 73
Jones, A.P. 460, 471
Jones, D.T. 254, 282
Jones, J.M. 34, 50
Jones, L.E. 96, 117
Jones, M.B. 303, 312
Jones, M.R. 33, 35, 50
Jones, S.D. 299, 312
Joyce, W.F. 460, 471
Judd, B.B. 232, 242
Judge, T.A. 346, 364
Juralewicz, R.S. 482, 499

Kabanoff, B. 96, 118
Kahn, R.L. 113, 118, 199, 202, 205, 222, 287, 312, 358, 364, 452, 458, 471, 508, 514, 527, 569, 577
Kahn, W.A. 560, 577
Kalleberg, A.L. 13, 20
Kanfer, R. 178, 184, 185
Kanki, B.B. 519, 529
Kanki, B.G. 103, 104, 115, 118
Kano, N. 228, 244
Kanter, R.M. 56, 58, 73, 126, 139, 144, 158, 176, 185, 379, 392, 395, 454, 457, 467, 468, 471
Karesek, R.A. 234, 241, 244, 345, 352, 364
Karsh, B. 412, 419
Kashima, Y. 481, 492, 499
Kasl, S.V. 349, 360, 364
Katelaar, T. 85, 92
Katerberg, R. 199, 206, 222
Katz, D. 113, 118, 199, 202, 205, 222, 452, 458, 471, 508, 527
Katz, P.A. 61, 73
Katz, R. 326, 341, 434, 448, 566, 577
Katzell, R.A. 13, 19, 236, 243, 299, 311
Katzenbach, J.R. 8, 20, 533, 536, 552
Kaufman, G.M. 358, 364
Keating, D.E. 239, 244
Keck, S.L. 73
Keeley, M.A. 301, 312
Keller, R.T. 356, 364, 515, 527
Keller, W.J. 171, 185
Kellett, S. 568, 572, 578
Kelley, J.R. 294, 313
Kelloway, E.K. 346, 364
Kelly, C. 408, 409, 410, 419
Kelly, J.R. 34, 35, 36, 47, 50, 51, 106, 112, 117, 118, 233, 244, 407, 408, 409, 410, 412, 413, 415, 419
Kemp, N.J. 257, 258, 259, 280
Kennedy, R. 131
Kenney, D.A. 304, 312
Kent, R.N. 96, 97, 118
Keppel, G. 136, 140
Kerr, N.L. 113, 116
Kerr, S. 67, 72, 191, 193, 198, 199, 202, 205, 222, 223, 239, 244
Kerschberg, L. 162, 187
Kerwin, A. 453, 471
Kidder, D.L. 435, 449
Kiesler, S.B. 132, 139, 324, 342, 564, 577
Kiggundu, M.V. 238, 244
Kiggundu, M.N. 287, 288, 293, 297, 300, 312, 350, 364
Kim, H. 191, 222
Kim, K.I. 480, 484, 499
Kincaird, D.L. 462, 473
King, N. 319, 333, 335, 340, 342, 351, 364
Kinlaw, D.C. 383, 395
Kirchmeyer, C. 483, 484, 499
Kirkbride, P. 411, 419
Kirkbridge, P.S. 496, 499
Kirsch, C. 264, 280
Kirshnan, A.R. 491, 498
Klandermans, B. 407, 419

AUTHOR INDEX

Klein, H.K. 177, 187
Klein, J.A. 237, 238, 244
Klein, K.J. 200, 202, 203, 209, 210, 217, 222
Klein, K.K. 13, 20
Klein, M. 147, 152, 158
Klimoski, R. 86, 87, 88, 90, 92
Knorr, K.D. 333, 342
Ko, J. 374, 396
Koenig, R. Jr. 160, 186
Kogan, N. 319, 343
Kolb, D.M. 402, 406, 407, 418, 419
Kolb, J.A. 333–4, 342
Kolodny, H.F. 287, 288, 293, 297, 300, 302, 312, 350, 364
Komaki, J.L. 520, 527
Koonce, R. 520, 527
Kopelman, R.E. 511, 527
Korsgaard, M.A. 373, 395
Kotter, J.P. 175, 185
Kötter, W. 255, 279, 280
Koopman, P.L. xxix, 162, 169, 170, 172, 173, 174, 182, 185, 187, 565
Kornhauser, A. 406, 419
Korteweg, S.M. 179, 185
Kozlowski, S.W.J. 304, 312, 380, 381, 382, 395, 425, 428, 432, 433, 443–4, 449, 519, 520, 527
Kraar, L. 127, 139
Krackhardt, D. 458, 471
Kraiger, K. 485, 499
Kraly, E.P. 61, 73
Kram, K.E. 64, 73
Kramer, R.M. 402, 418
Kraut, A.I. 390–1, 395
Kreeger, L. 153, 158
Krizner, I.M. 465, 471
Krueger, D.L. 483, 501
Kruger, L.J. 356, 365
Kuk, G. 571, 577
Kumar, K. 65, 75, 351, 367, 483–4, 485, 494, 501
Kurchner-Hawkins, R. 355, 367
Kurowski, L.L. 483, 501
Kwan, J. 133, 136, 140
Kwun, S.K. 239, 245
Kylen, S. 329, 330–1, 342

Labouvie-Vief 56
Labich, K. 127, 139
Lachman, R. 355, 361, 365
La Follette, M.C. 453, 471
Lalonde, R.M. 400, 420
Lamon, S.J. 57, 72

La Rocco, J.M. 358, 365
Landsberger, H.A. 108, 110, 118, 563, 577
Lane, H. 485, 499
Lane, I.L. 102, 109, 116
Lane, T. 412, 414, 419
Landy, F.J. 286, 305, 312
Lanzara, G.F. 175, 176, 183
Lanzetta, J.T. 104, 114, 118
Larsen, R.J. 85, 92
Larson, J.R. 101, 103, 107, 111, 118, 562, 577
Lase, 564
Latané, B. 292, 312, 479, 499
Latham, G.P. 106, 119, 129, 141, 162, 177, 178, 185, 241, 244
Laughlin, P.R. 61, 66, 73
Laurent, A. 491, 496, 499
La Voie, L. 304, 312
Lawler, E.E. 7, 20, 162, 172, 184, 186, 226, 227, 229, 230, 235, 239, 243, 244, 245, 251, 280, 533, 552
Lawler, E.J. 169, 182
Lawrence, B.S. 57, 58, 64, 73, 75, 324, 343
Lawrence, P.R. 398, 404, 419, 452, 458, 459, 463, 471
Lawson, M.B. 376, 394
Lazarus, R.S. 86, 92
Lazenga, E. 40, 50
Leary, M.R. 564, 577
Leavitt, H.J. 4, 7, 20, 165, 185
Ledford, G.E. 6, 7, 19, 20, 226, 244
Ledford, S.G. 231, 236, 237, 242
Lee, A.M. 457, 471
Lee, D.M. 295, 310
Leedom, D. 518–19, 527
Lehner, F. 277, 280
Leiba, S. 485, 499
Leiter, M.P. 349, 356, 358, 359, 361, 365, 366
Leitner, K. 268, 279, 280
Leyden, D.P. 384, 394
Lietner, K. 352, 365
Lerner, D. 192, 196, 222
Levacic, R. 465, 471
Leviatan, N. 191, 220
Levine, D.I. 13, 20
Levine, J.M. 9, 13, 20, 29, 40, 50, 51, 62, 63, 73, 103, 119, 126, 139, 424, 425, 436–8, 439, 448, 449, 534, 550, 552, 563, 564, 565, 577
Levine, R.V. 34, 50, 492, 499
Levy, L.H. 132, 139

Lewin, K. 255–6, 280, 352, 365, 398, 400, 401, 420, 490, 499, 534
Lewis, M. 80, 92
Lewis, R.S. 453, 472
Liang, D.W. 40, 50
Lieberman, M.A. 543, 552
Lieberman, S. 105–6, 118
Liebowitz, S.J. 359, 363, 515, 526
Liff, S. 410, 420
Likert, R. 198, 199, 202, 205, 222, 463, 472, 533, 552
Lillibridge, J.R. 235, 246
Lincoln, J.R. 64, 73
Linn, M.C. 57, 72
Little, B.R. 80, 90
Little, L. 232, 234, 244
Littlepage, G.E. 113, 118
Liverpool, P.R. 229, 242, 244
Lloyd, J. 414, 417
Lloyd, R.F. 228, 245
Lobel, S. 484, 498
Locke, E.A. 106, 111, 119, 120, 174, 177, 178, 185, 187, 241, 244, 482, 499, 563, 578
Lodahl, T.M. 67, 72
Lorsch, J. 398, 404, 419
Lord, R.G. 103, 119, 191, 195, 196, 203, 204, 207, 208, 221, 222, 306, 312
Lorenz, E.H. 465, 472
Lorge, I. 303, 312
Lorsch, J.W. 452, 458, 459, 463, 471
Lott, A.J. 63, 73, 351, 365
Lott, B.E. 63, 73, 351, 365
Louis, M.R. 380, 395, 424, 425, 426, 427, 429–31, 432, 435, 444, 448, 449, 450
Lovelace, R.F. 325, 342
Lowe, C.A. 564, 565, 578
Lucas, R. 460, 472
Lyles, M.A. 564, 565, 577
Lynn, 413, 420
Lynskey, M. 486, 498

Maass, A. 445, 449
Mabee, T. 459, 462, 470
Macduffie, J.P. 226, 244
Machatka, D.E. 36, 51
Machleit, V. 400, 419
Mackie, D.M. 402, 408, 420
Mackie, M. 491, 500
MacKenzie, S.B. 191, 222
Macy, B.A. 12, 13, 20, 523, 527, 272, 280
Mael, F. 377, 394, 411, 414, 416, 417
Magjuka, R.J. 505, 511, 528
Magro, A.P. 131, 140

Mahoney, T.A. 300, 312
Maier, N.R.F. 60, 67, 72, 109, 118, 129, 132, 139, 331–2, 332–3, 341, 342, 563, 564, 577
Maier, R.A. 563, 577
Main, J. 564, 577
Majchrzak, A. 233, 244
Major, B. 356, 357, 363
Malik, S.D. 29, 30, 52, 423, 424, 439–40, 450
Mann, L. 109, 118
Mann, R.D. 28, 38, 50
Manning, F.J. 356, 365
Mansfield, R. 460, 472
Manski, M.E. 132, 139
Manz, C.C. 200, 202, 210, 222, 235, 239, 241, 244, 482, 499
March, J.G. 457, 472
Mark, M.M. 302, 312
Markham, I.S. 200, 202, 204, 210, 211, 222
Markham, S.E. 191, 193, 194, 196, 199, 200, 202, 204, 206, 207, 208, 210, 211, 214, 216, 217, 220, 222, 224, 304, 315, 452, 469
Markoczy, L. 493, 498
Marks, M.L. 228, 244
Markus, H. 137, 139
Markus, M.L. 175, 185
Marrett, C.B. 458, 470
Marrow, A.J. 482, 500, 534, 552
Marshall, A.A. 453, 472
Martell, R.F. 306, 312, 313
Martin, E. 253, 278
Martin, J.N. 495, 498
Martin, R. 133, 139
Martin, T.N. 356, 365
Martineau, J.W. 506, 528
Maslach, C. 356, 365
Mason, P.A. 57, 59, 72
Mastenbroek, W.F.G. 179, 180, 185, 406, 420
Mathieu, J.E. 375, 395, 506, 528
May, K.E. 57, 59, 72, 132, 139
McCain, B.E. 67, 73, 351, 365
McCall, G.J. 403, 420
McCarrey, M.W. 319, 342
McCarthy, M.E. 356, 366
McClain, T.M. 89, 93
McClean Parks, J. 435, 448
McConkie, M.L. 514, 526
McCrae, R.R. 78, 79, 81, 91, 92
McDaniel, R.R. 173, 174, 175, 176, 182, 187

AUTHOR INDEX

McFarlan, F.W.   162, 173, 176, 185
McFarlane Shore, L.   435, 443, 449
McGrath, J.   xxviii, 5, 10, 11, 15, 20, 26, 27, 33, 34, 35, 36, 37, 38, 40, 42, 43, 44, 45, 47, 48, 49, 50, 51, 58, 65, 67, 68, 73, 96, 97, 98, 105, 106, 108, 112, 117, 118, 119, 133, 139, 285, 289, 294, 296, 297–8, 310, 313, 338, 342, 347, 359, 365, 399, 420, 488, 489, 515, 528, 547, 552, 556, 557, 559, 566
McGuinness, T.   465, 472
McIntyre, R.M.   520, 528
McKeen, J.D.   162, 186
McKersie, R.B.   415, 422
McLeod, P.L.   484, 498
McMillan, C.J.   162, 185
McMillian, J.J.   461, 469
McPherson, J.M.   63, 73
McShane, S.L.   379, 395
Mead, G.H.   403, 420
Medsker, G.J.   10, 11, 19, 236, 237, 242, 348, 351, 352, 354, 357, 358, 361, 363, 510, 522, 524, 526, 557, 575
Megaree, E.I.   62, 72
Meindl, J.R.   191, 222
Meissner, M.   104, 119
Menzies Lyth, I.   146, 147
Merrith, A.C.   486, 500
Messer, H.M.   173, 187
Messick, D.M.   402, 408, 420
Meyer, D.C.   386, 395
Meyer, H.D.   490, 500
Meyer, G.D.   399, 417
Meyer, G.J.   78, 92
Meyer, J.P.   299, 314, 373, 375, 376, 394, 395
Meyer, R.   485, 498
Miceli, M.P.   564, 577
Michael, R.   319, 342
Michaelsen, L.K.   351, 367, 483–4, 485, 949, 501
Milburn, T.W.   564, 565, 575
Miller, E.J.   155, 156, 158, 233, 245, 398, 405, 420
Miller, G.A.   100, 107, 119, 560, 577
Miller, J.G.   191, 192, 196, 222
Miller, V.D.   64, 73, 453, 472
Mills, T.M.   38, 51
Miner, J.B.   178, 185
Minor, M.J.   462, 472
Mintzberg, H.   103, 110, 119, 160, 161, 169, 172, 185, 399, 404, 420
Michaelson, L.K.   65, 75
Mischel, W.   79, 80, 92, 97, 119

Misumi, J.   479, 481, 492, 500
Mitchell, D.R.D.   350, 356, 363
Mitchell, J.C.   452, 462, 472
Mitchell, T.R. 199, 203, 206, 221
Mitroff, I.I.   563, 564, 577
Mobley, W.H.   80, 92
Moch, M.K.   350, 365, 463, 472
Moeller, A.   305, 313
Moghaddam, F.M.   400, 401, 402, 403, 407, 409, 411, 413, 420, 421
Mohammed, S.   86, 87, 88, 90, 92
Mohrman, A.M.   13, 20
Mohrman, S.A.   7, 13, 20, 226, 227, 229, 230, 244, 245
Molloy, E.S.   256, 258, 278
Monge, P.R.   452, 453, 459, 462, 466, 470, 472
Moody, J.W.   13, 20
Moreland, R.L.   9, 20, 29, 40, 50, 51, 62, 63, 73, 126, 103, 119, 139, 424, 425, 436–8, 439, 439, 448, 449, 534, 550, 552, 563, 564, 565, 577
Morgan, G.   456, 461, 472, 548, 549, 552
Morgan, R.M.   374, 395
Morgan, R.T.   485, 490, 500
Morley, I.   403, 415, 419, 420
Morris, C.G.   5, 20, 90, 92, 96, 102, 103, 117, 119, 133, 139, 160–1, 184, 338, 341, 345, 350, 355, 364, 536, 548, 551, 556, 562, 576
Morris, W.N.   89, 92
Morrison, E.W.   380, 395, 425, 433–4, 443, 449
Moscovici, S.   180, 186, 403, 418, 420
Mosier, K.   134–5, 140
Mossholder, K.W.   355, 357, 360, 365
Motowidlo, S.J.   512, 526
Mouton, J.S.   129, 138, 408, 409, 413, 417, 418
Mucchi-Faina, A.   445, 449
Mueller, G.F.   104, 119
Mueller, W.S.   6, 19, 236, 237, 243, 353, 354, 363, 532, 551
Mugny, G.   180, 186
Mullen, B.   294, 295, 313, 339, 342, 355, 365, 373, 395, 570, 577
Mumby, D.K.   461, 472
Mumford, E.   174, 186
Murnighan, J.K.   41, 48, 294, 310, 515, 528
Murray, N.   87, 92

Nadler, D.A.   172, 186
Nahavandi, A.   385, 395, 504, 523, 528
Nalbantian, H.   9, 20

Naughton, T.J. 216, 224, 304, 315, 356, 367
Naumann, J.D. 162, 186
Naylor, J.C. 98, 100, 119, 298, 313
Near, J.P. 564, 577
Neck, C.P. 200, 202, 204, 210, 211, 222
Neider, L.L. 205, 206, 208, 216, 217, 223, 520, 529
Neilsen, E.H. 540, 541–2, 546, 552
Nelson, D.L. 425, 430, 431, 449
Nelson, R.E. 381, 395, 408, 420
Nemeth, C.J. xxix, 63, 73, 125, 128, 133, 134–5, 136, 140, 180, 186, 445, 449, 494, 500, 562, 574
Neuman, G.A. 238, 245, 360, 365
Newell, A. 109, 119
Newman, J.R. 89, 93
Nicholls, J.G. 319, 342
Nicholson, N. 407, 409, 412, 414, 415, 419, 426, 436, 444, 449, 569, 577
Nieva, V.F. 287, 288, 290, 303, 313
Nijhof, H. 181, 186
Nkomo, D. 68
Noakes, J. xxxi, 215–16, 566
Nohria, N. 466, 472
Nolan, L.L. 515, 529
Norman, W.T. 81, 92
Novak, M. 194, 199, 202, 206, 221
Nowicki, C.E. 82, 93
Nowicki, G.P. 87, 92
Noyes, C. 133, 139
Numerof, R.E. 359, 365
Nystrom, H. 325, 333, 341, 342
Nystrom, P.. 564, 576

Obert, S.L. 540, 541–2, 546, 552
Obholzer, A. 153, 155, 158
O'Brien, G.E. 96, 118, 234, 245
Ochsenbein, G. 100, 101, 102, 103, 104, 105, 107, 113–14, 120
O'Connor, E. 292, 294, 313
O'Connor, K.M. xxviii, 37, 45, 49, 50, 515, 528, 359, 488, 489, 556, 557, 559, 566
Oesterreich, R. 101, 119, 256, 264, 268, 280
Offerman, L.R. 511, 512, 528
Ohmae, K. 491, 500
Oldham, G.R. 98, 105, 117, 235, 238, 240, 243, 245, 251, 275, 280, 291, 312, 351, 364
O'Leary, V.E. 57, 75
Olivas, L. 453, 471
Olson, E.E. 180, 186

Olson, M.H. 178, 171, 174, 175, 176, 177, 183, 184
Ondrack, D. 485, 499
O'Neill, B. 456, 472
Orasanu, J. 517, 528
O'Reilly, B. 520, 528
O'Reilly, C.A. 59, 63, 66, 67, 73, 74, 75, 126–7, 132, 140, 324, 342, 462, 463, 464, 467, 472, 473, 485, 501
O'Reilly, C.C. III. 351, 365
Osborn, A.F. 131, 140
Osborn, R.N. 191, 222
Osborne, D. 398, 420
Osborne, E. 151, 158
Osterman, P. 226, 239, 245
Ostroff, C. 304, 313, 380, 381, 382, 295, 425, 428, 432, 442, 443–4, 448, 449
Ourth, L. 299, 312
Owens, P. xxix, 562, 574

Packer, A.E. 61, 73
Pages, M. 544, 552
Park, H.J. 484, 499
Parker, S. 234, 235, 243
Parks, M.R. 462, 463, 469
Parsons, C.K. 350, 356, 363
Parsons, T.C. 28, 51
Pasmore, W.A. 234, 236, 245, 256, 257, 258, 280
Pascale, R.T. 515, 528
Patterson, M. 326, 342
Paul, C.F. 514, 528
Payne, R.L. 160, 186, 326, 342, 351, 365, 460, 472
Pearce, J.A. 6, 20, 60, 73, 231, 238, 245, 257, 258, 280, 287, 288, 291, 297, 300, 301, 302, 303, 309, 313, 352, 365
Pearce, J.L. 460–1, 473
Pearson, C.A.L. 236, 245, 353, 356, 365, 522, 528
Peiro, J.M. 355, 365
Pelz, D.C. 67, 74
Pennebaker, J.W. 78, 93
Pennings, J.M. 295, 302, 311
Perkins, D.V. 113, 119
Perrow, C. 161, 186, 572, 577
Perry, B.C. 111, 116
Pervin, L.A. 80, 92
Peters, L.H. 292, 313
Peters, T.J. 144, 158, 328, 342
Peterson, M.F. 479, 500
Pfaff, H. 356, 365

AUTHOR INDEX

Pfeffer, J. 59, 66, 67, 73, 74, 75, 132, 140, 162, 186, 290, 313, 351, 365, 456, 472, 485, 500
Pfeiffer, A.L. 453, 469
Pierson, H.D. 489, 500
Philip, H. 547, 552
Philipsen, H. 352, 366
Phillips, J.S. 191, 222
Pinto, J.K. 295, 313
Plovnick, M. 537-8, 551
Podsakoff, P.M. 191, 199, 203, 204, 206, 208, 209, 222, 223
Pondy, L.R. 405-6, 420, 467, 472
Pool, J. 169, 170, 173, 185
Poole, M.S. 9, 20, 38, 41, 51, 109, 119, 406, 420
Poppler, P. 102, 117
Porac, J.F. 60, 74
Porras, J.I. 359, 366
Porter, L.W. 460-1
Porter, M.E. 533, 552
Posner, B.Z. 380, 395, 425, 429-31, 432, 448, 449
Postman, L. 136, 140
Potter, J. 403, 420
Potter, L.W. 460-1, 473
Poulton, B.C. 301, 302, 313, 558, 568, 578
Pounds, W.F. 565, 578
Powell, G.N. 380, 395, 425, 429-31, 432, 448, 449
Powell, W.W. 454, 459, 465, 466, 468, 473
Pradhan, P. 106, 120
Prescott, J.E. 295, 313
Pressman, R.S. 295, 313
Pretty, G.M.H. 356, 366
Pribram, K.H. 100, 107, 119, 560, 577
Prince, C. 518, 528
Pringle, C.D. 234, 242
Pritchard, R.D. 98, 100, 106, 119, 179, 186, 286, 298, 299, 300, 305-6, 311, 313, 314, 386, 396, 567, 568, 578
Pruitt, D.G. 180, 186
Pulakos, E.G. 196, 204, 208, 233
Pun, A. 495, 500
Putai, J. 487, 500
Putman, L.L. 406, 420

Quick, J.C. 425, 430, 431, 449
Quinn, J.B. 70, 74

Rabbie, J.M. 176, 180, 186, 401-2, 404, 420
Raisinghani, D. 103, 110, 119
Raju, N.J. 360, 365

Rakestraw, T.L. 82, 93
Ramos, J. 355, 365
Rao, R. 43, 51
Rasmussen, J. 101, 119
Ratiu, I. 491, 500
Rau, R. 350, 366
Ravetz, J.R. 453, 473
Ravlin, E.C. 6, 20, 60, 73, 231, 238, 245, 257, 258, 280, 287, 288, 291, 297, 300, 301, 302, 303, 309, 311, 313, 350, 352, 363, 365, 373, 376, 394, 505-6, 527
Ray, S.P. 328, 341
Raymond, P. 40, 52
Rechner, P.L. 63, 74
Rees, A. 569, 579
Reichers, A.E. 29, 30, 52, 326, 343, 373, 375, 393, 396, 423, 424, 433, 439-40, 445, 449, 450
Reider, H.W. 106, 116
Reilly, N.P. 89, 92
Reis, H.T. 492, 499
Repetti, R.L. 347, 355, 357, 360, 361, 366
Rennie, D.L. 559-60, 578
Resnick, L.B. 87, 93
Retzlaff, R.D. 115, 119
Reynolds, E.V. 462, 463, 464, 468, 473
Rice, A.K. 233, 245, 248, 250, 251, 253, 254, 257, 258, 259, 280, 398, 405, 408, 420, 457, 471
Richardson, A.M. 359, 360, 366
Richman, J.M. 350, 366
Ridgeway, C.L. 61, 62, 74
Rieck, A. 287, 288, 290, 303, 313
Rigby, M. 496, 500
Ringenbach, K.L. 178, 183
Roberts, K.H. 86, 93, 412, 414, 419, 462, 463, 464, 473
Roberts, V.Z. 153, 155, 158
Robertson, I.T. 168, 178, 179, 182, 442, 448
Robertson, P.J. 359, 366
Robinson, J.P. 31, 51
Roby, T.B. 104, 114, 118
Rockart, J.F. 160, 186
Roese, N.J. 299, 314
Roethlisberger, F.J. 4, 20, 349, 366, 398, 420
Rogelberg, S.G. 564, 565, 578
Rogers, E.M. 452, 457, 462, 473
Rogers, J. 133, 135, 140
Rognes, J.K. 404, 411, 418
Rohrbaugh, J. 40, 49
Roloff, M.E. 64, 74
Romezek, B.S. 375, 396

Roos, D. 254, 282
Roos, L.L. 514, 528
Ropo, A. 191, 222
Ropp, V.A. 462, 469
Rosenberg, L. 162, 182
Ross, A. 406, 419
Rosenstiel, L.V. 255, 281
Rosier, G. 490, 500
Rosen, S. 564, 578
Ross, A. 406, 419
Ross, J. 564, 578
Ross, W.H. 180, 186
Rosse, J.G. 356, 357, 366
Rotchford, N.L. 33, 51
Roth, J. 38, 41, 51, 109, 119
Rouse, S.H. 454, 473
Rouse, W.B. 454, 473, 528
Rousseau, D.M. 236, 245, 304, 314, 326, 342, 434, 435, 443, 449, 453, 467, 473
Royce, J. 130, 140
Rubin, I. 537–8, 551
Rubin, J.Z. 180, 186
Rudolph, E. 350, 366
Ruhe, J. 483, 500
Russell, H. 452, 470
Rutenfranz, 255, 279

Saavedra, R. 239, 245
Sachdev, I. 413, 418, 420
Sader, M. 255, 281
Salancik, G.R. 290, 313
Salas, E. xxxii, 18, 19, 86, 90, 350, 366, 505, 506–8, 510, 514, 515, 517, 518, 520, 525, 526, 528, 529
Salzberger-Wittenberg, I. 151, 158
Sandberg, W.R. 63, 74
Sandelands, L.E. 88, 93, 467, 473
Sapienza, H.J. 373, 395
Sari, L.M. 106, 119
Sarocchi, F. 35, 52
Sato, K. 485, 501
Satow, T. 493, 501
Scandura, T.A. 194, 199, 202, 206, 216, 217, 221, 223
Schaalman, M.L. 564, 565, 575
Schachter, S. 64, 72, 106, 116, 128, 130, 140, 460, 473
Schaumann, L.J. 107, 111, 118
Scheier, M.F. 565, 575, 578
Schein, E.H. 126, 140, 425, 426, 427, 428–9, 434, 435, 439, 441, 442, 449, 450, 456, 473, 487, 500, 514, 528, 533, 547, 552
Schiffman, R. 404, 413, 420

Schlesinger, A.M., Jr. 131, 140
Schlesinger, L.A. 175, 185
Schmidt 406, 421
Schmidt, F.L. 304, 314, 511, 528
Schmidt, W.H. 63, 74
Schminke, M. 287, 297, 300, 311, 373, 376, 394, 505–6, 527
Schmitt, N. 510, 528
Schneider, B. 13, 20, 80, 93, 292, 314, 326, 343, 399, 420
Schneider, W. 100, 101, 119, 120
Schön, D.A. 160, 177, 182, 320, 321, 328, 340, 548, 552, 557, 558, 578
Schonberger, R.J. 162, 186
Schönfelder, E. 350, 366
Schoorman, F.D. 292, 314
Schneider, B. 428, 449
Schneider, H.D. 255, 281
Schriescheim, C.A. 193, 198, 199, 202, 203, 204, 205, 206, 207, 208, 209, 216, 217, 222, 223, 520, 529
Schultz, P. 566, 578
Schutz, W.C. 541, 546, 552
Schwartz, S.H. 480, 500
Schwartzman, H.B. 9, 21
Schweiger, D.M. 63, 74, 373, 395, 482, 499
Schweiger, U.M. 174, 185
Schwenk, C.R. 63, 70, 71, 74, 169, 186, 563, 564, 578
Scott, J. 459, 473
Scott, M. 486, 498
Scullion, H. 411, 412, 418
Seashore, S.E. 460, 473
Self, R.M. 438–9, 450
Semmer, N. 101, 119
Senge, P.M. 328, 343, 533, 552
Sevastos, P.P. 234, 235, 243
Shack, J.R. 78, 92
Shackleton, V.J. 436, 447
Shah, S. 384, 394
Shamir, B. 199, 200, 202, 203, 204, 209, 210, 211, 212, 221, 223
Shaw, K.N. 106, 119
Shaw, M.E. 66, 67, 74, 97, 103, 119, 132, 140, 399, 420, 458, 473
Shea, G.P. 4, 5, 7, 11, 19, 20, 98, 117, 160, 184, 286, 287, 288, 291, 293, 300, 301, 311, 314, 331, 338, 341, 345, 350, 352, 354, 355, 364, 366, 373, 394, 398, 419, 506, 527
Sheats, P. 547, 551
Sheffield, D.T. 227, 245
Shenkar, O. 229, 245

Shepard, H.A. 540, 541, 543, 546, 551
Shephard, H.A. 408, 418
Sherif, M. xxxi, 61, 74, 255, 281, 405, 408–9, 411, 412–13, 420, 421
Sherif, C. 255, 281, 405, 408–9, 420
Sherwood, J.J. 515, 529
Shiereck, J.J. Jr. 62, 71
Shiffrin, R.M. 100, 101, 119, 120
Shiflett, S. 562, 578
Shim, W. 376, 396
Shomenta, J. 162, 186
Short, J.E. 160, 186
Shotland, R.L. 302, 312
Shotter, J. 446, 448, 449, 552
Silver, S.D. 62, 74
Simmons, J.L. 403, 420
Simon, H.A. 60, 66, 74, 109, 119, 457, 458, 470, 472
Simon, R. 518–19, 527
Simpson, J.A. 345, 367
Simpson, M.J. 409, 419
Sims, H.P. 200, 202, 210, 222, 235, 241, 244
Sinclair, R.C. 87, 93
Sinha, J.B.P. 479, 500
Sivitanides, M.P. 131, 140
Skaret, D.J. 356, 366
Skell, W. 104, 117
Skinner, M. 409, 421
Skov, R. 199, 203, 207, 208, 222
Slater, J.A. 568, 572, 578
Slater, P.E. 534, 543, 552
Slevin, D.P. 295, 313
Slocum, J.W. 355, 364 460, 471
Sloma 418
Smeets, J.J. 177, 184
Smircich, L. 564, 578
Smith, C. 44, 51
Smith, D.A. 468, 470
Smith, D.K. 8, 20, 533, 557
Smith, E.M. 425, 433, 449
Smith, G.F. 565, 566, 578
Smith, K. 398, 399, 408, 410, 415, 417, 421
Smith, K.K. 535, 543–4, 552
Smith, K.G. 67, 74, 106, 111, 120, 563, 578
Smith, L.M. 6, 8, 19, 236, 237, 243, 353, 354, 363, 532, 551
Smith, M. 453, 473
Smith, P.B. xxxi, 215–16, 479, 480, 481, 484, 492–3
Smith, P.C. 286, 296, 314
Smith, R. 28, 51

Smith-Lovin, L. 63, 73
Smoll, F.L. 34, 51
Snell, S.A. 513, 528
Snow, C.C. 513, 528
Solem, A.R. 129, 139, 331, 342, 563, 577
Solomon, 353
Somers, M.J. 237, 245
Sommerkamp, P. 194, 199, 202, 206, 221
Sonnentag, S. xxx, 237, 240, 295, 314, 348, 357–8, 361, 366, 568, 569
Sonoda, S. 493–4, 500
Souder, W.E. 324, 343
South, S.J. 64, 74
Spangler, R. 229, 242
Spangler, W.D. 200, 202, 204, 207, 208, 209, 210, 211, 212, 216, 221, 224
Spector, B. 505, 525
Spector, P.E. 359, 366
Spencer, L.M. 512, 529
Spencer, S.M. 512, 529
Sproull, L. 564, 577
Srivastva, S. 540, 541–2, 546, 549, 551, 552
Stacey, R. 487, 501
Stagner, R. 409, 412, 421
Stahelski, A.J. 351, 366
Stalker, G.M. 399, 404, 418
Stankiewicz, R. 323, 343
Starbuck, W.H. 564, 576
Starke, F.A. 514, 528
Stasser, G. 40, 51, 52
Staw, B.M. 63, 73, 88, 93, 125, 140, 305, 306, 314, 467, 473, 564, 578
Stayer, R. 523, 529
Steel, R.P. 228, 245
Steers, 376, 396
Stefaniak, D. 81, 90
Stein, A.A. 408, 409, 421
Stein, B.A. 126, 139
Stein, M. xxix, 149–50, 153, 158, 564
Steiner, I.D. 5, 8, 21, 38, 52, 62, 74, 97, 98, 107, 120, 293, 296, 303, 314, 534, 536, 552
Stening, B.W. 491, 498
Sternberg, R.J. 434, 450
Stephan, W.G. 58, 74
Stephenson, G.M. 408, 417
Stevens, F. 352, 366
Stevens, M.J. 238, 245, 381, 383, 394, 396
Stevenson, W.B. 460–1, 473
Steward, T.A. 126, 140
Stocking, S.H. 453, 473
Stogdill, R.M. 199, 202, 205, 223
Stohl, C. 453, 472

Stolte-Heiskanen, V. 334, 343
Stone, D.N. 131, 140
Strobel, L.P. 453, 473
Strodtbeck, F.L. 28, 38, 48, 108, 116, 536, 551
Stroebe, W. 292, 311
Storey, J. 226, 245
Strohm, O. 264, 281
Stroop, R.J. 140
Sundstrom, E. 11, 14, 17, 21, 226, 231, 245, 286, 287, 288, 290, 291, 293, 298, 302, 314, 334, 338, 343, 350, 352, 359–60, 366, 515, 529, 556, 570, 578
Susman, G.I. 231, 234, 245, 246, 248, 257, 258, 259, 260–1, 161–2, 281, 353, 366
Sussman, L. 460, 467, 470, 471
Sutton, R.I. 429, 450
Suzuki, N. 484, 499
Sweeney, D.A. 571, 579
Swezey, R.W. 510, 517, 529
Swierczek, F. 486, 492, 495, 501
Swieringa, J. 177, 186
Syme, S.L. 358, 363
Symon, G. 173, 183

Tajfel, H. xxx, 105, 120, 378, 396, 399, 400, 409, 411, 413, 421
Talland, G.A. 108, 120
Tang, S. 496, 499
Tang, T.L. 230, 245, 505, 529
Tannenbaum, S.I. xxxii, 350, 366, 505, 506–7, 507–8, 510, 514, 515, 517, 528, 529, 570, 572
Taylor 144
Taylor, D.A. 61, 73
Taylor, D.W. 132, 140, 400, 401, 402, 403, 407, 409, 411, 413, 420, 421
Taylor, F.W. 274, 281
Taylor, J.C. 7, 19
Taylor, L. 40, 51
Taylor, M. 460, 473
Taylor, R.R. 386, 395
Taylor, S.E. 137, 140
Tellegen, A. 78, 79, 81, 83, 85, 86, 93
Terborg, R.R. 351, 366
Tesser, A. 564, 578
Tetlock, P.E. 131, 140
Tetrault, L.A. 520, 529
Tetrick, L.E. 435, 443, 449
Tett, R.P. 299, 314
Thayer, R.E. 89, 93
Theorell, T. 234, 241, 244, 345, 364
Theoret, A. 103, 110, 119
Thierry, H. 178, 179, 186

Thomas, H. xxxi, 564, 566, 578
Thomas, K. 406, 421
Thommen, B. 103, 120
Thompson, G. 466, 473
Thompson, J.D. 162, 163, 168, 186, 398, 421
Thompson, J. 238, 246
Thompson, V.A. 334–5, 343
Thorsrud, E. 251, 253, 254, 279
Tindale, R.S. 40, 52
Titus, W. 40, 51, 52
Tjosvold, D. 327, 343, 562–3, 578, 579
Todor, W.D. 199, 203, 204, 206, 208, 209, 223
Tollison, P.S. 230, 245, 505, 529
Tom, V.R. 80, 93
Tomaszewski, T. 251, 253, 281
Torrance, E.P. 61, 74, 106, 115, 120, 129, 140
Tosi, H.L. 191, 221, 223
Trevor, M. 487, 501
Triandis, H.C. 60, 67, 68, 74, 480, 483, 501
Trice, H.M. 399, 421
Trist, E.L. 6, 21, 233, 246, 248, 251, 253, 256, 257, 258, 281, 282, 349, 352, 353, 366
Trompenaars, F. 480, 495, 501
Trow, D.R. 42, 52
Tschan, F. xxviii, 100, 102, 110, 112, 114, 120, 338, 561
Tsui, A.S. 58, 59, 74, 485, 501
Tsukuda, R.A. 351, 366
Tubbs, M.E. 178, 186
Tuckman, B.W. 28, 29, 30, 46, 52, 294, 314, 343, 488, 501, 535, 541, 546, 552
Tuden, A. 162, 186
Turner, B. 565, 579
Turner, J.C. 58, 59, 74, 105, 120, 399, 402, 408, 409, 421
Tushman, M.L. 295, 310
Tuttle, J.M. 351, 363
Tziner, A.E. 511, 529

Uhl-Bien, M. 199, 202, 206, 210, 221
Ulich, E. xxx, 252, 253, 255, 256, 257, 258, 259, 260, 262, 263, 264, 267, 268, 270, 272, 278, 279, 281, 293, 314, 346, 362, 562, 571
Urwick, 144
Usunier, J. 31, 49

Vaas, S. 173, 175, 186, 187

AUTHOR INDEX

Valach, L. 100, 101, 102, 103, 104, 105, 107, 113, 120
Valacich, J.S. 36, 50
Valax, M.F. 35, 52
Vandenberg, R.J. 438–9, 450
van der Vliert, E. 406, 421
van de Ven, A.H. 160, 170, 187, 321, 343
Van Fleet, D.D. 190, 198, 224, 482, 501, 510, 520, 529
van Gils, M.R. 160, 184
van Maanen, J. 403, 420, 425, 426, 427, 439, 450
Van Offenbeek, M.A.G. xxix, 164, 169, 170, 173, 174–5, 176, 182, 187, 565
van Oostrum, J. 176, 180, 186
Vernon, P.E. 319, 343
Verbrugge, L.M. 63, 75
Vidmar, N. 96, 117
Vijlbrief, H.P.J. 170, 172, 182, 187
Villanova, P. 286, 297, 310
Vinsel, A.M. 128, 138
Viteles, M.S. 4, 21
Vogelman, L. 415, 421
Volpato, C. 445, 449
Volpert, W. 100, 111, 120, 249, 251, 253, 256, 264, 268, 280, 281
von Cranach, M. xxviii, xxix, 100, 101, 102, 103, 104, 105, 107, 111, 113, 114, 116, 120, 338, 561
von Hayek, F. 464, 473
Vroom, V.H. 162, 169, 174, 175, 176, 180, 187, 199, 202, 205, 206, 223

Wachtler, J. 128, 136, 140
Waddington, D. 412, 414, 421
Wagner, J. 490, 500
Wagner, R.K. 434, 450
Wagner, V. 400, 419
Wagner, W.G. 66, 67, 75
Wakabayashi, M. 494, 498
Waldman, D.A. 200, 216, 217, 223, 224
Wall, T.D. 6, 21, 231, 234, 236, 237, 238, 239, 240, 243, 246, 257, 258, 259, 281, 353, 354, 367, 523, 529
Wall, V.D. 515, 529
Wallas, G. 319, 343
Wallace, M. 579
Wallace, S.R. 309, 314
Wallach, M.A. 319, 343
Wallmark, J.T. 323, 343
Wallston, B.S. 57, 75
Walsh, J.P. 86, 88, 93
Walsh, J.O. 485, 500

Walton, R.E. 226, 232, 234, 237, 246, 392, 395, 415, 422
Wang, Z.M. 493, 501
Wanous, J.P. 29, 30, 52, 423, 424, 425, 426, 427, 429, 439–40, 441, 450
Warner, R.M. 34, 52
Warr, P.B. 234, 246, 346, 367, 569, 571, 579
Waterman, R.H. 144, 158, 328, 342
Watson, C.E. 564, 579
Watson, D. 78, 85, 86, 91, 93
Watson, M.D. 299, 314, 567, 568, 578
Watson, W.E. 65, 75, 351, 367, 483–4, 485, 494, 501
Wayne, S.J. 228, 246
Weber, W.G. xxx, 256, 264, 268, 280, 281, 293, 314, 562, 571
Wegner, D.M. 40, 52, 294, 314
Wehner, T. 255, 279
Weick, K.E. 15, 21, 42, 86, 93, 167, 180, 181, 183, 187, 468, 473
Weimann, G. 462, 473
Weiner, E.L. 519, 529
Weingart, L. 106, 111, 120, 287, 288, 292, 314
Weiss, J.A. 103, 111, 118, 563, 570
Weiss, H.M. 82, 93
Weiss, W. 128, 139
Weitzel, J.R. 162, 187
Weldon, E. 106, 120, 287, 288, 292, 314
Wellins, R.S. 231, 232, 246
Wendt, H. 127
Werner, C.M. 34, 36, 52
West, L.J. 492, 499
West, M.A. 235, 241, 291, 301, 302, 304, 313, 314, 319, 326, 327, 328, 331, 337, 338, 339, 340, 342, 343, 442, 448, 450, 501, 539, 552, 556, 558, 559, 562, 565, 567, 568, 569, 570, 571, 572, 575, 577, 578, 579
Wetherell, M. 403, 420
Wexley, K.N. 195, 196, 203, 204, 207, 208, 223
Whetten, M.G. 457, 470
Whipp, R. 32, 52
Whitaker, D.S. 543, 552
White, H. 465, 470
Whitehead, A.M. 532, 552
Whiteside, H.D. 230, 245, 505, 529
Whitney, K. 57, 59, 72
Whitsett, D.A. 240, 246
Whyte, W.F. 5, 21
Wible, D.S. 489, 501
Wicker, A.W. 113, 120

Wicklund, R.A. 404, 413, 420, 565, 576
Wiersma, M.F. 173, 177, 185, 186, 320, 325, 343, 511, 529
Wijers, G.J. 173, 187
Wilemon, D. 328, 341
Wilensky, H. 456, 459, 473
Willems, E.P. 67, 75
Williams, K. 235, 246, 292, 312, 479, 499
Williams, J. 410, 418
Williams, M.L. 199, 203, 204, 206, 209, 223
Williams, S. 102, 117
Williamson, 466
Williges, R.C. 104, 121, 564, 579
Willis, C.E. 306, 313
Wills, T.A. 358, 363, 569, 570
Wilson, A.T.M. 253, 283
Wilson, C. 520, 526
Wilson, J.M. 231, 232, 246
Wilson, M. 103, 121
Winograd, T. 549, 552
Winter, D.G. 320, 343
Winterton, J. 414, 422
Winterton, R. 414, 422
Wissema, J.G. 173, 187
Withey, M. 460, 473
Wolf, G. 83, 92, 304, 312
Womack, J.P. 254, 282
Won-Doornink, M. 490, 501
Wong, C.S. 354, 367
Wood, R.E. 98, 99, 100, 110, 121, 178, 187, 229–30, 235, 246
Wood, W. 67, 75, 345, 367
Wood-Harper, A.T. 162, 183
Woodman, R.W. 515, 529
Worchel, S. 28, 52, 345, 367, 399, 417
Worley, C.G. 482, 498
Woycke, J. 200, 202, 204, 209, 221
Wright, T.A. 571, 579

Wyer, R., Jr. 460, 473

Xin, K.R. 58, 74

Yamagishi, T. 481, 485, 501
Yammarino, F.J. xxix, 190, 191, 192, 193, 194, 195, 196, 197, 198, 199, 200, 202, 203, 204, 205, 206–7, 208, 209, 210, 211, 212, 214, 216, 217, 219, 220, 223, 224, 304, 315, 356, 367, 478, 574
Yarrow, M.R. 565, 579
Yerkes 133, 140
Yetton, P.W. 162, 180, 187, 199, 202, 205, 223, 563, 575
Yoon, J. 374, 396
Yorks, L. 240, 246
Yukl, G.A. 129, 141, 190, 191, 198, 200, 201, 202, 203, 204, 206, 207, 208, 209, 211, 212, 213, 222, 224, 333, 343, 479, 501, 510, 520, 529
Yuzl 174, 187

Zaccaro, S.J. 356, 367, 374, 396
Zajac, D. 375, 395
Zajonc, E.J. 456, 469
Zajonc, R.B. 137, 139
Zalesny, M.D. 355, 367
Zaltman, G. 335, 343, 467, 473
Zakay, D. 47, 52
Zamarripa, P.O. 483, 501
Zammuto, R.F. 302, 315
Zander, A. 4, 7, 21, 75, 129, 141
Zapf, D. 100, 101, 104, 107, 117, 293, 311, 350, 363, 561, 563, 576
Zautra, A.J. 79, 93
Zelditch, M. Jr. 58, 59, 61, 71
Zenger, T.R. 64, 75, 324, 343
Zhou, X. 62, 71
Zink, K. 274, 282

Subject Index

ad hoc groups 292
advanced manufacturing
    technologies xxvii, 234, 238
affective attachment 374–6, 388–9
affective commitment 374–7
affective measures 374
age 15, 55–7, 61–8, 132, 325, 483
assembly line
    automobile production 7
    work teams, 492, 556
anxiety 143, 146–50, 157, 319, 322, 346, 355, 357, 359, 365, 571
assessment centers 510, 513
authority 152–4, 216, 239, 477, 486
Autonomous Work Groups xxix, xxx, 225, 254–6, 259, 263–4, 345, 352, 360, 457, 510, 522, 524, 556, 572
    decisions 260–1
    goal settings 256
    work designs 234, 241
    work group effectiveness 233
autonomy xxx, 6, 8, 12, 42, 179, 232–5, 251–2, 260, 263, 271, 273, 275, 293, 334, 352, 524, 558, 568, 572
    collective 238, 256, 269, 270
    individual 259, 268–70
    individual and/or collective self-
        regulation 247

bi-national teams 487
boundaries xxviii, 10, 126, 148, 156, 225, 229, 267, 318, 335, 336, 414, 416
    control 6
    group 3, 14, 42, 338, 405
    maintenance 257, 259
    management 17, 239, 288–9, 536, 538, 547, 550
    membership 16
    spanning 507
    tasks 254
    team 12–16, 54, 58
brainstorming

groups 96, 131, 132
burnout 347, 349, 355, 357, 359, 453

circumplex model of group tasks 98
climate
    corporate 136
    for change 326
    for excellence 317, 327, 338
    for innovation 326
    for quality 326
    group xxv, xxx, 317–18, 326, 327, 330, 333, 335–40, 355, 569
    social 570
co-operation 18, 63, 69, 166, 180, 252–3, 398, 328, 334, 350–76, 484, 512
co-ordination 5, 17, 32, 34, 54, 126, 173, 257, 267–8, 288–290, 333–4, 386, 507, 518, 538
coaching/team building
    coaching 198, 510, 520
    consultants 143, 153–7, 163, 169
coal-mining 249, 262
cognitions
    group 402
cognitive knowledge, skills, abilities 57, 238, 308, 383, 404
cognitive learning 320–2
cognitive processes 86, 134, 319
cohesiveness xxvii, 16, 54, 55, 59, 63, 70, 323–4, 339, 347, 406, 409, 460, 507–10, 514–15, 570
    team 356
collaboration 200, 338, 397, 398, 417
collective performance strategies 290, 302
collective self-regulation 257, 259, 260
collective strategies 307
collective well-being levels of groups 90
collectivist cultures 215, 477, 482, 484
collectivist individualist and collectivist
    cultures 495
collectivist orientation 492

collectivist values   382, 482, 493
commitment   xxx, 165–6, 169, 173, 177, 179, 200, 216, 241, 256, 430, 432–3, 436–8, 442, 477, 481, 571
  group   288
communication   xxx, 102, 104, 115, 126, 128, 156, 166, 173, 229, 269, 270, 288, 295, 333, 335, 356–78, 403, 458, 510, 514, 517–18, 520, 523, 535, 538, 540, 547, 561, 564
  barriers   328
  climate for   163
  competence   484
  cycles   96, 112
  group   108
  horizontal   65
  networks   461, 464
  patterns   10, 14–15, 18, 31, 36–7, 55, 58, 62, 64
  structure   451, 445–56, 459, 464, 507
  style   293, 328, 490
  technologies   33, 47
  vertical   65
community psychiatric teams   558
competencies   179, 228, 240, 511–13, 519
competition   10, 18, 98, 334, 347, 357, 397–8, 409, 411, 484, 507
  between teams   417
complex decision-making
  group effectiveness in   3, 555, 558–9
  and groups   559, 569–74
composition   xxviii, 37–9, 351–2, 360, 536
  age diversity   55
  bi-polar teams   58
  change   26–9, 41–7, 160, 165, 320, 333
  characteristics of team members   566
  dispositional composition of the group   77, 84
  educational background   132, 134
  ethnicity   15, 55–7, 61–2, 68, 407, 414, 483, 485, 487
  group/team   43, 55–8, 64, 69, 99, 230, 307, 483, 496
  high ability   66
  individual differences   33, 207, 238, 240
  individual effectiveness   303
  multi-cultural   216
computer
  assisted groups   9–10, 15, 17, 18
  based network   160
  based team training   520
  mediated communication   37
  mediated work groups   37
conflict   xxix, xxviii, xxx, 6, 38, 63, 66, 102, 125–6, 132, 137, 148, 173–4, 179–80, 237, 241, 291, 299, 302, 324, 332, 355, 375, 392, 397, 404–17, 443, 564, 575
  and controversy   327, 330, 562
  intergroup   405–17
  and management skills   70
  management of   xxx, 407
  resolution   398, 492, 507, 509–10, 514–15, 519, 569
  unproductive   53–4
conformity   10, 60, 130–1, 428, 443, 478–9, 564
  peer pressure   5
constituency
  groups   65
  model   568
contingency
  approach   160, 162–6, 208
  reward/s   82, 203–4, 208–9
creativity   xxviii, 88, 96, 125–6, 130, 133, 136, 235, 331–4, 336, 351, 532, 562
  and ability   318, 337
  and decision-making   62, 67
  process   331–6, 340
  and production   317
cross-cultural teams   492, 495
cross-cultural training   495
cross-national differences   482
cross-sectional research   349, 352
culture   xxx, 7, 31–3, 55, 68–9, 130, 174, 216, 335, 382, 385, 387, 423, 460, 489
  corporate   56, 125–9, 137, 156, 487
  individualist   215, 481, 484, 490
  team/group   157, 384, 538
  differences in group processes   477–8
cultural differences in teamwork   481
cultural diversity   480, 485, 487
cultural heterogeneity   484, 566
cultural values   424, 483, 488
customers   8, 14, 53, 54, 232, 301, 533

decision-making   xxv, xxx, xxix, 12, 15, 55–64, 70, 86, 130, 159, 173, 225, 231, 236, 238, 241, 251–2, 268, 274, 327, 333, 414, 457, 468, 488, 507–10, 517–20, 522, 541, 561, 565
  collective   481
  effective   477, 535
  group effectiveness in   63, 555, 558, 559
  group/team   9, 58, 77, 88, 130, 235, 494, 492, 564
  majority   4, 10, 63, 125–37, 180, 483
  models   230
  participation in   174, 202, 205, 227, 255

SUBJECT INDEX

processes 110, 162, 169, 256, 263
quality of 130–6
and self-regulation 257–60
demands-constraints model 234, 241
dependence
  basic assumption 157
  mutual 213
depersonalization 356
depression 346, 355, 356, 361, 571
development 25–6, 30, 37, 41, 289, 539, 551
  mid-point transactions 294
  of intergroup relations 403
  of norms 294
  of team/group 148, 486, 494, 516
  team/group xxv, xxvii, xxx, 12, 26–31, 46–7, 294, 296, 334, 345, 351, 424, 439, 477, 490–1, 531, 535, 540–1, 543, 545, 556
diversity xxviii, 29, 53–70, 133, 318, 478, 494, 566–9
  in tenure 324
  managing 69
  race 56, 63–4, 407, 410, 414
  teams xxx, 47, 57, 59, 60, 65–6, 70, 477, 484
division of labour 43, 114, 398
dyads xxix, 34, 105, 112, 114, 189–219, 485

effectiveness xxviii, xxx, 3–5, 9, 13, 17, 65, 159, 170, 180, 205, 225, 227, 230, 240, 285–304, 334, 392, 486, 491, 493, 504–8, 515–20, 524–5, 533–9, 545, 557–65, 572, 573
  criteria 298, 302
  and decision-making 535
  dimensions 289, 290, 298
  group/team 11, 45, 194, 210, 287, 291, 295, 303, 328, 384, 531, 535, 555
  measures 44
  organizational 161, 162
  of innovation 166, 168
efficiency 4, 12, 44, 228, 300, 320, 328, 457, 467
employee
  self-esteem 228
  well-being 302
empowerment xxix, xxx, 144, 210, 262
  teams 231
environmental 6, 10, 25–6, 46, 47, 60, 110, 126, 181, 215, 404–5, 539, 555, 561
  constraints 290
  production uncertainty 234

stability or liability 274
uncertainty 292, 507, 556, 572
equal opportunities 410, 417
external relations 26, 59, 334

facilitators 550
feedback 37, 63, 65, 69, 101–6, 133–4, 171–2, 178, 235, 251–2, 273–98, 338, 352, 386, 463, 496, 507, 518, 520–1, 535, 538–40, 556, 561, 566
  negative 63, 306
  of results 253
  positive 179, 306
  system 299
  task performance and 573
focus group discussion 572
four-factor model 318, 337

gender xxx, 15, 31, 55–6, 61, 63, 68–9, 400, 407, 410, 414, 485
  balance 483
  composition 47
goals 62, 82, 99, 112–14, 127, 159, 160, 163–7, 169, 180, 190, 218, 261, 290, 291, 293, 300, 302, 329, 336–8, 381, 398, 406, 453, 456, 515, 546, 557
  attainment 38, 58, 235, 253, 570
  clarity 178, 537
  group 105, 129, 200–1, 241, 372, 376, 436
  oriented information 355
  setting 35, 106–7, 111, 174, 179, 198, 238, 251, 264, 359
  organizational 377
group
  abilities 230, 238
  affect 77–81, 86–7
  autonomy xxx, 67, 231, 234, 239, 247, 253, 256, 260, 285–6, 289, 293, 300, 307–8, 522–5, 556
  boundaries 3, 14, 42, 317, 334, 338, 405
  characteristics 96–7, 236, 328, 360, 400, 440, 443
  climate xxv, xxx, 317–18, 323, 326, 327, 330, 333–40, 355, 569
  cohesiveness 253, 237, 288, 290, 294, 352, 355, 358, 373
  consensus 299
  context xxviii, 11, 17, 37–47, 68, 161–2, 337, 427, 540
  definition 388, 401
  development xxx, 295
  dynamics 423
  discussion 33, 482, 495

effectiveness xxv, xxviii, 236, 291, 298–9, 302, 305, 331, 555–6
interaction 5, 15, 28–9, 32, 42, 291, 350, 355, 391, 408, 536
leader 81, 84, 332, 372, 377, 390–2, 574
leadership 190
level constructs 87
level wage plan 258, 259
life 535, 549
maintenance 29, 273
outcome 82, 283, 354, 556
problem-solving 26, 27, 38, 235
process skills 230
productivity and output xxv, 287, 305, 300, 323, 350, 445, 535, 564, 563
size 29, 254, 317–18, 347, 351, 401
socialization 423–46
viability 568, 569
group processes 6, 27, 43, 95–7, 106–8, 115, 323, 331, 345, 354, 355, 357, 378, 360, 361, 486, 532–5, 540, 556, 559, 561, 565, 574
group think 103, 241, 328, 398, 444, 494
heterogeneity 18, 165, 194, 210–13, 323, 351, 508, 511
  groups 132, 484, 498, 566
  member 509, 510
  teams 483, 485
hierarchical communication structures 458
hierarchical organizations 320
hierarchical levels 327
hierarchical task structure 112, 467
hierarchical team roles 524
homogeneity 56, 165, 211-13, 351, 325
  and abilities 62
  and members 507
  group 484, 566
  organizational 55
  team 57, 58, 63, 66, 70
hospital management team 557

impact of the group on individual members 10
individual
individual growth 66, 569
individual level of analysis 89, 216
individual performance 5, 178, 285–6, 292
individual satisfaction 105, 290, 303
individual self-regulation 260
individual well-being xxx, 345, 347, 352
industrial relations 247, 276, 278, 413, 414

influential group members 5, 8, 16, 17, 85
informal groups 4
informal leadership 201, 212, 213
informal processes 115
ingroup cohesion 484
ingroup favouritism 105, 412
ingroup harmony 216, 477
ingroup–outgroup 404
innovation xxix, xxx, 7, 12, 54, 125–9, 132, 160–78, 182, 226, 235, 288, 289, 308, 333–8, 351, 442, 451, 468, 487, 559, 568, 569
  abandoned 317
  acceptance of 166–8
  cycle 339
  group xxv
  implementation 291, 296, 307
  quality of 168
  research 162
  resistance to 330
  support for 317–329, 336, 482, 561
  task 167, 168
  team innovation 562
input–process–output framework 289, 296, 350, 556
inter-group collaboration 398
inter-group conflict 397–399, 405, 408–416
inter-group processes xxv, 397, 400, 407, 415
inter-group relations xxx, 8, 397, 403, 415, 507, 561
interdependence 8, 62, 179, 180, 238, 299, 398, 400, 406, 456, 505, 556, 573
interdependent tasks 231, 413
interpersonal conflicts 347, 355, 358, 359
interpersonal group relations 132, 407
interpersonal processes 486
interpersonal relationships xxviii, 34, 58, 189, 194, 197, 207, 480, 537, 538
interpersonal skills 357, 385
interpersonal trust 357, 490
intervention 12, 13, 40, 143, 145, 155, 178, 226, 359, 496, 503–507, 513, 516, 522, 532, 536, 547–550, 570, 574
  methods 154
  to promote effectiveness 510
  strategies 180
  team/group 508, 525, 546
  techniques 156
intragroup relations 398, 400
intragroup cohesion 415
intragroup communication 466
intragroup cooperation 228

SUBJECT INDEX

intragroup processes xxv, 3, 10, 11, 14, 351, 402

job
   characteristics model 238
   complexity 361
   design 12, 147, 346, 354, 522
   discretion 317, 318, 331, 335–8
   enrichment 275
   involvement 356–7

knowledge, skills and abilities xxx, 57, 59, 288–90

leader 18, 45–6, 70, 85, 131, 148, 150–4, 173–4, 189–90, 196–7, 216, 230, 290, 323–36, 340, 412–16, 535–8, 550
   charismatic 199, 202–4, 209–12
   elected and emergent 200–1, 212–13
   styles 162, 202, 210, 230, 333, 477, 520
   team 55, 172, 232, 510, 518–23
leadership xxix, xxx, 5, 26, 45–6, 154, 157, 200, 212, 261, 293, 318, 331–6, 405, 412–16, 478, 479, 483, 488, 494, 519, 535, 537
   abilities 67
   development and training 215, 503, 510, 520–1
   support 317
learning organization 69, 70, 533
life cycle
   team/group 25, 26, 83, 87, 516
longitudinal studies 215, 352, 362, 572
low ability members 66

majority
   dissent 134, 136
   power of the 128
management xxix, xxvii, xxx, 127, 129, 137, 159–71, 177, 181, 227–31, 299, 300, 331, 409–14, 452, 454, 456, 457, 459, 461, 464, 482, 505, 525, 533, 535, 567
   human resource 237, 239, 384
   practices 12, 13, 62, 226
   styles 276, 495
   support 11
   systems 241
   teams 18, 320, 325–6, 486, 490
   theorists 398, 404
medical team 54
meetings 14, 156, 173, 231, 359, 477, 486, 492, 494
   formal and informal 64

team/group 9, 148, 156, 174, 330
membership
   boundaries 16
   change 26, 42, 43, 566
   diversity in work groups 47
   stability 43, 59, 67, 68
mental health xxv, 241, 346, 347, 349, 353, 356, 357, 358, 559, 571
minority 63, 70
   dissent xxix, 125, 132, 133, 134, 135, 137, 323
   faction 58
   group members 483–7
   influence groups xxx, 14, 445, 494, 562, 574
   views 130, 333, 494
mission 4, 8, 505, 537
   clarity 295, 556
   group 200
mixed national teams 494
model
   of team effectiveness 503, 506, 555–9
   of work group socialization 425, 440, 441
   of decision-making 230
   universal models 161, 180
monocultural teams 477, 497
motivation xxx, 64, 105–6, 136–7, 162, 168, 225, 236, 251, 256, 289–91, 296–9, 306–8, 350, 487, 514, 536
multi-skilled employees 276
multicultural and multinational work teams xxx, 477, 478, 485–9, 495–7
multidisciplinary
   groups xxvi
   teams xxviii, 53–5, 59–60, 62, 65–70

natural groups 28, 39, 41, 42, 399
naturalistic observations 18
negotiating 61, 64–5, 67, 132, 160, 168–80, 397–9, 412, 415–16, 492, 496, 546
   bargaining 417
   identity 403
network xxx, 451, 459, 464, 466
   communication 463
   organizations 160
   relationships 455
new group members 267
newcomer 81–2, 380, 382–3, 389, 430–4, 439, 442–5, 566
   characteristics 440
   integration 425
   learning 431

socialization 424, 426, 428–9, 447
non-participative members 113
norms 16, 26, 40, 41, 70, 82, 125, 126, 127, 128, 129, 130, 177, 216, 237, 254, 255, 276, 317, 320, 336, 427, 428, 429, 443, 460, 487, 538
   group/team 5, 170, 201, 328, 424, 439, 467, 507–10, 514, 536, 556, 564
   support of innovation 338
nursing teams 558

objectives xxv, xxvi, xxvii, xxx, 54, 157, 190, 233, 334, 335, 555, 561, 565, 567, 573
   group 560, 574
opportunities for
   control 234
   learning 234, 251
orchestras 556
organizational attachment 241, 373
organizational change xxviii, 12, 165, 566
organizational climate 228, 229, 460, 507
organizational commitment 227, 237, 346, 373, 438–9, 481
organizational context 385
organizational culture 318, 406, 417, 460, 487, 556
organizational development 177, 482, 535
organizational effectiveness 3, 11–12, 17, 285, 301, 457
organizational goals xxvi, 291, 515
organizational hierarchy 55, 399, 401, 453, 456
organizational intervention 28, 240, 299
organizational learning 40, 177
organizational objectives xxvi, 561, 562, 574
organizational performance 13, 126, 236
organizational rewards 557
organizational structure 12, 160, 170, 182, 229, 249, 273, 379–400, 416, 459, 461, 524
organizational support system 11, 18
out-group 14, 194, 216, 412, 415, 477

participant observation 149
participation 26, 45–6, 55, 62, 64, 126, 160, 168–9, 173–4, 225, 227, 229, 236, 272–3, 299, 318, 327, 329, 352, 354, 453, 481, 483, 497, 522, 533, 559
   group 235, 482
   non-participative members 113

participative safety 149, 236, 240, 288, 317, 327, 336–8, 488–9, 949, 505
performance xxviii, xxx, 8, 18, 28, 45, 54, 64, 109–14, 126, 132–5, 168, 199, 207, 210, 227–8, 236, 238, 241, 264, 326, 332–45, 350–2, 355, 376, 392, 425, 430–1, 433, 443–55, 462, 477–8, 481, 494, 539, 570
   appraisal 232, 239
   effectiveness dimensions 300
   effectiveness 10–11, 13, 17, 229, 235, 239, 240, 298
   evaluation 385-7
   feedback 129
   goals 179
   group xxv, 5, 96–8, 102, 104–5, 107, 111, 115, 129, 205, 218, 286–7, 290, 305, 322, 331, 339, 511, 547, 556, 559, 563–4, 571
   individual job 5, 178, 285–6, 292
   low performing groups 77
   quality 125
   strategies 103, 178, 289, 306
   team 55, 58, 62, 66–8, 288, 324, 387, 445, 483, 493, 496, 506–23
planning 26, 31, 33, 108–14, 238, 252–3, 256, 263–4
   action plans 103, 107
   action processes 104–5
   action regulation theories 95, 97, 115–16, 268
   action theory xxvii, 100, 350, 533, 561
police crowd control teams 556
power xxix, xxvii, xxx 54, 67, 152, 159, 169, 180, 261, 301, 404–5, 411, 416–17, 457, 461, 567
primary health care team xxvi, 558, 568
problem solving 37–39, 55, 60–1, 63–4, 96, 173–4, 225–9, 331, 412, 454, 515, 520, 563
   groups 66, 108, 156, 226
   sequential model of 110
   skills 230, 233
   solving tasks 108, 109, 114
processes
   group 5–6, 27, 43, 95–7, 106–8, 115, 323, 331, 333, 345, 354–61, 486, 532–5, 540, 556, 559, 561, 565, 574
   interaction xxviii, xxx, xxix, 35, 37, 44–5, 61, 96, 159–61, 165, 167, 173, 175, 179–80, 182, 255, 294, 354, 359, 402–6, 410, 416, 463, 556, 573
   team 506–10, 516–20, 525

process losses 5, 38, 39, 62, 107, 114, 241, 293, 303, 536
production blocking 292
project manager 160, 162, 164, 168, 173
proMES 298, 299, 300
psychodynamic approach 329
punctuated equilibrium model 544, 566

quality 12, 35, 54, 165, 166, 170, 174, 227, 265, 266, 297, 301, 327, 507, 508
quality assurance 9, 231
quality auditing 232
quality circles xxix, 7, 153, 225, 273, 399, 482, 486, 505
quality decision-making 130, 132, 135, 136
quasi-groups 399

R&D teams 54, 62, 79
recruiting and selecting 29, 232, 262, 383, 436
  teams 510–11, 523
reflexivity 555, 558, 560
  group task 559, 562, 565, 569, 571, 573
  non-reflexive groups 561, 564–7, 574
  team/group 539, 546
research 10, 13, 16–18, 27, 37, 42, 107, 116, 534
  methods 9
resources xxv, 15, 26, 30, 39, 58, 59, 151, 227, 230, 294, 328, 385, 404, 406, 411, 507, 518, 539
  allocation 61, 182, 218, 231, 505, 536
  human resources 67, 86, 126, 248, 458
  inadequate/unavailable 292
  material 159, 167, 171, 274, 292
rewards 77, 84, 85, 136, 180, 198, 210, 251, 317, 334, 335, 336, 339, 349, 454, 459
  individual 481
  monetary 8
  pay practices 5, 8, 17, 179, 413
  performance 382
  systems 11, 229, 276, 318, 385, 427, 507, 525, 538, 556, 561
role
  clarity 228, 299, 434, 515, 524
  conflict 514, 524
  definition 537
  differentiation 481, 486
  team 517

sales teams 273, 292, 297, 528

satisfaction 34, 59, 126, 174, 218, 225, 234–6, 277, 288, 291, 297, 305, 346–51, 353–62, 429–33, 460, 463
  team 290
selection 218–19, 383, 387, 436, 442–43, 493, 503
  attraction, selection and attrition processes 80, 82, 276
  interviews 510–13
  teams xxx
self-directed teams 226
self-efficacy 179, 235, 240, 317, 319, 320, 328, 336, 338, 506
self-esteem 179, 350, 355, 409, 413, 416, 445
self-managed work team 79, 81, 482
self-regulating work groups 272, 276, 297, 352
self-reported effectiveness and satisfaction 306
semi-autonomous work groups xxvi, 352, 353, 398
senior management teams 155, 556
social identity theory 411, 412
social loafing 113, 292, 479, 482
social processes 241, 319, 478, 559, 562, 573, 573
social service teams 558
social support xxv, 7, 59, 236, 253, 347, 349, 350, 355, 358, 430, 431, 432, 442–9, 570
socialization xxx, 30, 77, 79, 81, 83, 423, 425, 431–9, 445–6
  entry and socialization into teams 442
  of members into groups 29
  of newcomers 380
  of the work group 439
  work group socialization model 425, 440–1
socio technical systems 25, 27, 233, 239, 248–9, 250, 257, 274
software development projects 295
sports teams 556
stakeholder group 166, 168, 301, 558
status xxviii, 70, 128, 200, 252, 335, 338, 404, 408, 486, 491, 567
  differences 115, 208
  differentiation inhibits creativity 62
  hierarchies 55, 59, 61
  power 61
stress 18, 43, 136, 252, 272, 345, 346, 375, 384, 453, 507, 517, 569

supervision 81, 82, 173, 175, 190, 191, 237, 239, 299, 333, 357, 358, 361, 430–2, 523
support 16, 64, 200, 230, 252, 328, 355, 505, 543, 556
surgical teams 556
synergy xxvi, 5, 536

T-group 534, 539, 540, 544
task
  activity 28, 38, 143
  analysis 95–9, 517
  commitment 288
  competence 511
  completion models of effectiveness 102, 112, 291, 296, 307, 308
  complexity 99, 165, 112, 241, 251, 468, 557, 573
  demands 96, 97, 102, 107, 111–15, 290, 295–6
  design 238, 252, 264, 275, 277, 338, 536, 556
  effectiveness 559, 564, 567–8, 570–3
  identity 235, 354
  interdependence 338, 433
  orientation 107, 247, 250–4, 272, 278, 317, 327, 336, 338, 482, 488, 522, 536, 562
  performance feedback 573
  performance strategies 556
  reflexivity 559, 562, 565–6, 569–70, 571, 573–4
  significance 235, 354, 522
  structure 114, 307, 333, 517
  team/group task xxix, xxviii, 15, 41, 43, 77, 79, 82, 97, 105, 201, 253, 273, 293, 345, 351, 352, 391, 425, 522, 525
Tavistock Institute 154, 155
team building xxx, 306, 360, 503, 508–13, 414, 516, 570
  based feedback systems 525
  coaching 198, 510, 520

consultants 143, 153–7, 163, 169
characteristics 507, 510, 520
climate 326, 339, 445, 510, 520
competencies 518–19
effectiveness xxx, 11, 17, 486, 493, 503–8, 515–20, 524, 525
incentive schemes 67
interventions 514–15
member interdependence 558
support 539
training xxx, 496, 503–21, 571–2
viability 301, 479, 568, 574
work 53–4, 77, 155, 225, 350, 372, 383, 504, 512, 516, 518–19, 531–2
Team Climate Inventory 326
temporal aspects of groups 308
temporal boundaries 15
temporal changes 285
temporal context 36
temporal development 403
temporal effects 37
temporal factors 30, 47
temporal work group functioning 293
theoretical model
  group performance 11, 285, 310
  leadership 202
top management teams 59, 65, 67, 68, 79, 325, 511
training 11, 105, 114–15, 154, 218–19, 230, 232, 267, 320, 382, 384–5, 387, 399, 495, 516–17, 523, 535, 556
  team xx, 496, 503–21, 571–2
trade union xxx, 412, 414, 482

vision 127, 155, 199, 200, 317, 327, 333, 335, 336, 337, 338, 482

well-being xxviii, xxx, 13, 34, 240, 304, 320, 345, 353, 357, 358, 361, 556, 573, 574
  effect of group work on 349–50
  group 38, 39, 347
  group member 77, 86, 89, 90, 571
women 55–6, 64, 69, 402

Related titles of interest from Wiley...

Handbook of Work and Health Psychology

Edited by **Marc. J. Schabracq, Jacques A.M. Winnubst** and **Cary L. Cooper**

A valuable resource and guide for psychologists and manager who need to understand and prevent, or minimise, work-related health problems.

0471 95789 5   504pp   1996   Hardback

Journal of Organizational Behavior

Editor-in-Chief: **Cary L. Cooper**

Reports and reviews the growing research in the industrial-organizational psychology and organizational behavior fields throughout the world.

Subscription rates include the current volume of **Trends in Organizational Behavior**, edited by **Cary L. Cooper** and **Denise Rousseau**, an annual series which provides a quick and up-to-date account of research on issues of relevance to industrial and organizational psychologists.

ISSN: 0894-3796

International Review of Industrial and Organizational Psychology

Edited by **Cary L. Cooper** and **Ivan T. Robertson**

This series of annual volumes provides authoritative reviews in the field of industrial and organizational psychology. Chapters in each volume are 'stand alone' reviews of important existing and new topics.

ISSN: 0886-1528

Creating Healthy Work Organizations

Edited by **Cary L. Cooper** and **Stephen Williams**

Brings together 'best practice' in the field of organizational health, drawing together chief medical officers and human resource executives from leading companies including ICI/Zeneca and Marks & Spencer who have all attempted to create healthy work organizations.

Wiley Series in Work, Well-Being and Stress
0471 94345 2   266pp   1994   Hardback